Congenital Heart Disease in Adolescents and Adults

Endorsed by

The ESC Working Group on Grown-up Congenital Heart Disease
AEPC Adult with Congenital Heart Disease Working Group .

Series Editors

Massimo Chessa
San Donato Milanese, Italy

Helmut Baumgartner
Münster, Germany

Andreas Eicken
Munich, Germany

Alessandro Giamberti
San Donato Milanese, Italy

The aim of this series is to cast light on the most significant aspects – whether still debated or already established – of congenital heart disease in adolescents and adults and its management. Advances in the medical and surgical management of congenital heart disease have revolutionized the prognosis of infants and children with cardiac defects, so that an increasing number of patients, including those with complex problems, can reach adolescence and adult life. The profile of the adult population with congenital heart disease (ACHD) is consequently changing, and in future many adult patients will present different hemodynamic and cardiac problems from those currently seen. A cure is rarely achieved, and provision of optimal care is therefore dependent on ongoing surveillance and management in conjunction with experts in this highly specialized field. Specialists in ACHD management need to have a deep knowledge not only of congenital cardiac malformations and their treatment in infancy and childhood, but of general medicine, too. A training in adult cardiology, including coronary artery disease, is also essential. Similarly, surgeons need to acquire expertise and good training in both adult and pediatric cardiosurgery. Readers will find this series to be a rich source of information highly relevant to daily clinical practice.

More information about this series at http://www.springer.com/series/13454

Eduardo da Cruz • Duncan Macrae
Gary Webb
Editors

Intensive Care of the Adult with Congenital Heart Disease

Springer

Editors
Eduardo da Cruz
Children's Hospital Colorado
University of Colorado Denver
Aurora, CO
USA

Duncan Macrae
Pediatric Intensive Care
Royal Brompton & Harefield NHS
Foundation Trust
London
United Kingdom

Gary Webb
Adult Congenital Heart Program
Heart Institute
Cincinnati Children Hospital Medical
Center
Cincinnati, OH
USA

ISSN 2364-6659 ISSN 2364-6667 (electronic)
Congenital Heart Disease in Adolescents and Adults
ISBN 978-3-319-94170-7 ISBN 978-3-319-94171-4 (eBook)
https://doi.org/10.1007/978-3-319-94171-4

Library of Congress Control Number: 2018960935

This Springer imprint is published by the registered company Springer Nature Switzerland AG
The registered company address is: Gewerbestrasse 11, 6330 Cham, Switzerland

I dedicate this book to my lovely family, to my co-editors, and to the distinguished authors, and mostly to all the patients with congenital heart disease, those who have reached adulthood and those who will. Sending a strong message of hope and great expectations for the future.

Eduardo da Cruz

I thank my wife Anne, family, colleagues, and friends for their continuing support and forbearance, and Drs. Frank Shann and Michael Scallan for inspiring me through their professionalism and humility.

Duncan Macrae

Dedicated to the patients I have cared for, the colleagues I have worked with, and my loving family.

Gary Webb

Preface to the Series

In Europe, we are currently faced with an estimated ACHD population of 4.2 million; adults with congenital heart disease now outnumber children (approximately 2.3 million). The vast majority cannot be considered cured but rather having a chronic heart condition that requires further surveillance and timely re-intervention for residual or consequent anatomical and/or functional abnormalities. ACHD patients have very special needs and the physicians taking care of them need expert training. Special health care organization and training programs for those involved in ACHD care are therefore required to meet the needs of this special population.

ACHD problems remain a small part of general cardiology training curricula around the world, and pediatric cardiologists are trained to manage children with CHD and may, out of necessity, continue to look after these patients when they outgrow pediatric age.

There are clearly other health issues concerning the adult with CHD, beyond the scope of pediatric medicine, that our patients now routinely face. Adult physicians with a non-CHD background are therefore increasingly involved in the day-to-day management of patients with CHD.

Experts in congenital heart disease should work to improve the health care system, so that teens and young adults have an easier time making the transition from receiving health care in pediatric cardiology centers to receiving care from specialists in adult cardiology.

The aim of this series is to cast light on the most significant aspects of congenital heart disease in adolescents and adults and its management, such as transition from pediatric to adulthood, pregnancy and contraception, sport and physical activities, pulmonary hypertension, burning issues related to surgery, interventional catheterization, electrophysiology, intensive care management, and heart failure.

This series wishes to attract the interest of cardiologists, anesthesiologists, cardiac surgeons, electrophysiologists, psychologists, GPs, undergraduate and postgraduate students, and residents, and would like to become relevant for courses of cardiology, pediatric cardiology, cardiothoracic surgery, and anesthesiology.

We thank both the wonderful groups of leading cardiovascular experts from around the world, for donating their precious time, producing excellent textbooks and making this book series a reality, and the members of the two Working Groups (ESC and AEPC ACHD/GUCH Working Group) for the invaluable suggestions and support without which this work would not be possible.

San Donato Milanese, Italy — Massimo Chessa
Münster, Germany — Helmut Baumgartner
Munich, Germany — Andreas Eicken
San Donato Milanese, Italy — Alessandro Giamberti

Foreword

The care of children with congenital heart disease has been without doubt one of the greatest achievements of cardiovascular medicine and surgery in the twentieth century. As a result, the number of adults with congenital heart disease has grown exponentially; there are currently more adults with congenital heart disease alive than children. This number has now exceeded one million in North America, with similar increases in Western Europe. In parallel, there are now more patients with complex congenital heart disease, who—with improved care—also survive to adulthood.

The net effect of this successful story of modern medicine is that there are ever-increasing needs and pressures for tertiary expertise to provide for this growing adult population with congenital heart disease. Many patients require re-interventions, catheter and/or surgical, whereas late complications such as arrhythmias, heart failure, and pulmonary hypertension are common among them. The spectrum of anatomic substrate, the range of cardiovascular physiology, and the dynamic and continuously evolving nature of catheter and surgical interventions, both at presentation—early in life—and thereafter, means that adults with congenital heart disease represent a very heterogeneous patient group in need of tertiary expertise and multidisciplinary care.

Our approach to diagnosis and management of adults with congenital heart disease has made great progress over the past 2–3 decades, improving the prospects for our patients. There are now worldwide units and teams with medical and surgical expertise to provide for patients with congenital heart disease and their life-long needs. There are still areas, however, where a better understanding, more evidence, and a consensus to adult congenital heart care are lacking. Intensive care (IC) is one of them; patients coming for cardiac reoperations, high-risk catheter or other intervention, management of decompensated heart failure or pulmonary arterial hypertension, and/or for mechanical support (as a bridge to transplantation or destination therapy) require tertiary expertise in the best possible environment. The textbook *Intensive Care of the Adult with Congenital Heart Disease: Interdisciplinary Concepts* edited by Eduardo M da Cruz, Duncan Macrae, and Gary Webb comes to cover this need. The three eminent editors have brought together an international panel of experts in their respective fields to contribute to this effort. The ideal intensive care setting is discussed; there are chapters on nomenclature, classification and risk score assessment, general IC management, pharmacological considerations, anesthesia, psychosocial preparation, and follow-up of the patient. There are specific challenges with this patient population requiring and receiving intensive care, namely ventricular fibrosis and dysfunction, low cardiac output, peri-procedural arrhythmia, cyanosis, and different adaptive mechanism/s to acute hemodynamic changes, compared to their pediatric counterparts. This necessitates intensive care adult expertise, ideally applied in an adult congenital heart disease health care environment. There are essential chapters on cardio-pulmonary interactions, critical care management of common conditions (tetralogy of Fallot, coarctation of the aorta, single ventricle, aortopathies, Eisenmenger syndrome), arrhythmias, endocarditis, heart failure, mechanical support, and transplantation. Last but not least, the textbook covers management of acquired cardiac disease, other noncardiac comorbidities, anticoagulation, nutrition, nursing, rehabilitation, and end of life issues. This rather comprehensive textbook, therefore, comes to fill in a knowledge gap and at the same time highlights research opportunities in this important field of IC, as pertains to the adult with congenital heart disease.

I believe that every physician, nurse, or health care professional—whether senior or junior—who works in our expanding field of adult congenital heart disease has much to gain from this book.

Royal Brompton and Imperial College
London, UK

Michael A. Gatzoulis

Preface

There are currently more adults than children with congenital heart disease in the developed world, and this trend will continue owing to improvements in the management of pediatric patients and notably those with complex congenital heart disease. This number has now exceeded one million in North America reflecting similar data in other developed countries. This growing adult population with congenital heart disease requires highly specialized and multidisciplinary follow-up, surgical and interventional procedures, and management of late complications related to the natural history of their primary disease, comorbidities, and acquired ailments. Resources needed to successfully manage this very heterogeneous patient group are onerous as the expert community endeavors to implement consistent and efficient models that serve patients within the frame of excellent quality and safety. Although much progress has been accomplished, there are areas such as intensive care that still need to evolve as a core of interdisciplinary and transdisciplinary close collaboration between professionals trained in both pediatric and adult internal medicine, cardiology, anesthesia, intensive care, nursing, pharmacology, psychology, and surgery, to name but a few. The need to integrate experts from multiple backgrounds into a horizontal line of collaboration is vital, with the common objective of compassionately and effectively serving patients and their families. This textbook's title *Intensive Care of the Adult with Congenital Heart Disease: Interdisciplinary Concepts* illustrates the need for this interaction that is the only way to ultimately provide the best possible care to adults with congenital heart disease.

This comprehensive book discusses the many challenges faced in the management of these patients and attempts to provide the first universal review of the practical management of patients with these complex conditions. It advocates for a consistent interaction and collaboration between several disciplines while offering concise and pragmatic recommendations and basic and advanced concepts that allow caregivers to anticipate, prevent, and effectively treat such pathologies. While bringing together top international experts who are leading reference programs around the globe, this book is an indispensable teaching tool for clinicians and caregivers involved in the management of critically ill adults with congenital heart disease.

Aurora, CO — Eduardo da Cruz
London, UK — Duncan Macrae
Cincinnati, OH — Gary Webb

Contents

About the Editors

Eduardo da Cruz was born in Lisbon, Portugal, and has had an international life career, having lived in Portugal, Costa Rica, France, United Kingdom, Switzerland, and the United States of America. He trained in medicine and then in pediatrics at the Universidad de Costa Rica and the Hospital Nacional de Niños in San José, Costa Rica, and then pursued a fellowship in pediatric cardiology and intensive care in Paris, France (Hôpital Necker-Enfants Malades, Université René Descartes-Paris V). After completion of his training, he stayed in Europe as an attending physician in pediatric cardiology and intensive care until 2007, when he joined the Heart Institute at Children's Hospital Colorado, University of Colorado Denver, School of Medicine, in Denver, USA. He currently holds the title of Tenured Full Professor of Pediatrics, Pediatric Cardiology and Intensive Care, Associate Medical Director of the Heart Institute, and Head of the Pediatric Cardiac Critical Care Program and Inpatient Services. He has extensive experience in the medical and perioperative management of neonates, children, and young adults with complex congenital or acquired heart disease, including heart transplant, pulmonary hypertension, heart failure, mechanical assistance and quality improvement, safety, clinical effectiveness, stewardship, and crew resource management. He is very actively involved in clinical and translational research and teaching in the fields of pediatric cardiology and cardiac intensive care, has delivered hundreds of international lectures, and is a reviewer for 24 peer-reviewed journals, and the co-editor of seven CICU textbooks, and the editor-in-chief of the recently published reference entitled *Pediatric and Congenital Cardiology, Cardiac Surgery and Intensive Care* (Springer-Verlag UK), a major textbook and e-book/e-reference with 6 volumes and close to 4000 pages. He has published more than 60 book chapters and close to 100 manuscripts in peer-reviewed journals. He is the founder and former chair of the Working Group on Pediatric Cardiac Intensive Care of the Association for the European Pediatric and Congenital Cardiology (AEPC), founder and chair of the Section of Pediatric and Congenital Cardiac Intensive Care and Mechanical Circulatory Assistance of the European Society of Pediatric and Neonatal Intensive Care (ESPNIC), a former board member of the Congenital Domain of the European Association for Cardio-Thoracic Surgery (EACTS), and member of the Society of Pediatric Research (SPR) and of multiple other international societies. Eduardo da Cruz is also an expert reviewer for the European Commission Horizon 2020 Project and the president and chair of the board of the Surgeons of Hope Foundation, a nongovernmental organization based in New York, USA.

Duncan Macrae is a pediatric intensivist at the Royal Brompton Hospital, London, UK, and also holds an academic appointment at Imperial College, London. He has worked in critical care for over 30 years, supporting the evolution of specialist congenital cardiac critical care. Dr. Macrae has made major contributions through research and teaching in areas such as ECMO, inhaled nitric oxide therapy, and glycemic control. He is a member of the editorial boards of several major journals including *Pediatric Critical Care Medicine*, *Intensive Care Medicine*, and the *World Journal for Pediatric and Congenital Heart Surgery*. He is a former president of the Pediatric Cardiac Intensive Care Society.

Gary D. Webb, M.D. is a professor of pediatrics and internal medicine at the University of Cincinnati College of Medicine and, until May 2016, the director of the Adult Congenital Heart Program at Cincinnati Children's Hospital Heart Institute. After receiving a B.Sc. and MDCM from McGill University in Montréal, Québec, he went on to intern at the Royal Victoria Hospital in Montréal, and then to training in internal medicine and cardiology at the University of Toronto. After 8 years as chief of cardiology at the Wellesley Hospital in Toronto, he moved back to Toronto General Hospital. Beginning in 1980, he was codirector and then director of the Toronto Congenital Cardiac Center for Adults. For several years, he directed the adult cardiology training program at the University of Toronto. He is a Fellow of the Royal College of Physicians and Surgeons of Canada in both internal medicine and cardiology. He is a Fellow of the American College of Cardiology and a life member of the European Society of Cardiology. In 2004, he relocated to Philadelphia, serving as director of the Philadelphia Adult Congenital Heart Center at the University of Pennsylvania. In 2009, he took up his position at Cincinnati Children's Hospital.

Part I

General Aspects

The Ideal Intensive Care Unit for Adults with Congenital Heart Disease

1

David Briston and Curt Daniels

The intensive care unit (ICU) represents the highest acuity of care available in the modern hospital setting. Various subspecialties have ICUs that focus on their specific practice area such as postoperative cardiac care, neurosurgical postoperative care, as well as many others. Altogether, millions of hospital admissions occur to various ICUs annually. Patients with congenital heart disease (CHD) are one such population who require high levels of care on a regular basis. Adults with CHD (ACHD) are a rapidly growing population with over 1.4 million ACHD patients estimated in the USA alone. These patients are not only relatively higher healthcare utilizers, but also when inpatients, they often require higher acuity care such as that offered in the ICU [1]. Demographic studies have shown that the ACHD population is aging [2, 3], suggesting the need for an ICU that not only provides expert care for complex of CHD but for adult comorbidities of an aging population.

Caring for patients with CHD requires a multidisciplinary team with skills and expertise in a variety of pre- and postsurgical anatomies and complex physiology as well as sufficient resources to properly do so [4]. ACHD patients often require catheter-based or surgical interventions that lead to post-procedural care in the intensive care unit (ICU) but also admissions for medical issues that necessitate advanced monitoring and high level of care. Senescence for CHD patients occurs sooner, and increased levels of interaction with the healthcare system and at higher acuity levels transpire at younger ages, further clarifying the need for specialized ICUs in this patient population.

While in the ICU, the ACHD population should have access to specialists who perform cardiac catheterizations and trans-catheter therapies, provide electrophysiologic advice and care, evaluate and treat advanced heart failure, and, at the same

D. Briston · C. Daniels (✉)
Nationwide Children's Hospital, The Ohio State University, Columbus, OH, USA
e-mail: David.Briston@nationwidechildrens.org; Curt.Daniels@nationwidechildrens.org

E. da Cruz et al. (eds.), *Intensive Care of the Adult with Congenital Heart Disease*, Congenital Heart Disease in Adolescents and Adults,
https://doi.org/10.1007/978-3-319-94171-4_1

time, understand congenital cardiac anatomy and physiology. The ICU should have additional specialists available who can evaluate the breadth of non-cardiac issues facing the ACHD patient in the ICU. The ACHD patient is unique in the ICU setting and to the ICU caregivers, bringing together the complexity of childhood CHD but also the medical issues of an adult patient.

The importance of a specialized ICU for the care of ACHD patients is underscored by the delicate nature of congenital heart surgery in adult patients. Many ACHD patients undergo reoperation, and the rate of cardiac injury—defined as entry into a cardiac chamber or vascular structure during repeat sternotomy or mediastinal dissection that required initiation of cardiopulmonary bypass for control or repair—has been reported to be as high as 6% with early mortality at 3.6% [5]. Caring for complications such as these in the ICU requires attentive and well-trained healthcare providers. Also, it has been noted that 24% of ACHD patients have severe perioperative complications such as arrhythmia, renal failure, stroke, or multiorgan system failure, and a significant percentage of ACHD patients die in the perioperative period [6, 7]. With complicated procedures being performed in the operating room and catheterization laboratory, morbidity is high in the ACHD cohort. This underscores the need for a wide range of appropriate services to be in place and available when caring for an ACHD patient in the ICU.

ICU admissions for ACHD patients are increasing, and it is anticipated that this trajectory will continue for the foreseeable future as more patients are reaching adult age than in the past [8] (Fig. 1.1). To provide the best outcomes, the ideal environment to care for ACHD patients in an ICU, whether in a children's hospital or a general hospital, must have complete medical teams composed of physicians, nurses, technicians, patient aides, and social work staff familiar with ACHD patients.

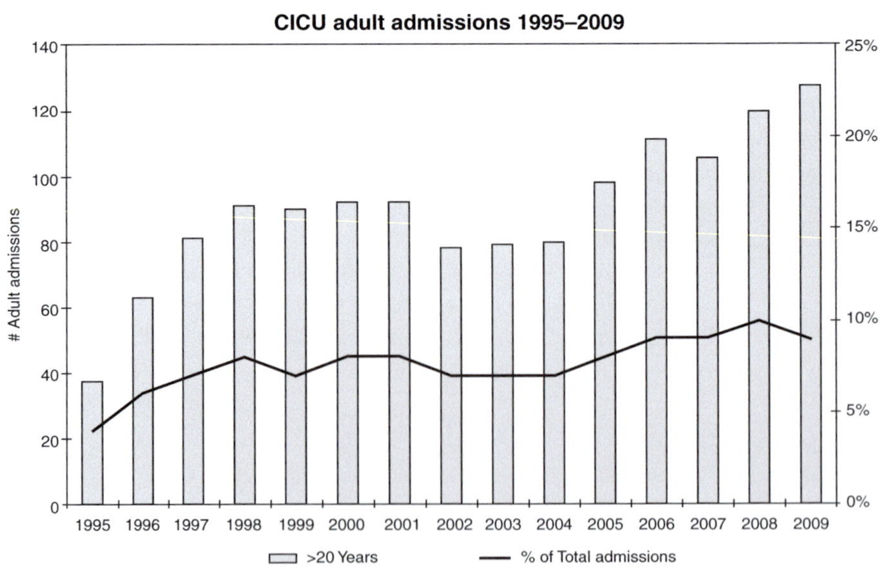

Fig. 1.1 Rising ACHD admissions to the ICU

ACHD patients are hospitalized at twice the frequency of age-matched controls and have double the number of days in a critical care bed [9, 10]. Among ACHD patients, those with heart failure are known to have significantly higher resource utilization rates compared to those who do not [1]. Because heart failure is the primary cause of death in the contemporary ACHD population, it is not surprising that overall higher resource utilization is seen [7]. Utilization of hospitals and ICU specifically in the final year of life has been well documented in Australia where 59% of decedents had been admitted to the hospital within their final year of life [11]. Among ACHD patients, unplanned admissions for medical reasons and surgical procedures as well as post-procedure are increasing (Fig. 1.2). With an increasing population who utilizes the healthcare system more often and has diagnoses associated with frequent hospitalization, the need for an appropriate ICU setting for ACHD patients is clear.

The comprehensive nature of the ideal ACHD ICU is hard to define by modern metrics. While many aspects of ICU care can be quantified, providing patient-specific ACHD care is complex, and a one-size-fits-all approach is neither feasible nor practical. Given how ACHD is not a single entity or disease process, no single characteristic defines this setting other than appropriate quality care being provided to the patient. Cardiothoracic surgical care as provided by congenitally trained vs. non-congenitally trained surgeons and whether performing procedures at adult and pediatric institutions for adult patients have been reviewed multiple times [12–15]. While some data show improved survival for ACHD patients at pediatric centers, the data are limited but reinforce the decision regarding where a patient should receive care is specific *to the patient* rather than generalized to all ACHD patients

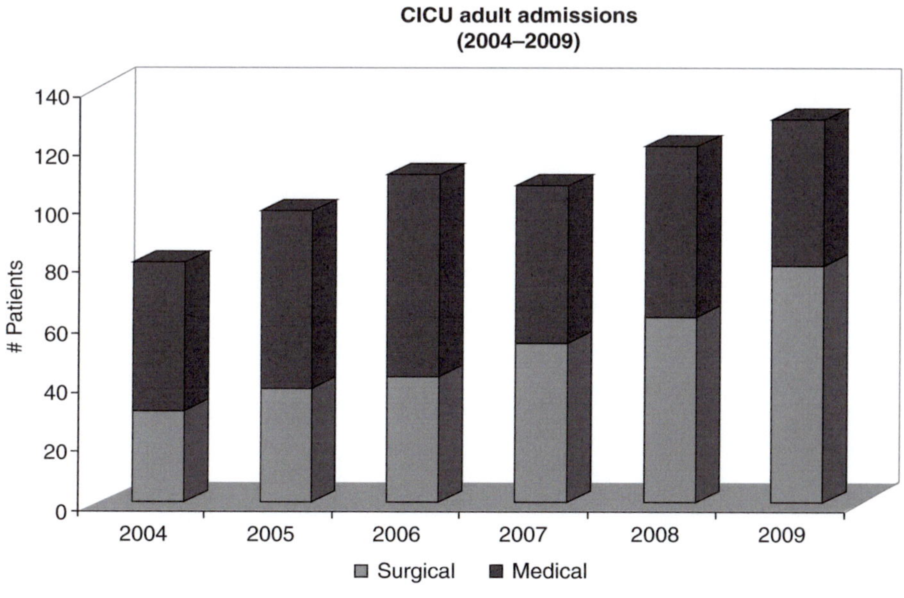

Fig. 1.2 ACHD admissions by type

[14]. The data seem to suggest that surgical outcomes are better in children's hospitals. This finding may be interpreted to imply that there are aspects to care that are optimized when the ICU team is experienced in CHD care as opposed to adult medicine care. However, the optimal disposition for critical care needs for ACHD patients is truly not well defined and continues to pose one of the most burdensome dilemmas for ACHD providers [16].

The location of the ideal ACHD ICU remains debatable, and the strengths and limitations of each setting are outlined herein (Table 1.1).

The pediatric intensive care unit (PICU) or pediatric cardiothoracic ICU (CTICU) offers many advantages as compared to other medical ICUs for the care of ACHD patients. Many patients and families are acquainted with the PICU/CTICU since the majority of ACHD patients have required invasive procedures in the past. The PICU/CTICU medical teams are experts in caring for patients with congenital heart issues. For instance, nurses who are familiar with CHD physiology may better understand the significance of low saturations and when to intervene. Advanced knowledge of complicated procedures and physiology in childhood makes understanding these in issues adulthood much simpler. Knowing the differences between pre- and post-ductal blood pressures and oxygen saturations in left- and right-sided aortic arches is critical basic knowledge for medical decision-making. Complex cardiac issues such as those seen in heterotaxy syndrome patients are important when interpreting imaging studies. Also, one must contemplate how basic ICU data are interpreted. Vital signs are core to the management of ICU patients. Right arm blood pressure readings are required for all patients with left-sided aortic arches as a true measure of carotid and coronary artery blood pressures except in special circumstances, which hopefully prior imaging will have elucidated. When addressing aortic arch abnormalities, the pre-ductal blood pressure should be compared with either of

Table 1.1 Strengths and weaknesses for caring for ACHD patients in various settings

Location of care	Strengths	Weaknesses
Children's hospital	Familiarity with CHD as it relates to anatomy, physiology, procedures, nursing care, diagnostic testing, and right ventricular disease	Lack of familiarity with adult-related comorbid conditions with possible decrease in access to adult-based consultative services familiar with treating them
	Availability of pediatric consultative services familiar with CHD patients	Environment not designed for adult patients
	Potential for patient and family familiarity with facilities and healthcare providers	Nursing and ancillary services accustomed to and credentialed to caring for children
Adult hospital	Familiarity within ICU for adult patients and their comorbid conditions	Limited exposure to and knowledge of CHD anatomy and physiology
	Environment and resources designed for adult care	Potential for errors in nursing procedures and diagnostic testing
	Availability of consultative services familiar with adult comorbidities	Lack of exposure to ACHD-specific complications

those in the leg and generally not with those obtained in the contralateral arm. This comparison is useful in determining adequacy of aortic flow. Interpretation of other common tests in the cardiac ICU such as electrocardiogram, echocardiogram, and chest X-ray also is different from those without congenital heart disease. Echocardiograms with structures being absent or on the opposite side from usual anatomy and with abnormal arterial and venous connections are difficult to interpret. Chest X-rays with abnormally positioned hearts or with pulmonary fields both appearing as if right-sided structures are sufficiently common that expertise in such pathology is mandatory. Familiarity with right-sided chest leads and V7 also is sometimes useful in patient management. Advanced life support devices such as extracorporeal membrane oxygenation units are available in most ICU settings, and their usage in CHD patients is more common in the PICU setting. Beyond familiarity with diagnostic testing, expert CHD care includes knowledge of how unique physiology affects other systems. For instance, avoidance of laparoscopic procedures that insufflate air into the abdomen, which might greatly reduce infra-diaphragmatic systemic venous return in patients living with central shunts, is an important clinical knowledge. Third, familiarity with right ventricle issues is typically higher in the PICU setting. Recently, a number of risk factors were identified for right ventricular dysfunction in an ACHD cohort, including preoperative right ventricular dysfunction, postoperative supraventricular tachycardia, and cardiopulmonary bypass time >150 min [17]. Even patients who were not undergoing surgery on the right side of the heart were at risk for RV dysfunction. ICU providers familiar with systemic right ventricles may better recognize and understand, for instance, the paradoxical response of a patient with an atrial switch palliation to inotropes. Fourth, PICUs caring for patients with CHD should have associated fully staffed pediatric consult services. This is particularly important for ACHD patients who are at risk for extra-cardiac complications both related and unrelated to their heart disease. Some centers have purposefully employed internal medicine-trained intensivists and hospitalists for the PICU/CTICU to better care for the ACHD population. Medical team familiarity with CHD, availability of consultants, and patient familiarity are all strengths associated with care of ACHD patients in the PICU.

While the PICU offers many advantages in caring for patients with CHD, there are certain limitations as well. First, the PICU is designed inherently for pediatric patients, and the physical space and equipment may not be conducive to properly care for adult patients. While certainly there are hospital beds available for patients of all sizes, the PICU may have numerous available cribs, warmers, and incubators but only a few beds designed for fully grown and even obese adults. Other aspects of the PICU environment such as room design, floor activities, space, and equipment for cardiac rehabilitation may not be appropriate or adequate for ACHD care. Second, the ability to provide high-quality way care rapidly for adult-specific medical or cardiac issues may not be available at a children's hospital PICU or CTICU. While the crossover in both pediatric and adult specialty care in various subspecialties is growing, it is not complete or universally available (Table 1.2). For instance, pediatric cardiologists do not often treat or manage atrial fibrillation, whereas it is a common clinical scenario for adult cardiologists. Also, pediatric neurologists are not trained

Table 1.2 Adult ICU consultative services and issues they handle

Specialty service	Comorbid condition
Cardiology	Atrial fibrillation
	Myocardial infarction
Neurology	Acute cerebrovascular accident
Hematology	Clotting disorder such as deep venous thrombosis
	Bleeding diathesis
Gastroenterology	Gastrointestinal bleeding
	Liver dysfunction

specifically in adult stroke management, whereas in adult care it is a core curriculum and training. Moreover, in gastroenterology, pediatrics rarely focuses on life-threatening GI bleeding. While pediatric providers are assuredly aware of such issues, their prior training often is insufficient to provide the level of expertise in providing clinical care. Third, nurses who work with children may not be as comfortable in caring for critically ill adult patients. They may not have received appropriate training for adult patients, have not been offered or completed ACLS, have not received ongoing credits for continuing nursing education for adult patients, and may not have nursing support when caring for adult patients such as might be available for physicians. Adults have different physiology and cannot be treated as big children, and pediatric-based ICU care in some ways is not ideal [18].

The alternative to the PICU/CTICU is to care for ACHD patients in the medical intensive care unit (MICU), cardiac surgical intensive care unit (CSICU), or the cardiac intensive care unit (CICU), depending on the hospital's organizational structure. First, the expertise in caring for adult patients is a significant advantage. All of the healthcare providers are comfortable caring for adult patients. Second, the non-CHD issues, both cardiac and non-cardiac complications, are well evaluated and treated in an adult ICU. The ICU team caring for ACHD patients must be skilled in the evaluation and treatment of not only the post-procedure patient but also in age-related comorbidities that are not specific to ACHD patients such as diabetes, obstructive lung disease, dementia, and renal insufficiency [19]. Third, arrhythmias are relatively more common in the ACHD patient population with most patients having had an atrial arrhythmia by age 65 [20, 21]. Arrhythmia was noted to be the primary cause of hospital admission among ACHD patients, so having specialists readily available who are familiar with them and confident in treating them is logical [10]. Having the necessary equipment readily available is necessary for all ACHD patients in the ICU. Fourth, extra-cardiac comorbidities associated with sequela of various ACHD lesions are often better treated in the adult setting, and some are listed below.

Renal dysfunction is relatively more common in patients with ACHD for a variety of reasons such as cyanosis, contrast administration, and cardiopulmonary bypass [22, 23]. A European study showed almost half of adults have some degree of renal dysfunction and that 20% have moderate or worse kidney failure [24]. This study shows that renal dysfunction is not unique to any one lesion or category of lesions, highlighting the need for providers being aware of such medical complexities of ACHD patients. It appears for many ACHD patients their kidneys are vulnerable to injury with a baseline level of renal dysfunction at much younger ages than expected. This is important especially when in the ICU wherein procedures may occur that are associated with contrast usage or where medications might be used that reduce renal blood flow. When grouped by use for diuretics, by heart failure classification, and by cyanosis, markedly worsened survivals are noted in patients with worse kidney function (Fig. 1.3)

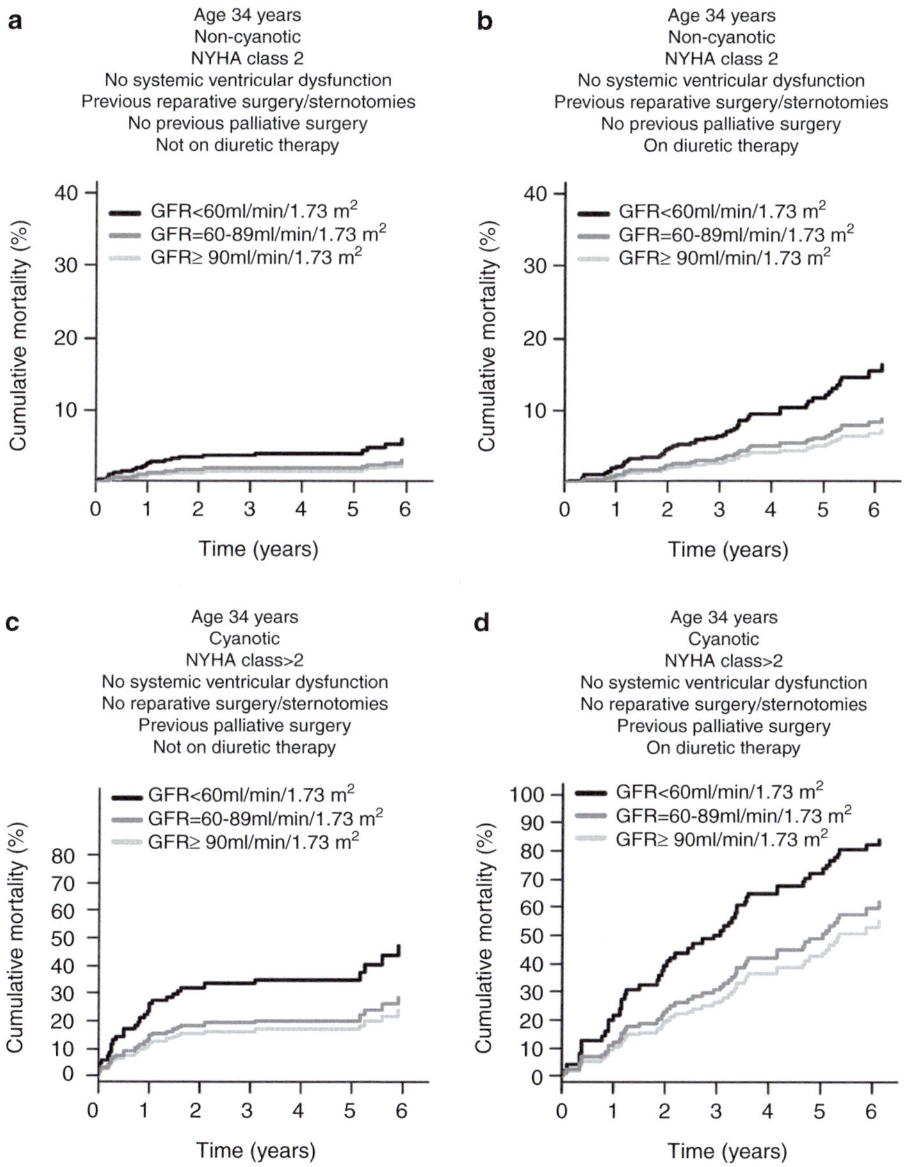

Fig. 1.3 Adjusted mortality curves for noncyanotic (**a** and **b**) and cyanotic (**c** and **d**) ACHD patients separated by those not receiving (**a** and **c**) or those receiving (**b** and **d**) diuretic therapy

[24]. Moreover, ACHD patients may be in the ICU after cardiopulmonary bypass or after an arrest, both of which are renal insults. Regiments to protect renal function such as avoidance of nephrotoxic agents, maintenance of adequate volume status, and vigilance to maintain hemodynamic parameters are important. The use of adequate hydration, sodium bicarbonate solutions, and *n*-acetylcysteine to prevent contrast-induced kidney injury is also a topic well known to adult providers. Familiarity with less commonly utilized medications such as with the use of fenoldopam, which is renal protective, may also be more commonplace in the MICU.

Hematologic considerations also are well cared for by adult centers. Many patients are on aspirin if not Coumadin therapy for mechanical valves, intracardiac pacing wires with residual shunt, atrial arrhythmias, and Fontan palliation with residual shunt. Also, ACHD patients are not only at risk for thromboembolic events but also bleeding complications. There are known risk factors for bleeding diatheses in CHD patients such as cyanosis and significant valvar disease independent of anticoagulation medication [25]. These issues can be assessed with preoperative hematologic studies, but sometimes even premedication or specific treatments cannot significantly mitigate operative bleeding risks. The concept of red blood cell shearing has most extensively been evaluated as it relates to aortic valve stenosis, and data regarding acquired von Willebrand disease are emerging as it relates to surgery in ACHD patients. Knowledge of bleeding risks prior to planned procedures is important and possibly can minimize complications.

Pulmonary considerations must be addressed when an ACHD patient is in the ICU. Restrictive lung disease is common after thoracotomies and can lead to respiratory insufficiency and is known risk factor for increased mortality [26]. It also may occur with lung hypoplasia as is seen in Scimitar syndrome or in those with significant vertebral anomalies such as kyphosis or scoliosis. Prior nerve damage that has affected diaphragmatic or vocal cord function can complicate recovery intubations related to planned procedures or from respiratory infections. The inability to move the vocal cords completely can markedly affect flow-volume loops and hinder recovery. Adult patients may also acquire diseases such as obstructive lung disease which also affects ICU management. Understanding how these multiple respiratory dysfunctions interact with ACHD is complicated and underscores the need for care by well-trained individuals.

Gastroenterology consultation is increasingly required as patients develop sequela of their heart disease. For instance, single ventricle patients have increased central venous pressures, leading to a congestive hepatopathy. Now termed Fontan-associated liver disease, this complicated disease process leads to portal hypertension, hepatic cirrhosis, and reduced survival for this population [27]. The potential for protein losing enteropathy, hepatocellular carcinoma, and other sequelae specific to the single ventricle population complicates ICU care. While no expert consensus yet exists, having awareness of these potential complications is desirable in the ICU setting. Gastrointestinal bleeds are also relatively more common as more patients are prescribed anticoagulation.

There are also disadvantages of the adult ICU setting for ACHD patients. Most striking is the lack of knowledge and familiarity with CHD. The understanding of where invasive monitors can be placed and where to avoid (such as subclavian or internal jugular central venous catheters in single ventricle patients) is imperative to appropriate treatment. Alterations in traditional treatment practices may be required. For instance, the use of filters on IV lines is necessary in patients with right-to-left shunts to prevent air emboli. The ability to interpret complex CHD imaging data may also be limited and require extensive consultation. Details of systemic right ventricles, ventricular interdependence and single ventricle physiology as they relate to the lungs are not as commonplace in adult hospitals. Issues such as these must be overcome for ACHD patients to receive adequate and high-quality care in an adult ICU.

Objective data in the ACHD population as it relates to ICU care is sparse. Outcomes for ACHD surgery were analyzed and showed improved survival in the hands of a congenitally trained heart surgeon [14]. Details regarding surgery type were not assessed. Another study identified relatively increased rates of complications among ACHD patients who had undergone prior surgery [28]. Another study reported a 4.9% mortality rate among a younger ACHD cohort, again without specifying the details regarding surgery type, location, and surgeon characteristics [29]. While risk factors for poor outcomes have been identified, many patients have such characteristics and still require interventions, further emphasizing the need for an ICU capable of caring for ACHD patients.

In the ideal situation, ACHD patients would be cared for in a hospital environment that has adult and pediatric services close at hand, preferably within the same building. The primary ICU staff would be dual trained with credentialing in both internal medicine and pediatrics, and subspecialty training would include cardiac ICU advance training with an interest or background in congenital cardiology. Primary and consultative services would be continuously available for any need that arises. The nurses would be equally familiar with and capable to treat adult patients and CHD-related problems. Programs would ideally be offered to medical professionals to address deficiencies and steps taken to modify the existing environment to make it more amenable for ACHD care (Table 1.3).

It is paramount to this population's survival that it receives high-quality care ideally by practitioners who have completed multiple credentialed programs to care for congenital patients within the ICU and who have familiarity with both children and adults alike. As ACHD patients continue to utilize the healthcare system, the need for a collaborative care environment with practitioners of all types with advanced training will only increase.

Table 1.3 Educational programs and resources that should be offered to caregivers in charge of ACHD patients

Location of care	Areas of targeted development
Children's hospital	Education • Nursing and specialized adult care • Physicians regarding adult care • Heart failure guidelines • Novel anticoagulation • Liver dysfunction in CHD patients • Familiarity with invasive monitoring devices
	Environment and resources • Ancillary service availability to help care for adults • Rooms designated as appropriate to care for adults • Guarantee of equipment able to perform diagnostics on patients of all adult sizes • Monitored telemetry
Adult hospital	Education • Specific CHD anatomy, physiology, and diagnostic testing • Right ventricular principles and ventricular interdependence • Single ventricle physiology • Pulmonary hypertension in various CHD scenarios • Restrictive lung disease, vocal cord dysfunction, and paralyzed hemidiaphragms
	Environment and resources • Use and placement of blood pressure cuffs and pulse oximeters • Family resources for patients with disabilities • Availability of 15 lead electrocardiograms • Availability of iv line filters

References

1. Bhatt AB, Rajabali A, He W, Benavidez OJ. High resource use among adult congenital heart surgery admissions in adult hospitals: risk factors and association with death and comorbidities. Congenit Heart Dis. 2015;10(1):13–20.
2. Marelli AJ, Ionescu-Ittu R, Mackie AS, Guo L, Dendukuri N, Kaouache M. Lifetime prevalence of congenital heart disease in the general population from 2000 to 2010. Circulation. 2014;130(9):749–56.
3. Gilboa SM, Devine OJ, Kucik JE, Oster ME, Riehle-Colarusso T, Nembhard WN, Xu P, Correa A, Jenkins K, Marelli AJ. Congenital heart defects in the United States: estimating the magnitude of the affected population in 2010. Circulation. 2016;134(2):101–9.
4. Webb G, Mulder BJ, Aboulhosn J, Daniels CJ, Elizari MA, Hong G, Horlick E, Landzberg MJ, Marelli AJ, O'Donnell CP, Oechslin EN, Pearson DD, Pieper EP, Saxena A, Schwerzmann M, Stout KK, Warnes CA, Khairy P. The care of adults with congenital heart disease across the globe: current assessment and future perspective: a position statement from the International Society for Adult Congenital Heart Disease (ISACHD). Int J Cardiol. 2015;195:326–33.
5. Holst KA, Dearani JA, Burkhart HM, Connolly HM, Warnes CA, Li Z, Schaff HV. Risk factors and early outcomes of multiple reoperations in adults with congenital heart disease. Ann Thorac Surg. 2011;92(1):122–8.
6. Berdat PA, Immer F, Pfammatter JP, Carrel T. Reoperations in adults with congenital heart disease: analysis of early outcome. Int J Cardiol. 2004;93(2–3):239–45.
7. Engelings CC, Helm PC, Abdul-Khaliq H, Asfour B, Bauer UM, Baumgartner H, Kececioglu D, Körten MA, Diller GP, Tutarel O. Cause of death in adults with congenital heart

disease—an analysis of the German National Register for Congenital Heart Defects. Int J Cardiol. 2016;211:31–6.
8. Allan C. Intensive care of the adult patient with congenital heart disease. Prog Cardiovasc Dis. 2011;53(4):274–80.
9. Mackie AS, Pilote L, Ionescu-Ittu R, Rahme E, Marelli AJ. Health care resource utilization in adults with congenital heart disease. Am J Cardiol. 2007;99(6):839–43.
10. Verheugt CL, Uiterwaal CS, van der Velde ET, Meijboom FJ, Pieper PG, Sieswerda GT, Plokker HW, Grobbee DE, Mulder BJ. The emerging burden of hospital admissions of adults with congenital heart disease. Heart. 2010;96(11):872–8.
11. Goldsbury DE, O'Connell DL, Girgis A, Wilkinson A, Phillips JL, Davidson PM, Ingham JM. Acute hospital-based services used by adults during the last year of life in New South Wales, Australia: a population-based retrospective cohort study. BMC Health Serv Res. 2015;15:537.
12. Kogon BE, Plattner C, Leong T, Kirshbom PM, Kanter KR, McConnell M, Book W. Adult congenital heart surgery: adult or pediatric facility? Adult or pediatric surgeon? Ann Thorac Surg. 2009;87(3):833–40.
13. Maxwell BG, Maxwell TG, Wong JK. Decentralization of care for adults with congenital heart disease in the United States: a geographic analysis of outpatient surgery. PLoS One. 2014;9(9):e106730.
14. Karamlou T, Diggs BS, Ungerleider RM, Welke KF. Adults or big kids: what is the ideal clinical environment for management of grown-up patients with congenital heart disease? Ann Thorac Surg. 2010;90(2):573–9.
15. Karamlou T, Diggs BS, Person T, Ungerleider RM, Welke KF. National practice patterns for management of adult congenital heart disease: operation by pediatric heart surgeons decreases in-hospital death. Circulation. 2008;118(23):2345–52.
16. Redington A. Intensive care in the adult with congenital heart disease. Pediatr Crit Care Med. 2016;17(8 Suppl 1):S377–82.
17. Schuuring MJ, van Gulik EC, Koolbergen DR, Hazekamp MG, Lagrand WK, Backx AP, Mulder BJ, Bouma BJ. Determinants of clinical right ventricular failure after congenital heart surgery in adults. J Cardiothorac Vasc Anesth. 2013;27(4):723–7.
18. Perry J, Lanzberg M, Franklin W, Webb G, Chang AC. Cardiac intensive care of the adult with congenital heart disease: basic principles in the management of common problems. World J Pediatr Congenit Heart Surg. 2011;2(3):430–44.
19. Giannakoulas G, Dimopoulos K, Engel R, Goktekin O, Kucukdurmaz Z, Vatankulu MA, Bedard E, Diller GP, Papaphylactou M, Francis DP, Di Mario C, Gatzoulis MA. Burden of coronary artery disease in adults with congenital heart disease and its relation to congenital and traditional heart risk factors. Am J Cardiol. 2009;103(10):1445–50.
20. Bouchardy J, Therrien J, Pilote L, Ionescu-Ittu R, Martucci G, Bottega N, Marelli AJ. Atrial arrhythmias in adults with congenital heart disease. Circulation. 2009;120(17):1679–86.
21. Diller GP, Giardini A, Dimopoulos K, Gargiulo G, Müller J, Derrick G, Giannakoulas G, Khambadkone S, Lammers AE, Picchio FM, Gatzoulis MA, Hager A. Predictors of morbidity and mortality in contemporary Fontan patients: results from a multicenter study including cardiopulmonary exercise testing in 321 patients. Eur Heart J. 2010;31(24):3073–83.
22. Buelow MW, Dall A, Bartz PJ, Tweddell JS, Sowinski J, Rudd N, Katzmark L, Earing MG. Renal dysfunction is common among adults after palliation for previous tetralogy of Fallot. Pediatr Cardiol. 2013;34(1):165–9.
23. Buelow MW, Cohen SB, Earing MG. Renal dysfunction in adults with congenital heart disease. Prog Pediatr Cardiol. 2016;41:47–9.
24. Dimopoulos K, Diller GP, Koltsida E, Pijuan-Domenech A, Papadopoulou SA, Babu-Narayan SV, Salukhe TV, Piepoli MF, Poole-Wilson PA, Best N, Francis DP, Gatzoulis MA. Prevalence, predictors, and prognostic value of renal dysfunction in adults with congenital heart disease. Circulation. 2008;117(18):2320–8.
25. Waldow HC, Westhoff-Bleck M, Widera C, Templin C, von Depka M. Acquired von Willebrand syndrome in adult patients with congenital heart disease. Int J Cardiol. 2014;176(3):739–45.

26. lonso-Gonzalez R, Borgia F, Diller GP, Inuzuka R, Kempny A, Martinez-Naharro A, Tutarel O, Marino P, Wustmann K, Charalambides M, Silva M, Swan L, Dimopoulos K, Gatzoulis MA. Abnormal lung function in adults with congenital heart disease: prevalence, relation to cardiac anatomy, and association with survival. Circulation. 2013;127(8):882–90.
27. Pundi K, Pundi KN, Kamath PS, Cetta F, Li Z, Poterucha JT, Driscoll DJ, Johnson JN. Liver disease in patients after the Fontan operation. Am J Cardiol. 2016;117(3):456–60.
28. Giamberti A, Chessa M, Abella R, Butera G, Carlucci C, Nuri H, Frigiola A, Ranucci M. Morbidity and mortality risk factors in adults with congenital heart disease undergoing cardiac reoperations. Ann Thorac Surg. 2009;88(4):1284–9.
29. Wauthy P, Massaut J, Sanoussi A, Demanet H, Morissens M, Damry N, Dessy H, Malekzadeh-Milani SG, Deuvaert FE. Ten-year experience with surgical treatment of adults with congenital cardiac disease. Cardiol Young. 2011;21(1):39–45.

Overview of the Intensive Care of the Adult with Congenital Heart Disease

2

Jeremy Nicolarsen and Joseph Kay

2.1 Introduction

Through improvements in prenatal diagnosis, surgical technique, perioperative care, and long-term medical management and surveillance, children with congenital heart disease are now routinely surviving into adulthood. In 2001, it was estimated that 95% would see their adult years [1] and an increasingly larger proportion would be adults with moderately to severely complex congenital heart disease (CHD). In fact, the number of adults living with *severe* congenital heart disease (defined as lesions associated with cyanosis or requiring intervention early in life) has risen by 85% from 1985 to 2000 [2]. By now, it is expected that the number of adults with moderately and severely complex CHD outnumbers children.

As our ability to prolong the lives of adult patients with CHD continues to improve, we will see an increasingly larger number of admissions to the intensive care unit (ICU) as many of these patients require re-interventions or surgeries or are faced with exacerbations of chronic diseases. From 1996 to 2000, of 22,096 adult congenital heart disease (ACHD) patients in Quebec, 51% of those with severe defects were hospitalized, and 16% were admitted to the ICU, with more days spent in critical care (RR 2.12, 95% CI: 1.80–2.50) than patients with less complex congenital cardiac lesions [3]. Compared to the general population, ACHD patients are admitted twice as often [4] and many times, emergently. In a multicenter European

J. Nicolarsen (✉)
Providence Adult and Teen Congenital Heart Program (PATCH), Providence Sacred Heart Medical Center and Children's Hospital, Spokane, WA, USA
e-mail: jeremy.nicolarsen@providence.org

J. Kay
Colorado's Adult and Teen Congenital Heart Program (CATCH), Department of Cardiology, University of Colorado Hospital and Children's Hospital Colorado, Aurora, CO, USA
e-mail: joseph.kay@ucdenver.edu

E. da Cruz et al. (eds.), *Intensive Care of the Adult with Congenital Heart Disease*, Congenital Heart Disease in Adolescents and Adults,
https://doi.org/10.1007/978-3-319-94171-4_2

study of 5 hospitals, within 1 year there were 1033 admissions of adults with congenital heart disease, and 201 (160 patients; age 16–71 years) were emergencies [5]. With an estimated growth of this patient population of 5% per year [2], a 102% increase in the number of ACHD hospitalizations from 1998 to 2005 [6], and increasingly complex older patients, intensivists in both pediatric and adult ICUs stand to shoulder a large burden of the care for ACHD patients.

Caring for an ACHD patient in the ICU requires a fundamental understanding of the underlying physiologic consequences of the repairs performed, a keen observance of potential risks associated with acquired heart diseases, and a multidisciplinary approach that involves specialists experienced with the many nuances of this complex subset of patients. It is the adult patient with chronic kidney disease and cirrhosis undergoing his fourth sternotomy and cardiopulmonary bypass, perhaps more so than the neonate with aortic coarctation and a first surgical repair, who requires progressive, prepared ICU teams capable of handling complex ACHD patients. The critically ill ACHD patient should be cared for in a center that is equipped with cardiologists trained in adult congenital heart disease, surgical support that includes the ability to utilize ventricular assist devices, extracorporeal membrane oxygenation (ECMO), and cardiac transplantation, and an ICU team adept at managing medical complications that may arise in the adult. Furthermore, it is important to recognize that non-cardiac comorbidities are common in ACHD patients and may become clinically significant in the setting of critical illness and also that low risk surgical procedures or hospital admissions may still be challenging in those with highly complex CHD. This report aims to introduce providers to many of the issues complicating the care of adults with congenital heart disease in the intensive care setting, including how variable care can be, even for patients with the same defect.

2.2 Monitoring and Access

Further details about monitoring will be discussed in another chapter in this book.

2.2.1 Blood Pressure Monitoring

Surgical management of most types of CHD has changed significantly over the past half century. Therefore, providers involved in the care of ACHD patients need to understand the various surgical approaches for particular defects and their impact on management. For example, in tetralogy of Fallot and other cyanotic CHDs with inadequate pulmonary blood flow, palliation in the 1950s–1980s frequently involved the use of the classic Blalock-Taussig shunt, in which the subclavian artery was transected and anastomosed to the pulmonary artery [7]. The subclavian artery was also sacrificed in subclavian flap repair of aortic coarctation in many centers [8]. Each of these techniques leaves the patient with only collateral blood flow to the ipsilateral arm and results in a lower blood pressure (and radial pulse intensity) than expected (Fig. 2.1). In today's repairs of these defects, modified Blalock-Taussig shunts (Gore-Tex graft from the subclavian artery to

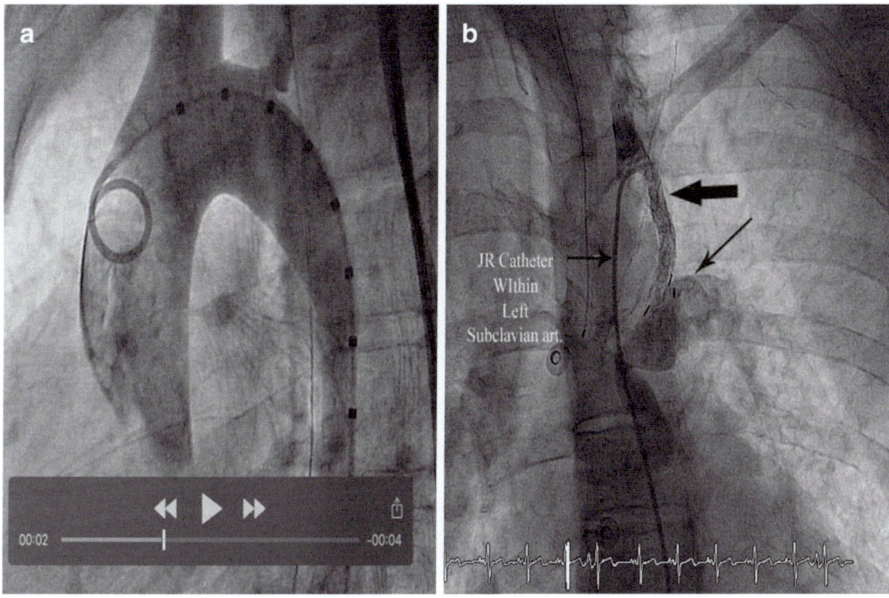

Fig. 2.1 (**a**) A patient after previous coarctation repair with subclavian flap. The first great vessel is the innominate artery and the second, a left carotid artery with no left subclavian artery seen. (**b**) Classic left Blalock-Taussig shunt (with stents) with the left subclavian artery anastomosed to a dilated left pulmonary artery

pulmonary artery) and extended end-to-end repairs of aortic coarctation obviate the use of the subclavian artery and ensure accurate blood pressure and pulse monitoring. If the patient entering the intensive care unit is not able to give a complete surgical history or is unaware of the details of his or her previous surgeries, a thorough physical exam is particularly important, including evaluation for a lateral thoracotomy scar, suggesting a previous shunt or coarctation repair. Blood pressure should be measured in both arms, and continuous or intermittent blood pressure assessment should then be obtained from the higher of the two sides.

2.2.2 Central Venous Access

Another issue faced by many ACHD survivors is systemic venous obstruction (femoral, subclavian, venae cavae, etc.) due to frequent cardiac catheterizations as a child, prolonged need for central venous access after surgical repair, or prolonged pacemaker/implantable cardioverter defibrillator use. Patients who have undergone a multistage palliation for single-ventricle physiology are the most common group to have venous obstruction, having had at least two to three cardiac catheterizations and prolonged recoveries after surgery, but venous obstruction can also be seen with moderately complex lesions such as tetralogy of Fallot. Therefore, providers should be careful when placing central venous catheters – if the wire does not pass easily, there needs to be a high index of suspicion of vascular occlusion with collaterals, and

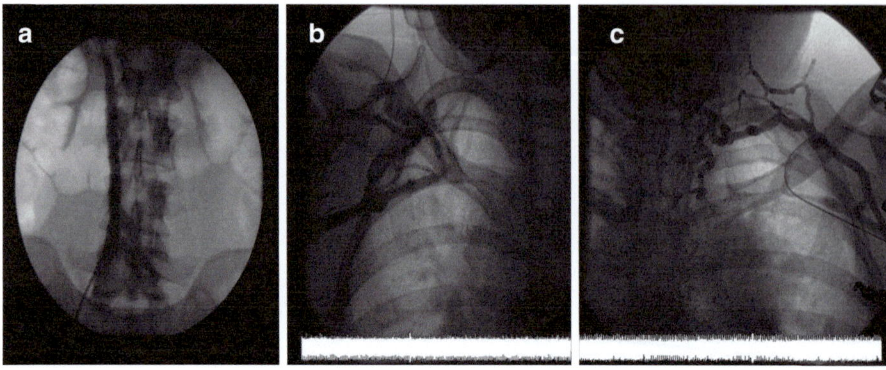

Fig. 2.2 (**a**) Adult with lateral tunnel Fontan with obstruction of the inferior vena cava above the iliac bifurcation. (**b**, **c**) Patient with pulmonary atresia/ventricular septal defect (late after repair) with occlusion of her right (panel **b**) and left (panel **c**) subclavian veins, requiring venoplasty prior to placement of pacemaker leads

alternate sites should be sought (Fig. 2.2). Ideally, vascular US should be performed in such patients in order to identify venous and arterial patency and flow patterns.

Providers should make every attempt to understand a patient's surgical and catheterization history before embarking on a procedure to obtain central venous access. For example, in patients palliated with a lateral tunnel or extracardiac Fontan, the superior vena cava and inferior vena cava are anastomosed directly to the pulmonary arteries with no pre-pulmonary pump or ventricle. While these patients can still undergo upper extremity placement of a peripherally inserted central catheter (PICC line), these lines and others placed via a subclavian or internal jugular vein communicate directly with the pulmonary arteries, and hence central venous pressure reflects mean pulmonary artery pressure.

2.2.3 Avoidance of Air Embolism

Normally, small air bubbles that may enter the circulation from central or peripheral venous catheters are routinely filtered out by the microvasculature in the lungs. However, in ACHD patients with residual intracardiac shunting, even small air bubbles can cross from the right to left side of the circulation and cause a stroke or distal embolism. Therefore, all patients with a congenital heart defects at risk of right-to-left shunting should have air filters placed on intravenous tubing to prevent inadvertent entrainment of air into the circulation, which could increase one's risk of stroke or other complication.

2.3 Congestive Hepatopathy and Hepatic Disease

Passive venous congestion of the liver can result from ventricular failure due to many congenital heart defects, such as pulmonary hypertension from chronic left-to-right shunting through a septal defect or as a result of a failing systemic ventricle in a patient with D-transposition of the great arteries who has undergone an atrial switch palliation. This congestive hepatopathy is especially common in patients with Fontan physiology, where the circulation depends on passive, nonpulsatile pulmonary blood flow through an intra- or extracardiac conduit connecting the venae cavae to the pulmonary circulation. Perturbations of flow, whether secondary to mechanics and compliance of the conduit, obstruction of the pulmonary arteries, or due to increased pulmonary vascular resistance from any number of cardiac or pulmonary causes, can result in impaired systemic venous flow and pressure transmission to the hepatic vascular bed. These elevated right-sided pressures can result in hepatic congestion and sinusoidal dilatation, inflammation, fibrosis, and eventually cirrhosis. Portal hypertension with gastroesophageal varices and gastrointestinal hemorrhage may also occur, as can protein-losing enteropathy. Furthermore, systemic ventricular dysfunction can result in decreased cardiac output and inadequate hepatic perfusion, which also plays a role in the development of liver disease in these patients.

While congestive hepatopathy is often a result of long-standing repaired or unrepaired congenital heart disease, problems like chronic viral hepatitis, transfusion or drug-related hepatitis, liver disease due to alcohol or obesity, and hepatocellular carcinoma may also be encountered in ACHD patients. Not surprisingly, the presence of chronic liver disease can heighten the risk of acute hepatic dysfunction in the postoperative or acutely ill patient and should be considered in every ACHD patient admitted to an ICU. Finally, a relatively common liver disease encountered in ACHD patients is hepatitis C, as older ACHD patients may have been exposed to this bloodborne infection before the era of routine pre-transfusion screening. In a 1992 cohort of 198 ACHD patients, 8.6% were positive for hepatitis C virus (HCV) antibody, up from 1.6% in the general population, and there was a direct correlation between the number of cardiac surgical procedures and the risk of HCV infection [9].

Whatever the cause of hepatic dysfunction in the ACHD patient, problems like ascites, coagulopathy, and hyperbilirubinemia can occur. In the critically ill ACHD patient, hemodynamic dysfunction can acutely impair hepatic venous drainage with worsening of ascites, abdominal compartment syndrome, and further impairment of cardiac preload, propelling the patient into a vicious cycle that can end in profound systemic tissue deoxygenation, acidemia, and impaired organ function or circulatory arrest.

Predicting which ACHD patients will be at greatest risk for hepatic dysfunction is not easy, but close monitoring of serum biomarkers in the pre- and postoperative period, as well as in those with known liver disease who are admitted to the ICU for other reasons, is important. Hepatic venous congestion most commonly manifests as an elevation in indirect bilirubin and mild prolongation of INR and less so as elevations of the aminotransferases [10]. Conversely, ischemic, drug, or viral hepatitis often results in acute increases in the transaminases. The rapidity of the return to normal of previously elevated transaminases also matters, such that an early drop in aspartate aminotransferase (AST) and alanine aminotransferase (ALT) suggests low cardiac output and hepatic ischemia [10]. Transaminase elevation in the immediate postoperative period is common, particularly in the setting of right-sided heart failure, and extreme elevations correlate negatively with postoperative survival [11]. Finally, serum albumin is usually preserved until the onset of decompensated cirrhosis, unless associated with protein-losing enteropathy [10], and may be a helpful biomarker in the newly admitted ICU patient with sequelae of chronic liver disease.

In addition to serologic markers of liver disease, new progress is being made in our understanding of the imaging of liver disease, both in its prognostic and diagnostic capabilities. Beyond simple liver ultrasound, there are now new techniques such as ultrasound or magnetic resonance elastography and multiphase liver computed tomography (CT). With these new techniques, however, comes uncertainty and variability in interpretation, and we are still far from widespread application and availability of novel imaging modalities. For the ACHD patient in the ICU, a better understanding of the underlying disease burden going into a critical illness, with any imaging modality locally available, is arguably more helpful than not having that information.

2.4 Renal Impairment

Chronic kidney disease (CKD) is one of the most common acquired diseases in the United States, affecting more than 20 million people, largely secondary to the growing burden of diabetes and hypertension. The presence of chronic kidney disease increases the risk of developing cardiovascular disease. In ACHD patients, whether a result of systemic venous congestion and increased renal vein hypertension, chronically impaired renal blood flow, or a concomitant acquired disease, it is fairly common for patients to be admitted to the ICU with underlying renal dysfunction. This places a greater importance on maintaining adequate circulating blood volume, cardiac output, and renal perfusion pressure to avoid further acute kidney injury. With each insult on the kidney that may be encountered while critically ill, the adult patient may experience earlier impairment in renal function and also be less likely to recover nephron quantity and function than before. This additive effect of recurrent renal injury can have important implications for the ACHD patient who is likely to require repeated ICU admissions during his or her lifetime.

In a study of 1102 ACHD patients, 9% had moderately or severely reduced estimated glomerular filtration rates (GFR) and with that a threefold higher 6-year mortality rate compared to those with a normal GFR [12]. Furthermore, there was an 18-fold higher prevalence of significant renal dysfunction in noncyanotic ACHD patients and a 35-fold higher prevalence in cyanotic ACHD patients compared to the general population [12]. This burden of antecedent renal dysfunction prior to cardiopulmonary bypass, combined with alterations in renal perfusion and use of nephrotoxic medications in the postoperative period, makes this a particularly important comorbidity that deserves close attention.

2.5 Arrhythmia

The most common reason for hospital admission for ACHD patients is arrhythmia [13]. Often the result of surgical scarring adjacent to the conduction system and/or atrial enlargement, arrhythmia in the ACHD patient can be challenging to manage, especially as the circulation may be abnormal at baseline and the arrhythmia, less well-tolerated. Furthermore, arrhythmia in the ACHD patient may be a sign of impending hemodynamic decompensation, something that is not universally well-known, and common antiarrhythmic therapies may actually be harmful in the ACHD patient due to negative inotropic effects. While not all patients with ACHD develop arrhythmia, the need for acute management and intervention is high among those that do. In a multicenter evaluation of 556 ACHD patients, 43.3% had a sustained arrhythmia or required an arrhythmia intervention [14]. This degree of disease burden in adults requires electrophysiologists adept at navigating the physiology and structure of complex congenital heart disease, and whether the patient is cared for in a children's or adult hospital, collaboration among specialists is often necessary.

Of particular importance in ACHD arrhythmia is the risk of sudden cardiac death. The lesions most commonly associated with late sudden cardiac death are tetralogy of Fallot (TOF), D-transposition of the great arteries (D-TGA), L-transposition of the great arteries with ventricular inversion (L-TGA) (congenitally corrected transposition of the great arteries, CC-TGA), aortic stenosis (AS), and univentricular heart (UVH) [15]. One particular defect that has been well studied is tetralogy of Fallot (TOF), in which 34% of adult patients with this lesion develop symptomatic supraventricular tachycardias, 8.5% develop high-grade ventricular tachycardia, and 2% develop sudden death [16]. With this lesion, QRS duration and right ventricular end-diastolic volume indexed to body surface area (RVEDVi) have been used to prognosticate and guide timing of surgical- or catheter-based intervention on the right ventricular outflow tract, which may then decrease this arrhythmia risk. Although there is some variability in the literature, and several criteria have been proposed, in patients with TOF and moderate to severe pulmonary insufficiency with a regurgitant fraction of >25%, QRS duration >140 ms and/or RVEDVi > 150 mL/m^2 by cardiac magnetic resonance imaging (MRI) represents conservative but reasonable thresholds above which to replace the pulmonary valve [17]. Criteria guiding if and when to place implantable cardioverter defibrillators (ICDs) in TOF patients are less well-defined but increasingly being performed for both primary and secondary prevention, making medical encounters and potential ICU admissions more common.

A second lesion among older patients that bears mention is the antiquated atriopulmonary Fontan, in which there is a 50% incidence of atrial tachycardia within 10 years of palliation. In many cases, these patients are now undergoing elective Fontan conversion to an extracardiac Fontan circuit, usually jointly with arrhythmia surgery. At one center where 133 Fontan conversion surgeries were performed between 1994 and 2011, freedom from arrhythmia recurrence was 85% at 10 years [18]. This circulation is an independent risk factor for atrial arrhythmias in patients with any type of Fontan circulation, as is heart failure requiring diuretic therapy, decreased heart rate reserve, and a prior history of clinically relevant arrhythmia [19].

2.6 Coagulopathy and Hematologic Disease

Bleeding and coagulopathy can frequently be encountered in the ACHD patient. Whether a result of impaired production of clotting factors such as that seen in pre-Fontan single ventricle patients [20], diminished clotting factor levels due to the

Fontan circulation itself [21], or secondary to impaired platelet function or an altered clotting cascade, bleeding in the ICU setting or post-procedural period can be problematic. Furthermore, bleeding can occur in the setting of normal platelet number or fibrinogen level, making this complication also unpredictable. In a study of patients with cyanotic congenital heart disease and elevated hematocrits (57 ± 8%), fibrinogen was dysfunctional, as evidenced by abnormal thromboelastography (TEG) and TEG fibrinogen function (TEG FF), despite its level being high [22]. This can result in impairment of clot formation and bleeding.

In addition to bleeding, ACHD patients are at risk of thrombosis. Those with Eisenmenger syndrome seem to be at the greatest risk of pulmonary vascular thrombosis, largely secondary to increased pulmonary vascular pressures, impaired pulmonary arterial flow, and iron-deficient erythrocytosis from chronic hypoxemia. Therefore, some have advocated for anticoagulation as primary prevention in these patients. However, doing so is not without risk, as patients with Eisenmenger syndrome have an increased risk of hemoptysis. In a recent retrospective review of Eisenmenger patients who have been followed for an average of 7 years, anticoagulation had no effect on long-term survival [23] and prophylactic use of anticoagulation in the acute setting in patients with Eisenmenger syndrome is not well-known. Another cause of thrombosis in ACHD patients is chronic venous insufficiency (CVI). In a multicenter trial of 159 adults with Fontan physiology, severe CVI (defined by skin changes beyond telangiectasias, varicose veins, or edema) was significantly higher in the Fontan group (22%; 95% CI: 16–29%) vs. the healthy controls (0%; 95% CI: 0–14%) ($p = 0.005$). Increased systemic venous pressure transmission to the calf veins, coupled with the inflammatory changes induced in the microcirculation, makes these patients prone to thromboembolism [24].

Lastly, barriers to transfusion secondary to antibody formation from multiple prior transfusions and anemia from chronic disease may also be encountered in the ACHD patient admitted to the ICU. In a study of 830 ACHD patients, there was a prevalence of anemia of 13% and a threefold increased risk of death compared to non-anemic patients [25]. Anemic patients were more likely to be receiving diuretics ($p < 0.0001$), have a lower mean corpuscular volume ($p = 0.0001$), and trend toward a higher New York Heart Association functional class ($p = 0.06$) [25]. Couple anemia with the aforementioned bleeding risks, and it becomes apparent just how important this problem can be. In an attempt to subvert the need for allogenic blood transfusions for the postoperative ACHD patient, some advocate pre-donation of autologous blood [21]. Furthermore, receiving blood transfusions from multiple donors leads to sensitization of the ACHD patient and a greater likelihood of allograft rejection or even the inability to undergo orthotopic heart transplantation. Desensitization protocols are used at some institutions, but this is far from universally available.

Conclusion

The field of adult congenital heart disease is ever-expanding and composed of a growing population of patients with inherent variability and complexity, unlike any other area of medicine. ACHD patients often have multi-system comorbidities that can be unpredictable and lead to or complicate critical illness. As this population of patients continues to grow, intensivists, whether in children's or adult hospitals or cardiac or combined ICUs, will need to work to understand the history of surgical repair of congenital heart disease and its resultant physiologies and prepare for the breadth of problems that come with caring for these interesting and challenging patients.

References

1. Warnes CA, Liberthson R, Danielson GK, Dore A, Harris L, Hoffman JI, et al. Task force 1: the changing profile of congenital heart disease in adult life. J Am Coll Cardiol. 2001;37(5):1170–5.
2. Marelli AJ, Mackie AS, Ionescu-Ittu R, Rahme E, Pilote L. Congenital heart disease in the general population: changing prevalence and age distribution. Circulation. 2007;115(2):163–72.
3. Mackie AS, Pilote L, Ionescu-Ittu R, Rahme E, Marelli AJ. Health care resource utilization in adults with congenital heart disease. Am J Cardiol. 2007;99(6):839–43.
4. Verheugt CL, Uiterwaal CS, van der Velde ET, Meijboom FJ, Pieper PG, Sieswerda GT, et al. The emerging burden of hospital admissions of adults with congenital heart disease. Heart. 2010;96(11):872–8.
5. Kaemmerer H, Bauer U, Pensl U, Oechslin E, Gravenhorst V, Franke A, et al. Management of emergencies in adults with congenital cardiac disease. Am J Cardiol. 2008;101(4):521–5.
6. Opotowsky AR, Siddiqi OK, Webb GD. Trends in hospitalizations for adults with congenital heart disease in the U.S. J Am Coll Cardiol. 2009;54(5):460–7.
7. Blalock A. The technique of creation of an artificial ductus arteriosus in the treatment of pulmonic stenosis. J Thorac Surg. 1947;16(3):244–57.
8. Pierce WS, Waldhausen JA, Berman W Jr, Whitman V. Late results of the subclavian flap procedure in infants with coarctation of the thoracic aorta. Circulation. 1978;58(3 Pt 2):I78–82.
9. Wang A, Book WM, McConnell M, Lyle T, Rodby K, Mahle WT. Prevalence of hepatitis C infection in adult patients who underwent congenital heart surgery prior to screening in 1992. Am J Cardiol. 2007;100(8):1307–9.
10. Asrani SK, Asrani NS, Freese DK, Phillips SD, Warnes CA, Heimbach J, et al. Congenital heart disease and the liver. Hepatology. 2012;56:1160.
11. Shteyer E, Yatsiv I, Sharkia M, Milgarter E, Granot E. Serum transaminases as a prognostic factor in children post cardiac surgery. Pediatr Int. 2011;53(5):725–8.
12. Dimopoulos K, Diller GP, Koltsida E, Pijuan-Domenech A, Papadopoulou SA, Babu-Narayan SV, et al. Prevalence, predictors, and prognostic value of renal dysfunction in adults with congenital heart disease. Circulation. 2008;117(18):2320–8.
13. Somerville J. Management of adults with congenital heart disease: an increasing problem. Annu Rev Med. 1997;48:283–93.
14. Khairy P, Aboulhosn J, Gurvitz MZ, Opotowsky AR, Mongeon FP, Kay J, et al. Arrhythmia burden in adults with surgically repaired tetralogy of Fallot: a multi-institutional study. Circulation. 2010;122(9):868–75.
15. Zipes DP, Camm AJ, Borggrefe M, Buxton AE, Chaitman B, Fromer M, et al. ACC/AHA/ESC 2006 guidelines for management of patients with ventricular arrhythmias and the prevention of sudden cardiac death—executive summary: a report of the American College of Cardiology/American Heart Association Task Force and the European Society of Cardiology Committee for Practice Guidelines (Writing Committee to Develop Guidelines for Management of Patients with Ventricular Arrhythmias and the Prevention of Sudden Cardiac Death) Developed in collaboration with the European Heart Rhythm Association and the Heart Rhythm Society. Eur Heart J. 2006;27(17):2099–140.

16. Lam W, Friedman RA. Electrophysiology issues in adult congenital heart disease. Methodist Debakey Cardiovasc J. 2011;7(2):13–7.
17. Geva T. Repaired tetralogy of Fallot: the roles of cardiovascular magnetic resonance in evaluating pathophysiology and for pulmonary valve replacement decision support. J Cardiovasc Magn Reson. 2011;13:9.
18. Backer CL. 12th annual C. Walton Lillehei memorial lecture in cardiovascular surgery: Fontan conversion—the Chicago experience. Cardiol Young. 2011;21(Suppl 2):169–76.
19. Diller GP, Giardini A, Dimopoulos K, Gargiulo G, Muller J, Derrick G, et al. Predictors of morbidity and mortality in contemporary Fontan patients: results from a multicenter study including cardiopulmonary exercise testing in 321 patients. Eur Heart J. 2010;31(24):3073–83.
20. Odegard KC, McGowan FX Jr, Zurakowski D, DiNardo JA, Castro RA, del Nido PJ, et al. Coagulation factor abnormalities in patients with single-ventricle physiology immediately prior to the Fontan procedure. Ann Thorac Surg. 2002;73(6):1770–7.
21. Odegard KC, McGowan FX Jr, Zurakowski D, Dinardo JA, Castro RA, del Nido PJ, et al. Procoagulant and anticoagulant factor abnormalities following the Fontan procedure: increased factor VIII may predispose to thrombosis. J Thorac Cardiovasc Surg. 2003;125(6):1260–7.
22. Jensen AS, Johansson PI, Bochsen L, Idorn L, Sorensen KE, Thilen U, et al. Fibrinogen function is impaired in whole blood from patients with cyanotic congenital heart disease. Int J Cardiol. 2013;167(5):2210–4.
23. Sandoval J, Santos LE, Cordova J, Pulido T, Gutierrez G, Bautista E, et al. Does anticoagulation in Eisenmenger syndrome impact long-term survival? Congenit Heart Dis. 2012;7(3):268–76.
24. Valente AM, Bhatt AB, Cook S, Earing MG, Gersony DR, Aboulhosn J, et al. The CALF (congenital heart disease in adults lower extremity systemic venous health in Fontan patients) study. J Am Coll Cardiol. 2010;56(2):144–50.
25. Dimopoulos K, Diller GP, Giannakoulas G, Petraco R, Chamaidi A, Karaoli E, et al. Anemia in adults with congenital heart disease relates to adverse outcome. J Am Coll Cardiol. 2009;54(22):2093–100.

Nomenclature, Classification, and Risk Score Assessment of the Adult with Congenital Heart Disease

3

Jeffrey P. Jacobs

3.1 Background

As of 2000, more adults than children are alive with congenital heart disease [1]. Many of these adults with congenital heart disease require cardiac surgery and reoperative cardiac surgery. In the specialty of cardiac surgery, multi-institutional databases are used for outcomes analysis, quality assessment, and quality improvement.

Founded in 1964, the Society of Thoracic Surgeons (STS) is the largest professional organization of cardiothoracic surgeons in the USA. The mission of STS is to enhance the ability of cardiothoracic surgeons to provide the highest-quality patient care through education, research, and advocacy. The STS Congenital Heart Surgery Database (CHSD) [2–4] is the largest database of pediatric and congenital cardiac operations in the world. The STS CHSD is a randomly audited, comprehensive database of patients who have undergone congenital and pediatric cardiac surgical operations at centers in the USA and Canada. The STS CHSD is a voluntary registry, which contains preoperative, operative, and outcomes data for all

J. P. Jacobs
Department of Surgery and Pediatrics, Johns Hopkins University, Baltimore, MD, USA

Division of Cardiovascular Surgery, Johns Hopkins All Children's Hospital, St. Petersburg, FL, USA

E. da Cruz et al. (eds.), *Intensive Care of the Adult with Congenital Heart Disease*, Congenital Heart Disease in Adolescents and Adults,
https://doi.org/10.1007/978-3-319-94171-4_3

patients undergoing congenital and pediatric cardiovascular operations at participating hospitals. The Report of the 2015 STS Congenital Heart Surgery Practice Survey estimates that 125 hospitals in the USA perform pediatric and congenital heart surgery [5]. In 2016, the STS CHSD included 114 pediatric heart surgery programs in the USA, representing 121 of these 125 hospitals (97% penetrance by hospital) in the USA.

In order for any multi-institutional databases including the STS CHSD to function as a platform for outcomes analysis, quality assessment, and quality improvement, the nomenclature, classification, and risk score assessment must be standardized across all participants. The purpose of this chapter is to review nomenclature, classification, and risk scores for adults with congenital heart disease.

3.2 Nomenclature and Classification

The choice of terminology and nomenclature is critical when analyzing outcomes of cardiac surgery, and this concept is especially true in the analysis of cardiac surgery in adults with congenital cardiac disease. STS CHSD utilizes the following age groupings: neonates (0–30 days), infants (31 days–1 year), children (>1 year to <18 years), and adults (18 years and above). Coding in the STS CHSD is accomplished by clinicians and highly trained database managers using the International Pediatric and Congenital Cardiac Code (IPCCC) [6, 7] and is entered into the contemporary version of the STS CHSD data collection form [8]. The definitions of all terms and codes in the STS CHSD have been standardized and published [8]. In congenital cardiac surgery, the use of this clinical nomenclature (IPCCC) is critical because several studies have documented that the nomenclature used in administrative databases (that are designed for billing and not quality assessment) is poor and prone to misclassification and error [9–12]. Therefore, the IPCCC is the standardized system of nomenclature for pediatric and congenital cardiac care. The IPCCC is the gold standard system of nomenclature and classification for the surgical treatment of both children and adults with congenital heart disease and is available for free download at [http://ipccc.net/].

3.3 Risk Score Assessment

Because of the large number of different types of pediatric and congenital cardiac operations (more than 200 individual procedure types, most often performed in various combinations), it is useful to stratify individual operations into groups or categories that are relatively homogeneous with respect to complexity or risk. This methodology, called risk stratification (or complexity stratification), has been used by STS CHSD since 2002. Complexity stratification is a method of analysis in which the data are divided into relatively homogeneous groups (called strata). The data are analyzed and reported within each stratum. STS CHSD has employed three methods of complexity stratification (Tables 3.1, 3.2 and 3.3) [13–15]:

Table 3.1 The *S*ociety of *T*horacic Surgeons—European *A*ssociation for Cardio-*T*horacic Surgery Congenital Heart Surgery Mortality Categories (STAT Mortality Categories) (2016)

Data version 3.22 procedure	Procedure	STAT Mortality Score	STAT mortality category
30	ASD repair, Patch	0.1	1
190	AVC (AVSD) repair, Partial (incomplete) (PAVSD)	0.1	1
10	PFO, Primary closure	0.2	1
20	ASD repair, Primary closure	0.2	1
110	VSD repair, Patch	0.2	1
570	DCRV repair	0.2	1
780	Aortic stenosis, Subvalvar, Repair	0.2	1
1210	Coarctation repair, End to end	0.2	1
1360	Vascular ring repair	0.2	1
1470	ICD (AICD) implantation	0.2	1
1480	ICD (AICD) ([automatic] implantable cardioverter defibrillator) procedure	0.2	1
2110[a]	ASD repair, Patch + PAPCV repair	0.2	1
100	VSD repair, Primary closure	0.3	1
180	AVC (AVSD) repair, Intermediate (transitional)	0.3	1
260	PAPVC repair	0.3	1
350	TOF repair, No ventriculotomy	0.3	1
360	TOF repair, Ventriculotomy, Nontransannular patch	0.3	1
580	Conduit reoperation	0.3	1
600	Valve replacement, Pulmonic (PVR)	0.3	1
680	Valve replacement, Aortic (AVR), Mechanical	0.3	1
690	Valve replacement, Aortic (AVR), Bioprosthetic	0.3	1
810	Sinus of Valsalva, Aneurysm repair	0.3	1
970	Fontan, TCPC, Lateral tunnel, Fenestrated	0.3	1
1250	Coarctation repair, Interposition graft	0.3	1
1460	Pacemaker procedure	0.3	1
1680	Glenn (unidirectional cavopulmonary anastomosis) (unidirectional Glenn)	0.3	1
2120[b]	PAPVC Repair, Baffle redirection to left atrium with systemic vein translocation (Warden) (SVC sewn to right atrial appendage)	0.3	1
520	1 1/2 ventricular repair	0.4	2
530	PA, Reconstruction (plasty), Main (trunk)	0.4	2
660	Valvuloplasty, Aortic	0.4	2
740	Ross procedure	0.4	2
820	LV to aorta tunnel repair	0.4	2
830	Valvuloplasty, Mitral	0.4	2
950	Fontan, Atrio-pulmonary connection	0.4	2
1330	PDA closure, Surgical	0.4	2
1365	Aortopexy	0.4	2
1450	Pacemaker implantation, Permanent	0.4	2
1500	Arrhythmia surgery—ventricular, Surgical ablation	0.4	2
1690	Bilateral bidirectional cavopulmonary anastomosis (BBDCPA) (bilateral bidirectional Glenn)	0.4	2
2130[c]	Superior cavopulmonary anastomosis(es) + PA reconstruction	0.4	2
210	AP window repair	0.5	2
370	TOF repair, Ventriculotomy, Transannular patch	0.5	2
510	RVOT procedure	0.5	2

(continued)

Table 3.1 (continued)

Data version 3.22 procedure	Procedure	STAT Mortality Score	STAT mortality category
590	Valvuloplasty, Pulmonic	0.5	2
620	Conduit placement, LV to PA	0.5	2
715	Aortic root replacement, Bioprosthetic	0.5	2
720	Aortic root replacement, Mechanical	0.5	2
790	Aortic stenosis, Supravalvar, Repair	0.5	2
930	Pericardiectomy	0.5	2
1070	Congenitally corrected TGA repair, VSD closure	0.5	2
1220	Coarctation repair, End to end, Extended	0.5	2
1291	Anomalous origin of coronary artery from pulmonary artery repair	0.5	2
1380	Aortic aneurysm repair	0.5	2
1670	Bidirectional cavopulmonary anastomosis (BDCPA) (bidirectional Glenn)	0.5	2
1730	Aneurysm, Ventricular, Left, Repair	0.5	2
1772	Conduit placement, Other	0.5	2
2760[d]	Hybrid approach, Transcardiac balloon dilation	0.5	2
2350[b]	Explantation of pacing system	0.5	2
50	ASD, Common atrium (single atrium), Septation	0.6	2
220	Pulmonary artery origin from ascending aorta (hemitruncus) repair	0.6	2
270	PAPVC, Scimitar, Repair	0.6	2
735	Aortic root replacement, Valve sparing	0.6	2
840	Mitral stenosis, Supravalvar mitral ring repair	0.6	2
1000	Fontan, TCPC, External conduit, Fenestrated	0.6	2
1010	Fontan, TCPC, External conduit, Nonfenestrated	0.6	2
1290	Coronary artery fistula ligation	0.6	2
1790	Ligation, Pulmonary artery	0.6	2
2770[d]	Hybrid approach, Transcardiac transcatheter device placement	0.6	2
2780[d]	Fontan, TCPC, Intra-/extracardiac conduit, Fenestrated	0.6	2
2790[d]	Fontan, TCPC, Intra-/extracardiac conduit, Nonfenestrated	0.6	2
3160[d]	Kawashima operation (superior cavopulmonary connection in setting of interrupted IVC with azygous continuation)	0.6	2
3180[d]	Intravascular stent removal	0.6	2
1305[b]	Anomalous aortic origin of coronary artery from aorta (AAOCA) repair	0.6	2
2100[b]	Aortic stenosis, Subvalvar, Repair, With myectomy for IHSS	0.6	2
2270[b]	Valvuloplasty converted to valve replacement in the same operation, Pulmonic	0.6	2
3310[e]	Fontan, TCPC, External conduit, hepatic veins to pulmonary artery, Fenestrated	0.6	2
3320[e]	Fontan, TCPC, External conduit, hepatic veins to pulmonary artery, Nonfenestrated	0.6	2
85	Atrial fenestration closure	0.7	2
130	VSD, Multiple, Repair	0.7	2
250	Valve replacement, Truncal valve	0.7	2
290	Cor triatriatum repair	0.7	2

Table 3.1 (continued)

Data version 3.22 procedure	Procedure	STAT Mortality Score	STAT mortality category
310	Atrial baffle procedure (non-Mustard, non-Senning)	0.7	2
340	Systemic venous stenosis repair	0.7	2
380	TOF repair, RV–PA conduit	0.7	2
460	Valvuloplasty, Tricuspid	0.7	2
470	Valve replacement, Tricuspid (TVR)	0.7	2
550	PA, reconstruction (plasty), Branch, Peripheral (at or beyond the hilar bifurcation)	0.7	2
910	Partial left ventriculectomy (LV volume reduction surgery) (Batista)	0.7	2
980	Fontan, TCPC, Lateral tunnel, Nonfenestrated	0.7	2
1230	Coarctation repair, Subclavian flap	0.7	2
1490	Arrhythmia surgery—atrial, Surgical ablation	0.7	2
3140[d]	Hepatic vein to azygous vein connection, Direct	0.7	2
3150[d]	Hepatic vein to azygous vein connection, Interposition graft	0.7	2
2240[b]	Valvuloplasty converted to valve replacement in the same operation, Aortic	0.7	2
3210[e]	Removal of transcatheter delivered device from blood vessel	0.7	2
150	Ventricular septal fenestration	0.8	3
170	AVC (AVSD) repair, Complete (CAVSD)	0.8	3
240	Valvuloplasty, Truncal valve	0.8	3
330	Anomalous systemic venous connection repair	0.8	3
450	Occlusion MAPCA(s)	0.8	3
540	PA, reconstruction (plasty), Branch, Central (within the hilar bifurcation)	0.8	3
750	Konno procedure	0.8	3
1110	Arterial switch operation (ASO)	0.8	3
1240	Coarctation repair, Patch aortoplasty	0.8	3
1410	Transplant, Lung(s)	0.8	3
1630	Shunt, Ligation, and Takedown	0.8	3
1700	Hemi-Fontan	0.8	3
1720	Aneurysm, Ventricular, Right, Repair	0.8	3
1740	Aneurysm, Pulmonary artery, Repair	0.8	3
1275[a]	Coarctation repair + VSD repair	0.8	3
2280[b]	Valvuloplasty converted to valve replacement in same operation, Tricuspid	0.8	3
3220[e]	Removal of transcatheter delivered device from heart	0.8	3
70	ASD partial closure	0.9	3
960	Fontan, Atrioventricular connection	0.9	3
1150	Rastelli	0.9	3
1774	Conduit placement, Ventricle to aorta	0.9	3
1802	Pulmonary embolectomy, Acute pulmonary embolus	0.9	3
700	Valve replacement, Aortic (AVR), Homograft	1	3
2290[b]	Valvuloplasty converted to valve replacement in the same operation, Truncal valve	1	3
420	Pulmonary atresia–VSD (including TOF, PA) repair	1.1	3
1140	Mustard	1.1	3
1160	REV	1.1	3
1370	Pulmonary artery sling repair	1.1	3

(continued)

Table 3.1 (continued)

Data version 3.22 procedure	Procedure	STAT Mortality Score	STAT mortality category
610	Conduit placement, RV to PA	1.2	3
1800	Pulmonary embolectomy	1.2	3
2310[b]	Valvuloplasty converted to valve replacement in the same operation, Aortic—with Ross procedure	1.2	3
2340[b]	Fontan + atrioventricular valvuloplasty	1.2	3
1145[e]	Atrial baffle procedure, Mustard or Senning revision	1.2	3
850	Valve replacement, Mitral (MVR)	1.3	4
920	Pericardial drainage procedure	1.3	4
2750[d]	Unifocalization MAPCA(s), Unilateral pulmonary unifocalization	1.3	4
2260[b]	Valvuloplasty converted to valve replacement in the same operation, Mitral	1.3	4
2300[b]	Valvuloplasty, Common atrioventricular valve	1.3	4
890	Transplant, Heart	1.4	4
1025	Fontan revision or conversion (redo Fontan)	1.4	4
1180	DORV, Intraventricular tunnel repair	1.4	4
1200	DOLV repair	1.4	4
1280	Aortic arch repair	1.4	4
1650	PA debanding	1.4	4
1760	Cardiac tumor resection	1.4	4
1120[a]	Arterial switch operation (ASO) and VSD repair	1.4	4
1123[a]	Arterial switch procedure + aortic arch repair	1.4	4
2330[b]	Superior cavopulmonary anastomosis(es) (Glenn or hemi-Fontan) + atrioventricular valvuloplasty	1.4	4
400	TOF—absent pulmonary valve repair	1.5	4
490	Valve excision, Tricuspid (without replacement)	1.5	4
1300	Coronary artery bypass	1.5	4
1590	Shunt, Systemic to pulmonary, Modified Blalock–Taussig shunt (MBTS)	1.5	4
2740[d]	Unifocalization MAPCA(s), Bilateral pulmonary unifocalization—incomplete unifocalization (not all usable MAPCA[s] are incorporated)	1.5	4
3200[e]	PA band adjustment	1.5	4
390	TOF–AVC (AVSD) repair	1.6	4
465	Ebstein's repair	1.6	4
760	Ross–Konno procedure	1.6	4
1130	Senning	1.6	4
2730[d]	Unifocalization MAPCA(s), Bilateral pulmonary unifocalization—complete unifocalization (all usable MAPCA[s] are incorporated)	1.6	4
3130[d]	Shunt, Systemic to pulmonary, Central (shunt from the aorta), Central shunt with an end-to-side connection between the transected main pulmonary artery and the side of the ascending aorta (i.e., Mee shunt)	1.6	4
430	Pulmonary atresia–VSD–MAPCA repair	1.7	4
440	Unifocalization MAPCA(s)	1.7	4
730	Aortic root replacement, Homograft	1.7	4
1080	Congenitally corrected TGA repair, VSD closure, and LV to PA conduit	1.7	4
1390	Aortic dissection repair	1.7	4

Table 3.1 (continued)

Data version 3.22 procedure	Procedure	STAT Mortality Score	STAT mortality category
1640	PA banding (PAB)	1.7	4
2710[d]	Pulmonary atresia–VSD–MAPCA repair, Status post prior complete unifocalization (includes VSD closure + RV to PA connection [with or without conduit])	1.7	4
1285[a]	Aortic arch repair + VSD repair	1.7	4
140	VSD creation/enlargement	1.8	4
280	TAPVC repair	1.9	4
880	HLHS biventricular repair	1.9	4
2230[b]	Valve replacement, Common atrioventricular valve	1.9	4
2250[b]	Valvuloplasty converted to valve replacement in the same operation, Common atrioventricular	1.9	4
2320[b]	Valvuloplasty converted to valve replacement in the same operation, Aortic—with Ross–Konno procedure	1.9	4
300	Pulmonary venous stenosis repair	2	4
3230[e]	Shunt, Systemic to pulmonary, Potts–Smith type (descending aorta to pulmonary artery)	2	4
1320	Interrupted aortic arch repair	2.1	4
1600	Shunt, Systemic to pulmonary, Central (from the aorta to the main pulmonary artery)	2.1	4
2720[d]	Pulmonary atresia–VSD–MAPCA repair, Status post prior incomplete unifocalization (includes completion of pulmonary unifocalization + VSD closure + RV to PA connection [with or without conduit])	2.1	4
2700[d]	Pulmonary atresia–VSD–MAPCA repair, Complete single-stage repair (one stage that includes bilateral pulmonary unifocalization + VSD closure + RV to PA connection [with or without conduit])	2.3	4
230	Truncus arteriosus repair	2.4	4
1125[a]	Arterial switch procedure and VSD repair + aortic arch repair	2.4	4
2190[b]	Aortic root translocation over the left ventricle (including Nikaidoh procedure)	2.4	4
2210[b]	TGA, Other procedures (Kawashima, LV-PA conduit, other)	2.4	4
60	ASD creation/enlargement	2.5	4
2170[b]	Hybrid approach “stage 1,” Stent placement in arterial duct (PDA)	2.5	4
80	Atrial septal fenestration	2.6	4
480	Valve closure, Tricuspid (exclusion, univentricular approach)	2.6	4
2160[b]	Hybrid approach “stage 1,” Application of RPA and LPA bands	2.6	4
1660	Damus–Kaye–Stansel procedure (DKS) (creation of AP anastomosis without arch reconstruction)	2.9	5
2200[b]	TAPVC repair + shunt—systemic to pulmonary	3	5
2180[b]	Hybrid approach “stage 1,” Stent placement in arterial duct (PDA) + application of RPA	3.1	5
900	Transplant, Heart and lung	3.2	5
1060	Congenitally corrected TGA repair, Atrial switch and Rastelli	3.2	5

(continued)

Table 3.1 (continued)

Data version 3.22 procedure	Procedure	STAT Mortality Score	STAT mortality category
1050	Congenitally corrected TGA repair, Atrial switch and ASO (double switch)	3.4	5
2755[d]	Conduit insertion of the right ventricle to the pulmonary artery + intraventricular tunnel left ventricle to neoaorta + arch reconstruction (Rastelli- and Norwood-type arch reconstruction) (Yasui)	3.6	5
2150[b]	Hybrid approach "stage 2," Aortopulmonary amalgamation + superior cavopulmonary anastomosis(es) + PA debanding + without aortic arch repair	3.6	5
870	Norwood procedure	4	5
2140	Hybrid approach "stage 2," Aortopulmonary amalgamation + superior cavopulmonary anastomosis(es) + PA debanding + aortic arch repair (Norwood [stage 1] + superior cavopulmonary anastomosis(es) + PA debanding)	4.1	5
2220[a]	Truncus + IAA repair	5	5

[a]Indicates a combined procedure (made up of two or more component procedures)

[b]Indicates that this procedure, score, and category were not included in the original JTCVS publication [14] but were subsequently assigned as part of the upgrade to version 3.0. The original list of procedure codes was based on version 2.5 of the STS Congenital Heart Surgery Database. These additional procedures represent the list of new procedure codes that were added to the STS Congenital Heart Surgery Database in 2010 as part of the upgrade to version 3.0 and have also been incorporated into the EACTS Congenital Heart Surgery Database and the Japan Congenital Cardiovascular Surgery Database (JCCVSD). To assign scores to these new procedures, a panel of highly experienced congenital heart surgeons from programs representing a variety of programmatic volume categories were surveyed and asked to provide an STS–EACTS Mortality Score for 26 procedures that were new to version 3.0, using the scores in the table of the JTCVS article [14] as a guide. The mean of the scores from these ten surgeons was then used to assign the STS–EACTS Mortality Score and STS–EACTS Mortality Category for these 26 new procedures (when the highest and lowest scores were discarded, the scores were essentially the same [9/23 scores did not change, 13/23 scores change by only 0.1, and 1/23 scores change by 0.2])

[c]Indicates a combined procedure and also a procedure for which the Score and Category were not part of the original JTCVS publication [14] and were assigned later as described above

[d]Indicates that this Procedure, Score, and Category were not included in the original JTCVS publication [14] but were subsequently assigned as part of the upgrade to version 3.22. The original list of procedure codes was based on version 2.5 of the STS Congenital Heart Surgery Database. These additional procedures represent the list of new procedure codes that were added to the STS Congenital Heart Surgery Database in 2014 as part of the upgrade to version 3.22 and have also been incorporated into the EACTS Congenital Heart Surgery Database and the Japan Congenital Cardiovascular Surgery Database (JCCVSD). To assign scores to these new procedures, a panel of highly experienced congenital heart surgeons from programs representing a variety of programmatic volume categories were surveyed and asked to provide an STS–EACTS Mortality Score for 16 procedures that were new to version 3.22, using the STAT scores provided in the STS Congenital Heart Surgery Database Spring 2014 Feedback Report as a guide. The mean of the scores from these 17 surgeons was then used to assign the STS–EACTS Mortality Score and STS–EACTS Mortality Category for these 16 new procedures (when the high and low scores were discarded, the STAT scores were essentially the same [12/16 scores did not change, and 4/16 scores change by only 0.1]; meanwhile, when the high and low scores were discarded, the STAT Categories were all unchanged)

(continued)

Table 3.1 (continued)

[e]Indicates that this Procedure, Score, and Category were not included in the original JTCVS publication [14] but were subsequently assigned as part of the upgrade to version 3.3. The original list of procedure codes was based on version 2.5 of the STS Congenital Heart Surgery Database. These additional procedures represent the list of new procedure codes that were added to the STS Congenital Heart Surgery Database in 2016 as part of the upgrade to version 3.3 and have also been incorporated into the EACTS Congenital Heart Surgery Database and the Japan Congenital Cardiovascular Surgery Database (JCCVSD). To assign scores to these new procedures, a panel of highly experienced congenital heart surgeons from programs representing a variety of programmatic volume categories were surveyed and asked to provide an STS–EACTS Mortality Score for seven procedures that were new to version 3.3, using the STAT scores provided in the STS Congenital Heart Surgery Database Spring 2016 Feedback Report as a guide. The mean of the scores from these 17 surgeons was then used to assign the STS–EACTS Mortality Score and STS–EACTS Mortality Category for these seven new procedures (when the high and low scores were discarded, the STAT scores were essentially the same)

Table 3.2 The Aristotle Basic Complexity Score (ABC Score) and the Aristotle Basic Complexity Levels (ABC Levels) (October 24, 2014)

	Score	Mortality	Morbidity	Difficulty	
	1 point	<1%	ICU 0–24H	Elementary	
	2 points	1–5%	ICU 1D–3D	Simple	
	3 points	5–10%	ICU 4D–7D	Average	
	4 points	10–20%	ICU 1W–2W	Important	
	5 point	>20%	ICU > 2W	Major	
	Complexity				
	1.5 to 5.9	1			
	6.0 to 7.9	2			
	8.0 to 9.9	3			
	10.0 to 15.0	4			
Procedures	**Total (basic score)**	**Complexity (basic level)**	**Mortality**	**Morbidity**	**Difficulty**
Pleural drainage procedure	1.5	1	0.5	0.5	0.5
Bronchoscopy	1.5	1	0.5	0.5	0.5
Delayed sternal closure	1.5	1	0.5	0.5	0.5
Mediastinal exploration	1.5	1	0.5	0.5	0.5
Sternotomy wound drainage	1.5	1	0.5	0.5	0.5
Intra-aortic balloon pump (IABP) insertion	2.0	1	0.5	1.0	0.5
Explantation of pacing system	2.5	1	1.0	1.0	0.5
PFO, Primary closure	3.0	1	1.0	1.0	1.0
ASD repair, Primary closure	3.0	1	1.0	1.0	1.0
ASD repair, Patch	3.0	1	1.0	1.0	1.0
ASD partial closure	3.0	1	1.0	1.0	1.0
Atrial fenestration closure	3.0	1	1.0	1.0	1.0
Pericardial drainage procedure	3.0	1	1.0	1.0	1.0
PDA closure, Surgical	3.0	1	1.0	1.0	1.0
Pacemaker implantation, Permanent	3.0	1	1.0	1.0	1.0

(continued)

Table 3.2 (continued)

	Score	Mortality	Morbidity	Difficulty	
Pacemaker procedure	3.0	1	1.0	1.0	1.0
Shunt, Ligation and takedown	3.5	1	1.5	1.0	1.0
ASD, Common atrium (single atrium), Septation	3.8	1	1.0	1.0	1.8
AVC (AVSD) repair, Partial (incomplete) (PAVSD)	4.0	1	1.0	1.0	2.0
Coronary artery fistula ligation	4.0	1	1.0	2.0	1.0
Aortopexy	4.0	1	1.5	1.5	1.0
ICD (AICD) implantation	4.0	1	1.5	1.0	1.5
ICD (AICD) (automatic implantable cardioverter defibrillator) procedure	4.0	1	1.5	1.0	1.5
Hybrid Approach, Transcardiac balloon dilation	4.0	1	1.5	1	1.5
Ligation, Thoracic duct	4.0	1	1.0	2.0	1.0
Diaphragm plication	4.0	1	1.0	2.0	1.0
ECMO decannulation	4.0	1	2.0	1.0	1.0
ASD creation/enlargement	5.0	1	2.0	2.0	1.0
Atrial septal fenestration	5.0	1	2.0	2.0	1.0
AVC (AVSD) repair, Intermediate (transitional)	5.0	1	1.5	1.5	2.0
PAPVC repair	5.0	1	2.0	1.0	2.0
Lung biopsy	5.0	1	1.5	2.0	1.5
Ligation, Pulmonary artery	5.0	1	1.5	2.0	1.5
Decortication	5.0	1	1.0	1.0	3.0
ASD repair, Patch + PAPVC repair	5.0	1	2.0	1.0	2.0
PAPVC Repair, Baffle redirection to left atrium with systemic vein translocation (Warden) (SVC sewn to right atrial appendage)	5.0	1	1.0	2.0	2.0
ECMO cannulation	5.0	1	2.0	1.0	2.0
Pectus repair	5.3	1	2.0	1.0	2.3
Aortic stenosis, Supravalvar, Repair	5.5	1	1.5	2.0	2.0
Valvuloplasty, Pulmonic	5.6	1	1.8	1.8	2.0
VSD repair, Primary closure	6.0	2	2.0	2.0	2.0
VSD repair, Patch	6.0	2	2.0	2.0	2.0
AP window repair	6.0	2	2.0	2.0	2.0
Valve replacement, Truncal valve	6.0	2	2.0	2.0	2.0
Cor triatriatum repair	6.0	2	2.0	2.0	2.0
Valve excision, Tricuspid (without replacement)	6.0	2	2.0	2.0	2.0
PA, reconstruction (plasty), Main (trunk)	6.0	2	2.0	2.0	2.0
Pericardiectomy	6.0	2	2.0	2.0	2.0
Coarctation repair, End to end	6.0	2	2.0	2.0	2.0
Coarctation repair, Subclavian flap	6.0	2	2.0	2.0	2.0

Table 3.2 (continued)

	Score	Mortality	Morbidity	Difficulty	
Coarctation repair, Patch aortoplasty	6.0	2	2.0	2.0	2.0
Vascular ring repair	6.0	2	2.0	2.0	2.0
PA banding (PAB)	6.0	2	2.0	2.0	2.0
PA debanding	6.0	2	2.0	2.0	2.0
ECMO procedure	6.0	2	2.0	3.0	1.0
Aortic stenosis, Subvalvar, Repair	6.3	2	2.0	1.8	2.5
Shunt, Systemic to pulmonary, Modified Blalock–Taussig shunt (MBTS)	6.3	2	2.0	2.0	2.3
RVOT procedure	6.5	2	2.0	2.0	2.5
Valve replacement, Pulmonic (PVR)	6.5	2	2.0	2.0	2.5
Shunt, Systemic to pulmonary, Central (from the aorta to the main pulmonary artery)	6.8	2	2.0	2.0	2.8
Shunt, Systemic to pulmonary, Central (shunt from aorta), Central shunt with an end-to-side connection between the transected main pulmonary artery and the side of the ascending aorta (i.e., Mee shunt)	7.0	2	3	2	2
Valvuloplasty, Truncal valve	7.0	2	2.0	2.0	3.0
Anomalous systemic venous connection repair	7.0	2	2.0	2.0	3.0
Occlusion MAPCA(s)	7.0	2	2.0	2.0	3.0
Valvuloplasty, Tricuspid	7.0	2	2.0	2.0	3.0
DCRV repair	7.0	2	2.0	2.0	3.0
Valve replacement, Aortic (AVR), Mechanical	7.0	2	2.0	2.0	3.0
Valve replacement, Aortic (AVR), Bioprosthetic	7.0	2	2.0	2.0	3.0
Atrial baffle procedure, Mustard or Senning revision	7.0	2	2.0	2.0	3.0
Aortic arch repair	7.0	2	2.0	2.0	3.0
Kawashima operation (superior cavopulmonary connection in setting of interrupted IVC with azygous continuation)	7.0	2	2.5	2	2.5
Bidirectional cavopulmonary anastomosis (BDCPA) (bidirectional Glenn)	7.0	2	2.5	2.0	2.5
Glenn (unidirectional cavopulmonary anastomosis) (unidirectional Glenn)	7.0	2	2.5	2.0	2.5
Hepatic vein to azygous vein connection, Interposition graft	7.0	2	2.5	2	2.5

(continued)

Table 3.2 (continued)

	Score	Mortality	Morbidity	Difficulty	
Hepatic vein to azygous vein connection, Direct	7.0	2	2.5	2	2.5
Right/left heart assist device procedure	7.0	2	2.0	3.0	2.0
Hybrid approach "stage 1," Stent placement in arterial duct (PDA)	7.0	2	1.5	1.5	4.0
VAD implantation	7.0	2	2.0	3.0	2.0
VAD explantation	7.0	2	2.0	3.0	2.0
Hybrid approach, Transcardiac transcatheter device placement	7.0	2	1.5	1.5	4
Intravascular stent removal	7.5	2	3	2	2.5
Ventricular septal fenestration	7.5	2	3.0	2.0	2.5
TOF repair, Ventriculotomy, Nontransannular patch	7.5	2	2.5	2.0	3.0
Valve replacement, Tricuspid (TVR)	7.5	2	2.5	2.0	3.0
Conduit placement, RV to PA	7.5	2	2.5	2.0	3.0
Sinus of Valsalva, Aneurysm repair	7.5	2	2.5	2.0	3.0
Valve replacement, Mitral (MVR)	7.5	2	2.5	2.0	3.0
Coronary artery bypass	7.5	2	2.5	2.0	3.0
Bilateral bidirectional cavopulmonary anastomosis (BBDCPA) (bilateral bidirectional Glenn)	7.5	2	2.5	2.0	3.0
Conduit placement, Other	7.5	2	2.5	2.0	3.0
Hybrid approach "stage 1," Application of RPA and LPA bands	7.5	2	2.5	2.5	2.5
Atrial baffle procedure (non-Mustard, non-Senning)	7.8	2	2.8	2.0	3.0
PA, reconstruction (plasty), Branch, Central (within the hilar bifurcation)	7.8	2	2.8	2.0	3.0
Coarctation repair, Interposition graft	7.8	2	2.8	2.0	3.0
PAPVC, Scimitar, Repair	8.0	3	3.0	2.0	3.0
Systemic venous stenosis repair	8.0	3	3.0	2.0	3.0
TOF repair, No ventriculotomy	8.0	3	3.0	2.0	3.0
TOF repair, Ventriculotomy, Transannular patch	8.0	3	3.0	2.0	3.0
TOF repair, RV–PA conduit	8.0	3	3.0	2.0	3.0
Conduit reoperation	8.0	3	3.0	2.0	3.0
Conduit placement, LV to PA	8.0	3	3.0	2.0	3.0
Valvuloplasty, Aortic	8.0	3	3.0	2.0	3.0
Aortic root replacement	8.0	3	2.5	2.0	3.5
Valvuloplasty, Mitral	8.0	3	3.0	2.0	3.0

Table 3.2 (continued)

	Score	Mortality	Morbidity	Difficulty	
Mitral stenosis, Supravalvar mitral ring repair	8.0	3	3.0	2.0	3.0
Coarctation repair, End to end, Extended	8.0	3	3.0	2.0	3.0
Arrhythmia surgery—atrial, Surgical ablation	8.0	3	3.0	2.0	3.0
Arrhythmia surgery—ventricular, Surgical ablation	8.0	3	3.0	2.0	3.0
Hemi-Fontan	8.0	3	3.0	2.0	3.0
Aneurysm, Ventricular, Right, Repair	8.0	3	3.0	2.0	3.0
Aneurysm, Pulmonary artery, Repair	8.0	3	3.0	2.0	3.0
Cardiac tumor resection	8.0	3	3.0	2.0	3.0
Pulmonary embolectomy	8.0	3	3.0	3.0	2.0
Pulmonary embolectomy, Acute pulmonary embolus	8.0	3	3.0	3.0	2.0
Aortic stenosis, Subvalvar, Repair, With myectomy for IHSS	8.0	3	2.0	2.0	4.0
Valvuloplasty converted to valve replacement in the same operation, Pulmonic	8.0	3	2.5	2.5	3.0
LV to aorta tunnel repair	8.3	3	3.0	2.3	3.0
Valve replacement, Aortic (AVR), Homograft	8.5	3	3.0	2.0	3.5
Aortic root replacement, Valve sparing	8.5	3	2.0	2.0	4.5
Senning	8.5	3	3.0	2.5	3.0
PA, Reconstruction (plasty), Branch, Peripheral (at or beyond the hilar bifurcation)	8.8	3	2.8	2.5	3.5
Unifocalization MAPCA(s), Unilateral pulmonary unifocalization	8.8	3	2.8	2.5	3.5
Aortic root replacement, Mechanical	8.8	3	3.3	2.0	3.5
Aortic aneurysm repair	8.8	3	3.0	2.8	3.0
VSD, Multiple, Repair	9.0	3	3.0	2.5	3.5
VSD creation/enlargement	9.0	3	3.0	3.0	3.0
AVC (AVSD) repair, Complete (CAVSD)	9.0	3	3.0	3.0	3.0
Pulmonary artery origin from ascending aorta (hemitruncus) repair	9.0	3	3.0	3.0	3.0
TAPVC repair	9.0	3	3.0	3.0	3.0
Pulmonary atresia–VSD (including TOF, PA) repair	9.0	3	3.0	3.0	3.0
Valve closure, Tricuspid (exclusion, univentricular approach)	9.0	3	4.0	3.0	2.0
1 1/2 ventricular repair	9.0	3	3.0	3.0	3.0

(continued)

Table 3.2 (continued)

	Score	Mortality	Morbidity	Difficulty	
Fontan, Atrio-pulmonary connection	9.0	3	3.0	3.0	3.0
Fontan, Atrioventricular connection	9.0	3	3.0	3.0	3.0
Fontan, TCPC, Lateral tunnel, Fenestrated	9.0	3	3.0	3.0	3.0
Fontan, TCPC, Lateral tunnel, Nonfenestrated	9.0	3	3.0	3.0	3.0
Fontan, TCPC, External conduit, Fenestrated	9.0	3	3.0	3.0	3.0
Fontan, TCPC, External conduit, Nonfenestrated	9.0	3	3.0	3.0	3.0
Fontan, TCPC, Intra-/extracardiac conduit, Fenestrated	9.	3	3.0	3.0	3.0
Fontan, TCPC, Intra-/extracardiac conduit, Nonfenestrated	9.	3	3.0	3.0	3.0
Congenitally corrected TGA repair, VSD closure	9.0	3	3.0	3.0	3.0
Mustard	9.0	3	3.0	3.0	3.0
Pulmonary artery sling repair	9.0	3	3.0	3.0	3.0
Aneurysm, Ventricular, Left, Repair	9.0	3	3.0	2.5	3.5
Conduit placement, Ventricle to aorta	9.0	3	3.0	3.0	3.0
Pulmonary embolectomy, Chronic pulmonary embolus	9.0	3	3.0	3.0	3.0
Valvuloplasty converted to valve replacement in the same operation, Truncal valve	9.0	3	2.5	3.0	3.5
Valvuloplasty, Common atrioventricular valve	9.0	3	3.5	2.5	3.0
TOF—absent pulmonary valve repair	9.3	3	3.0	3.0	3.3
Transplant, Heart	9.3	3	3.0	3.3	3.0
Aortic root replacement, Bioprosthetic	9.5	3	3.5	2.0	4.0
Aortic root replacement, Homograft	9.5	3	3.5	2.0	4.0
Pulmonary atresia–VSD–MAPCA repair, Status post prior complete unifocalization (includes VSD closure + RV to PA connection [with or without conduit])	9.5	3	3	3	3.5
Damus–Kaye–Stansel procedure (DKS) (creation of AP anastomosis without arch reconstruction)	9.5	3	3.0	3.0	3.5

Table 3.2 (continued)

	Score	Mortality	Morbidity	Difficulty	
Valvuloplasty converted to valve replacement in same operation, Tricuspid	9.5	3	3.0	2.5	4.0
Superior cavopulmonary anastomosis(es) (Glenn or hemi- Fontan) + atrioventricular valvuloplasty	9.5	3	3.0	3.0	3.5
Unifocalization MAPCA(s), Bilateral pulmonary unifocalization—incomplete unifocalization (not all usable MAPCA[s] are incorporated)	9.5	3	3	3	3.5
Unifocalization MAPCA(s), Bilateral pulmonary unifocalization—complete unifocalization (all usable MAPCA[s] are incorporated)	10.0	4	3.5	3	3.5
Ebstein's repair	10.0	4	3.0	3.0	4.0
Arterial switch operation (ASO)	10.0	4	3.5	3.0	3.5
Rastelli	10.0	4	3.0	3.0	4.0
Coarctation repair + VSD repair	10.0	4	2.5	3.5	4.0
Aortic arch repair + VSD repair	10.0	4	3.0	3.0	4.0
Anomalous origin of coronary artery from pulmonary artery repair	10.0	4	3.0	3.0	4.0
Superior cavopulmonary anastomosis(es) + PA reconstruction	10.0	4	3.5	3.0	3.5
Hybrid approach "stage 2," Aortopulmonary amalgamation + superior cavopulmonary anastomosis(es) + PA debanding + without aortic arch repair	10.0	4	2.5	3.5	4.0
Hybrid approach "stage 1," Stent placement in arterial duct (PDA) + application of RPA and LPA bands	10.0	4	3.0	3.0	4.0
Valve replacement, Common atrioventricular valve	10.0	4	3.5	3.5	3.0
Ross procedure	10.3	4	4.0	2.3	4.0
DORV, Intraventricular tunnel repair	10.3	4	3.3	3.0	4.0
Valvuloplasty converted to valve replacement in the same operation, Aortic	10.3	4	3.5	2.5	4.3
Ventricular septation	10.5	4	3.5	3.5	3.5

(continued)

Table 3.2 (continued)

	Score	Mortality	Morbidity	Difficulty	
Valvuloplasty converted to valve replacement in the same operation, Mitral	10.5	4	4.0	2.5	4.0
Interrupted aortic arch repair	10.8	4	3.8	3.0	4.0
Truncus arteriosus repair	11.0	4	4.0	3.0	4.0
TOF–AVC (AVSD) repair	11.0	4	4.0	3.0	4.0
Pulmonary atresia–VSD–MAPCA repair	11.0	4	4.0	3.0	4.0
Unifocalization MAPCA(s)	11.0	4	4.0	3.0	4.0
Konno procedure	11.0	4	4.0	3.0	4.0
Congenitally corrected TGA repair, Atrial switch and Rastelli	11.0	4	4.0	3.0	4.0
Congenitally corrected TGA repair, VSD closure and LV to PA conduit	11.0	4	4.0	3.0	4.0
Arterial switch operation (ASO) and VSD repair	11.0	4	4.0	3.0	4.0
REV	11.0	4	4.0	3.0	4.0
DOLV repair	11.0	4	4.0	3.0	4.0
Aortic dissection repair	11.0	4	4.0	3.0	4.0
TAPVC repair + shunt—systemic to pulmonary	11.0	4	4.0	3.5	3.5
Pulmonary atresia–VSD–MAPCA repair, Status post prior incomplete unifocalization (includes completion of pulmonary unifocalization + VSD closure + RV to PA connection [with or without conduit])	11.0	4	4	3.5	3.5
Pulmonary atresia–VSD–MAPCA repair, Complete single-stage repair (one stage that includes bilateral pulmonary unifocalization + VSD closure + RV to PA connection [with or without conduit])	11.5	4	4.5	3.5	3.5
Arterial switch procedure + aortic arch repair	11.5	4	4.0	3.5	4.0
Valvuloplasty converted to valve replacement in the same operation, Common atrioventricular valve	11.5	4	4.5	3.0	4.0
Fontan + atrioventricular valvuloplasty	11.5	4	4.0	3.5	4.0
Pulmonary venous stenosis repair	12.0	4	4.0	4.0	4.0

Table 3.2 (continued)

	Score	Mortality	Morbidity	Difficulty	
Partial left ventriculectomy (LV volume reduction surgery) (Batista)	12.0	4	4.0	4.0	4.0
Transplant, Lung(s)	12.0	4	4.0	4.0	4.0
Aortic root translocation over the left ventricle (including Nikaidoh procedure)	12.0	4	3.0	4.0	5.0
Valvuloplasty converted to valve replacement in the same operation, Aortic—with Ross procedure	12.0	4	4.0	3.5	4.5
Ross–Konno procedure	12.5	4	4.5	3.0	5.0
Fontan revision or conversion (redo Fontan)	12.5	4	4.0	4.0	4.5
Arterial switch procedure and VSD repair + aortic arch repair	13.0	4	4.5	4.0	4.5
Hybrid approach "stage 2," Aortopulmonary amalgamation + superior cavopulmonary anastomosis(es) + PA debanding + aortic arch repair (Norwood [stage 1] + superior cavopulmonary anastomosis(es) + PA debanding)	13.0	4	4.0	4.5	4.5
Transplant, Heart and lung(s)	13.3	4	4.0	5.0	4.3
Congenitally corrected TGA repair, Atrial switch and ASO (double switch)	13.8	4	5.0	3.8	5.0
Valvuloplasty converted to valve replacement in the same operation, Aortic—with Ross–Konno procedure	14.0	4	4.5	4.5	5.0
Conduit insertion of the right ventricle to the pulmonary artery + intraventricular tunnel left ventricle to neoaorta + arch reconstruction (Rastelli- and Norwood-type arch reconstruction) (Yasui)	14.5	4	5	4.5	5
Norwood procedure	14.5	4	5.0	4.5	5.0
HLHS biventricular repair	15.0	4	5.0	5.0	5.0
Truncus + interrupted aortic arch repair (IAA) repair	15.0	4	5.0	5.0	5.0
Interventional cardiology or not eligible (intentionally excluded from Aristotle) procedures					
ASD repair, Device					
VSD repair, Device					
PDA closure, Device					
ASD creation, Balloon septostomy (BAS) (Rashkind)					

(continued)

Table 3.2 (continued)

	Score	Mortality	Morbidity	Difficulty	
ASD creation, Blade septostomy					
Balloon dilation					
Stent placement					
Device closure					
RF ablation					
Coil embolization					
Pulmonary AV fistula repair/occlusion					
TGA, Other procedures (Kawashima, LV–PA conduit, other)					
Cardiovascular catheterization procedure, Therapeutic					
Echocardiography procedure, Sedated transesophageal echocardiogram					
Echocardiography procedure, Sedated transthoracic echocardiogram					
Non-cardiovascular, non-thoracic procedure on cardiac patient with cardiac anesthesia					
Radiology procedure on cardiac patient, Cardiac computerized axial tomography (CT scan)					
Radiology procedure on cardiac patient, Cardiac magnetic resonance imaging (MRI)					
Radiology procedure on cardiac patient, Diagnostic radiology					
Radiology procedure on cardiac patient, Noncardiac computerized tomography (CT) on cardiac patient					
Radiology procedure on cardiac patient, Noncardiac magnetic resonance imaging (MRI) on cardiac patient					
Radiology procedure on cardiac patient, Therapeutic radiology					
Cardiovascular catheterization procedure, Diagnostic					
Cardiovascular catheterization procedure, Diagnostic, Hemodynamic data obtained					

Table 3.2 (continued)

	Score	Mortality	Morbidity	Difficulty	
Cardiovascular catheterization procedure, Diagnostic, Angiographic data obtained					
Cardiovascular catheterization procedure, Diagnostic, Transluminal test occlusion					
Cardiovascular catheterization procedure, Diagnostic, Hemodynamic alteration					
Cardiovascular catheterization procedure, Diagnostic, Electrophysiology alteration					
Cardiovascular catheterization procedure, Therapeutic, Septostomy					
Cardiovascular catheterization procedure, Therapeutic, Balloon valvotomy					
Cardiovascular catheterization procedure, Therapeutic, Stent re-dilation					
Cardiovascular catheterization procedure, Therapeutic, Perforation (establishing interchamber and/or intervessel communication)					
Cardiovascular catheterization procedure, Therapeutic, Transcatheter Fontan completion					
Cardiovascular catheterization procedure, Therapeutic, Transcatheter implantation of the valve					
Cardiovascular catheterization procedure, Therapeutic adjunctive therapy					
Cardiovascular electrophysiological catheterization procedure					
Cardiovascular electrophysiological catheterization procedure, Therapeutic ablation					
Other miscellaneous, not scored					
(Either too vague or not a primary procedure)					
Atrial baffle procedure, NOS					
VSD repair, NOS					
Valve surgery, Other, Tricuspid					

(continued)

Table 3.2 (continued)

	Score	Mortality	Morbidity	Difficulty	
Valve surgery, Other, Pulmonic					
Valve surgery, Other, Mitral					
Valve surgery, Other, Aortic					
Tracheal procedure					
TOF repair, NOS					
Thoracotomy, Other					
Thoracic and/or mediastinal procedure, Other					
TGA, Other procedures (Nikaidoh, Kawashima, LV–PA conduit, others)					
Shunt, Systemic to pulmonary, Other					
Shunt, Systemic to pulmonary, NOS					
Pleural procedure, Other					
Peripheral vascular procedure, Other					
Pericardial procedure, Other					
PDA closure, NOS					
Palliation, Other					
PA, reconstruction (plasty), NOS					
Other					
Organ procurement					
Miscellaneous procedure, Other					
Mediastinal procedure					
Fontan, TCPC, Lateral tunnel, NOS					
Fontan, Other					
Fontan, NOS					
Esophageal procedure					
DORV repair, NOS					
Diaphragm procedure, Other					
Coronary artery procedure, Other					
Congenitally corrected TGA repair, Other					
Congenitally corrected TGA repair, NOS					
Conduit placement, NOS					
Coarctation repair, Other					
Coarctation repair, NOS					
Cardiotomy, Other					
Cardiac procedure, Other					
AVC (AVSD) repair, NOS					
ASD repair, NOS					
Arrhythmia surgery, NOS					
Other annular enlargement procedure					

Table 3.2 (continued)

	Score	Mortality	Morbidity	Difficulty	
Fontan, TCPC, External conduit, NOS					
VATS (video-assisted thoracoscopic surgery)					
Minimally invasive procedure					
Bypass for noncardiac lesion					
Valve replacement, Aortic					

Table 3.3 The Risk Adjustment for Congenital Heart Surgery (RACHS-1) Categories (October 24, 2014)

Procedure	RACHS-1 category
Aortopexy	1
ASD partial closure	1
ASD repair, Patch	1
ASD repair, Patch + PAPVC repair	1
ASD repair, Primary closure	1
Atrial fenestration closure	1
PAPVC repair	1
PAPVC Repair, Baffle redirection to the left atrium with systemic vein translocation (Warden) (SVC sewn to the right atrial appendage)	1
PAPVC, Scimitar, Repair	1
PFO, Primary closure	1
Aneurysm, Ventricular, Right, Repair	2
Aortic stenosis, Subvalvar, Repair	2
AP window repair	2
ASD, Common atrium (single atrium), Septation	2
AVC (AVSD) repair, Partial (incomplete) (PAVSD)	2
Bidirectional cavopulmonary anastomosis (BDCPA) (bidirectional Glenn)	2
Bilateral bidirectional cavopulmonary anastomosis (BBDCPA) (bilateral bidirectional Glenn)	2
Coronary artery fistula ligation	2
DCRV repair	2
Glenn (unidirectional cavopulmonary anastomosis) (unidirectional Glenn)	2
Hemi-Fontan	2
Kawashima operation (superior cavopulmonary connection in setting of interrupted IVC with azygous continuation)	2
Ligation, Pulmonary artery	2
PA, reconstruction (plasty), Branch, Central (within the hilar bifurcation)	2
PA, reconstruction (plasty), Branch, Peripheral (at or beyond the hilar bifurcation)	2
PA, reconstruction (plasty), Main (trunk)	2
PA, reconstruction (plasty), NOS	2
Pulmonary artery sling repair	2
RVOT procedure	2
Sinus of Valsalva, Aneurysm repair	2
Superior cavopulmonary anastomosis(es) + PA reconstruction	2
TOF repair, No ventriculotomy	2
TOF repair, Ventriculotomy, Nontransannular patch	2

(continued)

Table 3.3 (continued)

Procedure	RACHS-1 category
TOF repair, Ventriculotomy, Transannular patch	2
Valve replacement, Pulmonic (PVR)	2
Valve surgery, Other, Pulmonic	2
Valvuloplasty converted to valve replacement in the same operation, Pulmonic	2
Valvuloplasty, Pulmonic	2
Vascular ring repair	2
VSD repair, Patch	2
VSD repair, Primary closure	2
VSD, Multiple, Repair	2
Aortic aneurysm repair	3
Aortic arch repair + VSD repair	3
Aortic stenosis, Subvalvar, Repair, With myectomy for IHSS	3
Aortic stenosis, Supravalvar, Repair	3
Arterial switch operation (ASO)	3
Atrial baffle procedure (non-Mustard, non-Senning)	3
Atrial baffle procedure, Mustard or Senning revision	3
Atrial baffle procedure, NOS	3
Atrial baffle procedure, NOS	3
AVC (AVSD) repair, Complete (CAVSD)	3
AVC (AVSD) repair, Intermediate (transitional)	3
Cardiac tumor resection	3
Coarctation repair + VSD repair	3
Conduit placement, LV to PA	3
Conduit placement, RV to PA	3
Cor triatriatum repair	3
DORV repair, NOS	3
DORV, Intraventricular tunnel repair	3
Fontan + atrioventricular valvuloplasty	3
Fontan, Atrio-pulmonary connection	3
Fontan, Atrioventricular connection	3
Fontan, NOS	3
Fontan, Other	3
Fontan, TCPC, External conduit, Fenestrated	3
Fontan, TCPC, External conduit, Nonfenestrated	3
Fontan, TCPC, External conduit, NOS	3
Fontan, TCPC, Intra-/extracardiac conduit, Nonfenestrated	3
Fontan, TCPC, Intra-/extracardiac conduit, Fenestrated	3
Fontan, TCPC, Lateral tunnel, Fenestrated	3
Fontan, TCPC, Lateral tunnel, Nonfenestrated	3
Fontan, TCPC, Lateral tunnel, NOS	3
Hybrid approach "stage 1," Application of RPA and LPA bands	3
Hybrid approach "stage 1," Stent placement in arterial duct (PDA) + application of RPA and LPA bands	3
Mustard	3
PA banding (PAB)	3
Pulmonary artery origin from ascending aorta (hemitruncus) repair	3
Pulmonary atresia–VSD–MAPCA repair	3
Pulmonary atresia–VSD–MAPCA repair, Complete single-stage repair (one stage that includes bilateral pulmonary unifocalization + VSD closure + RV to PA connection [with or without conduit])	3

Table 3.3 (continued)

Procedure	RACHS-1 category
Pulmonary atresia–VSD–MAPCA repair, Status post prior complete unifocalization (includes VSD closure + RV to PA connection [with or without conduit])	3
Pulmonary atresia–VSD–MAPCA repair, Status post prior incomplete unifocalization (includes completion of pulmonary unifocalization + VSD closure + RV to PA connection [with or without conduit])	3
Pulmonary atresia–VSD (including TOF, PA) repair	3
Ross procedure	3
Senning	3
Shunt, Systemic to pulmonary, Central (from the aorta to the main pulmonary artery)	3
Shunt, Systemic to pulmonary, Central (shunt from the aorta), Central shunt with an end-to-side connection between the transected main pulmonary artery and the side of the ascending aorta (i.e., Mee shunt)	3
Shunt, Systemic to pulmonary, Modified Blalock–Taussig Shunt (MBTS)	3
Shunt, Systemic to pulmonary, NOS	3
Shunt, Systemic to pulmonary, Other	3
Superior cavopulmonary anastomosis(es) (Glenn or hemi-Fontan) + atrioventricular valvuloplasty	3
Valve closure, Semilunar	3
Valve excision, Tricuspid (without replacement)	3
Valve replacement, Aortic (AVR)	3
Valve replacement, Aortic (AVR), Bioprosthetic	3
Valve replacement, Aortic (AVR), Homograft	3
Valve replacement, Aortic (AVR), Mechanical	3
Valve replacement, Mitral (MVR)	3
Valve replacement, Tricuspid (TVR)	3
Valve surgery, Other, Aortic	3
Valve surgery, Other, Mitral	3
Valve surgery, Other, Tricuspid	3
Valvuloplasty converted to valve replacement in same operation, Tricuspid	3
Valvuloplasty converted to valve replacement in the same operation, Aortic	3
Valvuloplasty converted to valve replacement in the same operation, Aortic—with Ross procedure	3
Valvuloplasty converted to valve replacement in the same operation, Mitral	3
Valvuloplasty, Mitral	3
Valvuloplasty, Tricuspid	3
Aortic arch repair	4
Arterial switch operation (ASO) and VSD repair	4
ASD creation/enlargement	4
Conduit insertion of the right ventricle to the pulmonary artery + intraventricular tunnel left ventricle to neoaorta + arch reconstruction (Rastelli- and Norwood-type arch reconstruction) (Yasui)	4
Congenitally corrected TGA repair, Atrial switch and ASO (double switch)	4
Interrupted aortic arch repair	4
Konno procedure	4
Rastelli	4
Truncus arteriosus repair	4
Unifocalization MAPCA(s)	4

(continued)

Table 3.3 (continued)

Procedure	RACHS-1 category
Valvuloplasty converted to valve replacement in the same operation, Aortic—with Ross–Konno procedure	4
VSD creation/enlargement	4
Truncus + interrupted aortic arch repair (IAA) repair	5
Damus–Kaye–Stansel procedure (DKS) (creation of AP anastomosis without arch reconstruction)	6
Hybrid approach "stage 2," Aortopulmonary amalgamation + superior cavopulmonary anastomosis(es) + PA debanding + aortic arch repair (Norwood [stage 1] + superior cavopulmonary anastomosis(es) + PA debanding)	6
Norwood procedure	6
Coarctation repair, End to end	1 if > 30 days, 2 if ≤ 30 days
Coarctation repair, End to end, Extended	1 if > 30 days, 2 if ≤ 30 days
Coarctation repair, Interposition graft	1 if > 30 days, 2 if ≤ 30 days
Coarctation repair, NOS	1 if > 30 days, 2 if ≤ 30 days
Coarctation repair, Other	1 if > 30 days, 2 if ≤ 30 days
Coarctation repair, Patch aortoplasty	1 if > 30 days, 2 if ≤ 30 days
Coarctation repair, Subclavian flap	1 if > 30 days, 2 if ≤ 30 days
PDA closure, Surgical	1 if > 30 days, not eligible if ≤ 30 days
TAPVC repair	2 if > 30 days, 4 if ≤ 30 days
Valvuloplasty, Aortic	2 if > 30 days, 4 if ≤ 30 days
Ebstein's repair	3 if > 30 days, 5 if ≤ 30 days
TAPVC repair + shunt—systemic to pulmonary	3 if age > 30 days, 4 if age ≤ 30 days
Others, not categorized (eligible, but not assigned a category)	
1 1/2 ventricular repair	
Aneurysm, Pulmonary artery, Repair	
Aneurysm, Ventricular, Left, Repair	
Anomalous origin of coronary artery from pulmonary artery repair	
Anomalous systemic venous connection repair	
Aortic root replacement	
Aortic root replacement, Bioprosthetic	
Aortic root replacement, Homograft	
Aortic root replacement, Mechanical	
Aortic root replacement, Valve sparing	
Aortic root translocation over left ventricle (including Nikaidoh procedure)	
Arterial switch procedure + aortic arch repair	

Table 3.3 (continued)

Procedure	RACHS-1 category
Arterial switch procedure and VSD repair + aortic arch repair	
Atrial septal fenestration	
AVC (AVSD) repair, NOS	
Conduit placement, NOS	
Conduit placement, Other	
Conduit placement, Ventricle to the aorta	
Conduit reoperation	
Congenitally corrected TGA repair, Atrial switch and Rastelli	
Congenitally corrected TGA repair, NOS	
Congenitally corrected TGA repair, Other	
Congenitally corrected TGA repair, VSD closure	
Congenitally corrected TGA repair, VSD closure and LV to PA conduit	
Coronary artery bypass	
Coronary artery procedure, Other	
DOLV repair	
Fontan revision or conversion (redo Fontan)	
HLHS biventricular repair	
Hybrid approach "stage 1," Stent placement in arterial duct (PDA)	
Hybrid approach "stage 2," Aortopulmonary amalgamation + superior cavopulmonary anastomosis(es) + PA debanding + without aortic arch repair	
LV to aorta tunnel repair	
Mitral stenosis, Supravalvar mitral ring repair	
Occlusion MAPCA(s)	
Other annular enlargement procedure	
PA debanding	
Partial left ventriculectomy (LV volume reduction surgery) (Batista)	
Pulmonary AV fistula repair/occlusion	
Pulmonary embolectomy	
Pulmonary embolectomy, Acute pulmonary embolus	
Pulmonary embolectomy, Chronic pulmonary embolus	
Pulmonary venous stenosis repair	
REV	
Ross–Konno procedure	
Shunt, Ligation and takedown	
Systemic venous stenosis repair	
TGA, Other procedures (Kawashima, LV–PA conduit, others)	
TGA, Other procedures (Nikaido, Kawashima, LV–PA conduit, others)	
TOF–AVC (AVSD) repair	
TOF–Absent pulmonary valve repair	
TOF repair, NOS	
TOF repair, RV–PA conduit	
Valve closure, Tricuspid (exclusion, univentricular approach)	
Valve excision, Pulmonary (without replacement)	
Valve replacement, Common atrioventricular valve	
Valve replacement, Truncal valve	
Valvuloplasty converted to valve replacement in the same operation, Common atrioventricular valve	
Valvuloplasty converted to valve replacement in the same operation, Truncal valve	
Valvuloplasty, Common atrioventricular valve	
Valvuloplasty, Truncal valve	

(continued)

Table 3.3 (continued)

Procedure	RACHS-1 category
Ventricular septal fenestration	
Ventricular septation	
Hepatic vein to azygous vein connection, Direct	
Hepatic vein to azygous vein connection, Interposition Graft	
Hybrid approach, Transcardiac balloon dilation	
Hybrid approach, Transcardiac transcatheter device placement	
Intravascular stent removal	
Unifocalization MAPCA(s), Bilateral pulmonary unifocalization—complete unifocalization (all usable MAPCA[s] are incorporated)	
Unifocalization MAPCA(s), Bilateral pulmonary unifocalization—incomplete unifocalization (not all usable MAPCA[s] are incorporated)	
Unifocalization MAPCA(s), Unilateral pulmonary unifocalization	
Others, not eligible (intentionally excluded from RACHS-1)	
Aortic dissection repair	
Arrhythmia surgery—atrial, Surgical ablation	
Arrhythmia surgery—ventricular, Surgical ablation	
Arrhythmia surgery, NOS	
ASD creation, Balloon septostomy (BAS) (Rashkind)	
ASD creation, Blade septostomy	
ASD repair, Device	
ASD repair, NOS	
Balloon dilation	
Bronchoscopy	
Bypass for noncardiac lesion	
Cardiac procedure, Other	
Cardiotomy, Other	
Cardiovascular catheterization procedure, Diagnostic	
Cardiovascular catheterization procedure, Diagnostic, Angiographic data obtained	
Cardiovascular catheterization procedure, Diagnostic, Electrophysiology alteration	
Cardiovascular catheterization procedure, Diagnostic, Hemodynamic alteration	
Cardiovascular catheterization procedure, Diagnostic, Hemodynamic data obtained	
Cardiovascular catheterization procedure, Diagnostic, Transluminal test occlusion	
Cardiovascular catheterization procedure, Therapeutic	
Cardiovascular catheterization procedure, Therapeutic Adjunctive therapy	
Cardiovascular catheterization procedure, Therapeutic, Balloon valvotomy	
Cardiovascular catheterization procedure, Therapeutic, Perforation (establishing interchamber and/or intervessel communication)	
Cardiovascular catheterization procedure, Therapeutic, Septostomy	
Cardiovascular catheterization procedure, Therapeutic, Stent re-dilation	
Cardiovascular catheterization procedure, Therapeutic, Transcatheter Fontan completion	
Cardiovascular catheterization procedure, Therapeutic, Transcatheter implantation of the valve	
Cardiovascular electrophysiological catheterization procedure	
Cardiovascular electrophysiological catheterization procedure, Therapeutic ablation	

Table 3.3 (continued)

Procedure	RACHS-1 category
Coil embolization	
Decortication	
Delayed sternal closure	
Device closure	
Diaphragm plication	
Diaphragm procedure, Other	
Echocardiography procedure, Sedated transesophageal echocardiogram	
Echocardiography procedure, Sedated transthoracic echocardiogram	
ECMO cannulation	
ECMO decannulation	
ECMO procedure	
Esophageal procedure	
Explantation of pacing system	
ICD (AICD) ([automatic] implantable cardioverter defibrillator) procedure	
ICD (AICD) implantation	
Intra-aortic balloon pump (IABP) insertion	
Ligation, Thoracic duct	
Lung biopsy	
Lung procedure, Other	
Mediastinal exploration	
Mediastinal procedure	
Minimally invasive procedure	
Miscellaneous procedure, Other	
Non-cardiovascular, non-thoracic procedure on cardiac patient with cardiac anesthesia	
Organ procurement	
Other procedure	
Pacemaker implantation, Permanent	
Pacemaker procedure	
Palliation, Other	
PDA closure, Device	
PDA closure, NOS	
Pectus repair	
Pericardial drainage procedure	
Pericardial procedure, Other	
Pericardiectomy	
Peripheral vascular procedure, Other	
Pleural drainage procedure	
Pleural procedure, Other	
Radiology procedure on cardiac patient, Cardiac computerized axial tomography (CT scan)	
Radiology procedure on cardiac patient, Cardiac magnetic resonance imaging (MRI)	
Radiology procedure on cardiac patient, Diagnostic radiology	
Radiology procedure on cardiac patient, Noncardiac computerized tomography (CT) on cardiac patient	
Radiology procedure on cardiac patient, Noncardiac magnetic resonance imaging (MRI) on cardiac patient	
Radiology procedure on cardiac patient, Therapeutic radiology	
RF ablation	

(continued)

Table 3.3 (continued)

Procedure	RACHS-1 category
Right/left heart assist device procedure	
Stent placement	
Sternotomy wound drainage	
Thoracic and/or mediastinal procedure, Other	
Thoracotomy, Other	
Tracheal procedure	
Transplant, Heart	
Transplant, Heart and lung	
Transplant, lung(s)	
VAD explantation	
VAD implantation	
VATS (video-assisted thoracoscopic surgery)	
VSD repair, Device	
VSD repair, NOS	

1. The *S*ociety of *T*horacic Surgeons—European *A*ssociation for Cardio-*T*horacic Surgery Congenital Heart Surgery Mortality Categories (**STAT Mortality Categories**) (Table 3.1)
2. *A*ristotle *B*asic Complexity *L*evels (**ABC Levels**) (Table 3.2)
3. *R*isk *A*djustment for *C*ongenital *H*eart *S*urgery-1 Categories (**RACHS-1 Categories**) (Table 3.3)

STS CHSD initially used the Aristotle Basic Complexity Levels and the RACHS-1 Categories to stratify procedures according to the degree of complexity and risk. With the increasing availability of multi-institutional clinical data, the empirically based STAT Mortality Score and STAT Mortality Categories were introduced in STS CHSD in 2010. The STAT Mortality Categories [14, 15] are a tool for complexity stratification that is based on the risk of discharge mortality, which was developed from an analysis of 77,294 operations entered into the EACTS Congenital Heart Surgery Database (33,360 operations) and the STS Congenital Heart Surgery Database (43,934 patients). Procedure-specific mortality rate estimates were calculated using a Bayesian model that was adjusted for small denominators. Operations were sorted by increasing risk and grouped into five categories (the STAT Mortality Categories) that were designed to be optimal with respect to minimizing within-category variation and maximizing between-category variation. STAT Category 1 is associated with the lowest risk for mortality, and STAT Category 5 is associated with the highest risk for mortality.

In 2013, Hörer and Schreiber published a manuscript that sought to assess the potential risk factors for adverse outcome after cardiac operations in adults with congenital heart disease and to evaluate the predictive power of the Aristotle Basic Complexity (ABC) Score and the Aristotle Comprehensive Complexity (ACC) Score for hospital mortality in adults with congenital heart disease [16]. The ACC Score augments the ABC Score by adding procedure-dependent factors and procedure-independent factors. In this analysis, procedure-dependent factors, procedure-independent factors, and outcome factors of all consecutive patients aged 16 or more who underwent surgery for congenital heart disease between 2005 and 2008 at a single institution were evaluated according to the nomenclature and database standards of the European Association for Cardio-Thoracic Surgery Congenital Database. An ABC Score and an ACC Score were assigned to each operation. The discriminatory power of the scores was assessed using the area under the receiver operating curve (ROC). (The discrimination of a system of risk stratification or risk adjustment can be quantified by the area under the receiver operating characteristic curve [also known as the C-index]. The C-index is interpreted as the probability that a randomly selected patient who died [or had the outcome of interest] was considered to be higher risk than a randomly selected patient who survived. The C-index generally ranges from 0.5 to 1.0, with 0.5 representing no discrimination [i.e., a coin flip] and 1.0 representing perfect discrimination.) In this analysis by Hörer and Schreiber, during 542 operations, 773 procedures were performed, with an early mortality rate of 2.4% and an early complication rate of 53.7%. Risk factors for 30-day mortality were tricuspid valve replacement ($P = 0.009$), mitral valve replacement ($P < 0.001$), elevated lung resistances ($P = 0.002$), hypothyroidism ($P = 0.002$), and redo sternotomy ($P = 0.003$). Risk factors for complications were tricuspid valve replacement ($P < 0.001$), tricuspid valvuloplasty ($P = 0.006$), mitral valve replacement ($P = 0.003$), shunt implantation ($P = 0.009$), surgical ablation ($P = 0.024$), myocardial dysfunction ($P = 0.014$), elevated lung resistances ($P = 0.004$), hypothyroidism ($P = 0.002$), and redo sternotomy ($P < 0.001$). Mean ABC Score and ACC Score were 6.6 ± 2.3 and 9.0 ± 3.7, respectively. The C-index of the ABC Score and ACC Score for 30-day mortality were 0.663 ($P = 0.044$) and 0.755 ($P = 0.002$), respectively. The C-index of the ABC Score and ACC Score for complications were 0.634 ($P < 0.001$) and 0.670 ($P < 0.001$), respectively. The authors concluded that "Surgery for adults with congenital heart disease can be performed with low early mortality. However, complications are frequent, especially in patients who require repeat operations for atrioventricular valve incompetence. The ACC Score may be helpful to estimate the risk of early mortality."

In 2014, Kogon and Oster published a manuscript addressing the question of whether or not pediatric scoring systems were appropriate for assessing surgical risk for adults with congenital heart disease [17]. The authors acknowledged that at the time of their study, there were no validated risk scoring systems for adult congenital heart surgery, and predicting outcomes in these patients was challenging. Their study was designed to determine if commonly used pediatric congenital heart disease surgery risk scores were also applicable to adults. In their analysis, 458 adult cardiac surgical operations performed in adults (age ≥ 18 years) with congenital heart disease between 2000 and 2010 at a single institution were studied retrospectively. The scores evaluated were the RACHS-1 Categories, the ABC Score, and the STAT Mortality Score. Receiver operating characteristic (ROC) curves were generated to assess the ability of the three scoring systems to predict mortality, major adverse events (stroke, renal failure, prolonged ventilation, prolonged coma, deep sternal infection, reoperation, and operative mortality), and prolonged length of stay

(>7 days). Outcomes of the 458 operations in the analysis included 16 (3%) deaths, 94 (21%) major adverse events, and 90 (20%) prolonged lengths of stay. Four hundred thirty (94%) of the operations were included in all three scoring systems and the ROC analysis. For mortality, areas under the ROC curve were 0.91, 0.91, and 0.65 for the Aristotle, STAT, and RACHS-1 scores, respectively. For major adverse event, areas under the ROC curves were 0.81, 0.76, and 0.61 for the Aristotle, STAT, and RACHS-1 scores, respectively. For prolonged length of stay, areas under the ROC curve were 0.82, 0.76, and 0.61 for the Aristotle, STAT, and RACHS-1 scores, respectively. Kogon and Oster concluded that, "Pediatric risk scoring systems such as Aristotle, STAT, and RACHS-1 offer prognostic value in adults undergoing congenital heart surgery. The scores are predictive of mortality, major adverse events, and prolonged lengths of stay. The STAT and Aristotle systems fared best."

In 2016, Hörer, Schreiber, and Lange published an analysis that sought to evaluate whether the predictive power of the common pediatric scores is applicable for adults [18]. They also evaluated a new "grown-ups with congenital heart disease (GUCH) score" specifically designed for adults undergoing congenital heart surgery. In this analysis, data of all consecutive patients aged ≥ 18 years who underwent surgery for congenital heart disease between 2004 and 2013 at a single institution were collected. The authors evaluated the ABC Score, the ACC Score, the RACHS-1 Categories, and the STAT Mortality Score. Their proposed GUCH score consisted of the STAT Mortality Score, the procedure-dependent and procedure-independent factors of the ACC Score, and age. The discriminatory power of the scores was assessed using the area under the receiver-operating characteristics curve (C-index). The analysis included 830 operations with hospital mortality of 2.9%. C-indexes were 0.67, 0.80, 0.62, 0.78, and 0.84 for the ABC Score, ACC Score, RACHS-1 Categories, STAT Mortality Score, and GUCH Mortality Score, respectively. Hörer and colleagues concluded that "The evidence-based STAT Mortality Score outperforms the expert-based ABC Score. The expert-based ACC Score is superior to the evidence-based STAT Mortality Score because comorbidities are included. Our proposed GUCH Mortality Score outperformed all other scores because it integrates the advantages of the evidence-based STAT Mortality Score for procedures and the expert-based ACC Score for comorbidities. Evidence-based scores for adults with congenital heart disease should include comorbidities and patient ages."

Clearly, the adjustment for case mix is critical to accurate outcomes analysis in congenital heart surgery. The three previously described established tools encompass all age groups and are not specific to the growing population of adults undergoing congenital heart operations. Therefore, in 2015, Fuller and colleagues derived an empirically based Adult Congenital Heart Surgery (ACHS) Mortality Score [19]. In-hospital mortality was analyzed for the 152 most common procedures/procedural groups in adults 18 years of age and older in the STS CHSD using data from 2000 to 2013. Procedure-specific adult mortality rate estimates were calculated for procedures with 30 cases or more ($N = 52$) using Bayesian methods adjusting for small denominators. Each procedural group was assigned an ACHS Mortality Score ranging from 0.1 to 3.0 based on the estimated mortality rate. Discrimination was assessed using the C-index in a separate validation sample. During the development of the *ACHS Mortality Score*, a total of 12,513 procedures (116 centers) were analyzed (Table 3.4). Overall unadjusted mortality was 1.8%. Significant differences in mortality rates in adults compared with patients of all ages were seen for several procedures, including Ebstein's repair (0.7% versus 4.9%; $P = 0.003$) and Fontan operations (6.8% versus 1.4%; $P < 0.01$). The procedure with the lowest model-based estimate of mortality and accompanying ACHS Mortality Score was atrial septal defect repair (0.2%, 0.1), and the highest was Fontan revision (9.7%, 3.0). The C-index for the ACHS Mortality Score was 0.809 versus 0.777 for the "nonage-specific" STAT Mortality Score applied to adults. Fuller and colleagues concluded that "Risk estimation based on the aggregate of all age groups is suboptimal when analyzing outcomes specifically among adults. An empirically based *ACHS Mortality Score* can facilitate case-mix adjustment by providing accurate estimation of mortality risk for adults."

Table 3.4 Adult congenital heart surgery (ACHS) mortality score

Procedural group	*N*	Group unadjusted mortality estimate percentage (95% interval[a])	Group model-based mortality estimate percentage (95% interval[b])	ACHS mortality score
ASD	817	0.0 (0.0, 0.5)	0.2 (0.0, 0.5)	0.1
Pacemaker procedure	888	0.2 (0.1, 0.8)	0.3 (0.1, 0.8)	0.2
PAPVC repair	299	0.0 (0.0, 1.2)	0.4 (0.0, 1.1)	0.2
Aortic stenosis, subvalvar	244	0.0 (0.0, 1.5)	0.4 (0.0, 1.3)	0.2
Conduit reoperation	232	0.0 (0.0, 1.6)	0.4 (0.0, 1.4)	0.2
PV replacement	1110	0.5 (0.1, 1.0)	0.5 (0.2, 1.0)	0.2
Anomalous coronary from aorta repair	115	0.0 (0.0, 3.2)	0.7 (0.1, 2.3)	0.3
Explantation of pacing system	105	0.0 (0.0, 3.5)	0.7 (0.1, 2.4)	0.3
AICD procedure	88	0.0 (0.0, 4.1)	0.8 (0.1, 2.8)	0.3
Pacemaker implantation, permanent	631	0.8 (0.3, 1.8)	0.9 (0.3, 1.7)	0.3
AV repair	163	0.6 (0.0, 3.4)	0.9 (0.1, 2.6)	0.3
AICD implantation	267	0.7 (0.1, 2.7)	0.9 (0.2, 2.2)	0.3
Vascular ring repair	63	0.0 (0.0, 5.7)	0.9 (0.1, 3.4)	0.3
Ebstein's repair	152	0.7 (0.0, 3.6)	1.0 (0.1, 2.7)	0.3
MV repair	244	0.8 (0.1, 2.9)	1.0 (0.2, 2.5)	0.4
Konno procedure	54	0.0 (0.0, 6.6)	1.0 (0.1, 3.8)	0.4
PA reconstruction	464	1.1 (0.4, 2.5)	1.1 (0.4, 2.3)	0.4
Pulmonic valvuloplasty	43	0.0 (0.0, 8.2)	1.2 (0.1, 4.5)	0.4
Sinus of Valsalva aneurysm	40	0.0 (0.0, 8.8)	1.2 (0.1, 4.4)	0.4
RVOT repair	610	1.1 (0.5, 2.4)	1.2 (0.5, 2.2)	0.4
Anomalous coronary artery from pulmonary artery	41	0.0 (0.0, 8.6)	1.2 (0.1, 4.6)	0.4
Valve-sparing aortic root replacement	183	1.1 (0.1, 3.9)	1.3 (0.3, 3.1)	0.4
PAPVC sdiratar	34	0.0 (0.0, 10.3)	1.3 (0.1, 4.8)	0.4

(continued)

Table 3.4 (continued)

Procedural group	*N*	Group unadjusted mortality estimate percentage (95% interval[a])	Group model-based mortality estimate percentage (95% interval[b])	ACHS mortality score
Aortic stenosis, supravalvar	33	0.0 (0.0, 10.6)	1.3 (0.1, 5.2)	0.4
RV aneurysm	33	0.0 (0.0, 10.6)	1.3 (0.1, 5.2)	0.4
DCRV	33	0.0 (0.0, 10.6)	1.3 (0.1, 5.1)	0.4
VSD	230	1.3 (0.3, 3.8)	1.4 (0.4, 3.1)	0.5
Common AV canal repair (incomplete)	147	1.4 (0.2, 4.8)	1.5 (0.3, 3.7)	0.5
Aortic arch repair	79	1.3 (0.0, 6.9)	1.6 (0.2, 4.7)	0.5
AV replacement	482	1.7 (0.7, 3.2)	1.7 (0.8, 2.9)	0.6
Aortic aneurysm	288	1.7 (0.6, 4.0)	1.8 (0.6, 3.5)	0.6
TV repair	432	1.9 (0.8, 3.6)	1.9 (0.8, 3.3)	0.6
Systemic venous stenosis repair	60	1.7 (0.0, 8.9)	1.9 (0.2, 5.7)	0.6
TOP repair	58	1.7 (0.0, 9.2)	2.0 (0.2, 5.8)	0.6
Ross procedure	147	2.0 (0.4, 5.8)	2.0 (0.5, 4.7)	0.7
Conduit EV-PA	366	2.2 (0.9, 4.3)	2.2 (1.0, 3.8)	0.7
Arrhythmia, surgical ablation, ventricular	48	2.1 (0.1, 11.1)	2.2 (0.3, 6.6)	0.7
Pericardial drainage	44	2.3 (0.1, 12.0)	2.3 (0.3, 7.0)	0.8
Arrhythmia, surgical ablation, atrial	457	2.4 (1.2, 4.3)	2.4 (1.2, 3.9)	0.8
Coarctation repair	112	2.7 (0.6, 7.6)	2.6 (0.6, 5.8)	0.8
Conduit placement, other	34	2.9 (0.1, 15.3)	2.8 (0.3, 8.5)	0.9
TV replacement	245	2.9 (1.2, 5.8)	2.8 (1.2, 5.1)	0.9
Shunt, systemic to pulmonary	32	3.1 (0.1, 16.2)	2.8 (0.3, 9.0)	0.9
Aortic root replacement, non–valve-sparing	291	3.1 (1.4, 5.8)	3.0 (1.4, 5.2)	1.0
ASD creation or enlargement	214	3.3 (1.3, 6.6)	3.2 (1.3, 5.8)	1.0
MV replacement	332	4.8 (2.8, 7.7)	4.7 (2.7, 7.1)	1.5
Cardiac tumor resection	54	5.6 (1.2, 15.4)	4.7 (1.1, 10.9)	1.5
Coronary artery bypass	184	5.4 (2.6, 9.8)	5.1 (2.5, 8.7)	1.6
Fontan procedure	59	6.8 (1.9, 16.5)	5.7 (1.7, 12.3)	1.8
Lung transplantation	61	8.2 (2.7, 18.1)	7.1 (2.4, 14.2)	2.2
Heart transplantation	227	7.5 (4.4, 11.7)	7.1 (4.2, 10.8)	2.2
Fontan revision	155	10.3 (6.0, 16.2)	9.7 (5.6, 14.7)	3.0

Procedure and procedural group names, proposed adult congenital heart surgery (ACHS) mortality score

AICD automatic implantable cardioverter-defibrillator, *ASD* atrial septal defect, *AV* atrioventricular valve, *DCRV* double-chamber right ventricle, *MV* mitral valve, *PA* pulmonary artery, *PAPVC* partial anomalous pulmonary venous connection, *PV* pulmonary valve, *RV* right ventricle, *RVOT* right ventricular outflow tract, *TOP* tetralogy of Fallot, *TV* tricuspid valve, *VSD* ventricular septal defect

[a]Denotes 95% exact binomial confidence interval

[b]Denotes 95% Bayesian probability interval

3.4 Summary

Data about the outcomes of adults undergoing congenital heart surgery are limited. Analyses have been performed using administrative claims data or focused on outcomes at single centers. In 2011, Mascio and colleagues published an analysis of the STS CHSD and the STS Adult Cardiac Surgery Database (ACSD) in order to describe the most common operations, patient characteristics, and postoperative outcomes in adults with congenital heart disease undergoing cardiac surgery, using a multicenter clinical database [20]. Their analysis included adults (aged $\geq$ 18 years) listed in the STS CHSD from 2000 to 2009 and described patient characteristics and morbidity and mortality. Their analysis also examined congenital procedures in the STS ACSD "to permit consideration of the primary dataset within a broader context." In this study, 5265 patients from 68 centers from STS CHSD were included. The median age was 25 years with an interquartile range of 20–35. Common preoperative risk factors included noncardiac abnormalities (17%) and arrhythmia (14%). Overall, in-hospital mortality was 2.1%, 27% had one or more complication, and median length of stay was 5 days. Common operations included right ventricular outflow tract procedures (21%) and pacemaker/arrhythmia procedures (20%). An additional analysis was performed of operations utilizing cardiopulmonary bypass that were performed in more than 100 patients, and in this cohort, mortality ranged from 0% (atrial septal defect repair) to 11% (Fontan revision/conversion). A separate evaluation of STS ACSD revealed 39,872 adults undergoing congenital heart operations. Mascio and colleagues concluded that "Most adult congenital heart operations listed in STS CHSD are performed in the third to fourth decades of life and approximately half are for right heart pathology or arrhythmia. Many patients have complications, but mortality is low with the exception of those undergoing Fontan revision/conversion. Many more adults undergoing congenital heart surgery are entered into STS ACSD." This analysis by Mascio and colleagues demonstrates both the power and the potential of multi-institutional registries of adults who undergo surgery for congenial heart disease to function as a platform for outcomes analysis, quality assessment, and quality improvement.

This chapter has reviewed the nomenclature, classification, and risk scores for adults with congenital heart disease. These tools will facilitate multi-institutional initiatives to analyze outcomes and assess and ultimately improve the quality of care provided to adults who undergo surgery for congenial heart disease.

References

1. Dearani JA, Mavroudis C, Quintessenza J, Deal BJ, Backer CL, Fitzgerald P, Connolly HM, Jacobs JP. Surgical advances in the treatment of adults with congenital heart disease. Curr Opin Pediatr. 2009;21(5):565–72. https://doi.org/10.1097/MOP.0b013e3283303fa7.
2. Jacobs JP, Shahian DM, Prager RL, Edwards FH, McDonald D, Han JM, D'Agostino RS, Jacobs ML, Kozower BD, Badhwar V, Thourani VH, Gaissert HA, Fernandez FG, Wright CD, Paone G, Cleveland JC Jr, Brennan JM, Dokholyan RS, Brothers L, Vemulapalli S, Habib RH, O'Brien SM, Peterson ED, Grover FL, Patterson GA, Bavaria JE. The Society of Thoracic Surgeons National Database 2016 annual report. Ann Thorac Surg. 2016;102(6):1790–7. https://doi.org/10.1016/j.athoracsur.2016.10.015.

3. Jacobs JP, Mayer JE Jr, Mavroudis C, O'Brien SM, Austin EH 3rd, Pasquali SK, Hill KD, Overman DM, St Louis JD, Karamlou T, Pizarro C, Hirsch-Romano JC, McDonald D, Han JM, Becker S, Tchervenkov CI, Lacour-Gayet F, Backer CL, Fraser CD, Tweddell JS, Elliott MJ, Walters H 3rd, Jonas RA, Prager RL, Shahian DM, Jacobs ML. The Society of Thoracic Surgeons Congenital Heart Surgery Database: 2017 update on outcomes and quality. Ann Thorac Surg. 2017;103(3):699–709. https://doi.org/10.1016/j.athoracsur.2017.01.004.
4. Jacobs ML, Jacobs JP, Hill KD, Hornik C, O'Brien SM, Pasquali SK, Vener D, Kumar SR, Habib RH, Shahian DM, Edwards FH, Fernandez FG. The Society of Thoracic Surgeons Congenital Heart Surgery Database: 2017 update on research. Ann Thorac Surg. 2017;104(3):731–41. https://doi.org/10.1016/j.athoracsur.2017.07.001.
5. Morales DL, Khan MS, Turek JW, Biniwale R, Tchervenkov CI, Rush M, Jacobs JP, Tweddell JS, Jacobs ML. Report of the 2015 Society of Thoracic Surgeons Congenital Heart Surgery practice survey. Ann Thorac Surg. 2017;103(2):622–8. https://doi.org/10.1016/j.athoracsur.2016.05.108.
6. International Pediatric and Congenital Cardiac Code. http://www.ipccc.net/. Accessed 26 Aug 2017.
7. Franklin RCG, Jacobs JP, Krogmann ON, Béland MJ, Aiello VD, Colan SD, Elliott MJ, Gaynor JW, Kurosawa H, Maruszewski B, Stellin G, Tchervenkov CI, Walters HL 3rd, Weinberg P, Anderson RH. Nomenclature for congenital and paediatric cardiac disease: historical perspectives and The International Pediatric and Congenital Cardiac Code. In: Jacobs JP, editor. 2008 Supplement to cardiology in the young: databases and the assessment of complications associated with the treatment of patients with congenital cardiac disease, prepared by: The Multi-Societal Database Committee for Pediatric and Congenital Heart Disease. Cardiol Young. 2008;18(Suppl 2):70–80.
8. STS Congenital Heart Surgery Database v3.3. http://www.sts.org/sites/default/files/documents/CongenitalDataSpecsV3_3_Updated.pdf. Accessed 26 Aug 2017.
9. Cronk CE, Malloy ME, Pelech AN, Miller RE, Meyer SA, Cowell M, McCarver DG. Completeness of state administrative databases for surveillance of congenital heart disease. Birth Defects Res A Clin Mol Teratol. 2003;67(9):597–603.
10. Frohnert BK, Lussky RC, Alms MA, Mendelsohn NJ, Symonik DM, Falken MC. Validity of hospital discharge data for identifying infants with cardiac defects. J Perinatol. 2005;25(11):737–42.
11. Strickland MJ, Riehle-Colarusso TJ, Jacobs JP, Reller MD, Mahle WT, Botto LD, Tolbert PE, Jacobs ML, Lacour-Gayet FG, Tchervenkov CI, Mavroudis C, Correa A. The importance of nomenclature for congenital cardiac disease: implications for research and evaluation. In: Jacobs JP, editor. 2008 Supplement to cardiology in the young: databases and the assessment of complications associated with the treatment of patients with congenital cardiac disease, prepared by: The Multi-Societal Database Committee for Pediatric and Congenital Heart Disease. Cardiol Young. 2008;18(Suppl 2):92–100.
12. Pasquali SK, Peterson ED, Jacobs JP, He X, Li JS, Jacobs ML, Gaynor JW, Hirsch JC, Shah SS, Mayer JE. Differential case ascertainment in clinical registry versus administrative data and impact on outcomes assessment for pediatric cardiac operations. Ann Thorac Surg. 2013;95(1):197–203. https://doi.org/10.1016/j.athoracsur.2012.08.074.
13. Jacobs JP, Jacobs ML, Lacour-Gayet FG, Jenkins KJ, Gauvreau K, Bacha E, Maruszewski B, Clarke DR, Tchervenkov CI, Gaynor JW, Spray TL, Stellin G, O'Brien SM, Elliott MJ, Mavroudis C. Stratification of complexity improves the utility and accuracy of outcomes analysis in a Multi-Institutional Congenital Heart Surgery Database: Application of the Risk Adjustment in Congenital Heart Surgery (RACHS-1) and Aristotle Systems in the Society of Thoracic Surgeons (STS) Congenital Heart Surgery Database. Pediatr Cardiol. 2009;30:1117–30. https://doi.org/10.1007/s00246-009-9496-0.
14. O'Brien SM, Clarke DR, Jacobs JP, Jacobs ML, Lacour-Gayet FG, Pizarro C, Welke KF, Maruszewski B, Tobota Z, Miller WJ, Hamilton L, Peterson ED, Mavroudis C, Edwards FH. An empirically based tool for analyzing mortality associated with congenital heart surgery. J Thorac Cardiovasc Surg. 2009;138(5):1139–53.

15. Jacobs JP, Jacobs ML, Maruszewski B, Lacour-Gayet FG, Tchervenkov CI, Tobota Z, Stellin G, Kurosawa H, Murakami A, Gaynor JW, Pasquali SK, Clarke DR, Austin EH 3rd, Mavroudis C. Initial application in the EACTS and STS congenital heart surgery databases of an empirically derived methodology of complexity adjustment to evaluate surgical case mix and results. Eur J Cardiothorac Surg. 2012;42(5):775–80. https://doi.org/10.1093/ejcts/ezs026.
16. Hörer J, Vogt M, Wottke M, Cleuziou J, Kasnar-Samprec J, Lange R, Schreiber C. Evaluation of the Aristotle complexity models in adult patients with congenital heart disease. Eur J Cardiothorac Surg. 2013;43(1):128–34; discussion 134–5. https://doi.org/10.1093/ejcts/ezs143.
17. Kogon B, Oster M. Assessing surgical risk for adults with congenital heart disease: are pediatric scoring systems appropriate? J Thorac Cardiovasc Surg. 2014;147(2):666–71. https://doi.org/10.1016/j.jtcvs.2013.09.053.
18. Hörer J, Kasnar-Samprec J, Cleuziou J, Strbad M, Wottke M, Kaemmerer H, Schreiber C, Lange R. Mortality following congenital heart surgery in adults can be predicted accurately by combining expert-based and evidence-based pediatric risk scores. World J Pediatr Congenit Heart Surg. 2016;7(4):425–35. https://doi.org/10.1177/2150135116656001.
19. Fuller SM, He X, Jacobs JP, Pasquali SK, Gaynor JW, Mascio CE, Hill KD, Jacobs ML, Kim YY. Estimating mortality risk for adult congenital heart surgery: an analysis of the Society of Thoracic Surgeons Congenital Heart Surgery Database. Ann Thorac Surg. 2015;100(5):1728–36. https://doi.org/10.1016/j.athoracsur.2015.07.002.
20. Mascio CE, Pasquali SK, Jacobs JP, Jacobs ML, Austin EH 3rd. Outcomes in adult congenital heart surgery: analysis of the Society of Thoracic Surgeons Database. J Thorac Cardiovasc Surg. 2011;142(5):1090–7. https://doi.org/10.1016/j.jtcvs.2011.07.028.

4 Cardiac Surgical Challenges in Adults with Congenital Heart Disease

Arman Arghami, Joseph A. Dearani, M. Sertaç Çiçek, and Sameh M. Said

4.1 Introduction

With significant improvements in cardiac surgery and perioperative care for infants and children with congenital heart disease over the past few decades, the number of adults with congenital heart disease (CHD) has dramatically increased and is likely to grow more in the coming years [1]. Adults with CHD (ACHD) fall in to three categories: the first group, which is the majority, includes those who will need reoperation to fix residual or recurrent defects or treat long-term complications (e.g., native or prosthetic valve deterioration), and the second group includes those with previously undetected CHD who present or require surgery for the first time in adulthood. And as the patients with CHD age, a new category emerges of patients with acquired heart disease such as coronary artery disease requiring cardiac surgery which is not related to their underlying CHD. Although many CHD are "corrected" in childhood, except for a few instances such as ligation of a patent ductus arteriosus or atrial septal defect closure, many may require further intervention during adulthood, particularly for the development or progression of arrhythmias, which can occur even after simple lesions like atrial septal defect closure. The term "total correction" or "complete repair" refers to an operation that results in a two-ventricle circulation with closure of septal defects and repair of valvar abnormalities. Importantly, it does not preclude need for re-intervention. Conversely, palliative procedures refer to preliminary operations that may include shunts or bands or an eventual single-ventricle circulation, i.e., modified Fontan procedure. These patients

A. Arghami · J. A. Dearani (✉) · M. S. Çiçek · S. M. Said
Department of Cardiovascular Surgery, Mayo Clinic, Rochester, MN, USA
e-mail: Arghami.Arman@mayo.edu; jdearani@mayo.edu; cicek.m@mayo.edu; Said.Sameh@mayo.edu

E. da Cruz et al. (eds.), *Intensive Care of the Adult with Congenital Heart Disease*, Congenital Heart Disease in Adolescents and Adults,
https://doi.org/10.1007/978-3-319-94171-4_4

have chronic arterial desaturation and do not have separate systemic and pulmonary circulations. Consequently, all patients with CHD, "corrected" or "palliated," require lifelong surveillance.

In this chapter, we will review the issues that go through a surgeon's mind when preparing and planning either a primary or repeat operation. The importance of collaboration between surgeons, anesthesiologists, cardiologists, critical care specialists, radiologists, other physician subspecialists, and other allied healthcare personnel cannot be overemphasized.

4.2 General Considerations

It is worth emphasizing that surgery and perioperative care for ACHD presents different challenges than surgery for acquired heart disease and surgery for CHD in infants and children. According to the Society of Thoracic Surgeons (STS) database, early mortality following cardiac surgery for CHD is higher in adults than in children, although neonates and infants have the highest mortality [2]. This higher mortality seen in ACHD is multifactorial and includes the presence of comorbidities, e.g., renal or hepatic disease, diabetes, pulmonary hypertension, coronary artery disease, as well as the probability of many prior operations. In addition, formal postgraduate training programs are in evolution so clinical care pathways are not yet refined, and a proper transition from pediatric healthcare providers to properly trained adult CHD specialist is not always predictable and well organized. The Bethesda report recommends organizing care of adults with CHD within a regionalized system of specialized adult CHD units, with each unit providing education, care, and research for its designated region [3]. There is evidence obtained from an analysis of national practice patterns involving more than 40,000 patients that mortality following CHD surgery in adults is lower if the surgeon performing the operation is an experienced pediatric (congenital) heart surgeon [4].

4.3 Preoperative Evaluation

A proper preoperative evaluation that includes basic testing of chest X-ray, electrocardiogram, transthoracic echocardiography, and standard laboratory testing are the essential first steps. Acquisition and review of prior operative records, if possible, are of outmost importance and may provide vital information to the surgeon and the caring team. In addition, complementary imaging that is also applied in almost all circumstances includes cross-sectional imaging, CT, or MRI. Since there are typically one or more prior operations, the information gained from cross-sectional imaging with or without three-dimensional reconstruction can greatly facilitate the planning for reoperation. Oftentimes there is anterior displacement and adhesions of the innominate vein, right atrium or right ventricle, great arteries, or extracardiac conduits to the chest wall or sternum that can make sternal reentry difficult and hazardous. Knowledge of these anatomic relationships in advance is essential.

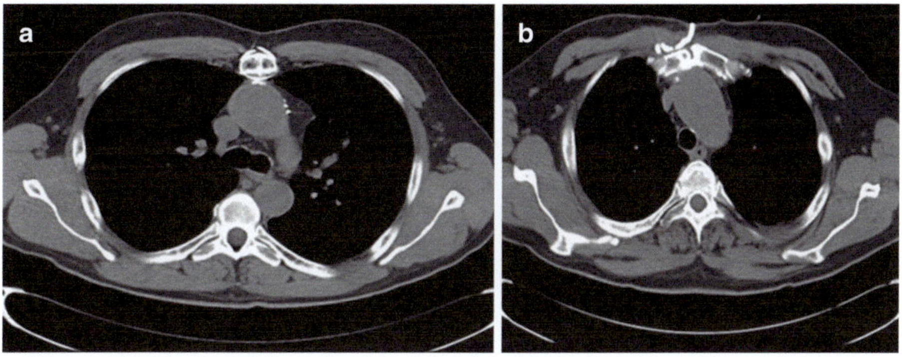

Fig. 4.1 Preoperative cross-sectional images demonstrating the relationship of the mediastinal structures to the underside of the sternum. In this particular case, the ascending aorta (**a**) and the aortic arch (**b**) are eroding into the sternum. Knowledge of this preoperatively is essential when planning redo sternotomy (Reprinted from *Cardiac CT and MRI for Adult Congenital Heart Disease*; Saremi F, editor; pp. 431–449, 2013, with permission from Springer [34])

Imaging such as computed tomography (CT) can delineate the relationships and proximity of structures making reentry safer and more predictable (Fig. 4.1). In general, echocardiography (transthoracic or transesophageal) provides the necessary detail about valvar anatomy, and CT or MRI provides anatomy about right and left ventricular size and function as well as details about cardiac anatomy, great vessel size and locations, and chest wall relationships. Three-dimensional reconstruction of the image is also invaluable in redo surgery as it provides the surgeon with an anatomic model of the heart and mediastinal structures, their relation to the sternum and location of extracardiac conduits, and anomalous course of major coronaries and facilitates operative planning (Fig. 4.2). In addition, the ability to print out a 3D model also provides the opportunity to practice the operation in advance of going to the operating room and better means of educating the patients and their families (Fig. 4.3).

Complete comparison of CT versus MRI is beyond the scope of this chapter, but a few advantages of MRI in the setting of adults with CHD are worth mentioning. MRI is usually preferred if feasible since the exposure to radiation is reduced and the need for multiple studies over a lifetime is common in this population. MRI is particularly helpful in providing additional information about cardiac chamber size and ventricular function, particularly anatomy and function of the right ventricle, which is not accomplished as well with echocardiography. The newest imaging technology adjunct is the three-dimensional (3D) printing. 3D printing in patients with CHD can help precisely visualize complex anatomy, plan surgical procedures, and teach trainees and patients [5].

Echocardiography is the mainstay of cardiac evaluation in adults with CHD. It provides accurate diagnosis, details about valve anatomy and function, the presence of septal defects, outflow tract anatomy, chamber dilations or hypertrophy, and ventricular function. For example, the presence of an intracardiac septal defect could increase the risk of air embolism if inadvertent cardiotomy occurs while the heart is

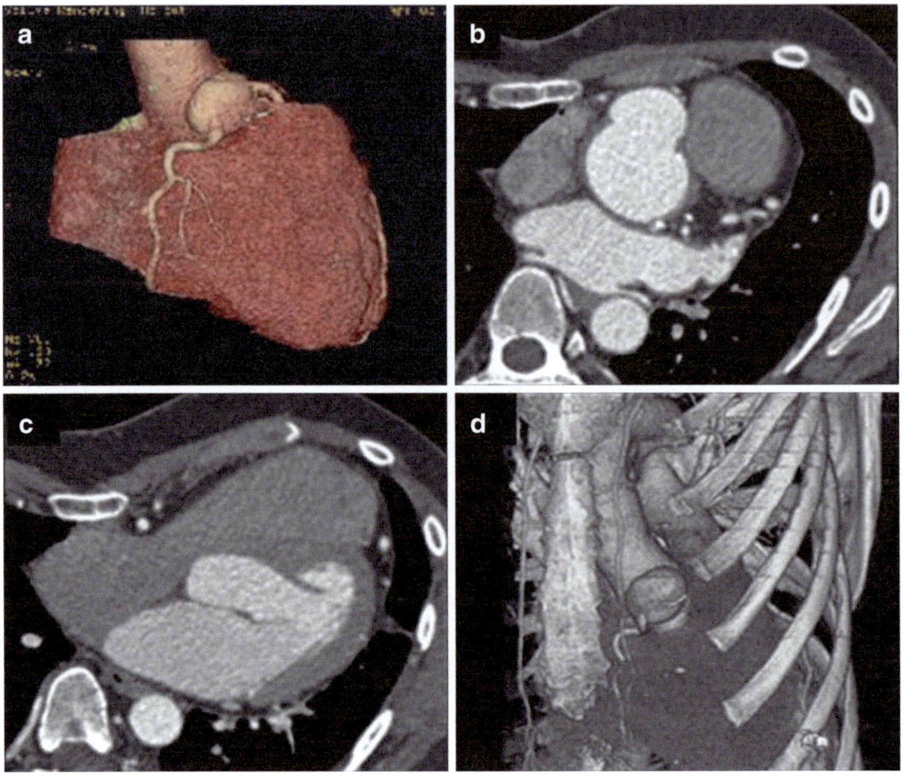

Fig. 4.2 Preoperative cross-sectional imaging with three-dimensional reconstruction demonstrating (**a**) a proximal right coronary artery aneurysm. (**b**, **c**) The same patient also has a severe pectus excavatum deformity with the mediastinal structures displaced into the left hemithorax. (**d**) Three-dimensional reformat showing the relationship of the leftward position of the right coronary artery aneurysm to the sternum (Reprinted from *Cardiac CT and MRI for Adult Congenital Heart Disease*; Saremi F, editor; pp. 431–449, 2013, with permission from Springer)

decompressed while on the cardiopulmonary bypass. In this situation, it is important to maintain a positive central venous pressure of at least 5 mmHg in order to avoid air entry into the right heart and subsequent systemic embolization through the intracardiac shunt. We routinely use an aortic root vent, Trendelenburg position, and carbon dioxide flooding of the field in all patients that will have cardiotomy without placement of an aortic cross clamp. Analysis of cardiac valves would also help plan your procedure even if they are not the focus of the operation. For example, mild to moderate aortic regurgitation may guide the surgeon to place a LV vent to prevent ventricular distention during hypothermic bypass. Intraoperative transesophageal echocardiogram is an essential tool and is used routinely. In addition to careful evaluation of the anatomy and the diagnosis, it can help with peripheral cannulation and ensure proper positioning of both arterial and venous cannula; it helps in evaluating collapse of the cardiac chambers after initiation of peripheral

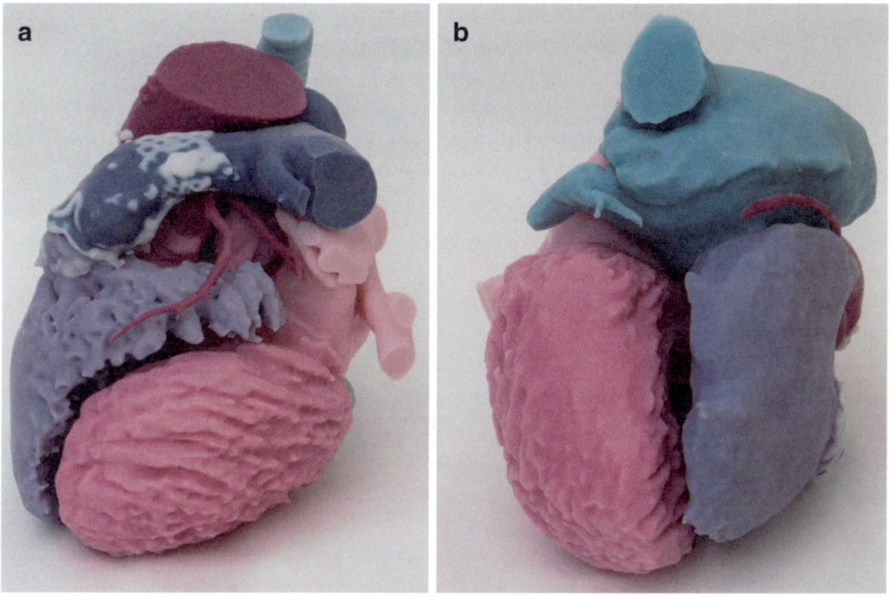

Fig. 4.3 3D-printed model of the heart and great arteries: (**a**) "front" and (**b**) "back" in a patient with multiple previous sternotomies and percutaneous stent placement in the right ventricular outflow tract who underwent a repeat sternotomy for right ventricular outflow tract reconstruction

CPB, providing continuous evaluation to the contractile status and distension of the ventricle, and guiding the de-airing process at the conclusion of bypass.

Cardiac catheterization may be required for hemodynamic analysis and to determine if there are any associated lesions that should be addressed before or at the same time of surgery [6]. Cardiac catheterization can also play a supplemental role in imaging, e.g., great vessel anatomy, pulmonary artery, and coronary artery anatomy. As many as 33% of selected adults with CHD may have an asymptomatic coronary artery disease or anomaly that is discovered with coronary angiography [7], e.g., anomalous course of the LAD across the right ventricular outflow tract reconstruction in the setting of pulmonary valve replacement after repair of tetralogy of Fallot. Other instances that coronary angiogram should be considered are the presence of risk factors such as angina, noninvasive evidence of ischemia, reduced systemic ventricular function, history of myocardial infarction, or for those patients with prior coronary, aortic root surgery, or other great artery surgery. There is a consensus that selective coronary angiography should be performed in men older than 40 years who have congenital heart disease and have been referred for surgery and in similar postmenopausal women [8, 9].

Analysis of peripheral vasculature, groin vessel and neck vessel patency, is necessary prior to going to the operating room. This can be accomplished with ultrasound, but if uncertainty remains, CT imaging of the abdomen and pelvis or neck can provide definitive results and can be obtained when thoracic imaging is being performed as described above.

Atrial and ventricular arrhythmias are the most common late complications in the adult with congenital heart disease [10]. The importance of a preoperative electrophysiological consultation and a low threshold for invasive electrophysiological study prior to surgery cannot be overemphasized. It is extremely important to consider both existing and potential arrhythmias in deciding an operative plan for patient with CHD because many techniques to address arrhythmias need to be performed using an operative approach. Although atrial arrhythmias are most common, the potential for ventricular arrhythmias must also be investigated. The management techniques are diverse, and caregivers should consider the best option or combination of some on a case by case basis. Such approaches can include surgical or percutaneous ablative approaches, pacing, and implantable cardioverter defibrillator. Timing of these approaches should be carefully planned. For example, it is important to consider percutaneous ablation therapy prior to surgical intervention if the surgery will limit access to the heart (such as in a cavopulmonary anastomosis) or to the tricuspid or mitral valve annulus (such as in a cone repair or atrioventricular valve replacement) [10].

4.4 The Surgeon and the Redo Sternotomy

The majority of cardiac surgery for adult CHD is "redo" operations. As mentioned in the previous section, planning is of utmost importance in these situations. Also communication with cardiology, anesthesia, perfusion, and the operating room team members is essential to the success of these challenging procedures. The following are a few technical considerations and pitfalls and our strategies:

- When there is a high possibility of injury to cardiac structures, peripheral cannulation of femoral, neck, or axillary vessels may be required. This risk is determined by preoperative studies, particularly the cross-sectional imaging. With the advent of percutaneous cannulation techniques and closure devices, one can obtain access via jugular, carotid or axillary artery, and femoral vein/artery cannulation with almost no need for an incision. This can be facilitated by placement of a catheter in the desired vessel using ultrasound guidance.
- Alternative peripheral cannulation sites include femoral arteries or veins, iliac arteries or veins, axillary arteries, innominate or carotid arteries, internal jugular vein (typically on the right), LV apex (via left thoracotomy), pulmonary artery (via left thoracotomy), and even the abdominal aorta [11].
- As the number of prior sternotomy and other procedures (e.g., cardiac catheterization, electrophysiological procedures, invasive monitoring, pacemaker insertion) increases, the risk of peripheral vessel complications and inadequacies increases. It is important, when suspected, to obtain a preoperative ultrasound or CT study of the arterial and venous system intended for use as peripheral cannulation sites.
- Vacuum-assisted venous drainage can facilitate the use of smaller cannula; however, they should be used selectively and with caution, especially in the presence

of intracardiac shunt(s). This point cannot be overemphasized since inadvertent injury to the right-sided structures (more common) may result in systemic air embolism.

- Initiation of CPB prior to sternotomy and during substernal dissection can be a valuable maneuver. By decompressing the heart and reducing the venous filling pressure, one can decrease the chances of a cardiac injury and, in case of an event, reduce the amount of blood loss and allow for a more controlled approach. This is particularly helpful when there is right heart enlargement or there are elevated right-sided pressures. The downside of this technique is that it does result in longer CPB time, which has been shown to be related to increase morbidity and mortality [12]. As a result, the operation should be orchestrated as such that the CPB time is as short, but as safe, as possible. One consideration is to separate from CPB after initial reentry and then perform the mediastinal dissection off bypass if possible. This can greatly reduce the total bypass time but does require a hemodynamic situation that allows initiation and separation from bypass without causing undo stress on the abnormal heart.
- Multiple techniques of resternotomy have been utilized. We use two techniques for resternotomy. The first is an air-driven microsagittal saw during repeat sternotomy to divide the anterior sternal table and followed by careful division of the posterior table with heavy scissors under direct vision with the help of Volkmann retractors that elevate the two halves of the sternum (Fig. 4.4). The microsagittal saw has the advantage of precise perpendicular division of the sternum, with relatively easy control of depth of blade penetration and the ability to feel the posterior sternal table [13]. The second approach is the use of a craniotome, which is an electric device that has no sharp edges that are in proximity to the heart (Fig. 4.5). This does require complete removal of old sternal wires. It has

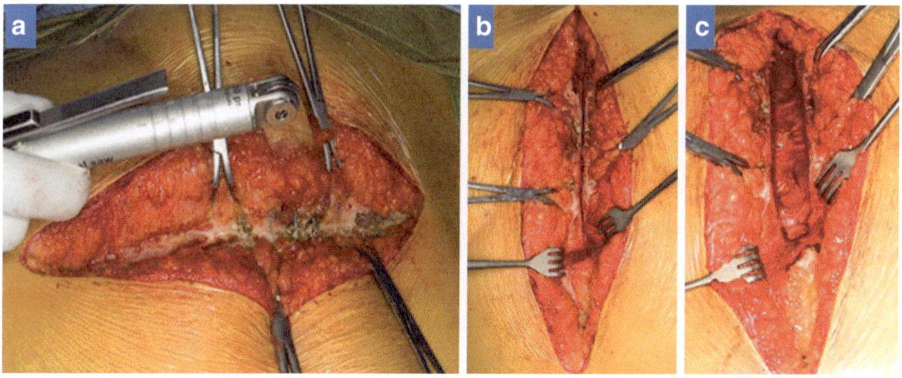

Fig. 4.4 Intraoperative photos demonstrating our technique of resternotomy when using a microsagittal saw. (**a**) The microsagittal saw. (**b**, **c**) Rake (Volkmann) retractors are placed at the level of the xiphoid, and towel clips are used on either side of the sternum to elevate the corresponding half during the resternotomy (Reprinted from *Cardiac CT and MRI for Adult Congenital Heart Disease*; Saremi F, editor; pp. 431–449, 2013, with permission from Springer)

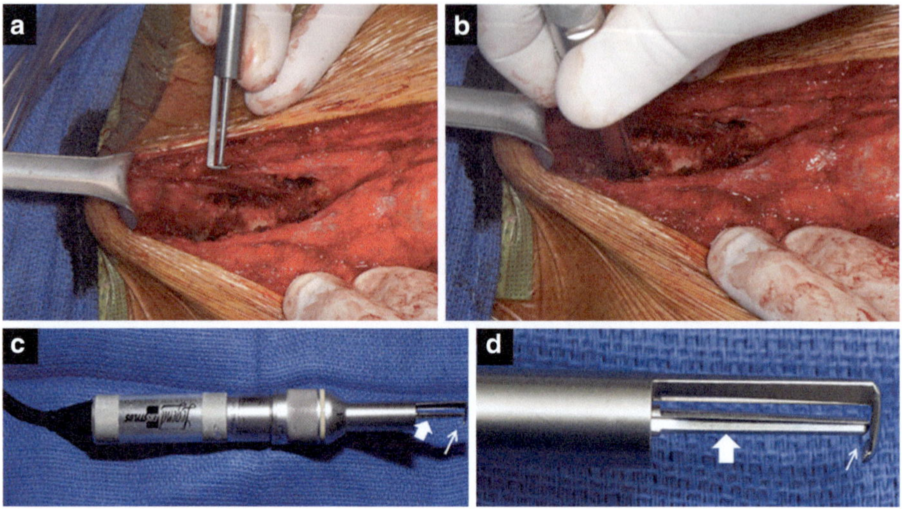

Fig. 4.5 Intraoperative photos showing the craniotome (**c**, **d**) (Midas Rex Microsaw) and its use (**a**, **b**) for safe reentry into the chest (Reprinted from *Cardiac CT and MRI for Adult Congenital Heart Disease*; Saremi F, editor; pp. 431–449, 2013, with permission from Springer)

the advantage of exceedingly low probability of cardiac injury (<0.05%) and allows steering away of structures that are adherent to the sternum.

- The heart and great vessels are gently released in stepwise fashion using scissors and very low-energy electrocautery. Due to the arrhythmogenic nature of the cautery, careful attention to the ECG monitor during this process by the anesthesia team is important, and the maintenance of low energy on the cautery is essential to minimize iatrogenic fibrillation. If ventricular arrhythmia occurs, DC cardioversion using external defibrillator pads, placed preoperatively, can be performed. Once the sternum has been divided and the pleural spaces have been entered, which we do routinely, internal-external defibrillator paddles can be utilized if necessary.
- Limiting the dissection to the areas required for a safe performance of the intended operation is suggested. This will reduce the unnecessary risk of injury to cardiac structures and also reduce postoperative bleeding.

Unique factors that are important in the adult CHD surgical patient include the systemic effects of chronic cyanosis, arrhythmia burden, presence of aortopulmonary collaterals, and ventricular dysfunction, particularly right ventricular dysfunction. Long-standing cyanosis results in intrinsic hemostasis abnormalities, and postoperative hemostasis may be difficult to achieve. Adult patients with CHD with chronic cyanosis often have multiple collateral vessels that are friable and difficult to coagulate. The difficulty in achieving perioperative hemostasis is exacerbated by long cardiopulmonary bypass times, which lead to a decrease in platelet number and activity through consumption coagulopathy and fibrinolysis.

When the preventive techniques described above are utilized, outcomes of multiple sternotomies are improved. We published our experience with 984 redo sternotomies in adult CHD and showed that the risk of early mortality was 3.6% and the risk of cardiac injury was 6% [14]. This risk has now been reduced to <1% from the lessons learned from this and similar studies. Although with increasing number of prior resternotomy the risk of cardiac injury during reentry was increased in our study, on multivariate analysis the number of prior resternotomy did not affect the early mortality. Early mortality was affected by the duration of cardiopulmonary bypass, urgent operation, and single-ventricle physiology. These findings have been helpful in terms of our overall approach to patients with CHD that will require multiple reoperations over their lifetime. We now orchestrate the percutaneous interventions and repeat operations for these lesions so that a patient rarely gets to operation number five and beyond. Selectively applying percutaneous procedures when feasible, and performing valve replacement when a durable valve repair(s) is not likely to be obtained, accomplish this.

The variables that have been found to be protective at the time of reoperation include increased ejection fraction preoperatively, and cardiac injury was less likely to occur when there was an increased time interval from the previous sternotomy [14]. In a multicenter study of 2012 adult CHD patients requiring surgery from 13 European countries, an early mortality risk of cardiac surgery after a prior corrective procedure was 4% [15]. In addition, in another study of 458 adult patients with CHD who underwent cardiac surgery, risk factors associated with early mortality were history of cerebrovascular disease, NYHA class 3 or 4, and surgery on the aorta or aortic valve [16].

4.5 Specific Pathologies

Here we review specific lesions and associated concerns with regard to preoperative planning and intraoperative considerations:

Tetralogy of Fallot/pulmonary atresia: Currently, patients with tetralogy of Fallot (TOF) undergo "complete repair" before the age of one. "Complete" surgical repair typically involves patch closure of the ventricular septal defect, relief of infundibular obstruction by muscular resection with or without a transannular right ventricular outflow tract patch. Common sequelae of this repair later in life may include residual right ventricular outflow tract obstruction, severe pulmonary regurgitation, residual ventricular septal defect, tricuspid regurgitation, right ventricular outflow patch aneurysm, and branch pulmonary artery stenosis (commonly at the insertion site of previously taken down systemic to pulmonary artery shunts). Many of these patients will require percutaneous intervention or reoperation later in life. Preoperative studies include transthoracic echocardiography and MR imaging. In general, we prefer echocardiography for details about valvar function and MR (or CT) imaging for ventricular dimensions and function. In addition, cross-sectional imaging with CT or MR (with or without three-dimensional reconstruction) also provides information about cardiac and great vessel (or conduit) anatomy and their respective relationship to the sternum and chest wall. In general, a right ventricle to pulmonary artery conduit is usually to the left of the midline with TOF and pulmonary atresia with ventricular septal defect. It is not uncommon for the ascending aorta to be dilated in TOF (or any other conotruncal anomaly), and this is typically immediately posterior to the sternum. Coronary artery anomalies which are not uncommon also should be assessed. As mentioned earlier in this chapter, it is important to know if there is an anomalous LAD arising from the right coronary artery and extending across the right ventricular outflow tract that could be injured with an incision during pulmonary valve replacement. In addition, the left anterior descending coronary artery may be very close to the left side of a RV-PA conduit.

Truncus arteriosus/transposition of great arteries: The Rastelli procedure has been the most common procedure to treat transposition with VSD and pulmonary stenosis. The RV to PA conduit is located anteriorly and either to the left (most common) or to the right of the ascending aorta. Similarly, complete repair of truncus arteriosus involves placement of a RV to PA conduit; it is typically positioned to the left of the ascending aorta. With both of these lesions, the conduit is invariably posterior to the sternum and vulnerable to injury at the time of resternotomy, and in some situations the conduit may be eroded into the back of the sternum.

In the setting of truncus arteriosus, the right coronary artery may arise high on the ascending aorta above the level of the sinotubular junction. Consequently, it may be at risk at the time of resternotomy when the ascending aorta is dilated, or it may be at risk at the time of aortotomy if truncal valve repair or replacement is required.

Bicuspid aortic valve (BAV) and Ross procedure: Patient with BAV presenting in adulthood can either be primary with no prior intervention or secondary after a childhood procedure such as the Ross procedure. Patients with primary or secondary disease often present with gradual stenosis and/or regurgitation that eventually leads to symptoms or physiologic criteria for surgical intervention. Less often, the primary presentation is ascending aorta dilatation and, rarely, aortic dissection, aneurysm, or rupture.

Reoperation after the Ross procedure is inevitable for the majority of patients and can be related to pulmonary homograft structural degeneration, autograft (neoaorta) valve regurgitation, autograft dilation, concomitant tricuspid or mitral valve regurgitation, and coronary artery abnormalities [usually button(s) or proximal segment]. The pulmonary autograft (neoaorta) is at risk of dilation in these patients; the dilation is usually confined to the proximal segment and a clear line of demarcation is often present at the location of anastomosis with the smaller native ascending aorta. The aneurysmal segment of the pulmonary autograft or neoaorta and the anterior- and cephalad-displaced right coronary bottom are both at risk during resternotomy as they are usually located underneath the sternum. Preoperative cross-sectional 3D imaging and the selective use of coronary angiography facilitate surgical planning to avoid life-threatening injuries to these structures.

Ebstein's anomaly: Ebstein's anomaly is one of a few CHD that can present both as primary diagnosis in adulthood or after initial reparative operation in childhood. Clinical presentation varies widely from a symptomatic neonate to an asymptomatic octogenarian. Three main factors affecting clinical features of the disease are RV abnormality, TV abnormality, and conduction abnormalities. Undiagnosed adolescent and adult patients can present with palpitations usually due to arrhythmia, exertional dyspnea and fatigue and eventually right-sided heart failure, or sometimes with paradoxical embolization [17, 18]. The natural history of unoperated adult patients with Ebstein's anomaly (with time zero at 25 years of age) demonstrated survival of 76% and 53% at 10 and 15 years, respectively [19]. Operation is offered when symptoms are present (fatigue most common), increasing cyanosis becomes evident, or if paradoxical embolism occurs. Operation is also advised if there is objective evidence of deterioration, such as decreasing exercise performance by exercise testing, progressive increase in heart size on chest radiography, progressive RV dilation or reduction of systolic RV function by echocardiography, or appearance of atrial or ventricular arrhythmias. For patients who had prior repair or replacement of the tricuspid valve, reoperation rate was 10–20% [20]. Reoperations typically are focused on the tricuspid valve—often replacement or re-repair and maze procedure for atrial fibrillation or flutter [21]. Specific considerations when planning surgery include a dilated and thinned out right atrium and right ventricle that could be injured at resternotomy. Knowledge of any residual intracardiac atrial level shunt is essential in the event that cardiopulmonary bypass is required during resternotomy for a right-sided cardiac injury that could result in paradoxical air embolism. Preoperative cross-sectional imaging and careful and meticulous handling of tissues can minimize the risk of potential injuries.

Cardiac arrhythmias including supraventricular (42%) and ventricular arrhythmias are common in adults with Ebstein's anomaly [22]. Preoperative electrophysiological studies are often necessary. Preoperative percutaneous ablation is performed for atrioventricular nodal reentry tachycardia and accessory conduction pathway, and concomitant maze procedure at the time of tricuspid valve surgery is usually recommended for atrial fibrillation or flutter.

Single-ventricle and Fontan conversion: Single-ventricle heart disease compromises only 1% of congenital heart diseases. The prognosis without surgical intervention in childhood is poor, although, in rare cases, patients with well-balanced circulations survive with reasonable functional capacity into adulthood [23].

The goal of Fontan operation is to divert the systemic venous return to the pulmonary circulation without the assistance of a ventricle. It was devised in 1971 for palliation of tricuspid atresia but since then has undergone multiple modifications [24]. The classic Fontan operation consisted of a valved conduit between the right atrium and main pulmonary artery [24]. Many of the current adults with single-ventricle physiology have a classic modified Fontan, which involves a direct anastomosis of the right atrium to the pulmonary artery. The "lateral tunnel" is another modification of the Fontan, which involves creation of an end-to-side anastomosis of the SVC to the undivided right pulmonary artery with an intra-atrial tunnel completed with a patch that tunnels the inferior vena caval blood through the tunnel to the transected SVC [25]. More recently, extracardiac conduit from the IVC to the right pulmonary artery has been performed [26].

In an analysis of 261 patients with Fontan physiology with a mean age at follow-up of 25 years, actuarial event-free survival rates were 75% at 10 years, 68% at

20 years, and 54% at 25 years. The causes of death were determined to be thromboembolic, heart failure related, and sudden death [27]. Patients with an atriopulmonary Fontan connection inevitably develop atrial dilatation, which is associated with atrial arrhythmias, atrial thrombus with possible pulmonary embolism, and right pulmonary venous obstruction. These complications are more commonly seen with early iterations of the Fontan procedure and can diminish cardiac output and exercise capacity and affect quality of life [28]. Low cardiac output is commonly associated with exercise intolerance, protein-losing enteropathy, hepatic congestion and dysfunction, peripheral edema, pleural effusion and ascites, and plastic bronchitis.

The strategy of Fontan conversion was introduced in the early 1990s in an effort to improve outcomes of adult survivors of atriopulmonary Fontan procedures [29]. The goals of Fontan conversion are to excise a portion of the massively dilated right atrium and eliminate underlying atrial arrhythmias. The Fontan anatomy is reconstructed with a lateral tunnel or, more commonly, an extracardiac conduit with bidirectional cavopulmonary shunt [30]. Proper selection of Fontan conversion candidates is critical. In review of 70 patient who underwent Fontan conversion, authors showed that concomitant arrhythmia operations are associated with improved survival, but older age and atrioventricular valve regurgitation increase the risk of poor outcome, and cardiac transplantation may be a better option [31].

Preoperative echocardiography, cross-sectional imaging, and hemodynamic cardiac catheterization are necessary in all patients. Ideal patients for Fontan revision include those with atrial tachyarrhythmias. It is important to demonstrate normal systolic (EF > 50–55%) and diastolic (LVEDP $\leq$ 12 mmHg) ventricular function and mild or less systemic atrioventricular valve regurgitation. Protein-losing enteropathy and liver cirrhosis are contraindications to proceed with Fontan conversion.

Liver problems have recently been investigated in adult patients with Fontan circulation. Wu and colleagues [32] in a multicenter cross-sectional study of 241 adults with Fontan circulation found the majority of tested patients, 94%, had abnormal liver biochemical markers, and all of the patients who underwent imaging by magnetic resonance imaging or computed tomography had abnormalities on imaging consistent with variable degrees of hepatic fibrosis. All 68 patients who received liver biopsies also had a degree of liver fibrosis. Patients with abnormal laboratory values had higher degrees of fibrosis compared with patients with normal laboratory values, in tested patients. Disappointingly, no imaging studies correlated with the degree of fibrosis seen on histologic examination. Due to known risk of hepatocellular carcinoma (HCC) in this group of patients [33], the authors advocate a proactive approach to surveillance of liver health in the Fontan population that involves some combination of regular laboratory work, hepatic imaging, and liver biopsy when appropriate [32].

4.6 Summary

With significant improvements in cardiac surgery and perioperative care for infants and children with CHD over the past few decades, the number of adults with congenital heart disease has dramatically increased and is likely to grow more in the coming years. The majority of cardiac surgery for adult patients with CHD is "redo" operations. Although operative risk associated with "redo" operations in this group of patients can be high, careful preoperative planning with the necessary imaging and choreography of the reoperation results in excellent early outcome. In addition, serial evaluation and thoughtful communication between cardiology and surgery in order to minimize the cumulative number of interventions over a patient's lifetime optimize long-term outcome.

References

1. Hoffman JI, Kaplan S, Liberthson RR. Prevalence of congenital heart disease. Am Heart J. 2004;147(3):425–39.
2. Kouchoukos NT, Kirklin JW. Kirklin/Barratt-Boyes cardiac surgery: morphology, diagnostic criteria, natural history, techniques, results, and indications. Philadelphia, PA: Elsevier/Saunders; 2013. https://www.clinicalkey.com/dura/browse/bookChapter/3-s2.0-C20091575843.
3. Warnes CA, Liberthson R, Danielson GK, Dore A, Harris L, Hoffman JI, et al. Task force 1: the changing profile of congenital heart disease in adult life. J Am Coll Cardiol. 2001;37(5):1170–5.
4. Karamlou T, Diggs BS, Person T, Ungerleider RM, Welke KF. National practice patterns for management of adult congenital heart disease: operation by pediatric heart surgeons decreases in-hospital death. Circulation. 2008;118(23):2345–52.
5. Anwar S, Singh GK, Varughese J, Nguyen H, Billadello JJ, Sheybani EF, et al. 3D printing in complex congenital heart disease: across a spectrum of age, pathology, and imaging techniques. JACC Cardiovasc Imaging. 2017;10(8):953–6.
6. Landzberg MJ. Catheterization of the adult with congenital heart disease (ACHD): beyond "shooting the coronaries". J Interv Cardiol. 2001;14(3):329–37.
7. Koifman B, Egdell R, Somerville J. Prevalence of asymptomatic coronary arterial abnormalities detected by angiography in grown-up patients with congenital heart disease. Cardiol Young. 2001;11(6):614–8.
8. Warnes CA, Williams RG, Bashore TM, Child JS, Connolly HM, Dearani JA, et al. ACC/AHA 2008 guidelines for the management of adults with congenital heart disease: a report of the American College of Cardiology/American Heart Association Task Force on Practice Guidelines (Writing Committee to Develop Guidelines on the Management of Adults With Congenital Heart Disease). Developed in collaboration with the American Society of Echocardiography, Heart Rhythm Society, International Society for Adult Congenital Heart Disease, Society for Cardiovascular Angiography and Interventions, and Society of Thoracic Surgeons. J Am Coll Cardiol. 2008;52(23):e143–263.
9. Therrien J, Dore A, Gersony W, Iserin L, Liberthson R, Meijboom F, et al. CCS consensus conference 2001 update: recommendations for the management of adults with congenital heart disease. Part I. Can J Cardiol. 2001;17(9):940–59.
10. Holst KA, Said SM, Nelson TJ, Cannon BC, Dearani JA. Current interventional and surgical management of congenital heart disease: specific focus on valvular disease and cardiac arrhythmias. Circ Res. 2017;120(6):1027–44.
11. Said SM, Dearani JA. Strategies for high-risk reoperations in congenital heart disease. Semin Thorac Cardiovasc Surg Pediatr Card Surg Annu. 2014;17(1):9–21.
12. Kirklin JK, Westaby S, Blackstone EH, Kirklin JW, Chenoweth DE, Pacifico AD. Complement and the damaging effects of cardiopulmonary bypass. J Thorac Cardiovasc Surg. 1983;86(6):845–57.
13. Akl BF, Pett SB Jr, Wernly JA. Use of a sagittal oscillating saw for repeat sternotomy: a safer and simpler technique. Ann Thorac Surg. 1984;38(6):646–7.
14. Holst KA, Dearani JA, Burkhart HM, Connolly HM, Warnes CA, Li Z, et al. Risk factors and early outcomes of multiple reoperations in adults with congenital heart disease. Ann Thorac Surg. 2011;92(1):122–8; discussion 9–30.

15. Vida VL, Berggren H, Brawn WJ, Daenen W, Di Carlo D, Di Donato R, et al. Risk of surgery for congenital heart disease in the adult: a multicentered European study. Ann Thorac Surg. 2007;83(1):161–8.
16. Kogon B, Grudziak J, Sahu A, Jokhadar M, McConnell M, Book W, et al. Surgery in adults with congenital heart disease: risk factors for morbidity and mortality. Ann Thorac Surg. 2013;95(4):1377–82; discussion 82.
17. Attenhofer Jost CH, Connolly HM, Scott CG, Burkhart HM, Ammash NM, Dearani JA. Increased risk of possible paradoxical embolic events in adults with Ebstein anomaly and severe tricuspid regurgitation. Congenit Heart Dis. 2014;9(1):30–7.
18. Celermajer DS, Bull C, Till JA, Cullen S, Vassillikos VP, Sullivan ID, et al. Ebstein's anomaly: presentation and outcome from fetus to adult. J Am Coll Cardiol. 1994;23(1):170–6.
19. Attie F, Rosas M, Rijlaarsdam M, Buendia A, Zabal C, Kuri J, et al. The adult patient with Ebstein anomaly. Outcome in 72 unoperated patients. Medicine (Baltimore). 2000;79(1):27–36.
20. Brown ML, Dearani JA, Danielson GK, Cetta F, Connolly HM, Warnes CA, et al. The outcomes of operations for 539 patients with Ebstein anomaly. J Thorac Cardiovasc Surg. 2008;135(5):1120–36, e1–7.
21. Dearani JA, Said SM, Burkhart HM, Pike RB, O'Leary PW, Cetta F. Strategies for tricuspid re-repair in Ebstein malformation using the cone technique. Ann Thorac Surg. 2013;96(1):202–8; discussion 8–10.
22. Hebe J. Ebstein's anomaly in adults. Arrhythmias: diagnosis and therapeutic approach. Thorac Cardiovasc Surg. 2000;48(4):214–9.
23. Poterucha JT, Anavekar NS, Egbe AC, Julsrud PR, Connolly HM, Ammash NM, et al. Survival and outcomes of patients with unoperated single ventricle. Heart. 2016;102(3):216–22.
24. Fontan F, Baudet E. Surgical repair of tricuspid atresia. Thorax. 1971;26(3):240–8.
25. de Leval MR, Kilner P, Gewillig M, Bull C. Total cavopulmonary connection: a logical alternative to atriopulmonary connection for complex Fontan operations. Experimental studies and early clinical experience. J Thorac Cardiovasc Surg. 1988;96(5):682–95.
26. Marcelletti C, Corno A, Giannico S, Marino B. Inferior vena cava-pulmonary artery extracardiac conduit. A new form of right heart bypass. J Thorac Cardiovasc Surg. 1990;100(2):228–32.
27. Khairy P, Fernandes SM, Mayer JE Jr, Triedman JK, Walsh EP, Lock JE, et al. Long-term survival, modes of death, and predictors of mortality in patients with Fontan surgery. Circulation. 2008;117(1):85–92.
28. Gelatt M, Hamilton RM, McCrindle BW, Gow RM, Williams WG, Trusler GA, et al. Risk factors for atrial tachyarrhythmias after the Fontan operation. J Am Coll Cardiol. 1994;24(7):1735–41.
29. Kao JM, Alejos JC, Grant PW, Williams RG, Shannon KM, Laks H. Conversion of atriopulmonary to cavopulmonary anastomosis in management of late arrhythmias and atrial thrombosis. Ann Thorac Surg. 1994;58(5):1510–4.
30. Backer CL, Deal BJ, Mavroudis C, Franklin WH, Stewart RD. Conversion of the failed Fontan circulation. Cardiol Young. 2006;16(Suppl 1):85–91.
31. Said SM, Burkhart HM, Schaff HV, Cetta F, Driscoll DJ, Li Z, et al. Fontan conversion: identifying the high-risk patient. Ann Thorac Surg. 2014;97(6):2115–21; discussion 21–2.
32. Wu FM, Kogon B, Earing MG, Aboulhosn JA, Broberg CS, John AS, et al. Liver health in adults with Fontan circulation: a multicenter cross-sectional study. J Thorac Cardiovasc Surg. 2017;153(3):656–64.
33. Asrani SK, Warnes CA, Kamath PS. Hepatocellular carcinoma after the Fontan procedure. N Engl J Med. 2013;368(18):1756–7.
34. Saremi F, SpringerLink (online service). Cardiac CT and MR for adult congenital heart disease. Available from: https://doi.org/10.1007/978-1-4614-8875-0.

Preparing Adults with Congenital Heart Disease for Surgery or Intervention

5

Lynda Shaughnessy and Rafael Alonso-Gonzalez

5.1 Introduction

Patients with congenital heart disease require lifelong follow-up and medical input. Due to the advances in medical and surgical treatment, we have seen an increase in survival of people with *severe* congenital heart disease. The median age of patients surviving with severe congenital heart disease in 1985 was 11 years of age; however, this had increased to 17 years of age by the year 2000 and 29 years of age by 2002 [1]. In 2002 the median age of survival of the total population with congenital heart disease was 40 years of age which would indicate that the overall survival rate for this population group is decreased when compared to the general population [2]. Somerville on that same year suggested that the patients with congenital heart disease that required on-going and repeated interventions were those at the severe end of the spectrum [3].

ACHD can be a challenging group of patients, and they require a multidisciplinary team approach with specialists working in collaboration in areas such as congenital cardiac imaging, cardiology, diagnostic and interventional catheterization, congenital cardiac surgery, anesthesia, heart failure, transplantation, electrophysiology, reproductive and high-risk pregnancy services, genetics, pulmonary hypertension, hepatology, nephrology, hematology [4], congenital cardiac intervention, vascular surgery, psychology, social work, and social services and specialist nurses including clinical nurse specialists, advanced nurse practitioners, operating room nurses, intensive care nurses, recovery nurses, and ward nurses. As the number of patients surviving with severe congenital heart disease increases, so does the

L. Shaughnessy (✉) · R. Alonso-Gonzalez
Adult Congenital Heart Disease Unit, Royal Brompton Hospital, London, UK
e-mail: L.Shaughnessy@rbht.nhs.uk; R.Alonso@rbht.nhs.uk

E. da Cruz et al. (eds.), *Intensive Care of the Adult with Congenital Heart Disease*, Congenital Heart Disease in Adolescents and Adults,
https://doi.org/10.1007/978-3-319-94171-4_5

complexity of the care required and the number of specialist practitioners involved with this group.

It is necessary to be prepared for what may occur with any intervention with ACHD patients. The medical team needs to be prepared as well as the patient. Many of the interventions in congenital heart disease patients are palliative rather than curative leading to the suboptimal cardiovascular physiology which with time can result in multi-organ system involvement [1]. In addition, these patients are likely to need several interventions throughout their lives, thus it is essential to be prepared before any intervention to reduce avoidable complications.

This chapter aims to address some of the specific areas that need to be prepared in order for adults with congenital heart disease to be cared for at the highest levels and minimizing the morbidities that occur with complex interventions.

5.2 Psychological Aspects

The hospitalization rates for adults with congenital heart disease are twice the expected figure for that of the general population, and in general most of these hospitalizations within the congenital heart disease cohort occur during the final year of life [5, 6].

People facing the prospect of admission to hospital and then further intervention have been shown to experience a multitude of emotions including fear, loss of control, decrease of self-esteem, and stress of social disruption [7–10]. These feelings can lead to an anxiety that is disproportionate to the patient's illness. Patients with congenital heart disease are rarely cured with most interventions being palliative. Therefore, many people with congenital heart disease face the prospect of multiple hospital admissions, and after surgical interventions they will be required to have a period of time monitored in the intensive care unit.

Many studies have shown that patient preparation can reduce the negative effects of hospitalization and also have some physiological benefits after an operation or intervention [11–17]. This is not a new concept; however, there are many different forms of patient preparation ranging from written leaflets, verbal information from specialists (i.e., nurses, doctors, surgeons giving procedural information and information regarding the hospital stay), coping strategies including sensation information, behavioral instruction, hypnotic/relaxation training, cognitive behavioral approaches, emotion focused or psychotherapeutic interventions, and a combination of more than one of these approaches [18].

Although there is no one gold standard preparation that can be consensual, it is generally agreed that providing patients with at least one method of preparation is better than no preparation at all [11–15]. Reports show that patients receiving the preparation information feel more satisfied with the care that they have received [11–15].

Other benefits of patient preparation include patients requiring less analgesia and a decreased length of hospital stay [19–21]. Recognizing and discussing the source of the anxiety have been shown to be helpful to patients [17]; however, it is also recognized that the patient that regularly avoids these discussions can have more negative outcomes related to anxiety, fear, loss of control, and lack of knowledge [16].

Mott in 1999 stated that "a person's cognitive processes can alter the perceived meaning of a threatening stimulus and reduce the psychological response of anxiety" [22]. Prolonged anxiety has been shown to lead to an increased breakdown of proteins, can lead to fluid and electrolyte imbalances, causes a decrease in the body's ability to heal leading to decreased wound healing, causes a decrease in the immune response, and increases the risk of infection [23].

Using this knowledge, preadmission or preoperative information can be developed to decrease the anxiety experienced by an individual when being admitted to hospital and furthermore when requiring surgical or cardiac intervention. Thus, preadmission or presurgical preparation can be used to minimize the negative effects that are associated with high anxiety levels.

As mentioned earlier preadmission or presurgical preparation can be performed in a variety of ways. It is important to have some preparation for the patients in order to minimize their stresses and therefore their anxiety levels. Various members of the multidisciplinary team can be involved in this process, and each individual center will differ in what can be offered. Some centers offer the patient some time with the surgeon or cardiologist to discuss the procedure; others offer time with the anesthetist and the intensivist to discuss the operating room and intensive care procedures; others offer a specialist nurse consultation. Ideally all three multidisciplinary team members would be involved. If we look again at the aspects of life that patients become anxious about when preparing to be admitted to hospital, then we can see how these members of the team are extremely important to alleviate these anxieties.

Fear, loss of control, decrease of self-esteem, and stress of social disruption [7–10] are emotions and concerns that can be addressed by giving the patient a leaflet describing the hospital stay, the series of events, expected length of stay, and then information related to discharge home. However, for a small number of patients the, preadmission leaflet can cause them to worry and increase their levels of anxiety [24]. Ideally, the information patients receive with a leaflet should also be reinforced by providing them with time with one or more members of the multidisciplinary team, so that any specific issues can be addressed prior to the procedure.

An example of this is the self-employed/contract builder as patients may be concerned about the amount of time they will be required to be off work and how quickly they will be able to resume all aspects of their role. There can be a financial burden to being in hospital, and this can be heightened if the hospital is not local to where the patient lives. Being aware of this and enabling the patient and/or the family to have specific advice on these issues can be of significant help. These interventions cannot alleviate all of the concerns, but, particularly in some countries, patients may be eligible to, and yet unaware of, benefits from some schemes that may help with loss of earnings. Social workers are instrumental in exploring these avenues with the patients, hence alleviating some of the stress.

5.3 Vascular Access: Challenges and Planning

Patients undergoing cardiac surgery or intervention will require peripheral and central line access to monitor pressures within the vessels and inside the heart and also to deliver medications. Adults with congenital heart disease need to be approached with caution as planning will be required to prevent potential problems during the perioperative phases. Many of these patients have undergone numerous interventions including open-heart surgeries with perioperative invasive monitoring, multiple cardiac catheterizations, and electrophysiology procedures [25]. Having multiple invasive procedures can lead to scarring as well as obstruction to vessels, which can make cannulation of such vessels difficult or sometimes impossible. The identification of which vessels are patent is important as this can lead not only to lines being placed in a timely and accurate manner but also can prevent further vessel injuries which is important for those patients who might require further procedures in the future.

Patients with complex congenital heart disease on occasion can have vessels that are not anatomically correctly positioned or running an anatomically expected route. Some patients have anomalous drainage of vessels, and others have vessels that have been rerouted in previous operations. Anticipation allowing an adequate knowledge of these details is required by the medical and surgical teams involved in the patients care to prevent any damage to these vessels, or any complications.

Reentry injury from repeat sternotomy is a well-defined risk of cardiac surgery. When planning surgery for patients requiring re-sternotomy, it is important to know specific information regarding the type of congenital heart defect and how the previous operations were performed. This information can be very useful to the surgeon when planning a further sternotomy as in some conditions such as in tetralogy of Fallot or pulmonary atresia where a conduit is used in the repair, the conduit typically lies left of the midline. Frequently, the aorta in these groups is enlarged and lies directly beneath the sternum. This can cause a problem for the surgeon when opening the chest as it can lead to the aorta accidentally being dissected.

For other conditions the conduit could be the vessel that is midline behind the sternum and that could also lead to the same problems with the surgeon accidentally dissecting the conduit if not aware of the relationship of the vessels to the sternum. Right ventricular enlargement is also common in this patient group due to the type of congenital heart defect [25]. If the procedure is deemed to have a high risk of injury to the vessels or to the right heart, then a decision might need to be made to expose the femoral vessels. Exposing and cannulating the femoral vessels in preparation to commence bypass can be used to prevent catastrophic complications with re-sternotomy.

Imaging can be a useful way of assessing the location of the vessels and also of the chambers of the heart in relation to the sternum. Cardiac magnetic resonance (CMR) scanning is now routinely used in the preparation of congenital heart disease patients for surgery or intervention. The main benefit of this type of imaging is that it does not deliver any radiation to the patient. This can be very important as these patients have a lifetime of care and often require regular imaging, and therefore reducing their exposure to radiation can become very important. Many congenital heart disease patients will have had multiple cardiac catheterization procedures and might have metal stents in situ. Although many of these stents are not a contraindication to a cardiac magnetic resonance scan, some are CMR-incompatible or else can sometimes distort the images.

If the image quality gained by the CMR scan is not satisfactory or if the coronary arteries need to be better visualized, then a computed tomography (CT) scan can be performed. It can be argued that CT scanning should be performed on all patients having had one previous sternotomy in order to reduce the risks of adverse events during further surgery. However, this really should not be a procedure that is performed using a protocol. Each individual case should be evaluated by the multidisciplinary team including the cardiologist, the imaging specialists, and the surgeon prior to deciding who requires advanced imaging. Routine CT scanning is not advisable as it exposes patients to radiation, which in some cases could and should be avoided.

5.4 Preoperative Pulmonary Reserve

Up to 30% of patients with congenital heart disease have significantly impaired lung function. Moderate-to-severe impairment of lung function relates to the complexity of the underlying cardiac defect, enlarged cardiothoracic ratio, previous thoracotomy/thoracotomies, body mass index, scoliosis, and diaphragm palsy, and it is an independent predictor of survival in this population. Patients with reduced force vital capacity of at least moderate severity have a 1.6-fold increased risk of death compared to patients with normal lung function [26].

Postoperative pulmonary complications are defined as postoperative pulmonary abnormality that produce identifiable disease or dysfunction that is clinically significant and adversely affects the clinical course [27]. Postoperative pulmonary complications contribute significantly to overall perioperative morbidity and mortality and include atelectasis, infection, respiratory failure (mechanical ventilation for >48 h after surgery or unplanned reintubation), and hypoxemia.

Factors that can contribute to pulmonary complications can be divided in patient-related factors and procedure-related factors. Smoking is one of the most important patient-related factors. Smoking significantly increases the risk of postoperative complications, which can be reduced by stopping smoking at least 4 weeks before the intervention. Obstructive sleep apnea is a common disease among patients with congenital heart disease, and it is a well-known factor for respiratory complications from procedures with sedation and/or anesthesia. Preoperative evaluation of patients with obstructed sleep apnea should specifically include assessment of severity and adequacy of management. In addition, patients with severe or poorly controlled obstructive sleep apnea may benefit from initiation or optimization of treatment before surgery. Although obesity reduces lung volumes and causes ventilation/perfusion mismatch and relative hypoxemia, several studies have shown that in the absence of obstructive sleep apnea or significant hypercapnia, pulmonary complications are not more frequent in obese patients. Age >50 years, chronic obstructive pulmonary disease, congestive heart failure, poor general health status, functional dependence, pulmonary hypertension, low oxygen saturation, and serum albumin <3.5 g/dL are also recognized risk factors to develop pulmonary complications in this population.

Preoperative lung function tests should only be performed in selected patients. A detailed clinical assessment and physical examination are more important to identify signs or symptoms of an undiagnosed lung disease.

5.5 Assessment of Atherosclerotic Coronary Disease

As mentioned above, the number of adult patients with congenital heart disease is already higher than the number of children. As these patients grow older, the risk of developing coronary artery disease increases. Giannakoulas et al. reported a prevalence of 9.2% of significant coronary artery disease in a cohort of 250 adults with congenital heart disease who underwent coronary angiograms for reasons other than suspected coronary artery disease. In this study, young patients (<40 year old) and cyanotic patients did not have coronary artery disease; and systemic hypertension and hypercholesterolemia were strong predictors of coronary artery disease [28]. A more recent study using the CONCOR registry identified 55 patients with coronary artery disease (mean age 55.1 ± 12.4 years, 80% male) and 56 patients with stroke (mean age 46.9 ± 15.2, 46% male), among 6904 adults with congenital heart disease. In this study, systemic hypertension (odds ratio (OR) 2.45; 95% confidence interval (CI) 1.15–5.23), hypercholesterolemia (OR 3.99; 95% CI 1.62–9.83), and smoking (OR 2.25; 95% CI 1.09–4.66) were risk factors for coronary artery disease. However, they were not associated with ischemic stroke, which was associated with previous interventions, residual/unrepaired shunts, and left-sided mechanical valves [29].

The current American College of Cardiology and American Heart Association valve guidelines give a class IIa recommendation for revascularization of >70% luminal reduction in major coronary arteries or >50% luminal reduction in the left main coronary artery at the time of valve surgery in patients with acquired heart disease [30]. The rationale for concomitant coronary artery bypass grafting at the time of surgery originates from limited surgical data in which patients undergoing surgical aortic valve replacement with unrevascularized coronary artery disease had poorer long-term outcomes compared with those that had a CABG [31]. Unfortunately, there is no data about the need for concomitant CABG at the time of cardiac surgery in patients with congenital heart disease; however, it seems reasonable to extrapolate the data from acquired heart disease patients.

Therefore, assessment of the coronary arteries prior to cardiac surgery should be considered in patients with adult congenital disease: (a) if there is clinical history of chest discomfort, ischemia by noninvasive imaging, or both, (b) and in patients free of chest pain but in an older age range (>40 years old for men and >50 years old for women) and/or more than one risk factor for coronary artery disease. The gold standard for coronary assessment is coronary angiography, although computed tomography coronary angiography (CTCA) has developed significantly over the past decade. CTCA provides information about both vessel lumen and information on the composition of plaques and the vessel wall as well as other cardiac structures. However, it is important to know that the spatial and temporal resolutions remain inferior to invasive coronary angiography, mainly when assessing small vessels. CTCA is also operator-dependent, and although it is a good technique to assess coronary artery disease, we need to be aware of its limitations.

5.6 Assessment of Arrhythmias

The prevalence of atrial arrhythmias in the adult congenital heart disease population is estimated to be 15%, with a lifetime risk of 50% [32]. As in the general population, the primary mechanisms of supraventricular tachycardia in patients with adult congenital heart disease include reentry, increased automaticity, and triggered activity. Intra-atrial reentry tachycardia is the most frequent supraventricular arrhythmia in patients with congenital heart disease, and postoperative factors, such as scarring and suture lines, are an ideal substrate. Patients with extensive atrial scarring, such as patients with transposition of the great arteries repaired with atrial switch (Mustard or Senning), or patients with a large atrium, such as patients with classic Fontan, have the highest risk of atrial arrhythmias. However, atrial tachycardias also occur in one-third of patients with repaired tetralogy of Fallot and are common in patients with repaired or unrepaired atrial septal defects [32]. In addition, the risk of postoperative arrhythmias in patients with congenital heart disease is increased almost threefold over the non-congenital patients [33]. Clinical atrial arrhythmias should be ruled out in all congenital patients with frequent episodes of palpitations prior to surgery. Should a paroxysmal atrial arrhythmia be confirmed we would recommend to perform an ablation before the surgical procedure to minimize the perioperative risk of arrhythmias. In addition, in patients with atrial septal defects and arrhythmias originated in the left atrium, an ablation before closing the defect is recommended.

Atrioventricular reentry tachycardia accounts for less than 8% of supraventricular tachycardia in patients with congenital heart disease [32]. Accessory pathways are present in 9% of patients with Ebstein's anomaly and 1.4% of patients with congenitally corrected transposition of the great arteries [32]. In patients with congenital heart disease and antegrade conduction across the accessory pathway, an electrophysiological study is recommended even in the absence of symptoms due to the high incidence of atrial arrhythmias and multiple pathways.

Sudden cardiac death is the leading cause of death in patients with tetralogy of Fallot, with an incidence of approximately 2% per decade in adults [34]. There are several risk factors related to ventricular arrhythmias and sudden cardiac death in patients with tetralogy of Fallot such as late repair, previous palliative shunt, ventriculotomy incision, QRS duration >180 ms, etc. However, no single factor, apart from severely impaired left ventricular function, seems to have strong enough predictive power to solely justify an ICD device [35]. Residual pulmonary regurgitation is the most common indication for surgery in patients with repaired tetralogy of

Fallot. Severe pulmonary regurgitation and right ventricular dysfunction correlate with higher risk of ventricular arrhythmias in patients with tetralogy of Fallot, but pulmonary valve replacement does not reliably protect against them. Different risk factors should be used to stratify patients into low, intermediate, and high risk of sudden cardiac death prior to surgery. Patients with high risk of sudden cardiac death will probably benefit from an ICD. This is usually performed after surgery for pulmonary valve replacement but prior to discharge home. An ICD is not indicated in patients with low risk of sudden cardiac death. In patients with intermediate risk, electrophysiological evaluation may be needed to further improve risk stratification. Inducible ventricular tachycardia is an independent risk factor for sudden cardiac death in this population. With the available evidence, it is difficult to decide whether this should be performed before or after surgery. Some centers perform an electrophysiological study prior to surgery in all patients with tetralogy of Fallot to do a prophylactic ablation of the anatomical isthmuses in order to reduce the risk of perioperative ventricular tachycardias. Although this approach sounds reasonable, one can argue that the substrate will change after the intervention, and therefore the potential benefit of the prophylactic ablation might disappear. An integrated approach to the electrophysiology and anatomical issues is important and must be tailored to the individual patient.

5.7 Informed Consent

Decision-making is a complex issue that encompasses a wide range of behaviors resulting in the input-process-output-feedback loop [26]. It is really important that adequate time is given to patients as well as adequate information in order to allow them to go through the decision-making process loop and to take a fully informed decision. Decision-making is not easy and requires individuals to go through various processes in order to reach their final decision. This decision will also be influenced by previous experiences; for example, if a patient had an unexpected side effect from a medication previously, then this might lead to him or her being less willing to try a new medication in the future. Therefore, it can be agreed that this level of decision-making involves both the cognitive and emotional aspects of the brain. These components, however, are subject to developmental changes.

Adolescents are often required to make complex decisions regarding their healthcare with consent being taken from patients as young as 16 years of age in some countries. Research into neurodevelopment has shown that during the adolescent phase, there is remodeling occurring in the prefrontal cortex, with a decline in the relative size of this area. This is an area of the brain that is involved with the learning of rules: the working memory and spatial learning [26]. It is believed that during this phase there is a change in the neurotransmitters involved in brain cell communication with a reduction of the neurotransmitter glutamate and gamma-aminobutyric acid but an increase in the dopamine levels [27]. These adjustments in dopamine level can also be seen elsewhere in the brain such as in the limbic brain regions [28]. It can therefore be argued that the changes in dopamine levels in the adolescent brain can account for their emotional, cognitive, and psychological responses.

It is therefore important to understand the patients and their developmental level when discussing any procedure with them. In order to gain informed consent, the individual must fully understand the consequences of his or her decision. Therefore, the information delivered to the patient should be age appropriate and developmentally appropriate. It should not be assumed that if patients have a lower than normal cognitive development, they will lack the ability to consent for themselves. Processes should be put in place to allow for information to be delivered to the individuals in a way that they can understand. It may be necessary on occasions for an advocate to make the decision on behalf of the patient. In these instances there should be a discussion to be sure that the decision made is in the best interest of the patient.

There are occasions when it is necessary to perform emergency procedures that may not allow time to discuss the procedure in great depth; however, this should be only the case when not performing the procedure would result in significant harm being caused to the patient. Preparing the patient psychologically as well as physically is extremely important in gaining the best possible outcomes for the patient not just from the current procedure but in order to aid them in any future decision they may be required to make in the future.

Conclusion

Preparing patients with congenital heart disease for any intervention involves a multidisciplinary team approach. This is a complex group of patients, and it is essential that all aspects of the intervention are appropriately planned. It is also essential that all practitioners have an in-depth knowledge of the anatomy and physiology for the individual patient. Complex imaging can assist with the planning of the intervention and, in many instances, is essential to facilitate a comprehensive understanding of the patient's anatomy.

Preoperative assessment cannot be underestimated as this has been shown to have huge benefits not only to the patient in their understanding of the intervention and the postoperative course but also in reducing anxiety. This patient group, as mentioned herein, is often subjected to multiple interventions throughout their lifetime, and some of these may not leave them with positive experiences. It is essential to have knowledge and understanding of this, to allow the patient time to discuss his/her feelings, and to refer the patient for specific assistance when required. Looking after the social and psychological health of the patients as well as their physical wellbeing can have a positive impact on the hospital length of stay. Moreover, it is likely that a well-thought-out and well-planned procedure will lead to a positive overall outcome for the patient.

References

1. Allan C. Intensive care of the adult patient with congenital heart disease. Prog Cardiovasc Dis. 2011;53:274–80.
2. Marelli A, Mackie A, Ionescu-Ittu R, Rahme E, Pilote L. Congenital heart disease in the general population: changing prevalence and age distribution. Circulation. 2007;115:163–72.

3. Somerville J. Report of the British Cardiac Society Working Party. Grown-up congenital heart (GUCH) disease: current needs and provision of service for adolescents and adults with congenital heart disease in the UK. Heart. 2002;88(Suppl 1):1–14.
4. Dearani J, Connolly H, Martinez R, Fontanet H, Webb G. Caring for adults with congenital heart disease: successes and challenges for 2007 and beyond. Cardiol Young. 2007;17(Suppl 4):87–96.
5. Verheugt C, Uiterwaal C, van der Velde E, Mejiboom F, Pieper F, Sieswerda G, Plokker H, Grobbee D, Mulder B. The emerging burden of hospital admissions of adults with congenital heart disease. Heart. 2010;96(11):872–8.
6. Mackie A, Pilote L, Ionescu-Ittu R, Rahme E, Marelli A. Health care resource utilisation in adults with congenital heart disease. Am J Cardiol. 2007;99(6):839–43.
7. Asiliogu K, Celik S. The effect of pre-operative education on anxiety of open cardiac surgery patients. Patient Educ Couns. 2002;53:65–70.
8. Viney C. Pain and sedation needs. Cited in: Nursing the critically ill. London: Bailliere Tindall; 1996.
9. Quinn S, Redmond K, Begley C. The needs of relatives visiting the adult intensive care units as perceived by relatives and nurses. Intensive Crit Care Nurs. 1996;12(3):168–72.
10. McGonigal K. The importance of sleep and the sensory environment to critically ill patients. Intensive Care Nurs. 1986;2(2):73–83.
11. Garbee D, Gentry A. Coping with the stress of surgery. AORN J. 2001;73:946–51.
12. Watts S. Patients' perceptions of the pre-operative information they need about events they may experience in the intensive care unit. J Adv Nurs. 1997;26:85–92.
13. Nelson S. Pre-admission education for patients undergoing cardiac surgery. Br J Nurs. 1996;5:335–40.
14. Wit P, Duivervoorden H, Dixhoorn J. More psychological preparation in heart surgery for certain patients is beneficial. Ned Tijdschr Geneeskd. 1996;140:1720–3.
15. Hathaway D. Effect of preoperative instruction on postoperative outcomes: a meta-analysis. Nurs Res. 1986;35:269–75.
16. Egbert L, Batit G, Welch C, Bartlett M. Reduction of post-operative pain by encouragement and instruction of patients. N Engl J Med. 1964;270:825–7.
17. Janis I. Psychological stress: psychoanalytical and behavioural studies of surgical patients. New York: Wiley; 1958.
18. Johnston M, Vögele C. Benefits of psychological preparation for surgery: a meta-analysis. Ann Behav Med. 1993;15(4):245–56.
19. Bysshe J. The effect of giving information to patients before surgery. Nursing. 1988;3(30):36–9.
20. Mott A. Psychologic preparation to decrease the anxiety associated with cardiac catheterisation. J Vasc Nurs. 1999;17:41–9.
21. Wicker P. Pre-operative visiting: making it work. Br J Theatr Nurs. 1995;5(7):16–9.
22. Webb R. Pre-operative visiting from the perspective of the theatre nurse. Br J Theatr Nurs. 1995;4(16):919–25.
23. Boore J, Champion R, Ferguson C, editors. Nursing the physically ill adult. Edinburgh: Churchill Livingstone; 1987.
24. Gillies M, Baldwin G. Do patients booklets increase preoperative anxiety. Eur J Anaesthesiol. 2001;18:620–2.
25. Brown M, Joseph D, Burkhart H. The adult with congenital heart disease: medical and surgical considerations for management. Curr Opin Pediatr. 2009;21:561–4.
26. Alonso-Gonzalez R, Borgia F, Diller G, Inuzuka R, Kempny A, Martinez-Naharro A, Tutarel O, Marino P, Wustmann K, Charalambides M, Silva M, Swan L, Dimopoulos K, Gatzoulis M. Abnormal lung function in adults with congenital heart disease: prevalence, relation to cardiac anatomy, and association with survival. Circulation. 2013;127(8):882–90.
27. O'Donohue W Jr. Postoperative pulmonary complications. When are preventive and therapeutic measures necessary? Postgrad Med. 1992;91:167.
28. Giannakoulas G, Dimopoulos K, Engel R, Goktekin O, Kucukdurmaz Z, Vatankulu M, Bedard E, Diller G, Papaphylactou M, Di Francis D, Mario C, Gatzoulis M. Burden of coronary artery

disease in adults with congenital heart disease and its relation to congenital and traditional heart risk factors. Am J Cardiol. 2009;103(10):1445–50.
29. Bokma J, Zegstroo I, Kuijpers J, Konings T, van Kimmenade R, van Melle J, Kiès P, Mulder B, Bouma B. Factors associated with coronary artery disease and stroke in adults with congenital heart disease. Heart. 2018;104(7):574–80.
30. Nishimura A, Otto C, Bonow R, Carabello B, Erwin J 3rd, Guyton R, O'Gara P, Ruiz C, Skubas N, Sorajja P, Sundt T 3rd, Thomas J. American College of Cardiology/American Heart Association Task Force on Practice Guidelines. 2014 AHA/ACC guideline for the management of patients with valvular heart disease: executive summary: a report of the American College of Cardiology/American Heart Association Task Force on Practice Guidelines. J Am Coll Cardiol. 2014;63(22):2438–88.
31. Thalji N, Suri R, Daly R, Greason K, Dearani J, Stulak J, Joyce L, Burkhart H, Pochettino A, Li Z, Frye R, Schaff H. The prognostic impact of concomitant coronary artery bypass grafting during aortic valve surgery: implications for revascularization in the transcatheter era. J Thorac Cardiovasc Surg. 2015;149(2):451–60.
32. Janson C, Shah M. Supraventricular tachycardia in adult with congenital heart disease: mechanisms, diagnosis and clinical aspects. Card Electrophysiol Clin. 2017;9:189–211.
33. Karangelis D, Mazine A, Narsupalli S, Medis S, Veldtman G, Nikolaidis N. Morbidity after cardiac surgery in patient with adult congenital heart disease in comparison with acquire heart disease. Heart Lung Circ. 2018;27(6):739–44.
34. Gatzoulis M, Balaji S, Webber S, Siu S, Hokanson J, Poile C, Rosenthal M, Nakazawa M, Moller J, Gillette P, Webb G, Redington A. Risk factors for arrhythmia and sudden cardiac death late after repair of tetralogy of Fallot: a multicentre study. Lancet. 2000;356(9234):975–81.
35. Avila P, Chaix M, Mondésert B, Khairy P. Sudden cardiac death in adult congenital heart disease. Card Electrophysiol Clin. 2017;9:225–34.

General Intensive Care Monitoring and Management

6

Joan Sánchez-de-Toledo, Lucas Sáenz, and Daniel Pereda

6.1 Introduction

Over the last two decades, advances in surgical techniques and postoperative care have made a major impact on survival among children with congenital heart disease (CHD). Clinicians have abandoned the times of expected mortality and are now facing expected survival. The majority of children with CHD are now entering adulthood, and currently in the USA and Europe, there are more adults with CHD than children (Fig. 6.1). It is expected that in this decade, 1 in 150 young adults will have CHD.

Advances in surgical, interventional, and anesthesia techniques and postoperative care have decreased associated mortality. Adults with CHD have become the focus of attention of the majority of programs treating congenital heart disease. Their complex anatomy and physiology and the commonly associated comorbidities have challenged cardiovascular teams.

As much as the care of children with CHD has been organized and structured and there are now subspecialized teams focused on the specific needs of these children (dedicated cardiologists, anesthesiologists, intensivists, highly specialized nurses, and clinical practitioners), the optimal organization of care for adults with CHD is

J. Sánchez-de-Toledo (✉)
Cardiac Intensive Care Division, Children's Hospital of Pittsburgh, Pittsburgh, PA, USA

Department of Pediatric Cardiology, Hospital Sant Joan de Déu, Barcelona, Spain

L. Sáenz
Cardiac Intensive Care Division, Children's Hospital of Pittsburgh, Pittsburgh, PA, USA

D. Pereda
Department of Cardiovascular Surgery and Adult Cardiac Intensive Care Unit, Hospital Clínic, Barcelona, Spain
e-mail: dpereda@clinic.cat

E. da Cruz et al. (eds.), *Intensive Care of the Adult with Congenital Heart Disease*, Congenital Heart Disease in Adolescents and Adults,
https://doi.org/10.1007/978-3-319-94171-4_6

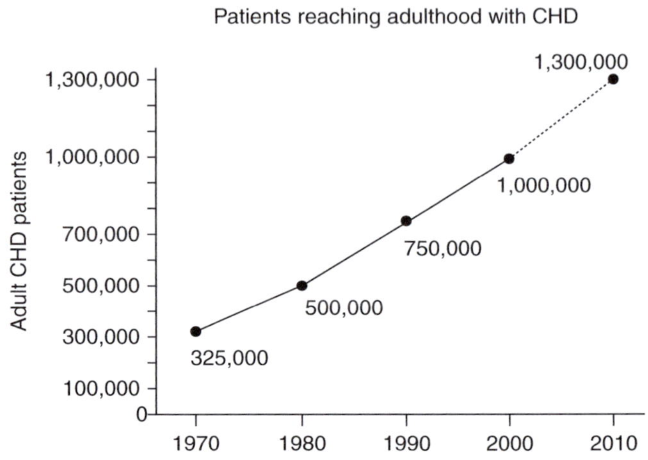

Fig. 6.1 Expanding population of adults with congenital heart disease by year. Moss and Adams' heart disease in infants, children, and adolescents, including the fetus and young adults, 7th edition

yet to be clearly defined. This challenge has been approached by advanced centers with dedicated teams working hand in hand with other specialties in a complex environment. Patients with adult congenital heart disease (ACHD) are not only facing unique challenges related to their heart disease and associated comorbidities due to surgical and nonsurgical interventions, but they are also aging and facing the burden of acquired heart disease as the normal population. These include COPD, cancer, renal and pulmonary diseases, and myocardial ischemia. Another special situation caregivers are now frequently facing with ACHD patients is the management of pregnancy and delivery in young women. ACHD programs are offering heart failure/transplant care, pulmonary vascular and outpatient follow-up clinics, and in some cases services supported by telemedicine. However, the proper surgical and postoperative care is still not well defined. The growing population of ACHD patients will generate new needs, and a dedicated model of care will be needed in the years ahead.

The proper organization and structure of the postoperative care of the ACHD will pose a big dilemma in the majority of institutions. As these teams are in development, ACHD patients surviving complex surgeries are also in need of more frequent evaluation, advanced multidisciplinary medical treatment, and multiple invasive and noninvasive diagnostic and procedural interventions.

ACHD programs are shifting from more invasive diagnostic interventions (such as cardiac catheterization) to less invasive diagnostic testing such as cardiac MRI and new echocardiographic techniques, leaving the most invasive procedures for the cases specifically in need of intervention.

Special consideration should be given to these patients before and after any intervention–evaluation, and careful consideration should be taken of preoperative risk factors, including those related to intrinsic heart disease and those associated with multiple interventions. Postoperative risk factors are prevalent in this population, and careful attention is needed. Special emphasis must be given to peripheral vascular system, renal and neurological sequelae.

During the past two decades, several task force guidelines have been developed as to how to approach the increasing demand of care for ACHD patients. ACC/AHA 2008 and the ESC/AEPC 2010 with their subsequent updates are worth mentioning.

The particular anatomy and physiology of ACHD patients determine the pathophysiological features of the organ dysfunction present in the intensive care unit.

6.2 Physiology

6.2.1 Single Ventricle

Unrepaired single ventricle young adult patients are uncommon. Usually by adulthood, these patients have received at least one palliative surgical procedure. Prognosis for those who have remained unrepaired is poor. In a report by Moodie et al., 50% of 83 adults with unrepaired less severe anatomical single ventricle physiology died at 14 years of diagnosis and 50% of those with more complex anatomical features died at 4 years of diagnosis [1]. In this cohort of patients, the most common causes of death were dysrhythmia, congestive heart failure, and sudden and unexplained death. Some anatomical and physiological features of unoperated single ventricle patients have been associated with extended survival [2]:

- Double-inlet LV with transposed great vessels
- Pulmonary stenosis
- Normal LV systolic function
- Less than mild AV valve regurgitation

6.2.1.1 Total Cavopulmonary Connections

Since the Fontan procedure was first performed in the 1970s, we are now facing a growing population of adult survivors from this palliative surgery.

The Fontan procedure merits special attention. The characteristic passive pulmonary flow in these patients is a factor that directly influences their systemic cardiac output. In order to secure systemic cardiac output, pulmonary pressures should be low. In the setting of elevated Fontan pressures and a low systemic cardiac output state, a proper estimation of the trans-pulmonary gradient (the difference between the atrial pressure and the pulmonary artery pressure) is key for their management. High trans-pulmonary gradients indicate a failure of cardiac function, whereas normal trans-pulmonary gradients indicate mechanical problems in the cavopulmonary connections, residual stenosis in the pulmonary tree, presence of aortopulmonary collaterals, or elevated pulmonary vascular resistances.

This passive pulmonary flow makes Fontan patients particularly vulnerable to the mechanical ventilation strategies. Early extubation, favoring spontaneous modes, and strategies aiming to minimize high peak inspiratory pressures are key to maintaining a proper pulmonary flow.

Moreover, the systemic venous congestion generated by the passive flow and increased venous pressures jeopardizes distal tissue perfusion. Organs such as the liver, kidneys, and intestines become particularly vulnerable in postoperative low-output states of Fontan patients.

6.2.2 Systemic Right Ventricular

Right ventricular dysfunction is a well-known predictive factor of bad outcomes in ACHD patients. Uncommonly seen nowadays in pediatrics, systemic right ventricles are frequently seen in adults with transposition of great arteries that were once palliated with atrial switch techniques. Another important group of patients with dysfunctional right ventricles are those with RVOT obstruction such as tetralogy of Fallot or pulmonary stenosis. Similar to patients with passive pulmonary blood flow, gentle ventilator strategies are key to minimizing the negative cardiopulmonary interactions generated by the increased pulmonary pressures.

6.2.3 Biventricular Failure

Chronic heart failure with biventricular dysfunction is a common scenario in our ACHD patient population. Appropriate inotropic selection with judicious use of noninvasive positive-pressure ventilation and diuresis are well-known strategies used in the adult units. Early recognition of failure, proper timing and allocation to mechanical circulatory support, and transplant list are key strategies. Major advances achieved in mechanical circulatory support in adults have helped to improve both the survival of critically ill patients and also the quality of life for those awaiting transplantation or those on destination therapy.

6.2.4 Left-to-Right Shunting Lesions

Early or later, detection of congenital heart diseases has brought a cohort of adults presenting with shunt lesions (repaired or unrepaired). Those who have been repaired as infants rarely present with pulmonary hypertension; however, those adults with unrepaired shunts will develop elevated pulmonary vascular resistances and subsequently Eisenmenger's syndrome.

6.2.4.1 Eisenmenger's Syndrome (ES)

Eisenmenger's syndrome is a multisystem disorder leading to multiple complications and reduced survival. The incidence and prevalence of Eisenmenger's syndrome are unknown. Historical data shows that 8% of patients with congenital heart disease developed ES and 11% of those had left-to-right shunts [3]. The development of ES is based on the size and location of the left-to-right shunt. Kidd et al. described ES in 3% of patients with small to moderate VSD, and in the same study, 50% of the patients with severe VSD (>1.5 cm) developed ES [4]. Saha et al. reported ES patient's survival rate of 80% at 10 years, 77% at 15 years, and 42% at 25 years. Patients with ES commonly survived into the third or fourth decade of life [5].

Eisenmenger's syndrome patients usually display a wide range of medical problems that include renal dysfunction, brain abscess, polycythemia, coagulopathy (the most common being platelet dysfunction), and cerebral microembolism. They can also have hyperuricemia. In the case of ES patients with symptomatic pulmonary vascular obstructive disease, phlebotomy should be considered. Nonetheless, special consideration is advised, since patients with multiple phlebotomies are at high risk of cerebral vascular accidents due to associated iron deficiency and microcytosis. Iron replacement with frequent monitoring of the hemoglobin level and mean corpuscular volume (MCV) is advised.

Medical therapy has become important as it improves exercise capacity and serves as a bridge for lung or heart-lung transplants. An RCT presented by Galiè et al. randomized 54 ES patients with either placebo (n = 17) or the endothelin-receptor antagonist, bosentan (n = 37). After 16 weeks, bosentan patients demonstrated a significant reduction in pulmonary vascular resistance index and an improved exercise capacity compared with the placebo patients [6]. Reports have demonstrated that advanced therapy (bosentan, treprostinil, sitaxsentan, beraprost, epoprostenol, and sildenafil) could significantly delay the need for heart-lung transplants in patients with unstable ES [7].

6.3 Lesion-Specific Considerations

6.3.1 Bicuspid Aortic Valve (BAV)

Congenital bicuspid aortic valve (BAV) is not an infrequent disease among ACHD patients, and it is estimated that approximately 2% of the general population is diagnosed with BAV [8]. A systolic ejection murmur is the most common sign. Patients with BAV and aortic stenosis or aortic insufficiency could present with exercise intolerance, dyspnea on exertion, or chest pain. Patients without significant aortic stenosis (a gradient <30 mmHg) and less than mild aortic insufficiency are not restricted. However, over time, the dysfunction can progress. Niaz et al. retrospectively analyzed young adult patients who were diagnosed with BAV from 1990 to 2015 and reported a higher incident of BAV among patients repaired of CoA (36%) and interrupted aortic arch (36%) [9]. Around the second decade of life, BAV patients are expected to develop aortic valve sclerosis. Progression to aortic calcification is not uncommon by the fourth decade.

6.3.2 Coarctation of the Aorta

Coarctation of the aorta repair has been performed since 1945, and since then, good short-term outcomes have been achieved. Nowadays, a large number of patients repaired of CoA are reaching adulthood; nonetheless, mortality in this group remains high compared to the normal population. Brown et al. reported an actuarial survival of 74% at 30 years of follow-up after surgery [10]. Recoarctation of the aorta is not an uncommon finding in adult patients and is mostly related with the age and technique used at the initial repair and the presence of an unrecognized hypoplastic arch. Therefore, proper identification and management of long-term complications is essential. There are a number or complications that need important consideration.

6.3.2.1 Systemic Hypertension

Approximately a third of patients with repaired CoA will develop residual hypertension in adulthood, and more than 60% of patients will present hypertension 25 years after repair [10]. Multiple studies have found a significant incidence of systemic hypertension following coarctation repair. Hypertension can occur with or without the presence of a residual gradient. If hypertension is detected at rest, recoarctation should be excluded. Doppler echocardiography, CMR, and cardiac CT imaging are radiological imaging studies useful to assess recoarctation. An aortic diameter narrowing of >50% and/or a systolic gradient of >20 mmHg measured noninvasively or during cardiac catheterization is considered indicative of significant recoarctation and may indicate the need for an intervention.

6.3.2.2 Aortic Aneurysm and Dissection

Dilation and aneurysm formation around the surgical repair can occur years after CoA repair [11]. These complications are often recognized too late, and by the time they are detected, there has already been aortic rupture, aortobronchial fistula, or sudden death. Aortic aneurysm and pseudoaneurysm can occur without recurrent coarctation or systemic hypertension. Aneurysm is more common after cardiac catheterization compared to surgical interventions. Patients presenting with chest pain and hemoptysis should not be ignored. Active screening and early management are paramount to prevent further life-threatening complications. Pseudoaneurysms carry a higher risk of rupture; therefore, surgical intervention should be considered at time of diagnosis. Some cases would benefit from an endovascular repair with a covered stent.

In recent years, evidence has shown that patients with CoA are at high risk of intrinsic aortic abnormalities despite repair. Coronary artery disease is not uncommon in this group and, together with BAV dysfunction and ascending aorta dilatation, represents the most commonly associated conditions requiring concomitant treatment at the time of reintervention [12].

Lifelong surveillance and follow-up are crucial in patients with aortic coarctation. Prevention and treatment of possible complications are key components for the management of this population [12].

6.3.3 Tetralogy of Fallot (TOF)

Survival after surgical correction of TOF has improved a lot since the earliest surgical era. It is estimated that more than 90% of the patients that underwent surgical repair 30 years ago are still alive [13]. Since the first surgical approach for TOF has been described, various techniques have been used. It is of paramount importance to determine with high accuracy the surgical history of the ACHD patients with TOF repair.

In a typical case, a TOF-ACHD patient will have undergone complete repair, and this technique would probably have involved VSD patch closure, pulmonary valvectomy, transannular patch, and possibly sub-pulmonic infundibulectomy. Patients with TOF and complete repair should be evaluated for right ventricular dysfunction, pulmonary valve insufficiency, residual shunts or right ventricular outlet tract obstruction, pulmonary stenosis, arrhythmias, and risk of sudden death [14].

Arrhythmias ought to be considered at all times. The incidence of life-threatening ventricular arrhythmias is around 6%. QRS duration is a strong predictor of sustained ventricular tachycardia [15].

Pulmonary valve replacement is now used as an acceptable surgical therapy to treat moderate to severe pulmonary insufficiency and RV dysfunction and is one of the most common procedures performed in ACHD programs [16]. In several reports, cardiac MRI has been used to follow RV size and pulmonary valve integrity.

Other problems that need to be addressed and considered are pulmonary stenosis and aortic root dilation.

6.3.4 D-Transposition of the Great Arteries

6.3.4.1 Atrial Switch Operation

Dr. Ake Senning performed the first atrial switch operation in 1957. In 1963, Dr. William Mustard also performed a similar procedure using prosthetic material [17]. Long-term complications for these patients include RV failure, atrial arrhythmias, and sudden cardiac death. In one series, Mustard patients had an 80% survival rate at the 20-year follow-up and 68% at 39 years. Survival free of events, including heart transplantation, arrhythmias, reintervention, or heart failure, was only 19% at 39 years [18].

Special consideration should be given to arrhythmias: atrial and ventricular tachyarrhythmias, heart block, and sudden cardiac death [18]. Other commonly seen complications after these procedures are systemic ventricular failure, systemic (tricuspid) atrioventricular valve regurgitation, and baffle obstruction including systemic and pulmonary venous obstruction. Cardiac MRI, computed tomography, and catheterization have a higher sensitivity to detect baffle obstruction than conventional transthoracic echocardiogram. Baffle leaks could also be present, and angiography is the most sensitive imaging modality of diagnosis [19].

Since sick sinus node syndrome is highly associated with this procedure, cautious selection of antiarrhythmic therapy is recommended. ICD therapy may be considered depending on individual sudden death risk assessment.

6.3.4.2 Arterial Switch Operation (ASO)

Nowadays, the majority of adolescents and young adults presenting to intensive care with a repaired transposition of the great arteries undergo an arterial switch operation. Long-term common complications that might present in these patients are described below:

Coronary Artery Stenosis

Patients who undergo ASO are at risk of coronary complications. Coronary event patterns follow a bimodal distribution. Coronary event-free initial survival was 93%

at 59 months and 88% at 15 years [18]. Single coronary patterns and intramural coronary arteries have the highest mortality. It is unknown at what time patients develop inadequate perfusion; however, myocardial perfusion scans have shown perfusion defects after surgery [20].

Neo-aortic Root Dilation

The anastomosis site and new location of the aorta are associated with either coarctation or dilation. There are multiple surgical factors that could lead to compression during the translocation of the aortic arch. In one study, aortic root dilation is present in more than half of the patients studied [21].

Pulmonary Artery Stenosis

Reintervention secondary to supravalvar pulmonary artery (PA) stenosis is well documented. Up to one-third of patients in some series needed reintervention. Stenosis usually occurs at the level of the main pulmonary artery or at its bifurcation. This complication has been associated with several factors including (1) patch reconstruction of the PA after the coronaries are harvested, (2) the use of a PA banding in staged repairs, and (3) Lecompte maneuver technique. If severe pulmonary stenosis is present, patients may have clinical signs of RV failure [22].

6.3.5 Congenitally Corrected Transposition of the Great Arteries

In the natural history of patients with congenitally corrected transposition of the great arteries (ccTGA), associated lesions are the predictors of outcomes. Usually, patients without any other associated lesion could survive until their fourth or fifth decades [23]. The highest frequency of nonsurgical mortality is described in patients under 5 years with associated lesions (VSD, LVOTO, and tricuspid valve abnormalities). Heart block, tricuspid regurgitation, and heart failure are common complications within these patients.

Some patients with ccTGA will continue to do well beyond age 60; however, this circumstance is probably the exception rather than the rule. Systemic ventricular dysfunction and clinical congestive heart failure are extremely common in middle-aged adults. Ventricular enlargement and early symptoms are a target for aggressive medical treatment, including afterload reduction. The benefits of the prophylactic use of vasodilators are unproven but deserve further studies in an attempt to delay or prevent systemic ventricular dysfunction [24].

6.4 Organ-Specific Considerations

6.4.1 Cardiopulmonary Interactions

Understanding of cardiopulmonary interactions is paramount to the management of patients with ventricular dysfunction [25]. Positive-pressure ventilation (PPV) produces characteristic changes in cardiac performance, including reduced left ventricular afterload, reduced right ventricular preload by hindering venous return, and increased right ventricle afterload secondary to increased pulmonary vascular resistance. These two latter effects are particularly deleterious in patients with cavopulmonary connections (CPC). Passive venous blood return and flow through the lungs, which is characteristic in patients with CPC, is limited by the impact of PPV. Early extubation in these patients facilitates venous return and pulmonary flow, with a consequent improvement in systemic cardiac output. The population of patients with single ventricle physiology with CPC palliative surgery continues to grow. It is highly possible that CPC patients with parenchymal lung disease will have to be mechanically ventilated. In acute respiratory distress syndrome (ARDS) in both children and adults, high mean airway pressures (MAP) might be used to improve oxygenation. High-frequency oscillatory ventilation (HFOV) may be used in ARDS to improve alveolar recruitment and improve oxygenation by applying continuously higher MAP levels [26]. However, HFOV use in Fontan patients has not produced uniform results. Similar incongruous or negative results have been obtained in studies evaluating other strategies such as negative pressure ventilation, hyperventilation-induced respiratory alkalosis, hypoventilation with buffered pH, and adjuvant treatment with inhaled nitric oxide, sildenafil, nesiritide, or milrinone.

Special care must be placed in the avoidance and aggressive management of pleural effusions after surgery and minimization of the risk of phrenic nerve dysfunction.

6.4.2 Kidneys

Cardiorenal syndrome (CRS) is a pathophysiologic state where heart and kidney dysfunctions coexist. Five subtypes of cardiorenal syndrome are typically described as follows: in CRS type 1, an acute worsening of cardiac function results in acute kidney injury (AKI) [27]. Ample literature exists reporting an incidence of AKI up to 53% in adults with acute heart failure [28]. AKI is associated with poor clinical outcomes, prolonged hospital stays, and increased morbidity and mortality. Multiple pathophysiologic mechanisms are involved in the development of postoperative AKI. Low cardiac output syndrome and secondary renal vasoconstriction are well-known risk factors for AKI. Fluid overload and increased filling pressures, resulting in renal congestion and consequently decreased kidney perfusion pressure, are also important pathophysiologic mechanisms [29].

Prevention and early diagnosis of postoperative AKI should improve clinical outcomes. In adults with postoperative AKI, an association between early institution of renal replacement therapies (RRT) and better clinical outcomes has been reported [30]. Recent data suggests that earlier initiation of RRT secondary to AKI in children and neonates undergoing cardiac surgery can be associated with improved survival [31, 32].

6.4.3 Central Nervous System

A recent study performed by our team shows an incidence of acute neurologic events of 8.6% among patients admitted to the CICU. Patients who develop an acute neurologic event have a higher mortality and a higher hospital and CICU length of stay. Literature has shown that survivors of congenital heart disease have neurodevelopmental delays, and much work has been invested to help determine the best way to identify risk factors that could be contributing to these deficits. Current evidence has shown a multifactorial etiology due to intrauterine conditions, genetic abnormalities, severity of cardiac lesion, pre- and postsurgical course, and intraoperative factors. Overall, ICU mortality remains low; however, there is evidence to suggest that with decreasing mortality, there is now an increase in new morbidity among survivors. Neurologic complications have been found to be prevalent in the general intensive care population with brain injury contributing to death in 65% of cases.

6.5 Monitoring

The adult cardiac intensive care unit should be able to manage and provide both noninvasive and invasive monitoring for all the common organ system functions.

6.5.1 Basic Monitoring

A proper clinical examination is a key component of patient monitoring. Our current era, which focused in advances and new technology, has moved our trainees away from the patient bedside. Electronic medical records including vital signs [33], laboratory data, and reports of imaging studies have replaced the physical examination. A close bedside observation of our patients is still key to identify problems and to intervene in a timely fashion. Accompanying the physical examination, monitoring devices are needed to adequately maintain patient stability and to anticipate changes in their status [34].

6.5.1.1 Electrocardiography (ECG)

A three-lead cardiographic monitor connected to a central monitoring system able to store and retrospectively analyze rhythm abnormalities is mandatory. A 12-lead surface ECG accompanied with an atrial ECG should be used if the patient has temporary epicardial pacing. Temporary epicardial atrial wires provide a reliable and rapid method of detecting atrial electrical activity. Atrial ECGs are used to magnify P-waves. Therefore, using an atrial ECG facilitates the diagnosis of atrial dysrhythmias [34].

6.5.1.2 Pulse Oximetry

The pulse oximetry noninvasively measures the percentage of hemoglobin (Hb) saturated with oxygen. Pulse oximetry reads peripheral oxygen saturation (SpO_2), and even though it is not always identical to the desirable measure of arterial oxygen saturation (SaO_2) obtained via arterial blood gas, it correlates well enough to be a reliable method for noninvasively estimating oxygen saturation. The pulse oximeter uses two light-emitting diodes, one red (wavelength of 660 nm) and another infrared (wavelength of 940 nm). Absorption of light at these wavelengths differs based on the total amount of blood loaded with oxygen. Deoxygenated blood absorbs more red light and leaves the infrared light to pass through. The ratio of the red/infrared light measurement is calculated by a processor and then converted to SpO_2 using a table based on the Beer-Lambert law. The oximeter is dependent on a pulsatile flow and produces a graph of the quality of flow. Pulse oximetry detects hypoxia before the patient becomes clinically cyanosed.

Reliability of pulse oximetry at saturations below 80% is reduced. Thirty percent of values were found to be in error by more than 5%. For cyanotic congenital heart disease, therefore, the value of the pulse oximeter is always to be compared with blood gas analysis [35].

6.5.2 Blood Pressure Monitoring

6.5.2.1 Noninvasive Blood Pressure Monitoring

Oscillometry is the most commonly used method. It is based on the principle that pulsatile blood flow through an artery creates oscillations of the arterial wall. Oscillometric devices can noninvasively determine blood pressure and pulse rate. Accuracy of this technique is related to the correct size of the cuff. If the cuff is too narrow, the pressure recorded will be erroneously high and if too wide it may be too low. Noninvasive blood pressure monitoring is inadequate in patients with low cardiac output, hypotension, arrhythmias with beat-to-beat changes in blood pressure, vasoconstriction, and significant edema. Due to these limitations in patients after cardiopulmonary bypass, intravascular arterial blood pressure measurement is mandatory [36].

6.5.2.2 Invasive Blood Pressure Monitoring

Continuous monitoring of systemic arterial blood pressure facilitates identification of fluctuations in arterial pressure and also offers the opportunity for intermittent arterial blood gas analysis. Invasive arterial blood pressure measurement reveals systolic, diastolic, and mean pressure values, and the shape of the pressure curve provides important additional information [36].

6.5.2.3 Central Venous Pressure Monitoring

Central venous catheters (CVC) are used to measure central venous pressure, for administration of vasopressors, inotropes, and fluids, and to monitor venous oxygen saturation (SvO_2).

Analysis of CVP alone is helpful to diagnose right-sided AV valve regurgitation or rhythm abnormalities in the perioperative period. Bimodal normal CVP waveform is associated with normal AV synchrony. The presence of cannon A waves are diagnostic of AV asynchrony. CVP alone has been shown not to be a reliable method for estimation of preload. Transmural pressure is the only value related to preload. Transmural pressure is not commonly measured, and it takes into account variations in intrathoracic pressure caused by mechanical ventilation. Although changes in CVP correlate poorly with preload and changes in CO, they can be used to assess fluid responsiveness or severe cardiac dysfunction and cardiac tamponade [37, 38].

6.5.2.4 Pulmonary Artery Pressure Monitoring

Less commonly used nowadays, a bedside inserted pulmonary artery Swan-Ganz catheter gives the bedside physician the capability of direct intracardiac measurements. Pulmonary artery catheters allow direct, simultaneous measurement of right atrial, right ventricular, pulmonary arterial, and pulmonary capillary wedge pressure. Moreover, pulmonary artery catheters can be used to estimate the cardiac output via thermodilution technique as explained below [39]. It also allows the diagnosis of oximetric fluctuations and the monitoring of mixed venous oxygen saturation.

6.5.2.5 Cardiac Output (CO) Monitoring

Adequate tissue oxygen delivery (DO_2) must be ensured in any intensive care patient. The components of DO_2 include cardiac output, blood hemoglobin concentration, and the degree of oxygen saturation of the hemoglobin molecule [40].

$$DO_2 = \text{Cardiac output} \times 1.34 \times \text{hemoglobin concentration} \times \text{oxygen saturation}$$

There are several methods of CO monitoring based on thermodilution, Fick's principle, Doppler, pulse contour analysis, and bioimpedance. CO monitoring methods are classified as invasive (pulmonary artery thermodilution), minimally invasive (pulse contour analysis or lithium dilution and esophageal Doppler), or noninvasive (thoracic bioimpedance, transthoracic Doppler, and plethysmography).

6.5.3 Invasive Methods for Cardiac Output Monitoring

6.5.3.1 Pulmonary Artery Pressure Monitoring

Less commonly used nowadays due to the associated complications (pneumothorax, arrhythmia, infection, pulmonary artery rupture, etc.), a bedside inserted pulmonary artery Swan-Ganz catheter is still considered the gold standard method to measure and monitor CO using thermodilution technique [39].

All dilution techniques are of limited value in the cardiac patient, because they are not accurate in the presence of intracardiac shunts or significant valvar regurgitation and some forms of mechanical circulatory support.

On the other hand, estimation of CO using the Fick's principle can be used when an intracardiac shunt is present. Using the Fick's principle, cardiac output can be calculated using the following equation:

$$\text{CO} = \text{Systemic oxygen consumption} / \left(\text{systemic arterial } O_2 \text{ saturation} - \text{systemic venous } O_2 \text{ saturation}\right)$$

This technique is limited by the difficulty of measuring oxygen consumption in the intubated and ventilated patient. Indirect assessment of cardiac output can be accomplished by following mixed venous saturation, using a fiber-optic catheter for continuous measurement of venous oxygen saturation placed either in the pulmonary artery or right atrium. In the presence of intracardiac shunts, the saturation in the superior vena cava can be monitored to estimate cardiac output.

A simple reorganization of the Fick equation gives us an easy method to estimate the CO using venous oxygen saturation (SvO_2):

$$SvO_2 = SaO_2 - \left(VO_2 / [CO \times Hb \times C]\right)$$

Central venous oxygen saturation ($ScvO_2$) measured at the right atrium to superior vena cava junction is used as a surrogate of SvO_2. Lower values of $ScvO_2$ have been associated with more complications in patients undergoing cardiothoracic surgery. In patients undergoing elective cardiac surgery, administration of intravenous fluid and inotropic therapy to attain a target SvO_2 of at least 70% in the first 8 h after surgery was associated with fewer complications and a shorter hospital stay.

6.5.4 Minimally Invasive Methods for Cardiac Output Monitoring

6.5.4.1 Pulse Contour Analysis

These so-called minimally invasive techniques are based on the principle that the area under the systolic portion of the arterial pressure waveform is proportional to the stroke volume (SV). These methods also measure SV variation and pulse pressure variation over the respiratory cycle, both useful parameters to predict fluid responsiveness. The PICCO, FloTrac, pressure recording analytic method (PRAM) Most Care system, and the EV100/Volume view system, among others, are commercialized methods using pulse contour analysis.

6.5.4.2 Pulse Power Analysis

Pulse contour analysis is based on the simple principle that changes in blood pressure are directly related to the SV. The LiDCO system combines pulse contour analysis and a lithium indicator dilution for continuous monitoring of SV. The accuracy of this method is grossly affected by cardiac surgery and the presence of shunts [41, 42].

6.5.5 Noninvasive Cardiac Output Monitoring

6.5.5.1 Doppler Methods

This technique uses the Doppler principle and pulse contour analyzing for the estimation of blood flow in the aorta via different techniques.

The transthoracic or transesophageal approach uses echocardiographic views to measure the area of the left ventricular outflow tract (LVOT) and the cross-sectional area (cm^2) of the LVOT to estimate the CO. The area under the curve is in fact a distance, the VTI (velocity time integral). Together, the VTI distance and the cross-sectional area (CSA) describe the cylinder of blood that will be traveling across the aorta with each contraction, thus defining the SV.

$$SV = VTI \times CSA$$

Finally, recording heart rate (HR) and multiplying SV times HR will give the estimation of CO.

Continuous transesophageal Doppler has also been used to continuously monitor CO. A transesophageal probe furnished with a pulsed-wave of continuous-wave Doppler is positioned in the mid-esophagus approximately 30–40 cm from the insertion point at the oral cavity. Using the same principle aforementioned, the VTI and the CSA of the descending aorta are measured. Aortic aneurysms, dissections, and the presence of aortic balloon counterpulsation are common contraindications of this technique [43, 44].

6.5.5.2 Thoracic Bioimpedance

Initially used by astronauts, in this technique, voltage sensing and current transmitting electrodes are placed on the chest, measuring the electrical resistance of the thorax to a high-frequency, low-amplitude current. The utility of this technique in the postoperative cardiac patient is limited due to the presence of the sternal incision and skin edema [45].

6.5.5.3 Impedance Plethysmography

This technique has also been used to measure CO. It is also based on the bioimpedance principle, and the current is passed through electrodes attached to the endotracheal tube. Changes of impedance due to aortic blood flow are detected and measured by the electrodes in the endotracheal tube. This technology is costly and has not yet been validated in humans [46].

6.5.5.4 Near-Infrared Spectroscopy (NIRS)

Determining regional SO_2 (rSO_2) in somatic organs has become a surrogate marker for resuscitation during shock and its resolution. Several groups have correlated cerebral NIRS (cNIRS) readings with important, available hemodynamic parameters. Some have correlated rSO_2 from cNIRS with arterial saturations, mixed venous oxygen saturation ($SmvO_2$) both in adult and pediatric patients, and jugular venous oxygen saturations ($SjvO_2$) with some success [47, 48]. Nevertheless, in a recent prospective observational study including pediatric patients undergoing heart surgery, Bhalala et al. did not find splanchnic and/or renal hypoxemia (as detected by NIRS) as an accurate indicator of low cardiac output after surgery for congenital heart disease [49]. Similarly, Fellahi et al., in a prospective observational study including 50 consecutive adult patients after cardiac surgery, found no correlation between brain and somatic rSO_2 and central venous oxygen saturation ($ScVO_2$) [50].

Conclusions

Managing critically ill ACHD patients in a modern interdisciplinary environment requires the integration of basic clinical evaluation with sophisticated advanced technology in order to successfully identify patient needs and responsiveness to therapy. This approach increases the odds of providing goal-oriented therapy while decreasing risks of complications and causing harm to this very complex patient group.

References

1. Moodie DS, Ritter DG, Tajik AJ, O'Fallon WM. Long-term follow-up in the unoperated univentricular heart. Am J Cardiol. 1984;53(8):1124–8.
2. Ammash NM, Warnes CA. Survival into adulthood of patients with unoperated single ventricle. Am J Cardiol. 1996;77(7):542–4.
3. Kaemmerer H, Mebus S, Schulze-Neick I, Eicken A, Trindade PT, Hager A, Oechslin E, Niwa K, Lang I, Hess J. The adult patient with Eisenmenger syndrome: a medical update after Dana point the adult patient with Eisenmenger syndrome: part I: epidemiology, clinical aspects and diagnostic options. Curr Cardiol Rev. 2010;6:343.
4. Kidd L, Driscoll DJ, Gersony WM, et al. Second natural history study of congenital heart defects. Results of treatment of patients with ventricular septal defects. Circulation. 1993;87(Suppl):138–51.
5. Saha A, Balakrishnan KG, Jaiswal PK, et al. Prognosis for patient with Eisenmenger syndrome of various aetiology. Int J Cardiol. 1994;45(3):199–207.
6. Galiè N, Beghetti M, Gatzoulis MA, Granton J, Berger RMF, Lauer A, Chiossi E, Landzberg M. Bosentan therapy in patients with Eisenmenger syndrome. Circulation. 2006;114:48–54.
7. Adriaenssens T, Delcroix M, Van Deyk K, Budts W. Advanced therapy may delay the need for transplantation in patients with the Eisenmenger syndrome. Eur Heart J. 2006;27(12):1472–7.
8. Braverman AC, Güven H, Beardslee MA, Makan M, Kates AM, Moon MR. The bicuspid aortic valve. Curr Probl Cardiol. 2005;30(9):470–522.
9. Niaz T, Poterucha JT, Johnson JN, Craviari C, Nienaber T, Palfreeman J, Cetta F, Hagler DJ. Incidence, morphology, and progression of bicuspid aortic valve in pediatric and young adult subjects with coexisting congenital heart defects. Congenit Heart Dis. 2017;12(3):261–9. https://doi.org/10.1111/chd.12429.
10. Vonder Muhll IF, Sehgal T, Ian Paterson D. The adult with repaired coarctation: need for lifelong surveillance. Can J Cardiol. 2016;32:1038.e11.
11. Torok RD, Campbell MJ, Fleming GA, Hill KD. Coarctation of the aorta: management from infancy to adulthood. World J Cardiol. 2015;7(11):765–75.
12. Roifman I, Therrien J, Ionescu-Ittu R, Pilote L, Guo L, Kotowycz MA, Martucci G, Marelli AJ. Coarctation of the aorta and coronary artery disease fact or fiction? Circulation. 2012;126:16–21.
13. Cuypers JAAE, Menting ME, Konings EEM, Opić P, Utens EMWJ, Helbing WA, Witsenburg M, van den Bosch AE, Ouhlous M, van Domburg RT, Rizopoulos D, Meijboom FJ, Boersma E, Bogers AJJC, Roos-Hesselink JW. Unnatural history of tetralogy of Fallot prospective follow-up of 40 years after surgical correction. Circulation. 2014;130:1944–53.
14. Dennis M, Moore B, Kotchetkova I, Pressley L, Cordina R, Celermajer DS. Adults with repaired tetralogy: low mortality but high morbidity up to middle age. Open Heart. 2017;4:e000564.
15. Knauth AL, Gauvreau K, Powell AJ, Landzberg MJ, Walsh EP, Lock JE, del Nido PJ, Geva T. Ventricular size and function assessed by cardiac MRI predict major adverse clinical outcomes late after tetralogy of Fallot repair. Heart. 2008;94:211–6. https://doi.org/10.1136/hrt.2006.104745.

16. Dobbels B, Herregods M-C, Troosta E, Van De Bruaene A, Rega F, Budts W, De Meester P. Early versus late pulmonary valve replacement in patients with transannular patch-repaired tetralogy of Fallot. Interact Cardiovasc Thorac Surg. 2017;25:427–33.
17. Haeffele C, Lui GK. Dextro-transposition of the great arteries long-term sequelae of atrial and arterial switch. Cardiol Clin. 2015;33:543–58.
18. Sarkar D, Bull C, Yates R, Wright D, Cullen S, Gewillig M, Clayton R, Tunstill A, Deanfield J. Comparison of long-term outcomes of atrial repair of simple transposition with implications for a late arterial switch strategy. Circulation. 1999;100(Suppl II):II-176–81.
19. Kammeraad JAE, van Deurzen CHM, Sreeram N, Bink-Boelkens MTE, Ottenkamp J, Helbing WA, Lam J, Sobotka-Plojhar MA, Balaji ODS. Predictors of sudden cardiac death after mustard or Senning repair for transposition of the great arteries. J Am Coll Cardiol. 2004;44:1095–102.
20. Lui GK, Fernandes S, McElhinney DB. Management of cardiovascular risk factors in adults with congenital heart disease. J Am Heart Assoc. 2014;3:e001076.
21. Schwartz ML, Gauvreau K, del Nido P, Mayer JE, Colan SD. Long-term predictors of aortic root dilation and aortic regurgitation after arterial switch operation. Circulation. 2004;110(Suppl II):II-128–32.
22. Safi LM, Bhatt AB. Update on the management of adults with arterial switch procedure for transposition of the great arteries. Curr Treat Options Cardiovasc Med. 2017;19:4.
23. Flack EC, Kaushik N, Graham TP. Congenitally corrected transposition of the great arteries (Chapter 7). In: Vijayalakshmi IB, Syamasundar Rao P, Chugh R, editors. A comprehensive approach to congenital heart disease. 1st ed. New Delhi: Jaypee Brothers Medical Publishers; 2013. isbn:978-93-5090-267-7.
24. Graham TP Jr, Bernard YD, Mellen BG, Celermajer D, Baumgartner H, Cetta F, Connolly HM, Davidson WR, Dellborg M, Foster E, Gersony WM, Gessner IH, Hurwitz RA, Kaemmerer H, Kugler JD, Murphy DJ, Noonan JA, Morris C, Perloff JK, Sanders SP, Sutherland JL. Long-term outcome in congenitally corrected transposition of the great arteries: a multi-institutional study. J Am Coll Cardiol. 2000;36(1):255–61.
25. Monnet X, Teboul JL, Richard C. Cardiopulmonary interactions in patients with heart failure. Curr Opin Crit Care. 2007;13(1):6–11.
26. Bojan M, Gioanni S, Mauriat P, Pouard P. High-frequency oscillatory ventilation and short-term outcome in neonates and infants undergoing cardiac surgery: a propensity score analysis. Crit Care. 2011;15(5):R259.
27. Valika AA, Costanzo MR. The acute cardiorenal syndrome type I: considerations on physiology, epidemiology, and therapy. Curr Heart Fail Rep. 2014;11(4):382–92.
28. Pickering JW, James MT, Palmer SC. Acute kidney injury and prognosis after cardiopulmonary bypass: a meta-analysis of cohort studies. Am J Kidney Dis Off J Natl Kidney Found. 2015;65(2):283–93.
29. Mariscalco G, Lorusso R, Dominici C, Renzulli A, Sala A. Acute kidney injury: a relevant complication after cardiac surgery. Ann Thorac Surg. 2011;92(4):1539–47.
30. De Vecchis R, Esposito C, Ariano C. Efficacy and safety assessment of isolated ultrafiltration compared to intravenous diuretics for acutely decompensated heart failure: a systematic review with meta-analysis. Minerva Cardioangiol. 2014;62(2):131–46.
31. Bojan M, Gioanni S, Vouhé PR, Journois D, Pouard P. Early initiation of peritoneal dialysis in neonates and infants with acute kidney injury following cardiac surgery is associated with a significant decrease in mortality. Kidney Int. 2012;82(4):474–81.
32. Ronco C, Ricci Z, Goldstein SL. (R)evolution in the management of acute kidney injury in newborns. Am J Kidney Dis Off J Natl Kidney Found. 2015;66(2):206–11.
33. May L, Longhurst CA, Pageler NM, Wood MS, Sharek PJ, Zebrack CM. Optimizing care of adults with congenital heart disease in a pediatric cardiovascular ICU using electronic clinical decision support. Pediatr Crit Care Med. 2014;15(5):428–34.
34. Huygh J, Peeters Y, Bernards J, Malbrain MLNG. REVIEW. Hemodynamic monitoring in the critically ill: an overview of current cardiac output monitoring methods. F1000Research. 2855;5(F1000 Faculty Rev):2016.

35. Poets CF, Southall DP. Noninvasive monitoring of oxygenation in infants and children: practical considerations and areas of concern. Pediatrics. 1994;93(5):737–46.
36. Tavernier B, Makhotine O, Lebuffe G, Dupont J, Scherpereel P. Systolic pressure variation as a guide to fluid therapy in patients with sepsis-induced hypotension. Anesthesiology. 1998;89(6):1313–21.
37. Rivers E, Nguyen B, Havstad S, et al. Early goal-directed therapy in the treatment of severe sepsis and septic shock. N Engl J Med. 2001;345(19):1368–77.
38. Kern JW, Shoemaker WC. Meta-analysis of hemodynamic optimization in high-risk patients. Crit Care Med. 2002;30(8):1686–92.
39. Swan HJ, Ganz W, Forrester J, et al. Catheterization of the heart in man with use of a flow-directed balloon-tipped catheter. N Engl J Med. 1970;283(9):447–51.
40. Vermeij CG, Feenstra BW, Adrichem WJ, Bruining HA. Independent oxygen uptake and oxygen delivery in septic and postoperative patients. Chest. 1991;99(6):1438.
41. Marik PE, Cavallazzi R, Vasu T, Hirani A. Dynamic changes in arterial waveform derived variables and fluid responsiveness in mechanically ventilated patients: a systematic review of the literature. Crit Care Med. 2009;37(9):2642–7.
42. Boyle M, Lawrence J, Belessis A, Murgo M, Shehabi Y. Comparison of dynamic measurements of pulse contour with pulsed heat continuous cardiac output in postoperative cardiac surgical patients. Aust Crit Care. 2007;20(1):27–32.
43. Dark PM, Singer M. The validity of trans-esophageal Doppler ultrasonography as a measure of cardiac output in critically ill adults. Intensive Care Med. 2004;30(11):2060–6.
44. Manasia AR, Nagaraj HM, Kodali RB, et al. Feasibility and potential clinical utility of goal-directed transthoracic echocardiography performed by noncardiologist intensivists using a small hand-carried device (SonoHeart) in critically ill patients. J Cardiothorac Vasc Anesth. 2005;19(2):155–9.
45. Shoemaker WC, Beizberg H, Wo CC, et al. Multicenter study of noninvasive monitoring systems as alternatives to invasive monitoring of acutely ill emergency patients. Chest. 1998;114(6):1643–52.
46. Porter JM, Swain ID. Measurement of cardiac output by electrical impedance plethysmograph. J Biomed Eng. 1987;9(3):222–31.
47. Gomez H, Torres A, Polanco P, et al. Use of non-invasive NIRS during a vascular occlusion test to assess dynamic tissue O_2 saturation response. Intensive Care Med. 2008;34(9):1600–7.
48. Santora RJ, Moore FA. Monitoring trauma and intensive care unit resuscitation with tissue hemoglobin oxygen saturation. Crit Care. 2009;13(Suppl 5):S10.
49. Bhalala US, Nishisaki A, McQueen D, Bird GL, Morrison WE, Nadkarni VM, Nathan M, Starr JP. Change in regional (somatic) near-infrared spectroscopy is not a useful indicator of clinically detectable low cardiac output in children after surgery for congenital heart defects. Pediatr Crit Care Med. 2012;13(5):529–34.
50. Monthé-Sagan K, Fischer MO, Saplacan V, Gerard JL, Hanouz JL, Fellahi JL. Near-infrared spectroscopy to assess microvascular dysfunction: a prospective pilot study in cardiac surgery patients. J Crit Care. 2016;31(1):264–8.

Cardiovascular Anesthesia for Adults with Congenital Heart Disease

7

Mark Twite, Richard Ing, and Lawrence Schwartz

7.1 Introduction

Congenital heart disease (CHD) affects 1% of live births, with a stable prevalence over time [1]. There is a large variety of congenital heart defects, ranging from simple to severe (Table 7.1). With significant medical and surgical advances over the past decades, most affected patients are now expected to survive to adulthood [2]. The number of adults with congenital heart disease (ACHD) now surpasses the number of children with CHD. The most recent estimates are that 2.4 million people (1.4 million adults, 1 million children) were living with CHD in the United States in 2010. Around 300,000 of these individuals had severe CHD [3]. The median age of patients with severe CHD has increased from 11 years in 1985 to 25 years in 2010. More than a third of ACHD patients are at least 45 years old [4]. The quality of life in adults with CHD is reported as generally good, and the care of ACHD patients is a rapidly growing field [5]. The growing population of adults with CHD means that the anesthesiologist providing anesthesia for non-cardiac surgery will provide perioperative care for adults who may have previously undergone surgery for even complex CHD.

In the developed world, children with CHD are either repaired, palliated, or undergo heart transplantation. Adults presenting with CHD are usually childhood survivors but occasionally may have a new diagnosis of CHD made. As surgical techniques have improved over time, there is a generational effect of adults with palliated heart defects. For example, the approach to transposition of the great arteries (TGA) was very different 40 years ago with intracardiac baffles to redirect blood

M. Twite (✉) · R. Ing · L. Schwartz
Department of Anesthesiology, Children's Hospital Colorado, University of Colorado Denver, Anschutz Medical Campus, Aurora, CO, USA
e-mail: Mark.Twite@childrenscolorado.org; Richard.ing@childrenscolorado.org; Lawrence.schwartz@childrenscolorado.org

E. da Cruz et al. (eds.), *Intensive Care of the Adult with Congenital Heart Disease*, Congenital Heart Disease in Adolescents and Adults,
https://doi.org/10.1007/978-3-319-94171-4_7

Table 7.1 Classification of CHD

Simple	Moderate	Severe
Long-term survival 95%	Long-term survival 90%	Long-term survival 80%
Atrial septal defect	Anomalous pulmonary venous drainage	Single ventricle palliation
Ventricular septal defect	Atrioventricular canal defect	Transposition of the great arteries
Patent ductus arteriosus	Coarctation of the aorta	Truncus arteriosus
	Tetralogy of Fallot	Tricuspid atresia
		Pulmonary atresia
		Eisenmenger syndrome

Simple defects have a favorable natural history unless they are unrepaired with a significant left-to-right shunt, which may then develop Eisenmenger syndrome
Long-term survival is >20 years

flow, originally described by Mustard and Senning, compared to the arterial switch procedure which is the surgical repair of choice today. Anesthetic management of CHD varies as much as the variety of heart defects. The anesthesiologist caring for adults with CHD must understand the anatomy and pathophysiology of the original heart defect and how it was repaired or palliated [6–9]. The effects of anesthetic drugs in congenital heart disease should also be fully appreciated (Table 7.2) [10].

ACHD is a risk factor for adverse outcomes at the time of cardiac and non-cardiac surgery [11]. In a study using the national anesthesia closed claims database, the most common factors contributing to the adverse event in cardiac cases were surgical technique and intraoperative anesthetic care, whereas in non-cardiac cases, postoperative monitoring and care, the type of congenital heart defect, and nature of the preoperative assessment were most common. Non-cardiac cases frequently involved orthopedic surgery and occurred in outpatient surgery centers [12]. Current consensus guidelines recommend that all surgical procedures that require general anesthesia in adults with moderate or complex CHD should be performed in a regional center with an anesthesiologist familiar with ACHD [13, 14]. However, many anesthesia providers report low levels of knowledge about CHD and are uncomfortable when asked to care for ACHD patients presenting for non-cardiac surgery [15]. The lack of specialized centers and providers familiar with CHD is known to be a serious problem in the delivery of care to ACHD patients [16].

One approach for the anesthesiologist providing perioperative care for an ACHD patient is to take a logical stepwise approach (Fig. 7.1). First consider the atria, ventricles, and great arteries and the various valvar connections. Specifically, consider valve stenosis or regurgitation. Second, consider the sequelae of CHD, specifically arrhythmias, cyanosis, thromboembolism, pulmonary hypertension, and heart failure. Finally, consider lesion-specific problems, especially with palliated single ventricle anatomy, transposition of the great arteries, and tetralogy of Fallot and any special situations such as pregnancy, laparoscopic surgery, or regional and neuraxial anesthesia. Endocarditis prophylaxis with an appropriate choice of antibiotics must also be considered. Some of these sequelae and specific conditions are reviewed in this chapter.

Table 7.2 Hemodynamic effects of anesthetic drugs

	Contractility	MAP	SVR	PAP	PVR	HR
Isoflurane	→	↓	↓↓	↓	↓	↑
Sevoflurane	↓	↓	↓	↓	↓	↑
Desflurane	→	↓	↓	↓	↓	↑
Propofol	↓	↓↓	↓↓	↓	↓	↓
Ketamine	→[a]	→	↑	↑→	↑→	↑
Etomidate	→	→	→	↑	↑	→
Dexmedetomidine	→	↑[b]	↑	→	→	↓↓
Opioids	→	→	→	→	→	↓
Benzodiazepines	→	→	→	→	→	→

MAP mean arterial pressure, *SVR* systemic vascular resistance, *PAP* pulmonary artery pressure, *PVR* pulmonary vascular resistance, *HR* heart rate, ↓ decrease, ↑ increase, → no significant change
[a]Ketamine can depress contractility in vitro and in catecholamine-depleted patients
[b]Dexmedetomidine can increase MAP during loading dose administration

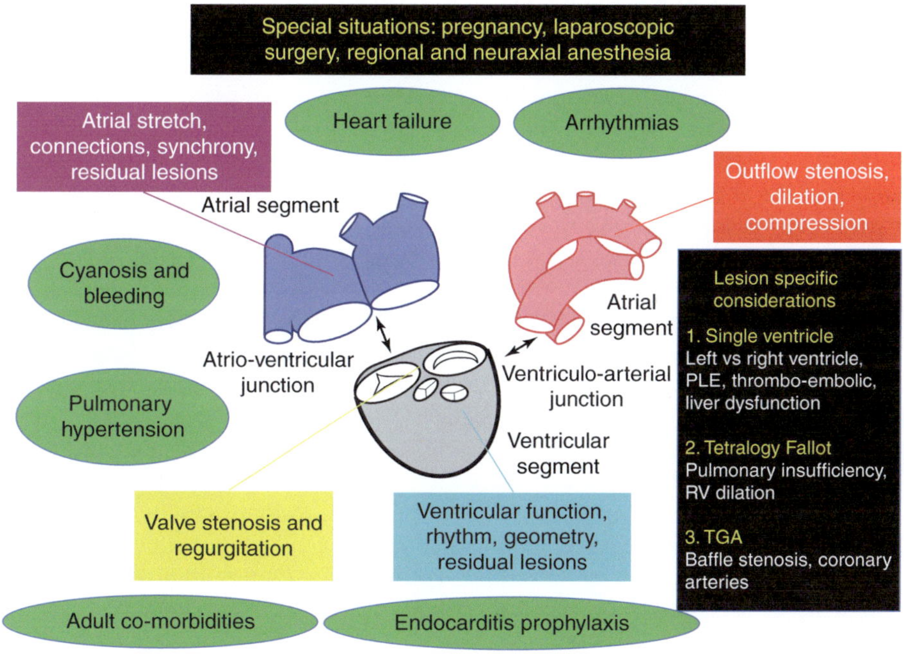

Fig. 7.1 An approach to congenital heart disease for the anesthesiologist

7.2 Sequelae of Congenital Heart Disease

7.2.1 Arrhythmias and Pacemakers

As patients with congenital heart disease live longer, their risk of developing abnormal cardiac dysrhythmia increases. There are a number of pathophysiologic factors that lead to arrhythmias in adult CHD patients. Preoperative factors include abnormal sinus and atrioventricular node positioning, atrial distention, cardiac valve regurgitation, cyanosis, hypoxemia, acidosis, ventricular hypertrophy or dilation, and abnormal coronary arteries. Postoperative factors include sinus and AV node dysfunction, atrial and ventricular scarring, and valvar abnormalities. Additionally, medications, electrolyte disturbances, systemic illness, and inflammation can also contribute to arrhythmias [17].

Arrhythmias associated with ACHD cover the full spectrum of abnormal rate and rhythm; bradyarrhythmias, atrial tachycardia, and ventricular dysrhythmia. While a history of simple CHD can lead to cardiac conduction abnormalities, patients with complex CHD, such as single ventricle, transposition of the great arteries, and tetralogy of Fallot, are at the highest risk of developing arrhythmias. The prevalence of different types of arrhythmias in the ACHD population is illustrated in Table 7.3. About 50% of 20-year-old patients with CHD will develop atrial tachyarrhythmia [18]. In a large database study of over 109,000 ACHD patients admitted to hospital, 25% had a history of arrhythmia. The most common arrhythmia was atrial fibrillation (85.7%), followed by atrial flutter (19.5%), and then paroxysmal ventricular tachycardia (5.4%). Aside from disease complexity, increasing age, heart failure, obstructive sleep apnea, and history of an atrial septal defect may also be independent risk factors for arrhythmia [19].

Next to heart failure, sudden cardiac death (SCD) is a leading cause of death among adults with congenital heart disease. Approximately 19–26% of late mortality in ACHD is due to SCD [20]. Ventricular arrhythmia is the leading cause of SCD in ACHD, with an overall risk that is 100-fold higher that in age-matched controls [21]. Complex CHD patients are most at risk for SCD. Patients with tetralogy of Fallot, TGA following atrial baffle surgery, and univentricular hearts with Fontan physiology are particularly at risk for SCD due to arrhythmia [22]. Prolonged QRS duration, progression of QRS duration, and progression of ventricular dysfunction can serve to identify those patients at increased risk of SCD [23].

With the increased likelihood of having a cardiac rhythm disturbance, adult patients with CHD often require ablation therapy in the catheterization suite, including prior to surgery. However, because of abnormal anatomy, shunts, scar tissue, and difficult vascular access, ablation of abnormal conduction pathways may be technically challenging or unsuccessful. Patients may require drug therapy with anti-arrhythmic agents. These medications may also be problematic for the anesthesiologist caring for ACHD. First, the arrhythmias may be refractory to therapy. Therefore, maintaining a physiologic milieu of homeostasis is imperative. Appropriate management of electrolytes, acid-base status, oxygenation, ventilation, and thermoregulation are important to minimize the risk of intraoperative arrhythmia. Second, many anti-arrhythmic agents will have adverse effect that can impact perioperative care. Some of the more common agents used to control dysrhythmias are listed in Table 7.4.

ACHD patients frequently require implantation of a pacemaker and/or internal cardioverter/defibrillator (ICD). The indications for permanent pacemaker and ICD placement have recently been published in a detailed consensus statement developed by the Pediatric and Congenital Electrophysiology Society in partnership with

Table 7.3 Risk estimates for arrhythmias and complexity of CHD

Complexity of CHD	Type of CHD	Prevalence (In CHD population)	Atrial arrhythmia			Ventricular arrhythmia	Other pacing needs		
			AT	AF	Other		SND	AV block	Dyssynchrony, heart failure
Simple	Patent ductus arteriosus	6–8%							
	Pulmonary stenosis	6–8%							
	Ventricular septal defect	30–32%							
	Secundum atrial septal defect	8–10%							
Moderate	Aortic coarctation	5–7%							
	Anomalous pulmonary venous return	0.5–2.5%							
	Atrioventricular septal defect	3–5%							
	Aortic stenosis	3–5%							
	Ebstein anomaly	0.5–1.5%							
	Tetralogy of Fallot	8–10%							
	Primum atrial septal defect	2–3%							
Severe	Truncus arteriosus	1.5–2%							
	Pulmonary atresia	2–2.5%							
	Double outlet right ventricle	1.5–2%							
	d-transposition of the great arteries	6–7%							
	l-transposition of the great arteries	1–2%							
	Hypoplastic left heart syndrome	3–4%							
	Other (heterotaxy, other single ventricles)	7–10%							

Approximate risk estimates for atrial tachycardia (AT), atrial fibrillation (AF), other supraventricular arrhythmias, ventricular arrhythmia, sinus node dysfunction (SND), atrioventricular (AV) block, and ventricular dyssynchrony are shown across various congenital heart defects (CHD) of simple, moderate, and severe complexity. The color-coded pattern ranges from minimal (no shading) to mild (light blue), moderate (medium blue), and high (dark blue) risk. Used with permission from the Heart Rhythm Society (2014;11(10):e102–65)

Table 7.4 Common anti-arrhythmic medications

	Class 1	Class 2	Class 3	Class 4
Mechanism of action	Sodium channel blockade	Beta-adrenergic receptor blockade	Potassium channel blockade	Calcium channel blockade
Examples	Procainamide Flecainide Propafenone	Atenolol Nadolol Propranolol Metoprolol Carvedilol	Amiodarone Sotalol	Verapamil Diltiazem
Practical uses	AF, SVT, VT	Rate control Nodal-dependent reentrant tachycardias VT Long QT syndrome	VT, SVT, AF	VT, SVT Nodal-dependent tachycardias
Adverse reaction	QTc prolongation QRS prolongation GI symptoms Proarrhythmia	Hypotension Bradycardia CHF exacerbation Bronchospasm Fatigue	Thyroid Lung toxicity Hepatotoxicity Prolong QTc Bradycardia	Hemodynamic depression

Adapted from Cecchin [103]

the Heart Rhythm Society [20]. Complex congenital heart lesions are most commonly associated with the need for a pacemaker and include repaired tetralogy of Fallot, transposition of the great arteries, single ventricle lesions post-Fontan completion, congenital conduction disorders, and surgeries involving the interventricular septum [24]. Patients with implanted cardiac devices present for a myriad of surgical interventions. Prior to induction, the preoperative evaluation should include gathering information on the type and manufacturer of the device, the functional capability, and the patient's dependency on the device [25]. Once the procedure has begun, electromagnetic interference (EMI) with radiofrequency waves of 50–60 Hz can disrupt the function of the pacemaker/ICD. Sources of EMI include electrocautery, therapeutic radiation, transthoracic defibrillation, radiofrequency ablation, shock wave lithotripsy, MRI, nerve stimulators, muscle fasciculation, shivering, and large tidal volume ventilation [26]. Implanted cardiac devices which are affected by EMI may cause inappropriate triggering or over pacing, inhibition of pacemaker triggering, asynchronous pacing, an inappropriate shock from an ICD, electrical discharge to the myocardium, and arrhythmias and patient burns. While technological advances, such as bipolar leads, insulation, and noise protection programming, have made modern devices less susceptible to EMI, adverse events have not been eliminated. Using bipolar diathermy can reduce the risk of patient injury further. The cutting mode creates less EMI than coagulation. It is advisable to use short, intermittent, irregular bursts of diathermy. The diathermy pad should be grounded, with excellent skin contact, and maximize the distance from the implanted device. It is always recommended that electrical current should not cross the implanted device. The American Society of Anesthesiologists recommends that if there is significant risk of EMI in a pacer-dependent patient, the device should be reprogrammed to asynchronous pacing. ICDs should be turned off, and external-defibrillating pads placed on the patient. Standard monitors should be used. Alternative means of temporary pacing should also be readily available [25].

Magnets are made primarily for device interrogation, not for emergency use. However, placing a magnet over a pacemaker will switch the mode to asynchronous pacing. The manufacturer of the device determines the default rate, which may not be high enough to provide appropriate cardiac output for a given patient. The magnet may also decrease the function of the pacemaker with a waning battery life. When applied to an ICD, the magnet will turn off the anti-tachycardia function and will not alter the pacemaker settings [24]. Best anesthesia practice is to have the pacemaker interrogated prior to surgery with the necessary adjustments made in consultation with a cardiologist.

The three most common causes of pacemaker failure are lead failure, generator failure, and a failure to capture. Preoperative interrogation should detect the first two causes. While commonly used anesthetic drugs are not believed to directly affect pacemaker function, the sequelae of undergoing general anesthesia for surgery can do so. Hyperkalemia, acidosis, alkalosis, hypothermia, hyperglycemia, hypovolemia, bleeding and transfusions, hypoxemia, and myocardial ischemia can all affect lead thresholds and cause failure of the pacemaker to capture [26]. Reprogramming a device preoperatively does not guarantee protection from damage during the procedure. The implanted cardiac device must be re-interrogated and programmed as necessary in the immediate postoperative period. Patients should receive appropriate observation and monitoring to assure proper device function.

7.2.2 Cyanosis, Thrombosis, and Embolism

With the improvements in surgical and medical therapy, patients born with cyanotic congenital heart disease are generally acyanotic in adulthood. Still, patients with long-standing left-to-right shunts develop pulmonary hypertension and reversal of the shunt, resulting in Eisenmenger's syndrome and chronic hypoxemia. Additionally, there are many patients with residual right-to-left intracardiac and intrapulmonary shunts who have long-term cyanosis. Fontan patients represent a unique group who may also live with chronic hypoxemia. Chronic cyanosis is a multi-organ system disease with the pathophysiology occurring mainly via two mechanisms: hyperviscosity and dysfunction of the endothelium. The primary response of the body to chronic hypoxemia is to increase erythropoietin production from the kidneys, which results in an increase in the production of red blood cells in the bone marrow. This is an attempt to maintain oxygen delivery in the face of low hemoglobin oxygen saturation. Blood viscosity rises, and flow through the microcirculation becomes impaired. When hematocrit levels exceed 65%, the high blood viscosity may actually decrease oxygen delivery to the tissues. The management of hyperviscosity in adults with cyanotic congenital heart disease is controversial. Limited data suggests that phlebotomy may be beneficial to reduce the symptoms of hyperviscosity such as headache, dizziness, and fatigue [27]. However, the resulting iron deficiency from excess blood removal results in microcytic erythrocytes that are less deformable for passage through the microcirculation and may further increase the risk for veno-occlusive events. There is some evidence that phlebotomy with iron supplementation may attenuate the hypocoagulable state of cyanotic CHD patients and decrease the risk of bleeding [28]. On the contrary, dehydration can both increase hematocrit and hyperviscosity and exacerbate bleeding and thromboembolic events. Therefore, prolonged fasting should be avoided in patients with cyanotic CHD. These patients should be encouraged to continue with oral clear liquids up until 2 h prior to surgery.

Patients with chronic cyanosis and associated elevated hematocrit develop hypocoagulation and increased risk of bleeding. This increased bleeding tendency is attributed to various hemostatic defects including thrombocytopenia, shortened platelet lifetime, suppressed platelet aggregation due to platelets which have already been activated as well as platelet microparticles, and deficiency of clotting factors such as von Willebrand factor [29, 30].

Chronic cyanosis and hyperviscosity are associated with injury to the vascular endothelium. Altered shear forces and changes in nitric oxide and prostacyclin release may modify the balance between vasodilators and vasoconstrictors and affect systemic endothelial function. Dysfunction of the endothelium may play an important role in the pathogenesis of hemostatic disorders and thrombotic events, as well as conditions such as hypertension and cardiac failure [31, 32].

Arrhythmia and chronic cyanosis place adults with congenital heart disease at risk of thromboembolism. Thromboses can occur in the peripheral, pulmonary, and cerebral circulation. Intracardiac thrombosis can embolize to vital organs causing ischemic injury. Intracardiac shunts further increase the risk of embolic events from the right side of the heart to the systemic circulation. The complexity of congenital heart disease has been shown to be independently associated with thromboembolic events [33]. In order to reduce the risk of these complications, many adults with congenital heart disease receive thromboprophylaxis therapy. Guidelines for thromboprophylaxis are widely published, including recommendations for ACHD [20, 34]. This means many ACHD patients will present to surgery with a history of taking anticoagulation medications including warfarin and newer oral anticoagulant drugs (NOACs). Table 7.5 lists some of the more commonly used agents. The crux of the perioperative management of these drugs relates to balancing thromboembolic risk with bleeding risk. The decision to continue, hold, or use a bridging agent, such as heparin, should be made after multidisciplinary discussion weighing the relative risks of bleeding versus thrombosis and tailored to each individual patient.

7.2.3 Pulmonary Hypertension

The growing ACHD population often presents complex and unique medical problems. Pulmonary hypertension (PH) is a well-recognized complication limiting the survival and functional capacity of patients with surgically unrepaired, palliated,

Table 7.5 Anticoagulant medications

	Warfarin	Dabigatran	Rivaroxaban	Apixaban
Mechanism of action	Vitamin K epoxide reductase inhibitor	Direct thrombin inhibitor	Factor Xa inhibitor	Factor Xa inhibitor
Plasma protein binding (%)	100	35	95	40–60
Renal excretion (%)	Liver metabolized Renal excretion, 92	80	35	25
Major drug interactions	Amiodarone, mexiletine, propafenone, and verapamil Antifungals NSAIDs, ASA	Rifampin Quinidine Anticoagulants	Antivirals Antifungals Anticoagulants	Antivirals Antifungals Anticoagulants
Adverse effects	Bleeding Rare skin necrosis	Dyspepsia Bleeding (GI)	Bleeding	Bleeding

and in some cases repaired CHD. Unique patient cohorts include those with Down syndrome and those with single ventricles palliated with total cavopulmonary anastomoses [35]. The prevalence of PH varies in different CHD populations, with estimates from 5% to 10% [36]. In ACHD, the additional diagnosis of PH increases the mortality twofold and morbidity complications, including heart failure and arrhythmia, threefold compared to ACHD without PH. Moreover, adults with CHD and PH have an increased utilization of inpatient and outpatient services, especially cardiac catheterization and intensive care unit hospitalizations [37].

Pulmonary hypertension is defined as elevated pulmonary artery pressure (PAP), with a mean PAP >25 mmHg. Appropriate diagnosis and management of PH associated with CHD (PH-CHD) depends on identifying the cause of elevated PAP: high pulmonary venous pressure, high pulmonary vascular resistance, high pulmonary flow, or some combination of these factors. Classification schemes in PH represent clinical perspectives of underlying pathophysiology. It is most helpful to consider the pulmonary vascular resistance (PVR) equation:

$$\text{PVR} = (\text{meanPAP} - \text{PAOP}) / \text{Qp}$$

Pulmonary artery occlusion pressure (PAOP) approximates pulmonary venous pressure, and Qp is pulmonary blood flow. Rearranging this equation:

$$\text{MeanPAP} = (\text{PVR} \times \text{Qp}) + \text{PAOP}$$

Elevated PAP, therefore, can result from an increase in PVR, Qp, or PAOP. An increase in PAOP is due to elevated left-sided filling pressures and may be due to obstruction to left heart inflow (pulmonary vein stenosis, cor triatriatum, mitral stenosis) or obstruction to outflow (aortic stenosis). An increase in Qp is often due to left-to-right shunts, which if left untreated may result in severe PH with PAP at a systemic BP level, attributable to high PVR (>10 Wood units) and consequently reversed or bidirectional shunt, so-called Eisenmenger syndrome [38].

Appropriate therapy for PH-CHD varies by underlying lesion, degree of pulmonary vascular remodeling, and associated pathophysiology. Medical therapies are continually evolving and mainly target remodeling of the pulmonary vascular bed. Atrial septostomy performed in the cardiac catheterization laboratory should be considered in the patient with worsening PH despite optimal medical therapy. The resulting improvement in cardiac output with decompression of the right heart is at the expense of hypoxemia. Features of a high-risk patient for this procedure include high right atrial pressure and low cardiac output, both of which increase mortality (5–15%) [39]. Atrial septostomy may be considered as an initial procedure or as a bridge to lung transplantation. An alternative procedure is the creation of a palliative Potts' Shunt (descending aorta to left pulmonary artery). This may be performed surgically or in the cardiac catheterization laboratory [40]. The optimal timing of these procedures is difficult to determine. End-stage options for worsening PH unresponsive to therapy are lung or heart-lung transplantation.

It is common for adults with CHD and PH to need anesthesia for procedures. The most important aspects of anesthetic management are thoughtful preparation regarding the choice of anesthetic drugs, airway management, avoidance of triggering stimuli, prophylactic pulmonary vasodilators, and appropriate monitoring. The ideal anesthetic drug for patients with PH would have pulmonary vasodilating effects, would not depress cardiac contractility, would maintain systemic vascular resistance and cardiac output, and would be short lasting and easy to titrate. Such an anesthetic agent, unfortunately, does not exist. Most anesthetics are associated with undesirable hemodynamic effects—depending on dosage and speed of administration—by altering heart rate or rhythm, cardiac contractility, SVR, or PVR. To minimize the undesired hemodynamic effects of a full anesthetic dose of a single anesthetic drug, it is preferable to utilize a balanced anesthetic technique. Balanced administration of sub-anesthetic doses of several anesthetics can achieve an adequate depth of anesthesia without the marked hemodynamic changes that can be associated with a high dose of a single drug. The cardiovascular effects of anesthetic drugs are summarized in Table 7.2. Of note, fentanyl does not affect PVR [41]. Ketamine despite earlier concerns can be used and carefully titrated [42, 43]. Dexmedetomidine has been used effectively in PH and has not been shown to increase PVR [44].

Cardiac arrest in patients with PH is often immediately preceded by an acute pulmonary hypertensive crisis, in which an acute increase in PVR leads to right ventricular failure, myocardial ischemia, and a decrease in cardiac output. The right ventricle dilates and encroaches on the left ventricle, thus decreasing left ventricular stroke volume, cardiac output, and mean systemic arterial pressure (MAP). Systemic hypotension then causes a decrease in coronary perfusion pressure, which exacerbates right ventricular failure and causes biventricular ischemia. Monitors will demonstrate an increase in PAP accompanied by decreases in SpO_2 and systemic blood pressure due to inadequate pulmonary blood flow and left heart filling. The self-perpetuating cycle of biventricular failure associated with a pulmonary hypertensive crisis is illustrated in Fig. 7.2.

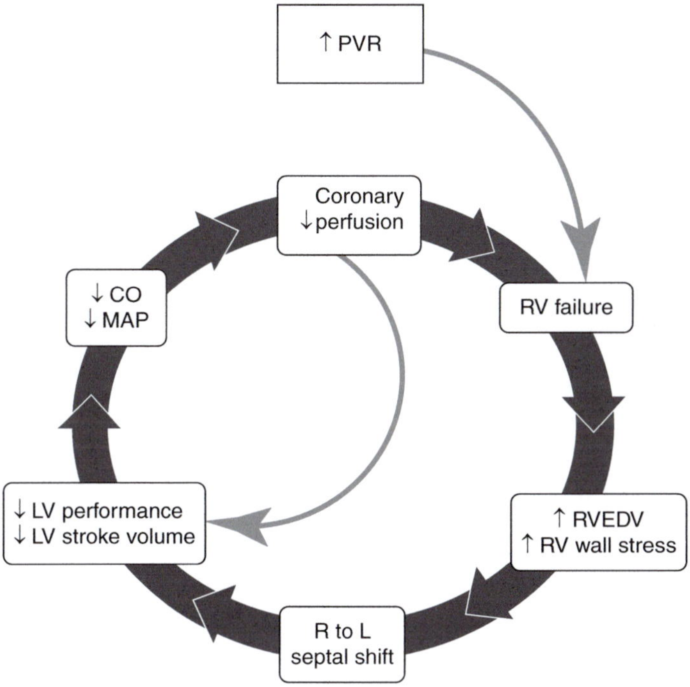

Fig. 7.2 The self-perpetuating cycle of a pulmonary hypertensive crisis. The cycle can be entered at any point and culminates with cardiac arrest

A pulmonary hypertensive crisis can be triggered by several stimuli that directly affect PVR or ventricular function. The best-known stimuli to increase PVR are hypoxia, acidosis, and hypercarbia [45–47]. Noxious tracheal stimulation is another known trigger. Tracheal suctioning in the postoperative intensive care unit triggered a 70% increase in PVR and PAP in children with a history of pulmonary hypertension [48]. Systemic hypotension, caused by a decrease in SVR, stroke volume, or myocardial contractility, can lead to inadequate coronary perfusion and right ventricular failure, thus triggering a pulmonary hypertensive crisis at another point in the cycle.

Treatment of a pulmonary hypertensive crisis is directed toward ameliorating the stimulating event and stabilizing hemodynamics (Table 7.6). Moderate hyperventilation with 100% oxygen, treatment of both respiratory and metabolic acidosis, and removal or attenuation of precipitating stimuli should be undertaken. A pulmonary vasodilator should be administered. Acute intravenous administration of pulmonary vasodilators can be associated with systemic hypotension, which may worsen coronary perfusion, so calcium channel blockers, sildenafil, and magnesium are generally not indicated for emergent treatment. Furthermore, pulmonary hypertensive crises have been observed to follow initiation of treatment of pulmonary hypertension with intravenous prostacyclin analogues. Therefore, it is preferable in an urgent setting to administer pulmonary vasodilators by inhalation. This reduces the risk of

Table 7.6 Treatment of pulmonary hypertensive crisis

Treatment	Rationale
Administer 100% O_2	↑ P_AO_2 and P_aO_2 can ↓ PVR
Hyperventilate	PVR is directly related to P_aCO_2
Exclude pneumothorax	Optimize ventilation
↓ Mean airway pressure	Avoid $P_{alv} > P_{art}$
Correct metabolic acidosis	PVR is directly related to H^+ level
Administer pulmonary vasodilators	iNO
Support cardiac output	Adequate preload and inotropic support, ECMO
Support coronary perfusion	Maintain SVR with epinephrine or NE
Analgesia	Decrease sensory/sympathetic mediated ↑ PVR

P_AO_2 alveolar oxygen pressure, P_aO_2 arterial oxygen pressure, *PVR* pulmonary vascular resistance, P_aCO_2 arterial carbon dioxide pressure, P_{alv} alveolar pressure, P_{art} arterial pressure, H^+ hydrogen ion, *iNO* inhaled nitric oxide, *ECMO* extracorporeal membrane oxygenation, *SVR* systemic vascular resistance, *NE* norepinephrine

systemic hypotension and coronary hypoperfusion by delivering the drug to the target pulmonary vasculature. The standard for inhaled pulmonary vasodilators is iNO, but inhaled prostacyclin analogues may also be effective in this setting [49].

Early treatment of bradycardia with atropine or another chronotropic drug can be helpful. If systemic hypotension persists following administration of pulmonary vasodilators, inotropic support is indicated. Since isoproterenol, dobutamine, and milrinone can decrease SVR, and dopamine can increase the PVR/SVR ratio [50], many clinicians prefer epinephrine or norepinephrine for inotropic support during emergent treatment of a pulmonary hypertensive crisis, as these will generally increase SVR and decrease PVR, thus decreasing the PVR/SVR ratio [51, 52]. In addition to inotropic support, a systemic vasopressor can improve coronary perfusion and ventricular function by supporting SVR and may avert cardiac arrest. For this purpose, epinephrine and norepinephrine, because they increase SVR while decreasing PVR, are preferable to phenylephrine, which is both a pulmonary and systemic vasoconstrictor [53, 54]. Limited clinical reports suggest that arginine vasopressin and its synthetic analogue, terlipressin, may increase SVR but not PVR in PAH patients [55, 56].

Optimizing the care of the patient with PH-CHD demands a comprehensive team approach in an ACHD center which offers contemporary medical, catheter-based, and surgical treatments.

7.2.4 Heart Failure

Heart failure (HF) is the leading cause of death in 27–38% of ACHD patients followed over 5 years [57–59]. The burden of HF in ACHD results in over 12,000 hospital admissions annually in the United States, and these admissions have doubled between 1998 and 2010 [60, 61]. A lifetime of structural heart disease, in the absence of symptoms, often results in difficulty describing a universally applicable definition of HF in ACHD. Recently, the Heart Failure Society of America endorsed by the American Heart Association defined HF in ACHD patients as, "a syndrome characterized by either or both pulmonary and systemic venous congestion and/or inadequate peripheral oxygen delivery at rest or during stress, caused by cardiac dysfunction" [57, 62]. There are other definitions of HF in ACHD. Norozi and colleagues define HF in physiological and pathophysiological terms as a peak oxygen consumption (VO_2) >25 mL/kg/min as measured by exercise testing, in combination with an n-terminal pro-brain natriuretic peptide (NT-pro-BNP) plasma level >100 pg/mL. Using this definition, they found HF in 26% of ACHD patients [63]. The probability of developing HF is related to the underlying diagnosis of the specific CHD lesion as shown in Fig. 7.3. Patients with more complex CHD including the diagnoses of tetralogy of Fallot (TOF), single ventricle anatomy, and following the Mustard operation for transposition of the great arteries (TGA) will develop HF sooner than patients with simpler left-to-right shunts [63]. Over time, most ACHD will develop HF due to several reasons, such as myocardial injury during the primary surgery [57, 63]. Myocardial injury over time leads to a decrease in cardiac output which may often be compensated for by the release of excess catecholamines, and activation of the renin–angiotensin–aldosterone (RAA) system. This leads to increased myocardial contractility and maintenance of systemic blood pressure but at the expense of an increased systemic vascular resistance. This leads to further myocardial injury, greater myocardial fibrosis, and worsening of systolic and diastolic dysfunction and a progressive fall in cardiac output and increase in pulmonary vascular resistance. This cycle of heart failure is shown in Fig. 7.4 [64].

The anesthetic care of ACHD patients with HF requires a thorough understanding of their medical management and any associated comorbidities [65]. Comorbidities

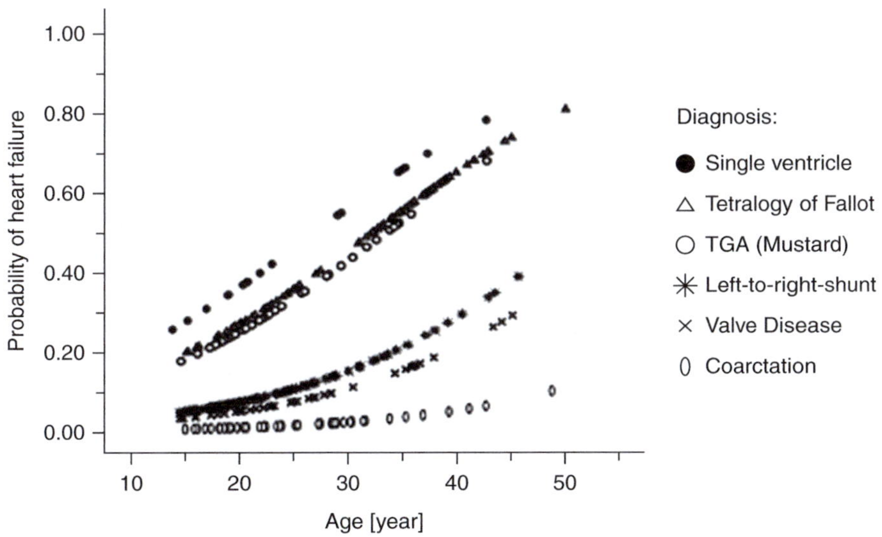

Fig. 7.3 The probability of heart failure bases on complexity of congenital heart lesion. Used with permission from Norozi [63]

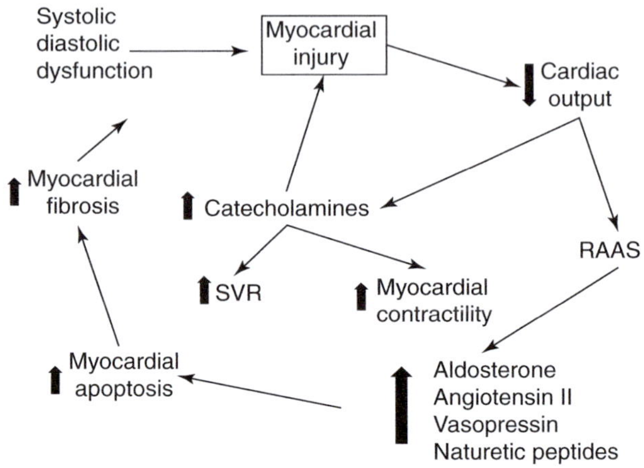

Fig. 7.4 The cycle of heart failure

are common in ACHD patients with HF and include hypertension, obesity and insulin resistance, and renal dysfunction. Hypertension is more common in adult males especially with previous repair of coarctation of the aorta. Hypertension is also more common in ACHD patients with renal disease associated with cyanosis. Obesity, hypertension, dyslipidemia, and insulin resistance are present in 20–54% of the ACHD population with a body mass index >25 kg/m^2. Some degree of renal dysfunction has been found to be present in 50% of elderly ACHD patients [66]. Medical therapy for HF can be difficult in ACHD because commonly prescribed medications for other forms of HF may not always be effective. The activation of the RAA system may not always be the dominant pathophysiological contributor [62]. Additionally, the benefit of β-blocking agents is highly uncertain especially in patients with the Fontan circulation and single ventricle physiology, where a β-blocker-induced reduction in heart rate and cardiac output is seldom tolerated [65].

Biomarkers are beginning to be monitored more frequently in ACHD patients, and their levels should be assessed preoperatively in anesthetic planning [67]. Brain natriuretic peptide (BNP) and NT-proBNP, which are hormones secreted from cardiac myocytes in response to ventricular wall stretch from pressure or volume overload, are often measured. These hormones have been found to be robust markers of ventricular function and functional status in ACHD [68]. On average, NT-proBNP is elevated in 50% of patients with ACHD and is typically fivefold higher compared to adults without CHD [69, 70]. Measurement of these biomarkers must always be correlated with myocardial performance by echocardiography especially in the Fontan patient, with normal ventricular function, where an elevated BNP result may reflect good myocardial performance in the presence of increased preload [67].

Options after failure of medical therapy for HF in ACHD have mirrored therapeutic options for HF in patients without CHD, namely, mechanical assist devices and heart transplantation, but with some significant differences. Only 2–4% of patients listed for heart transplantation during 2000–2009 were adult survivors of CHD [71]. Furthermore, adults with CHD listed for heart transplantation were delisted more commonly due to clinical deterioration compared to adults without CHD [72].

Implanted myocardial mechanical assist devices are not used as frequently in ACHD as they are in patients without CHD [73–75]. Implanted mechanical assist devices require careful planning and consideration in ACHD patients because their HF pathophysiology often comprises more than just myocardial systolic dysfunction.

7.2.5 Endocarditis Prophylaxis

Infective endocarditis (IE) is a rare but potentially devastating condition. The decline of rheumatic heart disease has greatly decreased the incidence of IE. Adults with certain types of congenital heart disease are in a high-risk patient population for IE and to suffer high morbidity and mortality due to the disease [76, 77]. The pathophysiology of infective endocarditis in congenital heart disease patients is multifactorial, but dependent on valvular or mural endocardial damage and bacteremia. The pathway includes endothelial injury which promotes platelet and fibrin deposition leading to nonbacterial thrombotic endocarditis. A transient bacteremia provides the source for bacterial adherence and proliferation within the vegetation. Patients with cyanotic heart disease and those with shunts and foreign materials implanted provide the milieu for this process to occur. Patients with CHD-associated endocarditis carry a high risk of thromboemboli including stroke, long-term antibiotic therapy, additional surgery, as well as death.

The prevention of IE during surgical procedures has been a high priority for decades, and the American Heart Association has been making recommendations since 1955. Prior to 2007, the recommendations for antibiotic prophylaxis were based on expert opinion, but little evidence. In 2007, the AHA published revised guidelines for the prevention of infective endocarditis. The rationale for the revision was that (1) infective endocarditis is an uncommon but life-threatening disease, and prevention is preferable to treatment; (2) certain underlying cardiac conditions predispose to IE; (3) bacteremia with organisms known to cause IE commonly occur in certain invasive procedures; (4) antimicrobial prophylaxis was proven to be effective in animal experiment; but (5) there is no clear evidence that antibiotic prophylaxis prevents infective endocarditis associated with dental, respiratory tract, gastrointestinal, or genitourinary surgery [78]. It was also felt that transient bacteremia is much more likely to occur during routine activities of daily living than during invasive procedures and that optimal oral hygiene may be more important than antibiotic therapy. Additionally, the exceedingly few cases of IE that may be prevented by antibiotic prophylaxis were outweighed by the risk of adverse drug reactions and the development of highly drug-resistant organisms. The guidelines restricted the routine use of antibiotic prophylaxis for invasive dental procedures to patients who not only had the high risk of developing infective endocarditis but also carried the highest risk of the most devastating outcomes.

No published data has linked respiratory tract procedures with infective endocarditis. Therefore, antibiotic prophylaxis is recommended only in patients listed in Table 7.7 who are having a respiratory tract procedure in which the respiratory tract mucosa is violated. This includes tonsillectomy and adenoidectomy. Drug

Table 7.7 Cardiac population recommended for antibiotic prophylaxis

Cardiac conditions associated with the highest risk of adverse outcome from endocarditis for which prophylaxis with dental procedures is reasonable (*AHA guidelines*)
Prosthetic cardiac valve or prosthetic material used for cardiac valve repair
Previous infective endocarditis
Congenital heart disease
Unrepaired cyanotic CHD, including palliative shunts and conduits
Completely repaired CHD with prosthetic material or device, whether placed by surgery or catheter intervention, during the first 6 months after procedure
Repaired CHD with residual defects at the site or adjacent to the site of a prosthetic patch or device
Cardiac transplantation recipients who develop valvulopathy

Except for the conditions listed, antibiotic prophylaxis is no longer recommended for any other form of CHD

Table 7.8 Antibiotic regimens for dental procedures

Situation dose	Agent	Adult dose	Pediatric
Oral	Amoxicillin	2 g po	50 mg/kg po
Unable to take oral medications			
IM/IV	Ampicillin	2 g IM/IV	50 mg/kg
	OR		
	Cefazolin or Ceftriaxone	1 g IM/IV	50 mg/kg
Allergic to PCN or AMP			
IM/IV	Cephalexin[a]	2 g po	50 mg/kg po
	OR		
	Clindamycin	600 mg po	20 mg/kg po
	OR		
	Azithromycin or clarithromycin	500 mg po	15 mg/kg po
Allergic to PCN or AMP and IM/IV	Cefazolin or ceftriaxone	1 g IM/IV	50 mg/kg
	OR		
Unable to take oral medication			
IM/IV	Clindamycin	600 mg IM/IV	20 mg/kg

Single dose 30–60 min prior to procedure
IM intramuscular, *IV* intravenous
[a]Cephalosporins should not be used in an individual with a history of anaphylaxis, angioedema, or urticaria with penicillins or ampicillin

regimens listed in Table 7.8 are appropriate for these procedures as well. Antibiotic prophylaxis is not appropriate for bronchoscopy, unless the airway mucosa is incised. The administration of prophylactic antibiotics solely to prevent endocarditis is no longer recommended for patients who undergo GU or GI tract procedures, including diagnostic endoscopy and cystoscopy. If there are surgical indications for antibiotic use, it is reasonable to include drugs that will also cover for endocarditis [78].

In addition to the AHA, the National Institute for Health and Care Excellence (NICE) and the European Society of Cardiology (ESC) also released recommendations in 2008 and 2009, respectively [79, 80]. The ECS recommendations were very much in line with those of the AHA. However, NICE recommended the cessation of antibiotic prophylaxis for all invasive procedures in the United Kingdom, and subsequent studies have noted a significant increase in IE cases, and there have been calls for adherence to the US and European guidelines [81]. Recent studies in the United States and Europe are not definitive as to the effect of the decrease in antibiotic prophylaxis on the incidence of IE. Several studies reveal that despite the new guidelines and decrease use of prophylactic antibiotics, there has been no increase in the incidence of endocarditis in the general population or in patients with congenital heart disease [82, 83]. However, these studies have their limitations including underpowered population sizes, heterogeneous patient populations in regard to risk factors, short follow-up periods, and diagnostic and treatment inconsistencies. Therefore, firm conclusions regarding cause and effect cannot be made [84]. More recently, studies by Dayer and Mackie have suggested an increase in IE in the United Kingdom and Canada since the most recent limitation on antibiotic prophylaxis; although, again a causation link cannot be made [85, 86]. With these reports in hand, the ECS released new antibiotic guidelines in 2015, which remain in line with AHA 2007 Guidelines [87]. NICE continues to recommend the routine use of antibiotic prophylaxis against IE (www.nice.org.uk/guidance/cg64).

7.3 Special Considerations

7.3.1 Fontan Circulation

In 1971, Fontan and Baudet described the first successful surgical palliation strategy for patients with tricuspid atresia and sub-pulmonary stenosis. Prior to this surgical intervention, 90% of these patients died before the end of the first year of life [88]. This was a major surgical breakthrough in terms of management of patients with single ventricle anatomy. The modern definition of single ventricle anatomy defines patients with CHD that are born with a diminutive size of either the right or left ventricle. These patients may have any one of several anatomical diagnoses, but they all undergo a series of three-staged surgical palliations usually within the first 4–5 years of life. The final stage is the Fontan circulation or total cavopulmonary anastomosis. The essential feature of the Fontan circulation is the lack of a ventricle to pump blood to the lungs, and all deoxygenated blood returns passively to the lungs from the superior and inferior vena caval connections to the pulmonary artery.

In 1990, Fontan and colleagues described the outcomes of 344 patients who had undergone a “perfect” Fontan operation. Two surgical cohorts of patients were followed until 1990, and in this study, there was a survival rate of approximately 50% at 15 years of follow-up [89]. However, Fontan pointed out that the total cavopulmonary anastomosis imposes a gradual declining functional capacity and premature death after an initial period of often excellent palliation, but he also speculated that changes in surgical technique may reduce the prevalence of sudden death and improve outcomes. This has indeed come to pass with several modifications to the original Fontan operation over the past three decades, which have redefined long-term outcomes [90]. The current 10-year survival rate after completion of the extra-cardiac Fontan procedure is now 85–95% [91]. However, patients with the Fontan circulation remain at significant risk for long-term morbidity and mortality. At 10-year follow-up, these complications include atrial dysrhythmias (46%), myocardial dysfunction and grade II heart failure (70%), and thromboembolic events (32%), of which 25% may be fatal. Additionally, a progressive increase in pulmonary vascular resistance (PVR) over time may result in right atrial enlargement, hepatic dysfunction, and protein losing enteropathy in 13% of Fontan patients [90–92].

Preoperative considerations for the Fontan patient include a thorough review of the medical chart, history, and physical examination directed at determining the presence of any complications associated with the Fontan circuit. It is important to determine the patient's exercise capacity, myocardial functional status, and presence or absence of arrhythmias and to determine if the PVR is elevated. Recurrent pleural effusions, hepatomegaly, a history of coughing up bronchial casts (plastic bronchitis) due to a raised Fontan pressure, and a low peripheral oxygen saturation due to pulmonary arteriovenous malformations are all significant complications. These place the patient at greater risk for arrhythmias, heart failure, oxygen desaturation, and thrombotic complications perioperatively [93].

Maintaining spontaneous ventilation when under general anesthesia preserves cardiorespiratory interactions. However, if endotracheal intubation and mechanical ventilation are required, peak airway pressures should ideally be kept below 30 cm H_2O and mean airway pressures less than 10 cm H_2O, with a long expiratory time. This helps optimize passive pulmonary blood flow returning to the lungs. An adequate preload is required, and systemic vascular resistance (SVR) should be normalized to optimize coronary perfusion. These patients are at risk for perioperative thrombosis due to low flow states and venous stasis. Excellent forward blood flow in these patients depends on ensuring an adequate trans-pulmonary pressure gradient. Any increase in PVR will prevent adequate filling of the systemic ventricle and a fall in cardiac output.

Patients with Fontan physiology often present to the cardiac catheterization laboratory for surveillance, assessment of PVR, coiling of collaterals, and ablation procedures for arrhythmias. Vascular access is often difficult. Many of the patients who received a cavopulmonary anastomosis in the 1970s–1980s have developed arrhythmias leading to reduced functional status and poor hemodynamics at cardiac catheterization. These older Fontan patients may present for Fontan conversion surgery in which the original systemic venous-to-pulmonary artery anastomosis is taken down and a modified pathway is constructed to decompress the right atrium in order to enhance forward flow through the passive Fontan circuit. This should decrease the risk of arrhythmias and thromboembolic events and improve survival. However, Fontan conversion surgery is high risk due to multiple factors including repeat sternotomy, advanced heart failure, and significant arrhythmias. It is commonly accompanied by intraoperative cryoablation of the atrial endocardium in a maze procedure. Fontan conversion surgery carries a 10% 30-day mortality [94, 95].

7.3.2 Pregnancy

As medical and surgical treatments of congenital heart disease continue to improve, an increased number of young women with CHD are now contemplating pregnancy. Between 1998 and 2007, annual deliveries for women with CHD in the United States increased 35% [96]. In fact, CHD has become the most common form of heart disease complicating pregnancy in the Western World [97, 98]. Most of these patients tolerate pregnancy well; however, those with complex disease may not tolerate the significant physiological changes that occur during pregnancy, labor, and delivery (Table 7.9) [99]. Women with complex CHD are at an increased risk of maternal complications including heart failure, arrhythmias, stroke, thromboembolic events, and death [96].

The World Health Organization has classified maternal cardiovascular risk into four categories. Women with mechanical heart valves, systemic right ventricles, Fontan circulation, unrepaired cyanotic CHD, and aortic dilation are considered at significant increased risk for morbidity and mortality. Patients with pulmonary arterial hypertension, severe systemic ventricular dysfunction, severe mitral or aortic stenosis, or severe aortic dilation are at extremely high maternal mortality risk, and pregnancy should be considered as contraindicated [99]. Maternal risk factors for poor fetal outcomes include poor functional status, cyanosis, maternal smoking, left-sided obstructive lesions, mechanical valves, anticoagulation, single ventricle physiology, and pulmonary hypertension. Fetal morbidity includes prematurity, low birth weight, respiratory distress, and fetal demise [100].

The anesthetic management of women with CHD for labor and delivery should be tailored to the individual patient [101, 102]. Patients with complex disease should be managed in an institution familiar with caring for adult CHD and require a multidisciplinary approach which includes anesthesiology, obstetrics, and cardiology. Some broad principles can be applied. Generally, volume-overloaded hearts tolerate the hemodynamics of pregnancy better than pressure-overloaded hearts. Vaginal delivery is often preferred, with the use of assist devices to minimize Valsalva. Epidural anesthesia can be used carefully with judicious use of crystalloids. The lowering of systemic vascular resistance may be beneficial for regurgitant lesions like tetralogy of Fallot with pulmonary insufficiency. Spinal anesthesia is typically unsuitable for adult CHD. Patients with complex disease will not tolerate the sudden hemodynamic changes, and right-to-left shunts can be exacerbated. When indicated, caesarian sections are usually performed under

Table 7.9 Normal cardiovascular changes associated with pregnancy

Parameter	Change
Blood volume	Increases by 30%
Plasma volume	Increases by 45%
Cardiac output	Increases by 30–50%
Stroke volume	Increases by 25%
Heart rate	Increases by 15–25%
Peripheral vascular resistance	Decreases by15–20%
CVP	Unchanged

general anesthesia. Indications for caesarian section include ascending aortic dilation, preterm labor in patients taking oral anticoagulants, symptomatic aortic stenosis, and severe heart failure [100].

Conclusion

The perioperative management of ACHD patients may be complex. The anesthesiologist should approach such patients in a stepwise manner. First, consider the underlying cardiac morphology and how any cardiac surgeries and interventions have changed this and the flow of blood through the heart, lungs, and systemic circulations. Second, consider the sequelae of having CHD such as arrhythmias, pacemakers and ICDs, heart failure, pulmonary hypertension, cyanosis, and coagulation issues leading to thromboembolism. Third, consider any lesion-specific issues such as the Fontan circulation. Finally, consider special circumstances related either to the patient, such as pregnancy, or to the procedure such as using neuraxial anesthesia techniques or laparoscopic surgical techniques. A balanced anesthetic approach is necessary to avoid any detrimental side effects of any single anesthetic agent. Successful perioperative management requires a team approach in a center experienced in caring for patients with adult congenital heart disease.

References

1. Egbe A, Uppu S, Lee S, Stroustrup A, Ho D, Srivastava S. Temporal variation of birth prevalence of congenital heart disease in the United States. Congenit Heart Dis. 2015;10(1):43–50.
2. Ntiloudi D, Giannakoulas G, Parcharidou D, Panagiotidis T, Gatzoulis MA, Karvounis H. Adult congenital heart disease: a paradigm of epidemiological change. Int J Cardiol. 2016;218:269–74.
3. Gilboa SM, Devine OJ, Kucik JE, Oster ME, Riehle-Colarusso T, Nembhard WN, et al. Congenital heart defects in the United States: estimating the magnitude of the affected population in 2010. Circulation. 2016;134(2):101–9.
4. Marelli AJ, Ionescu-Ittu R, Mackie AS, Guo L, Dendukuri N, Kaouache M. Lifetime prevalence of congenital heart disease in the general population from 2000 to 2010. Circulation. 2014;130(9):749–56.
5. Apers S, Kovacs AH, Luyckx K, Thomet C, Budts W, Enomoto J, et al. Quality of life of adults with congenital heart disease in 15 countries: evaluating country-specific characteristics. J Am Coll Cardiol. 2016;67(19):2237–45.
6. Baehner T, Ellerkmann RK. Anesthesia in adults with congenital heart disease. Curr Opin Anaesthesiol. 2017;30(3):418–25.
7. Rouine-Rapp K, Russell IA, Foster E. Congenital heart disease in the adult. Int Anesthesiol Clin. 2012;50(2):16–39.
8. Nasr VG, Kussman BD. Advances in the care of adults with congenital heart disease. Semin Cardiothorac Vasc Anesth. 2015;19(3):175–86.
9. Cannesson M, Earing MG, Collange V, Kersten JR. Anesthesia for noncardiac surgery in adults with congenital heart disease. Anesthesiology. 2009;111(2):432–40.
10. Friesen RH. Anesthetic drugs in congenital heart disease. Semin Cardiothorac Vasc Anesth. 2014;18(4):363–70.
11. Maxwell BG, Wong JK, Kin C, Lobato RL. Perioperative outcomes of major noncardiac surgery in adults with congenital heart disease. Anesthesiology. 2013;119(4):762–9.

12. Maxwell BG, Posner KL, Wong JK, Oakes DA, Kelly NE, Domino KB, et al. Factors contributing to adverse perioperative events in adults with congenital heart disease: a structured analysis of cases from the closed claims project. Congenit Heart Dis. 2015;10(1):21–9.
13. Warnes CA, Williams RG, Bashore TM, Child JS, Connolly HM, Dearani JA, et al. ACC/AHA 2008 guidelines for the management of adults with congenital heart disease: executive summary: a report of the American College of Cardiology/American Heart Association Task Force on Practice Guidelines (writing committee to develop guidelines for the management of adults with congenital heart disease). Circulation. 2008;118(23):2395–451.
14. Bhatt AB, Foster E, Kuehl K, Alpert J, Brabeck S, Crumb S, et al. Congenital heart disease in the older adult: a scientific statement from the American Heart Association. Circulation. 2015;131(21):1884–931.
15. Maxwell BG, Williams GD, Ramamoorthy C. Knowledge and attitudes of anesthesia providers about noncardiac surgery in adults with congenital heart disease. Congenit Heart Dis. 2014;9(1):45–53.
16. Greutmann M, Tobler D, Kovacs AH, Greutmann-Yantiri M, Haile SR, Held L, et al. Increasing mortality burden among adults with complex congenital heart disease. Congenit Heart Dis. 2015;10(2):117–27.
17. Escudero C, Khairy P, Sanatani S. Electrophysiologic considerations in congenital heart disease and their relationship to heart failure. + 2013;29(7):821–829.
18. Bouchardy J, Therrien J, Pilote L, Ionescu-Ittu R, Martucci G, Bottega N, et al. Atrial arrhythmias in adults with congenital heart disease. Circulation. 2009;120(17):1679–86.
19. Loomba RS, Buelow MW, Aggarwal S, Arora RR, Kovach J, Ginde S. Arrhythmias in adults with congenital heart disease: what are risk factors for specific arrhythmias? Pacing Clin Electrophysiol. 2017;40(4):353–61.
20. Khairy P, Van Hare GF, Balaji S, Berul CI, Cecchin F, Cohen MI, et al. PACES/HRS expert consensus statement on the recognition and management of arrhythmias in adult congenital heart disease: developed in partnership between the Pediatric and Congenital Electrophysiology Society (PACES) and the Heart Rhythm Society (HRS). Endorsed by the governing bodies of PACES, HRS, the American College of Cardiology (ACC), the American Heart Association (AHA), the European Heart Rhythm Association (EHRA), the Canadian Heart Rhythm Society (CHRS), and the International Society for Adult Congenital Heart Disease (ISACHD). Heart Rhythm. 2014;11(10):e102–65.
21. Silka MJ, Hardy BG, Menashe VD, Morris CD. A population-based prospective evaluation of risk of sudden cardiac death after operation for common congenital heart defects. J Am Coll Cardiol. 1998;32(1):245–51.
22. Avila P, Chaix MA, Mondesert B, Khairy P. Sudden cardiac death in adult congenital heart disease. Card Electrophysiol Clin. 2017;9(2):225–34.
23. Koyak Z, de Groot JR, Bouma BJ, Zwinderman AH, Silversides CK, Oechslin EN, et al. Sudden cardiac death in adult congenital heart disease: can the unpredictable be foreseen? Europace. 2017;19(3):401–6.
24. Navaratnam M, Dubin A. Pediatric pacemakers and ICDs: how to optimize perioperative care. Paediatr Anaesth. 2011;21(5):512–21.
25. Crossley GH, Poole JE, Rozner MA, Asirvatham SJ, Cheng A, Chung MK, et al. The Heart Rhythm Society (HRS)/American Society of Anesthesiologists (ASA) expert consensus statement on the perioperative management of patients with implantable defibrillators, pacemakers and arrhythmia monitors: facilities and patient management this document was developed as a joint project with the American Society of Anesthesiologists (ASA), and in collaboration with the American Heart Association (AHA), and the Society of Thoracic Surgeons (STS). Heart Rhythm. 2011;8(7):1114–54.
26. Stone ME, Salter B, Fischer A. Perioperative management of patients with cardiac implantable electronic devices. Br J Anaesth. 2011;107(Suppl 1):i16–26.
27. DeFilippis AP, Law K, Curtin S, Eckman JR. Blood is thicker than water: the management of hyperviscosity in adults with cyanotic heart disease. Cardiol Rev. 2007;15(1):31–4.

28. Jensen AS, Johansson PI, Idorn L, Sorensen KE, Thilen U, Nagy E, et al. The haematocrit—an important factor causing impaired haemostasis in patients with cyanotic congenital heart disease. Int J Cardiol. 2013;167(4):1317–21.
29. Tempe DK, Virmani S. Coagulation abnormalities in patients with cyanotic congenital heart disease. J Cardiothorac Vasc Anesth. 2002;16(6):752–65.
30. Horigome H, Hiramatsu Y, Shigeta O, Nagasawa T, Matsui A. Overproduction of platelet microparticles in cyanotic congenital heart disease with polycythemia. J Am Coll Cardiol. 2002;39(6):1072–7.
31. Cordina RL, Celermajer DS. Chronic cyanosis and vascular function: implications for patients with cyanotic congenital heart disease. Cardiol Young. 2010;20(3):242–53.
32. Oechslin E, Kiowski W, Schindler R, Bernheim A, Julius B, Brunner-La Rocca HP. Systemic endothelial dysfunction in adults with cyanotic congenital heart disease. Circulation. 2005;112(8):1106–12.
33. Khairy P, Aboulhosn J, Broberg CS, Cohen S, Cook S, Dore A, et al. Thromboprophylaxis for atrial arrhythmias in congenital heart disease: a multicenter study. Int J Cardiol. 2016;223:729–35.
34. Jensen AS, Idorn L, Norager B, Vejlstrup N, Sondergaard L. Anticoagulation in adults with congenital heart disease: the who, the when and the how? Heart. 2015;101(6):424–9.
35. Krieger EV, Leary PJ, Opotowsky AR. Pulmonary hypertension in congenital heart disease: beyond Eisenmenger syndrome. Cardiol Clin. 2015;33(4):599–609, ix.
36. Opotowsky AR. Clinical evaluation and management of pulmonary hypertension in the adult with congenital heart disease. Circulation. 2015;131(2):200–10.
37. Lowe BS, Therrien J, Ionescu-Ittu R, Pilote L, Martucci G, Marelli AJ. Diagnosis of pulmonary hypertension in the congenital heart disease adult population impact on outcomes. J Am Coll Cardiol. 2011;58(5):538–46.
38. Roth TS, Aboulhosn JA. Pulmonary hypertension and congenital heart disease. Cardiol Clin. 2016;34(3):391–400.
39. Bhamra-Ariza P, Keogh A, Muller D. Percutaneous interventional therapies for the treatment of patients with severe pulmonary hypertension. J Am Coll Cardiol. 2014;63(7):611–8.
40. Baruteau AE, Serraf A, Levy M, Petit J, Bonnet D, Jais X, et al. Potts shunt in children with idiopathic pulmonary arterial hypertension: long-term results. Ann Thorac Surg. 2012;94(3):817–24.
41. Hickey PR, Hansen DD, Wessel DL, Lang P, Jonas RA. Pulmonary and systemic hemodynamic responses to fentanyl in infants. Anesth Analg. 1985;64(5):483–6.
42. Williams GD, Philip BM, Chu LF, Boltz MG, Kamra K, Terwey H, et al. Ketamine does not increase pulmonary vascular resistance in children with pulmonary hypertension undergoing sevoflurane anesthesia and spontaneous ventilation. Anesth Analg. 2007;105(6):1578–84, table of contents.
43. Berman W Jr, Fripp RR, Rubler M, Alderete L. Hemodynamic effects of ketamine in children undergoing cardiac catheterization. Pediatr Cardiol. 1990;11(2):72–6.
44. Friesen RH, Nichols CS, Twite MD, Cardwell KA, Pan Z, Pietra B, et al. The hemodynamic response to dexmedetomidine loading dose in children with and without pulmonary hypertension. Anesth Analg. 2013;117(4):953–9.
45. Chang AC, Zucker HA, Hickey PR, Wessel DL. Pulmonary vascular resistance in infants after cardiac surgery: role of carbon dioxide and hydrogen ion. Crit Care Med. 1995;23(3):568–74.
46. Morray JP, Lynn AM, Mansfield PB. Effect of pH and PCO_2 on pulmonary and systemic hemodynamics after surgery in children with congenital heart disease and pulmonary hypertension. J Pediatr. 1988;113(3):474–9.
47. Rudolph AM, Yuan S. Response of the pulmonary vasculature to hypoxia and H+ ion concentration changes. J Clin Invest. 1966;45(3):399–411.
48. Hickey PR, Hansen DD, Wessel DL, Lang P, Jonas RA, Elixson EM. Blunting of stress responses in the pulmonary circulation of infants by fentanyl. Anesth Analg. 1985;64(12):1137–42.

49. Ivy DD. Prostacyclin in the intensive care setting. Pediatr Crit Care Med. 2010;11(2 Suppl):S41–5.
50. Barrington KJ, Finer NN, Chan WK. A blind, randomized comparison of the circulatory effects of dopamine and epinephrine infusions in the newborn piglet during normoxia and hypoxia. Crit Care Med. 1995;23(4):740–8.
51. McGovern JJ, Cheifetz IM, Craig DM, Bengur AR, Quick G, Ungerleider RM, et al. Right ventricular injury in young swine: effects of catecholamines on right ventricular function and pulmonary vascular mechanics. Pediatr Res. 2000;48(6):763–9.
52. Jaillard S, Elbaz F, Bresson-Just S, Riou Y, Houfflin-Debarge V, Rakza T, et al. Pulmonary vasodilator effects of norepinephrine during the development of chronic pulmonary hypertension in neonatal lambs. Br J Anaesth. 2004;93(6):818–24.
53. Koizumi T, Hermo CI, Bjertnaes LJ, Banerjee M, Newman JH, Kubo K. Nitric oxide and nitroglycerin reversal of pulmonary vasoconstriction induced by alpha-activation during exercise. Am J Phys. 1996;270(3 Pt 2):H875–80.
54. Kondo U, Kim SO, Nakayama M, Murray PA. Pulmonary vascular effects of propofol at baseline, during elevated vasomotor tone, and in response to sympathetic alpha- and beta-adrenoreceptor activation. Anesthesiology. 2001;94(5):815–23.
55. Mastropietro CW, Clark JA, Delius RE, Walters HL 3rd, Sarnaik AP. Arginine vasopressin to manage hypoxemic infants after stage I palliation of single ventricle lesions. Pediatr Crit Care Med. 2008;9(5):506–10.
56. Kalambokis GN, Pappas K, Tsianos EV. Terlipressin improves pulmonary pressures in cirrhotic patients with pulmonary hypertension and variceal bleeding or hepatorenal syndrome. Hepatobiliary Pancreat Dis Int. 2012;11(4):434–7.
57. Alshawabkeh LI, Opotowsky AR. Burden of heart failure in adults with congenital heart disease. Curr Heart Fail Rep. 2016;13(5):247–54.
58. Engelings CC, Helm PC, Abdul-Khaliq H, Asfour B, Bauer UM, Baumgartner H, et al. Cause of death in adults with congenital heart disease—an analysis of the German National Register for Congenital Heart Defects. Int J Cardiol. 2016;211:31–6.
59. Tutarel O. Acquired heart conditions in adults with congenital heart disease: a growing problem. Heart. 2014;100(17):1317–21.
60. O'Leary JM, Siddiqi OK, de Ferranti S, Landzberg MJ, Opotowsky AR. The changing demographics of congenital heart disease hospitalizations in the United States, 1998 through 2010. JAMA. 2013;309(10):984–6.
61. Opotowsky AR, Siddiqi OK, Webb GD. Trends in hospitalizations for adults with congenital heart disease in the U.S. J Am Coll Cardiol. 2009;54(5):460–7.
62. Stout KK, Broberg CS, Book WM, Cecchin F, Chen JM, Dimopoulos K, et al. Chronic heart failure in congenital heart disease: a scientific statement from the American Heart Association. Circulation. 2016;133(8):770–801.
63. Norozi K, Wessel A, Alpers V, Arnhold JO, Geyer S, Zoege M, et al. Incidence and risk distribution of heart failure in adolescents and adults with congenital heart disease after cardiac surgery. Am J Cardiol. 2006;97(8):1238–43.
64. Rosenthal DN, Hammer GB. Cardiomyopathy and heart failure in children: anesthetic implications. Paediatr Anaesth. 2011;21(5):577–84.
65. Bouma BJ, Mulder BJ. Changing landscape of congenital heart disease. Circ Res. 2017;120(6):908–22.
66. Afilalo J, Therrien J, Pilote L, Ionescu-Ittu R, Martucci G, Marelli AJ. Geriatric congenital heart disease: burden of disease and predictors of mortality. J Am Coll Cardiol. 2011;58(14):1509–15.
67. Rajpal S, Alshawabkeh L, Opotowsky AR. Current role of blood and urine biomarkers in the clinical care of adults with congenital heart disease. Curr Cardiol Rep. 2017;19(6):50.
68. Eindhoven JA, van den Bosch AE, Jansen PR, Boersma E, Roos-Hesselink JW. The usefulness of brain natriuretic peptide in complex congenital heart disease: a systematic review. J Am Coll Cardiol. 2012;60(21):2140–9.

69. Eindhoven JA, van den Bosch AE, Boersma E, Roos-Hesselink JW. The usefulness of brain natriuretic peptide in simple congenital heart disease—a systematic review. Cardiol Young. 2013;23(3):315–24.
70. Popelova J, Kotaska K, Cerny S, Prokopova M, Rubacek M. Range and distribution of NT-proBNP values in stable corrected congenital heart disease of various types. Can J Cardiol. 2012;28(4):471–6.
71. Davies RR, Russo MJ, Yang J, Quaegebeur JM, Mosca RS, Chen JM. Listing and transplanting adults with congenital heart disease. Circulation. 2011;123(7):759–67.
72. Alshawabkeh LI, Hu N, Carter KD, Opotowsky AR, Light-McGroary K, Cavanaugh JE, et al. Wait-list outcomes for adults with congenital heart disease listed for heart transplantation in the U.S. J Am Coll Cardiol. 2016;68(9):908–17.
73. Dinardo JA. Heart failure associated with adult congenital heart disease. Semin Cardiothorac Vasc Anesth. 2013;17(1):44–54.
74. Harper AR, Crossland DS, Perri G, O'Sullivan JJ, Chaudhari MP, Schueler S, et al. Is alternative cardiac surgery an option in adults with congenital heart disease referred for thoracic organ transplantation? Eur J Cardiothorac Surg. 2013;43(2):344–51.
75. Joyce DL, Crow SS, John R, St Louis JD, Braunlin EA, Pyles LA, et al. Mechanical circulatory support in patients with heart failure secondary to transposition of the great arteries. J Heart Lung Transplant. 2010;29(11):1302–5.
76. Baumgartner H, Bonhoeffer P, De Groot NM, de Haan F, Deanfield JE, Galie N, et al. ESC guidelines for the management of grown-up congenital heart disease (new version 2010). Eur Heart J. 2010;31(23):2915–57.
77. Knirsch W, Nadal D. Infective endocarditis in congenital heart disease. Eur J Pediatr. 2011;170(9):1111–27.
78. Wilson W, Taubert KA, Gewitz M, Lockhart PB, Baddour LM, Levison M, et al. Prevention of infective endocarditis: guidelines from the American Heart Association: a guideline from the American Heart Association Rheumatic Fever, Endocarditis, and Kawasaki Disease Committee, Council on Cardiovascular Disease in the Young, and the Council on Clinical Cardiology, Council on Cardiovascular Surgery and Anesthesia, and the Quality of Care and Outcomes Research Interdisciplinary Working Group. Circulation. 2007;116(15):1736–54.
79. Habib G, Hoen B, Tornos P, Thuny F, Prendergast B, Vilacosta I, et al. Guidelines on the prevention, diagnosis, and treatment of infective endocarditis (new version 2009): the Task Force on the Prevention, Diagnosis, and Treatment of Infective Endocarditis of the European Society of Cardiology (ESC). Endorsed by the European Society of Clinical Microbiology and Infectious Diseases (ESCMID) and the International Society of Chemotherapy (ISC) for Infection and Cancer. Eur Heart J. 2009;30(19):2369–413.
80. Richey R, Wray D, Stokes T, Guideline Development G. Prophylaxis against infective endocarditis: summary of NICE guidance. BMJ. 2008;336(7647):770–1.
81. Thornhill MH, Dayer M, Lockhart PB, Prendergast B. Antibiotic prophylaxis of infective endocarditis. Curr Infect Dis Rep. 2017;19(2):9.
82. Duval X, Delahaye F, Alla F, Tattevin P, Obadia JF, Le Moing V, et al. Temporal trends in infective endocarditis in the context of prophylaxis guideline modifications: three successive population-based surveys. J Am Coll Cardiol. 2012;59(22):1968–76.
83. Pasquali SK, He X, Mohamad Z, McCrindle BW, Newburger JW, Li JS, et al. Trends in endocarditis hospitalizations at US children's hospitals: impact of the 2007 American Heart Association Antibiotic Prophylaxis Guidelines. Am Heart J. 2012;163(5):894–9.
84. Dayer M, Thornhill M. Antibiotic prophylaxis guidelines and infective endocarditis: cause for concern? J Am Coll Cardiol. 2015;65(19):2077–8.
85. Dayer MJ, Jones S, Prendergast B, Baddour LM, Lockhart PB, Thornhill MH. Incidence of infective endocarditis in England, 2000–13: a secular trend, interrupted time-series analysis. Lancet. 2015;385(9974):1219–28.
86. Mackie AS, Liu W, Savu A, Marelli AJ, Kaul P. Infective endocarditis hospitalizations before and after the 2007 American Heart Association Prophylaxis Guidelines. + 2016;32(8): 942–948.

87. Habib G, Lancellotti P, Antunes MJ, Bongiorni MG, Casalta JP, Del Zotti F, et al. 2015 ESC guidelines for the management of infective endocarditis: the Task Force for the Management of Infective Endocarditis of the European Society of Cardiology (ESC). Endorsed by: European Association for Cardio-Thoracic Surgery (EACTS), the European Association of Nuclear Medicine (EANM). Eur Heart J. 2015;36(44):3075–128.
88. Fontan F, Baudet E. Surgical repair of tricuspid atresia. Thorax. 1971;26(3):240–8.
89. Fontan F, Kirklin JW, Fernandez G, Costa F, Naftel DC, Tritto F, et al. Outcome after a "perfect" Fontan operation. Circulation. 1990;81(5):1520–36.
90. Walker F. Pregnancy and the various forms of the Fontan circulation. Heart. 2007;93(2):152–4.
91. d'Udekem Y, Iyengar AJ, Galati JC, Forsdick V, Weintraub RG, Wheaton GR, et al. Redefining expectations of long-term survival after the Fontan procedure: twenty-five years of follow-up from the entire population of Australia and New Zealand. Circulation. 2014;130(11 Suppl 1):S32–8.
92. Alsaied T, Alsidawi S, Allen CC, Faircloth J, Palumbo JS, Veldtman GR. Strategies for thromboprophylaxis in Fontan circulation: a meta-analysis. Heart. 2015;101(21):1731–7.
93. Gnanappa GK, Celermajer DS, Sholler GF, Gentles T, Winlaw D, d'Udekem Y, et al. The long-term management of children and adults with a Fontan circulation: a systematic review and survey of current practice in Australia and New Zealand. Pediatr Cardiol. 2017;38(1):56–69.
94. Sridhar A, Giamberti A, Foresti S, Cappato R, Garcia CR, Cabrera ND, et al. Fontan conversion with concomitant arrhythmia surgery for the failing atriopulmonary connections: mid-term results from a single centre. Cardiol Young. 2011;21(6):665–9.
95. Mossad EB, Motta P, Vener DF. Anesthetic considerations for adults undergoing Fontan conversion surgery. Anesthesiol Clin. 2013;31(2):405–19.
96. Opotowsky AR, Siddiqi OK, D'Souza B, Webb GD, Fernandes SM, Landzberg MJ. Maternal cardiovascular events during childbirth among women with congenital heart disease. Heart. 2012;98(2):145–51.
97. Roos-Hesselink JW, Ruys TP, Stein JI, Thilen U, Webb GD, Niwa K, et al. Outcome of pregnancy in patients with structural or ischaemic heart disease: results of a registry of the European Society of Cardiology. Eur Heart J. 2013;34(9):657–65.
98. Siu SC, Sermer M, Colman JM, Alvarez AN, Mercier LA, Morton BC, et al. Prospective multicenter study of pregnancy outcomes in women with heart disease. Circulation. 2001;104(5):515–21.
99. Canobbio MM, Warnes CA, Aboulhosn J, Connolly HM, Khanna A, Koos BJ, et al. Management of pregnancy in patients with complex congenital heart disease: a scientific statement for healthcare professionals from the American Heart Association. Circulation. 2017;135(8):e50–87.
100. Greutmann M, Pieper PG. Pregnancy in women with congenital heart disease. Eur Heart J. 2015;36(37):2491–9.
101. Fernandes SM, Arendt KW, Landzberg MJ, Economy KE, Khairy P. Pregnant women with congenital heart disease: cardiac, anesthetic and obstetrical implications. Expert Rev Cardiovasc Ther. 2010;8(3):439–48.
102. Ortman AJ. The pregnant patient with congenital heart disease. Semin Cardiothorac Vasc Anesth. 2012;16(4):220–34.
103. Cecchin F, Halpern DG. Cardiac arrhythmias in adults with congenital heart disease: pacemakers, implantable cardiac defibrillators, and cardiac resynchronization therapy devices. Card Electrophysiol Clin. 2017;9(2):319–28.

Sedation in ACHD

8

Wolf B. Kratzert and Johanna C. Schwarzenberger

8.1 Introduction

One of the key elements in critical care medicine remains the management of analgesia and sedation of the critically ill. Since the establishment of intensive care units, the management of sedation has been driven by the limitations of mechanical ventilators, pharmacologic agents, and patients' pathophysiology. Historically, sedation and analgesic strategies have varied greatly based on individual practitioner preference and institutional bias. In the last two decades, advancements in technology and pharmacology have made it possible to reevaluate sedation strategies in the ICU. With more focus on the impact of sedation and early mobilization on ICU outcomes, significant progress has been made over the last couple of years, and recommendations defining the current approach to the management of pain, agitation, and delirium (PAD) have been published [1].

Adults with congenital heart disease are a particular patient population with unique physiologic and psychological characteristics. With improvement in surgical and interventional techniques and advanced understanding of pathophysiologic mechanisms as well as disease progression, survival of patients with congenital heart disease has significantly improved. Consequently, an increased number of this unique patient population is seen in the critical care setting challenging the ICU practitioner. Even though little to nothing is known about the specific effects and outcomes of sedation on ACHD patients, novel drugs and better overall strategies of sedation and analgesia offer opportunities to optimize sedation management in this specific patient group. In this chapter we will focus on the trends and advances in

W. B. Kratzert (✉) · J. C. Schwarzenberger
Department of Anesthesiology, Ronald Reagan UCLA Medical Center,
Los Angeles, CA, USA
e-mail: WKratzert@mednet.ucla.edu; jschwarzenberger@mednet.ucla.edu

E. da Cruz et al. (eds.), *Intensive Care of the Adult with Congenital Heart Disease*,
Congenital Heart Disease in Adolescents and Adults,
https://doi.org/10.1007/978-3-319-94171-4_8

critical care sedation in general and how this applies to the ACHD population. We will discuss pathologic aspects of the ACHD patient in detail and how these interact with specific sedation regimens in the ICU.

8.2 Current Trends in Critical Care Sedation

The key goals of sedation in the ICU aim to permit mechanical ventilation and invasive procedures, while mitigating agitation and anxiety and ensuring patient safety. Agitation and anxiety are associated with adverse outcomes of patients in the ICU [2–4], and practitioners are increasingly aware of potentially causing harm due to long-acting sedatives contributing to ICU delirium, psychological trauma, and immobilization. Modern practices now include the use of standardized assessment scores for anxiety and sedation, daily interruption of sedation, early mobilization, sleep hygiene measures, and more specific pharmacologic regimens to minimize drug-induced adverse effects. Furthermore, with advances in clinical care and extended survival of complex patients, the use of mechanical circulatory and respiratory support by extracorporeal membrane oxygenators (ECMO) is more frequent. This warrants more individualized use of sedatives with distinct pharmacologic profiles.

8.2.1 General Principles

The physiological stress response triggered by critical illness and ICU-related factors causes a variety of functional changes within the body, including tachycardia, increased oxygen consumption, hypermetabolic state, and systemic inflammatory response. Sedation in combination with analgesia is aimed at alleviating this negative response, but all currently used sedatives have intrinsic effects on the cardiovascular and respiratory system and can potentially harm the critically ill patient. The most commonly encountered adverse effects are respiratory depression, hypotension, and bradycardia. Hypotension is caused by vasodilation and drug-induced sympathectomy, whereas bradycardia is caused either by direct or indirect depression of sympathetic tone [5]. Even though mitigation of sympathetic tone blunts the hemodynamic response to intubation [4] and may provide positive effects on agitation and anxiety, in the ACHD patient with marginal hemodynamic reserve this suppression may be detrimental.

8.2.2 Common Drugs

Benzodiazepines in combination with opiates have been the mainstay of sedation in the ICU for decades. While the longer-acting lorazepam is moving out of common usage, midazolam infusions remain in use, especially in patients with substance abuse history, significant anxiety, or severe hemodynamic instability. The most commonly used sedative in the western world today is propofol, due to its short half-life, ease of titration, and minimal lasting neurocognitive depression.

Dexmedetomidine has emerged as a valuable agent with significant benefits due to its lack of respiratory depression [5]. With better understanding of the relationship between pain, agitation, and delirium, the modern pharmacologic approach to sedation has become multimodal, and opiates are an integral part of sedation regimens. As some patients do not require anxiolytic or hypnotic components provided by sedatives, or they are sensitive to the minimal sedative effects of narcotics, short-acting opiate infusions, such as fentanyl, are occasionally used as the sole agent to accomplish sedation.

8.2.3 Common Practice

Over the past decade, several sedation-associated adverse effects have been identified, including prolonged and oversedation, immobilization, and drug-induced delirium and neurocognitive dysfunction. Various approaches have been outlined to improve outcomes, and the current recommendations to manage agitation and sedation in the ICU are to maintain a light level of sedation, to continuously monitor depth of sedation and neurocognitive status, to utilize non-benzodiazepine sedatives, and to optimize delirium prevention. In addition, implementing integrative strategies for the management of pain, agitation and delirium is endorsed as a multidisciplinary approach [1].

It is well recognized that oversedation leads to prolonged mechanical ventilation, patient immobility, prolonged ICU stay, and worse clinical outcomes. In particular, benzodiazepines have the potential for oversedation due to their pharmacokinetic properties. Multiple studies comparing commonly used sedatives show prolonged time to extubation with benzodiazepines [6, 7]. Currently the most commonly used and best-validated sedation-agitation assessment scales are the Richmond Agitation-Sedation Scale (RASS) [8, 9], the Riker Sedation-Agitation Scale (SAS) [10], and the Confusion Assessment Method for the ICU (CAM-ICU) [11] (Tables 8.1 and 8.2). The RASS and SAS are mainly used to determine sedation, whereas the CAM-ICU is widely implemented as delirium screening tool [12]. Tighter therapeutic sedation management by protocolized light sedation [13, 14] and daily interruption of sedation, often in combination with daily spontaneous breathing trials [15, 16], have become standardized practice in many ICUs. These strategies result in decreased time of mechanically ventilation and improve patient outcomes.

Neuromuscular abnormalities from immobility occur within days in ICU patients, and the rate of decline in muscle strength can be up to 5% per day [17]. The incidence of ICU-acquired weakness is exceedingly high and associated with poor short- and long-term outcomes. Strategies to lessen sedation and increasing whole-body physical activity and rehabilitation of patients in the ICU, whether intubated or not, improve outcomes and can be done safely [18–20]. Decreasing sedation leads to improved mobilization, and early mobilization itself is one of the strongest components associated with a reduction in ICU delirium [21].

Aside from the secondary harm of sedatives described above, direct drug-induced adverse effects have been recognized to significantly impact ICU outcomes. Sedatives, by definition, are neurocognitive depressants and are believed to play a major role in the emergence of ICU delirium and prolonged neurocognitive

Table 8.1 Sedation assessment scales

		Richmond agitation-sedation scale (RASS)
+4	Combative	Violent, immediate danger to staff
+3	Very agitated	Pulls tubes or catheters, aggressive
+2	Agitated	Frequent non-purposeful movements, fights ventilator
+1	Restless	Anxious, apprehensive, movements not aggressive or vigorous
0	Alert and calm	
−1	Drowsy	Not fully alert, sustained awakening to voice (eye opening and contact >10 s)
−2	Light sedation	Briefly awakens to voice (eye opening and contact <10 s)
−3	Moderate sedation	Movement or eye opening to voice (no eye contact)
−4	Deep sedation	No response to voice, movement or eye opening to physical stimulation
−5	Unarousable	No response to voice or physical stimulation
		Riker Sedation-agitation scale (SAS)
7	Dangerous agitation	Trying to get out of bed, pulling out tubes, thrashing
6	Very agitated	May require physical restraint, unable to calm with verbal instructions
5	Agitated	Mild agitation or anxiety, calms with verbal instruction
4	Calm and cooperative	Easy arousal, follows commands
3	Sedated	Arousal to verbal or stimuli, follows simple commands
2	Very sedated	Arousal to physical stimuli, does not follow commands
1	Unarousable	Little or no response to noxious stimuli

Richmond Agitation-Sedation Scale (RASS) and Riker Sedation-Agitation Scale (SAS). Adapted from Sessler et al. [8] and Riker et al. [10]

Table 8.2 CAM-ICU delirium assessment scale

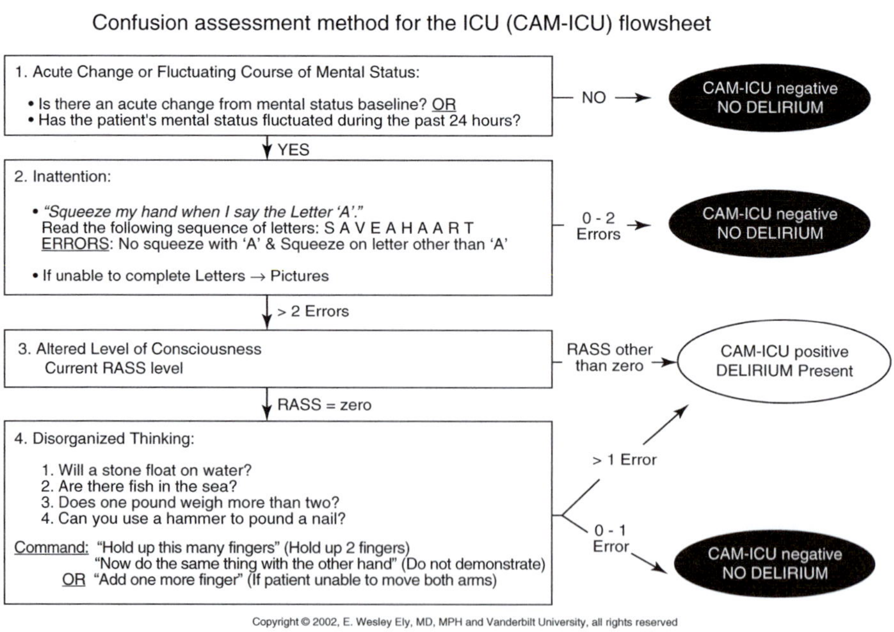

Brummel et al. [12], with permission

dysfunction. The prevalence of delirium in the ICU is high and significantly worsens patient's morbidity and mortality [22, 23]. Despite an occurrence of 60–80% in ventilated patients, ICU delirium is often overlooked, and the use of assessment tools like the CAM-ICU is imperative [11, 24]. Risk factors currently identified with the development of ICU delirium are as follows: preexisting dementia, hypertension, alcoholism, high severity of illness on admission to the ICU, and coma. The discrimination between specific etiologies of coma associated with delirium has not yet been established, but some sedatives and opiates have been implicated [25]. Long-acting benzodiazepines are associated with higher incidence of delirium [26–28], while propofol has not shown any significant association to delirium by itself, and dexmedetomidine may even have a preventive effect [29–32]. Prevention and management strategies for ICU delirium continue to emerge and are mainly based on non-pharmacologic methods. These include early mobilization, keeping the patient orientated to place and time, sleep hygiene measures, and maintaining a regular day-night cycle. Pharmacologic interventions that may have an effect on delirium duration are atypical antipsychotics and dexmedetomidine [33, 34]. To change overall poor outcomes from ICU delirium, a significant change in ICU culture is required: identification of patients at risk, regular delirium assessment, implementation of prevention strategies, and aggressive management of delirium have to become an integral multidisciplinary approach in current ICUs [12, 21, 35].

Cognitive impairment after critical illness and prolonged ICU stay has been described in up to 25% of patients. While pathophysiologic mechanisms are not fully understood, ICU-related factors are hypoxia, hypotension, and derangement of inflammatory and coagulation system. The only clearly identified risk factor for cognitive impairment is delirium. Even though sedatives and especially benzodiazepines are associated with prolonged sedation and delirium, a direct detrimental effect of these on cognitive impairment has yet to be shown [25, 36].

With emerging awareness of psychosocial trauma experienced during ICU stays, the occurrence of depression and posttraumatic stress disorder (PTSD) has been found to be a common long-term result after critical illness [37, 38]. Depending on patient demographics, the incidence is 40% or higher and is often associated with experience of pain, dyspnea, muscle weakness, decreased daily activity, and mechanical ventilation during the ICU stay [39, 40]. The role of sedatives in the development of mental health problems after critical illness, such as depression and PTSD, has not been defined [41]. The lack of sedation during critical illness and mechanical ventilation can be significantly traumatizing to the patient, but overt sedation with development of subsequent delirium may have similar long-term psychological effects. Given these factors, the ACHD patient seems particularly vulnerable.

8.2.4 Sedation in Patients on ECMO

With improving technology and mounting expertise from pediatric critical care management, veno-veno (VV) and veno-arterial (VA) ECMO has resurfaced in the adult population over the last decade. With its growing use, sedation management of these severely ill patients poses a significant challenge to the intensivist. Aside from the often coexisting multi-organ failure (MOF) affecting drug metabolism, ECMO itself changes the pharmacodynamics of many drugs, including sedatives and analgesics. The main alterations are due to an increased volume of distribution with hemodilution, drug sequestration by the ECMO circuit, and increased drug clearance from augmented circulation. All these aspects can potentially lead to therapeutic failure of sedatives during ECMO initiation, make sedation and analgesic management difficult to titrate, and pose the risk of prolonged sedation and oversedation, especially during the weaning process from ECMO. Data on most appropriate sedative and analgesic regimens is just emerging. The initial concern of propofol affecting the life-span of the membrane oxygenator due to its lipid emulsion has not been confirmed, and the drug appears to be safe in patients on ECMO [42]. When measuring drug concentrations after 24 h of ECMO, studies of fentanyl, midazolam, propofol, and dexmedetomidine all have shown a significant reduction in plasma concentration up to 90% from baseline. Whether overall drug dosing is increased due to intrinsic factors of ECMO is difficult to determine, as many patients on ECMO initially require deeper sedation levels. At this point, no specific sedative or analgesic drug can be recommended over others, and no data on adverse effects of prolonged ventilation, length of ICU and hospital stay, and outcomes is available. The use of modern practices to manage sedation and PAD has to be applied to minimize the risk of adverse effects of sedation in ECMO patients. This includes appropriate analgesia, use of short-acting sedatives, and daily interruption of sedation [43–45].

8.3 Predisposing Pathophysiology of ACHD and Sedation

With advances in diagnosis, palliative and corrective surgical interventions, and medical management of CHD, close to 90% of children survive into adulthood [46]. This adult population lives not only with their primary cardiovascular abnormalities but also with significant non-cardiovascular morbidities. These comorbidities may be related to the initial CHD lesion, subsequent repairs, medical management, or sequelae of chronic structural and hemodynamic alterations, and they carry a high incidence of morbidity and mortality by themselves. Complications can manifest in any of the major organ systems, including psychiatric, neurocognitive, cardiovascular, pulmonary, hepatic, renal, hematologic, and musculoskeletal. A complex CHD lesion is often associated with increase in comorbidities. Medical and interventional ICU management of critically ill patients significantly affects the same organ systems, and ACHD patients with their preexisting pathologies represent a challenging and particularly high-risk population when hospitalized. Little is known about the specific interaction between ICU management and ACHD pathophysiology, and outcome measures of critically ill ACHD patients are limited, except that these patients often develop complex multi-organ system failure (MOF) and their morbidity and mortality increases with an increase in complexity of their disease [47]. How ICU sedation intersects with the complex predisposing pathophysiology of ACHD and alters morbidity and mortality is unknown. Even with knowing the specific side effects of certain sedatives, practitioners can only infer their effects on ACHD pathophysiology and have to be cautious with the potential amplified response. To which extent ACHD and grades of its complexity combined with coexisting organ dysfunction worsen adverse effects of ICU sedation can only be surmised. While applying modern concepts of general adult critical care management to ACHD patients, an exceptional understanding of these patients' pathophysiology and recognition of the potential interactions is imperative to provide optimal sedation in the ICU. The key components of ACHD that interact with ICU sedation management are psychosocial, psychological, neurocognitive, pulmonary, cardiovascular, metabolic, endocrine, and musculoskeletal aspects (see Table 8.3).

8.3.1 Psychosocial

Patients with CHD who require critical care pose a particular challenge in the ICU setting. During their childhood these patients are cared for in the pediatric ICU, but once they reach adulthood, the optimal location for their care becomes uncertain [48]. While the challenges when admitting an ACHD patient to an adult ICU mainly lie in the inexperience of providers with complex CHD pathophysiology or interference in care by overprotective parents, many of the challenges when admitting ACHD patients to the pediatric ICU are posed by the sedation and analgesic management. These patients are often highly guarded by their family members who have long-standing experience and expectations from the pediatric critical care surrounding. It is important to recognize that some of the preconceived expectations stem from a certain era of ICU practices that have since been abandoned. Once in the adult critical care surrounding, and potentially decades after the patient's initial ICU care, this can cause difficulties as family members may interfere with weaning protocols, analgesic regimens, early mobilization, or other management aspects. Additionally, the use of non-pharmacologic methods useful to approach anxiety and agitation in developmentally delayed ACHD patients with syndromes like Down may not be as available or familiar in the adult ICU setting. On the other hand, when practitioners who are accustomed to the pediatric population manage adult patients, unfamiliarity with the sedation and pain assessment and medication requirements of adults can easily lead to under- and overdosing of drugs with subsequent adverse effects.

8.3.2 Neuropsychiatric

Most of the ACHD patients have a long history of hospitalization and ICU stays. These can result in long-term psychological conditioning which often leads to reduced pain tolerance, chronic pain syndromes, tachyphylaxis to analgesics and sedatives, and increased incidence of psychiatric disorders and their associated increased adverse effects [49]. Cardiac and non-cardiac surgical interventions, especially when associated with hypoxia, further impair neurodevelopment in CHD

Table 8.3 ACHD-associated pathophysiology and sedation management

Pathophysiology	Sedation concerns	Sedation-management strategies
Psychosocial	– Family interference with sedation strategies – Unfamiliarity of ICU provider with age-appropriate management resulting in over- or under-sedation	– Including family in defining goals and strategies of sedation management – Use of age-appropriate sedation
Neuro/Psych	– Tachyphylaxis to sedatives, anxiolytics, and analgesics – Drug interaction resulting in adverse effects (e.g. oversedation) – Unrecognized neurologic insult – Exacerbation of neurocognitive impairment – Delirium	– Use of non-pharmacologic methods to mitigate anxiety – Use of sedation and delirium scales – Frequent neurologic assessment
Pulmonary	– Inadequate oxygen delivery – Central or peripheral induced hypoventilation resulting in hypercarbia- and hypoxia-associated complications – Prolonged mechanical ventilation and immobilization	– Close monitoring of ventilation and oxygenation – Monitor for adequate D02 (e.g. SV02 or ScV02) – Daily SAT and SBT
CV—Pulmonary HTN	– Increase in PVR – RV failure	– Provide adequate sympathectomy – Minimize anxiety, agitation, and coughing – Avoid sedation-induced hypercarbia or hypoxia
CV—RV dysfunction	– Exacerbation of RV dysfunction or RV failure by RV ischemia, RV volume- or pressure-overload	– Avoid hypotension and bradycardia – Caution with overt sympathectomy – Avoid increase in PVR
CV—Cardiomyopathy	– Exacerbation of myocardial dysfunction or acute heart failure by volume- or pressure-overload	– Avoid hypotension and bradycardia – Caution with overt sympathectomy – Avoid hypertension
CV—Arrhythmias	– Exacerbation of tachy- or bradyarrhythmias – PM dysfunction	– Avoid sedation-induced hypercarbia or hypoxia
Metabolic—Hepatic	– Exacerbation of organ dysfunction – Prolonged pharmacologic effects	– Avoid hypotension-induced organ ischemia – Adjust drug dosing – Monitor for drug primary- and side-effects
Metabolic—Renal	– Exacerbation of organ dysfunction – Prolonged pharmacologic effects	– Avoid hypotension-induced organ ischemia – Adjust drug dosing – Monitor for drug primary- and side-effects

Table 8.3 (continued)

Pathophysiology	Sedation concerns	Sedation-management strategies
Musculoskeletal	– Prolonged mechanical ventilation and immobilization – Exacerbation of musculoskeletal weakness	– Minimize sedation, daily SAT, SBT – Early mobilization

NEURO neurologic, *PSYCH* psychologic, *CV* cardiovascular, *HTN* hypertension, *ICU* intensive care unit, DO_2 oxygen delivery, SvO_2 mixed venous oxygenation, $ScvO_2$ central venous oxygenation, *SAT* spontaneous awakening trials, *SBT* spontaneous breathing trials, *RV* right ventricle, *PVR* pulmonary vascular resistance

[50]. During childhood and adolescence, the prevalence of attention deficit hyperactivity disorder (ADHD) is 40–50% in patients with CHD [51]. Mental disorders like severe anxiety and depression have been described in 30–50% of patients [52, 53]. Emotional trauma from recurring critical illness, hospitalization, and procedures during childhood is associated with an increased incidence of PTSD. Deng et al. found that up to 21% of ACHD patients exhibit symptoms of PTSD, which was associated with a higher occurrence of stroke and depression. Many ACHD patients take a list of psychotropic medications on a regular basis and subsequently develop a higher tolerance to sedatives and anxiolytics. Additionally, practitioners have to be aware of possible drug interactions of central acting medications. Continuation of patients' antipsychotic medications is commonly warranted, in addition to ICU sedation regimens. Finding the correct balance between adequate sedation, anxiolysis, and analgesia, while avoiding oversedation, can be challenging, and utilization of a sedation-agitation scale is crucial.

8.3.3 Neurologic and Neurocognitive

CHD may be associated with congenital syndromes, and early childhood surgical management is associated with structural abnormalities of the brain, intracranial aneurysms, increased incidence of seizure and stroke, and cognitive deficiencies. Altered cerebral blood flow due to the CHD lesion and surgical interventions during the neonatal and early childhood period may lead to impaired brain development. Structural abnormalities of the circle of Willis, cerebellum, and parietal lobe are seen in patients with left ventricular outlet lesions and Williams syndrome [54, 55]. In particular cyanotic lesions, accompanied with hypoxia and high complexity, have a high prevalence of stroke [56]. When screened by brain MRI, half of CHD patients show signs of multiple previous strokes, with only 13% reporting clinical symptoms, suggesting that a large proportion have had silent cerebral events [57]. Interestingly, prior beliefs that erythrocytosis and hypercoagulability are the cause of higher thrombosis risks are not confirmed, and the etiology of CHD-associated coagulation abnormalities is currently unclear.

Multiple surgeries for CHD lesions during childhood increase the risk for seizures [58]. With an incidence of two to three times as often as seen in the general pediatric population, the prevalence of epilepsy in the ACHD population remains increased, and many patients take anti-seizure medications.

A significant proportion of children with CHD grow up with neurodevelopmental impairments affecting cognition, motor and language development, and higher-order cognitive functions, and many of these are associated with congenital syndromes affecting multiple organ systems including the brain. Neurodevelopmental impairment and mood disorders have been associated with syndromes like Noonan's or DiGeorge syndrome, trisomy 21, and q22 deletion [59]. With increasing complexity of the CHD lesion, prevalence of neurological abnormalities has been described in up to 70% of children [60]. Exposure to abnormal hemodynamics and deep hypothermic circulatory arrest (DHCA) as a neonate has also been implicated in the development of neurocognitive dysfunction [61]. Repeated exposure to anesthetics in childhood causing neurocognitive dysfunction has recently led to an FDA black box warning for the use of general anesthetics and sedatives in children less than 3 years of age.

In summary, currently identified key risk factors for neurological impairments in the ACHD patient are cyanotic lesions with chronic hypoxia and exposure during the neonatal and early childhood period to abnormal hemodynamics, DHCA, anesthesia, and multiple surgeries for CHD lesions. In many ACHD patients, neurologic or neurocognitive abnormalities persist and play a major role in their daily life. Critical illness and sedation management pose an increased risk for exacerbation of neurocognitive events. A history of cerebrovascular accident (CVA) increases the risk for recurrent insults due to sedation-induced hypotension. Also, preexisting stroke or neurocognitive dysfunction increases the likelihood of developing delirium during hospitalization. Since sedation management is often more difficult in the ACHD patient, the risk for failed recognition of new neurological insult is high, and vigilance by the ICU provider is prudent. Many of the centrally acting medications have intrinsic sedative attributes or affect the cardiovascular system. When sedating these patients in the ICU, common side effects of oversedation, arrhythmias, or hemodynamic instability need to be taken into account.

8.3.4 Pulmonary

Up to half of ACHD patients have lung disease with abnormal lung function and primarily a restrictive pattern, which represents an independent predictor for mortality [62, 63]. The etiology is multifactorial: principal CHD lesions with decreased pulmonary blood flow, primary or secondary arteriovenous malformations (AVMs) at the level of the lungs, and long-standing persistent abnormal physiology after surgical interventions all change the pulmonary vascular bed and are intrinsic causes for restrictive lung disease. In addition, congenital chest wall and spinal deformations like scoliosis, preexisting muscle weakness, and history of multiple thoracotomies have an extrinsic effect on pulmonary mechanics [63]. Moreover, early childhood hospitalization and critical illness with prolonged mechanical ventilation and associated tracheostomy, chronic aspiration, poor nutrition, and acquired muscle weakness, leads to additional impaired pulmonary function.

Most CHD lesions, whether surgically corrected or palliated, result in decreased ability of maximal oxygen consumption (VO_2) in the long term. The etiology of decreases in VO_2 is poorly understood. Pulmonary hypertension (pHTN) in ACHD causes inefficient pulmonary gas exchange and right ventricular (RV) dysfunction. This causes an inability to increase pulmonary blood flow in response to increased oxygen demand [64]. Heart failure by itself is associated with abnormal ventilatory patterns [65]. Increased V/Q mismatch from persistent right to left shunts and inadequate compensation by cardiac output with subsequent increase in carbon dioxide production (VCO_2) in the setting of anaerobe metabolism lead to increased carbon dioxide (CO_2) content in the blood. Many ACHD patients adjust for this by hyperventilating even at rest [66]. Patients with cyanotic lesions compensate their decrease in oxygen delivery (DO_2) by chronically increasing their hemoglobin (Hgb) level, changing blood viscosity. All these factors result in limited exercise capacity and stress tolerance. Many ACHD patients are deconditioned at baseline, thereby increasing their disease severity, which is independently associated with increased morbidity and mortality [67, 68].

Changes in pulmonary function and mechanics, as well as an overall decreased oxygen reserve, make ACHD patients vulnerable to complications during high metabolic states such as critical illness. As sedatives and analgesics affect central and peripheral respiratory mechanisms, small changes in respiratory drive and mechanics can have a significant impact on the well-being of ACHD patients. Drug interference with marginal baseline oxygenation and ventilation results in hypoxia and hypercarbia and thus reduces the patient's ability to provide adequate oxygen delivery. Hypoxic and hypercarbic respiratory failure in the setting of sedation and analgesic can lead to hemodynamic compromise either from arrhythmias or due to pulmonary vasoconstriction in patients predisposed with pulmonary hypertension and right ventricular dysfunction. With often preexisting musculoskeletal weakness and baseline high ventilatory requirements in ACHD, the risk of prolonged mechanical ventilation and immobilization with subsequent physical deconditioning and critical illness myopathy is high. Meticulous monitoring of oxygenation and ventilation in these patients and use of additional parameters to assess adequate end-organ oxygen delivery and hemodynamics are required to ensure adequate pulmonary mechanics while being sedated. Incorporation of baseline optimal parameters of specific ACHD lesions and measurement of mixed and central venous oxygenation and the use of a pulmonary artery catheter, if possible, can be helpful to guide management. Proactive sedation management to minimize the duration of mechanical ventilation is required to avoid adverse effects of sedation in these patients.

8.3.5 Cardiovascular

The majority of ACHD patients have persistently abnormal cardiovascular physiology with altered hemodynamics at baseline and reduced cardiovascular reserve to stress or pharmacological interference. The etiology of reduced cardiac output and adaptation to stress is plenty: unaltered CHD lesion, need for repetitive palliative surgical repair, or sequelae of living into adulthood with "fixed but not cured" lesions. Cardiovascular states most important in the setting of sedation are pHTN with associated RV dysfunction, cardiomyopathies, arrhythmias, chronotropic incompetence, abnormal coronaries predisposing to myocardial ischemia, persistent intracardiac shunts, and hypertension (HTN).

PHTN with a prevalence of up to 28% in patients with CHD amounts to increased morbidity and mortality. Its presence leads to more hospitalizations and ICU admissions [56]. Most common clinical symptoms are decreased exercise capacity, stress intolerance, and signs of chronic RV dysfunction. Key physiologic aspect for clinical management of patients with pHTN is the reactivity of the pulmonary vasculature to triggers of vasoconstriction and vasodilation.

Global cardiomyopathy due to inherent myocardial problems, underlying CHD, systemic RV, chronic myocardial ischemia, arrhythmias, as well as history of multiple cardiac surgeries predisposes ACHD patients to heart failure (HF) [69]. HF is now the leading cause for mortality in this patient population and a significant risk for hospital admission [70, 71]. A prior history of HF, atrial arrhythmias, and pHTN are specific risk factors for acute decompensation. There is a lesion-specific distribution of HF occurrence with right ventricular abnormalities greater than left ventricular abnormalities greater than univentricular physiology [72].

Arrhythmias in CHD are very common and have significant influence on the management of ACHD. While they can be associated with intrinsic lesions like Ebstein's anomaly or congenitally corrected transposition of the great arteries (TGA), most arrhythmias in ACHD are acquired from scarring after surgical intervention or from living with long-standing abnormal volume and pressure loads or cyanosis. Supraventricular tachyarrhythmias, in particular intra-atrial reentry tachycardia (IART), are most common, while serious ventricular tachycardia (VT) emerges later in life. With the onset of VTs, sudden death becomes a threat. The most common bradyarrhythmias are dysfunction of the sinus node (SN) due to surgical trauma and abnormal atrioventricular (AV) conduction. Abnormal AV conduction exists in up to 5% of CHD at birth, while the majority with up to 20% develops over time [73, 74]. Hemodynamics in ACHD are often tenuous, and low heart rates and arrhythmias are poorly tolerated. For these reasons, many of these patients have a permanent pacemaker placed.

Chronotropic incompetence (CI), defined as incompetence to mount an adequate HR response to exercise, has a high prevalence in ACHD [75]. Initially described in chronic heart diseases like congestive heart failure (CHF), dilated cardiomyopathy (DCM), or coronary artery disease (CAD), it is associated with a decreased exercise tolerance and VO_2 [76, 77].

All sedatives can have positive and negative effects on marginal hemodynamic profiles of critically ill patients with ACHD, and it is not always clear where benefits and risks intersect. Adding critical illness with changes in hemodynamics and metabolism to the often fragile hemodynamics of ACHD poses a significant risk for poor outcomes. Vigilance of a balanced sedation regimen is necessary to optimize patients' safety. Potential hemodynamic benefits come from suppression of anxiety and sympathetic stimulation resulting in decreases in myocardial oxygen consumption.

Suppression of cough reflex and patient-ventilator dyssynchrony mitigates the risk of harmful increases in intrathoracic pressures. However, several significant adverse hemodynamic effects can be caused by sedatives. When sedating patients with pHTN, key aspects to know are whether their pulmonary vasculature is reactive to triggers of vasoconstriction and vasodilation and whether RV dysfunction and the risk of exacerbation of RV failure exist. Sympathectomy, suppression of anxiety, and avoidance of elevated intrathoracic pressures are all beneficial to avoid exacerbation of pulmonary vasoconstriction, but overt sedation resulting in ventilatory compromise and acid-base abnormalities has the opposite effect. In patients with reactive pulmonary vasculature, sedation needs to be tailored to balance adequate reduction of sympathetic stimulation during mechanical ventilation, endotracheal suction, bedside procedures, etc. and ought to avoid respiratory depression causing hypoxemia or hypercarbia. Many of these patients have ischemia-prone hypertrophied right ventricles, and avoidance of hypotension with sedation is crucial. In patients with RV dysfunction, where maintenance of higher heart rates supports right-sided cardiac output and circulation, sedation-induced sympathectomy with subsequent bradycardia can result in failure of the right heart. Hypotension and bradycardia as a consequence of sedation in general pose a particular risk in ACHD. Aside from hypertrophied cardiac muscles, these patients often have abnormal coronary anatomy or elevated baseline blood pressures requiring maintenance of perfusion pressures to avoid myocardial and end-organ ischemia. Similarly, augmented bradycardia can compromise cardiac output of both ventricles, increasing the risk for heart failure. Many of these patients have chronotropic insufficiency resulting in an inadequate stress response; sympathetic suppression and even small decreases in HR are poorly tolerated. Most sedatives cause sympathectomy via direct or indirect mechanisms. While benzodiazepines in general have the least hemodynamic effects, propofol and particularly opiates cause significant sympathectomy as well as suppression of the ventilatory function. Dexmedetomidine represents a unique agent, as it has intrinsic characteristics affecting hemodynamics by causing strong presynaptic suppression of sympathetic drive resulting in bradycardia, hypotension, and sometimes hypertension. Bradycardia is especially seen due to its intrinsic negative chronotropic and dromotropic properties. These attributes may provide a benefit particularly in patients at high risk of tachyarrhythmias [78–80]. Even though commonly used sedatives don't have inherent arrhythmogenic properties, sedation-induced inadequate ventilation can worsen existing acid-base abnormalities in critically ill patients. This can result in arrhythmias but also in intermittent or complete loss of pacemaker (PM) function in patients with implantable rhythm devices. While complete loss of PM function can be detrimental, even occasional irregular function can cause hemodynamic compromise in marginal patients.

8.3.6 Metabolic

As a result of chronic hypoxia, poor cardiac output and systemic perfusion, and right-sided venous congestion, as well as from prior transfusions and medication toxicity, liver and kidney dysfunction is common in ACHD. The associated abnormal metabolic function affects multiple medications including sedatives used in the ICU. Additionally, sedation-induced hypotension can lead to acute liver or kidney failure, especially in organs with preexisting insults.

Aside from a few intrinsic liver diseases associated with congenital syndromes, the majority of liver dysfunction is due to chronic hemodynamic changes and non-specific to the CHD lesion [81]. Right-sided congestion predisposes the liver to injury from decreased hepatic blood flow, decreased arterial oxygen saturation, and increased hepatic venous pressures [82]. Especially Fontan physiology, with the multitude of insults from persistent congestive hepatopathy, hypoxia, and ischemic hepatitis, has a high incidence of liver dysfunction [83, 84]. These abnormalities eventually lead to changes on the cellular level ranging from chronic inflammation to cirrhosis and portal hypertension with subsequent effects on liver metabolic function. While hepatic dysfunction in critically ill patients leads to prolonged length of stay and decrease survival, consequences on outcomes of specific mechanisms in ACHD, like congestive hepatopathy, are unknown [85, 86].

Abnormal renal function exists in up to 50% of ACHD and is a highly prognostic marker for mortality. Depending on severity of disease, mortality ranges from three- to fivefold as compared to patients with normal renal function [87, 88]. Heart and kidney function is closely linked to maintaining normal physiology of hemodynamic parameters like vascular tone or blood volume. Abnormalities in this balance, termed cardiorenal syndrome (CRS), come from altered renal blood flow, increased central venous pressures, anemia, cyanosis, neurohormonal changes, oxidative stress, and renal sympathetic activity [88, 89]. Cyanosis in CHD results primarily in decreased oxygen supply to the kidneys and, secondarily, in erythrocytosis and hyperviscosity leading to increased pressures across the glomerulus. Both mechanisms damage renal cell tissue. The main adverse effect of anemia on renal function comes from its worsening effects on heart failure (HF) with resulting decrease in renal perfusion and reactive renal vasoconstriction. Similarly, activation of the sympathetic system and renin-angiotensin-aldosterone system (RAAS) in the setting of HF will cause decreased renal perfusion and fluid retention. Also, chronic increase in central venous pressures with decrease in transrenal gradient is a constant insult to renal function. In particular, the combination of acute decreases in renal perfusion with simultaneous increased elevation of right-sided pressures, such as in a failing Fontan physiology, poses a significant risk for acute renal failure.

Liver and kidney disease in ACHD is multifactorial due to chronically existing strain and intermittent acute insults to these organs. Exacerbation of organ dysfunction or acute organ failure is a constant risk in these patients. Key aspects with regard to sedation are twofold. For one, underlying chronic organ dysfunction and marginal baseline hemodynamics make the liver and kidneys highly vulnerable to sedation-induced hypotension and low cardiac output. Patients with HF in general are at increased risk for ischemic hepatitis from hypotension [90], but no defined information exists on sedation-induced hypotension and its effect on ACHD with liver disease. Propofol and dexmedetomidine with their significant vasodilatory and negative chronotropic effects should be used cautiously in this setting. Secondly, drug effects of sedatives may be augmented or prolonged by abnormal capacity of renal or liver metabolism. Hepatic blood flow is altered which may lead to changes in the extraction ratio of certain drugs, enzyme activity for direct drug metabolism is often impaired, and liver dysfunction can affect the binding of drugs to plasma proteins [91, 92]. Benzodiazepines, especially midazolam, may have a prolonged half-life by decreased liver extraction ratio with hypotension. Renal dysfunction leads to decreased extraction of midazolam's active metabolites. Propofol is generally well tolerated and commonly used in liver and renal failure, without prolongation of sedation. The use of dexmedetomidine in liver failure may cause significant bradycardia. However, little adverse effects have been described so far, and we have used it safely in our institution in ACHD patients demonstrating liver dysfunction.

8.3.7 Musculoskeletal

Peripheral and respiratory muscle dysfunction is often seen in long-term diseases like chronic obstructive pulmonary disease (COPD), chronic heart failure (HF), or end-stage renal disease (ESRD) and is associated with adverse outcomes [93–95]. Skeletal muscle atrophy is commonly seen in ACHD, and an increased incidence of respiratory and skeletal muscle weakness in these patients has been described [96]. Exact mechanisms are not well understood. Some are believed to be similar to muscle-wasting syndrome seen in chronic heart failure [97]. Particularly patients with cyanotic lesions have reduced physical exercise capacity as well as chronic insufficient perfusion and oxygenation of skeletal muscles leading to underdevelopment of musculature [98]. During critical illness, sedation-related prolonged ventilation and immobility are a constant threat to muscular well-being. Patients with preexisting poor musculoskeletal strength and exercise reserve like in ACHD may further decondition in a much faster and more pronounced way than the previously healthy, and acquired ICU myopathy may worsen preexisting weakness. Early mobilization and early initiation and continuance of physical and occupational therapy in these patients play an important role throughout their entire hospital stay. To minimize the risk of worsening musculoskeletal deficiencies in ACHD, sedation management in the ICU has to be closely monitored and adjusted to reduce immobility and mechanical ventilation.

8.4 Specific Pharmacologic Agents

Understanding in depth the clinical pharmacology of individual sedatives is important to balance risks and benefits of sedation strategies in ACHD. As described above, these patients have multiple comorbidities that are sensitive to sedation interaction, and their margin of error where the medication can adversely affect patient outcome is narrow. Currently, three main drug classes are used for sedation of critically ill patients in the ICU (see Table 8.4). Benzodiazepines and propofol are γ-aminobutyric acid (GABA) receptor agonists, dexmedetomidine acts as an alpha-2 receptor agonists, and short-acting narcotics such as fentanyl and remifentanil act

Table 8.4 Common drugs used for sedation in the ICU

Common drugs	Advantages/disadvantages	Dosing	Onset	Elimination half-life
Fentanyl	+ No hypnotic effects, no amnesia – Prolonged with hepatic impairment – Sympathectomy	0.7–10 μg/kg/h	1–2 min	2–4 h
Remifentanyl	+ No hypnotic effects, no amnesia + No prolongation with renal/hepatic impairment – Sympathectomy – Chest rigidity	0.5–15 μg/kg/h	1–3 min	3–10 min
Midazolam	+ Hemodynamic stability + Amnesia	0.02–0.1 mg/kg/h	2–5 min	3–11 h
Lorazepam	– Prolonged neurocognitive impairment – Prolonged with renal/hepatic impairment	0.01–0.1 mg/kg/h	15–20 min	8–15 h
Propofol	+ Short acting + Amnesia – Hypotension second to vasodilation	5–50 μg/kg/min	1–2 min	3–12 h
Dexmedetomidine	+ No respiratory depression + No amnesia – Sympathectomy – Bradycardia and hypotension	0.1–1.2 μg/kg/h	5–10 min	1.5–3 h
Ketamine	+ No respiratory depression + No hemodynamic compromise + Analgesic properties – Neurocognitive impairment/nightmares	0.05–0.4 mg/kg/h	30–40 s	2–3 h

on the opioid receptors. Ketamine, an *N*-methyl-D-aspartate (NMDA) receptor agonist, is another drug with sedating effects, but its use is mainly procedural or in chronic pain patients. Advancements in critical care have made utilization of these drugs more sophisticated and specific. Integrative management of analgesia, sedation, and agitation is now key element. As all sedatives act on the central nervous system (CNS), caution has to be taken with regard to the interaction with commonly prescribed drugs in ACHD for mood disorders, PTSD, or seizures.

8.4.1 Short-Acting Opiates (Fentanyl, Remifentanil)

Opioids are a key element for controlling pain in critically ill patients through their action on central and peripheral opioid receptors. In addition these drugs exhibit sedative properties, although the mechanism is not well understood [99]. Much of the anxiety and agitation of ICU patients are triggered by pain and irritation from

ICU-related devices such as the endotracheal tube (ETT), feeding tube, or central venous and arterial access. Suppression of these irritants, including the cough reflex caused by the ETT, is well achieved by opiates, and some patients tolerate sedation management based on pure analgesic regimens. In particular elderly patients or patients with underlying depressed mental status fit into this category. Given the lack of hypnotic and amnestic properties when using sole narcotic regimens, monitoring for agitation not relieved by opioids is important to avoid traumatic experiences. Two of the main synthetic opioids used as continuous infusion in the ICU for sedation are fentanyl and remifentanil. Both drugs have similar pharmacologic profiles in terms of onset, hemodynamics, and side effects, with fentanyl lasting significantly longer than remifentanil. Fentanyl is metabolized by the liver, via N-dealkylation and the CYP3A4 enzymatic pathway. Even though minimal when compared to long-acting opioids, accumulation over time causes prolonged fentanyl effect. Remifentanil has the great advantage of being ultrashort acting due to hydrolytic metabolism by plasma cholinesterase. Both drugs cause significant respiratory depression and chest wall rigidity; the latter is more common with remifentanil. Both drugs suppress the sympathetic nervous system, have negative chronotropic effects, and cause less histamine release as compared to morphine. Reminfentanil's half-life is maximal at 10 min; thus, the risk for hyperalgesia, especially during drug cessation, is high [100, 101]. In younger ACHD patients with a long history of ICU sedation or narrow hemodynamic margins, the use of opioid infusions as sole sedative often poses an increased risk for inadequate sedation or hemodynamic compromise due to augmented sympathectomy.

8.4.2 Benzodiazepines

Benzodiazepines exhibit their sedative effects centrally through action on the GABA system. They result in potent anxiolysis, sedation, hypnosis, and amnesia, without providing analgesia or causing significant hemodynamic changes. In high doses they can cause respiratory depression. Midazolam is the most frequently used drug as it has the shortest half-life and is easier to titrate [102]. Its primary metabolism by the liver results in the active metabolite 1-hydroxymidazolam, which then undergoes renal clearance. Therefore, prolonged drug effect in patients with renal impairment is a significant risk [103]. Lorazepam is metabolized in its entirety by the liver; thus, caution must be taken in patients with altered liver function. Even with normal liver function tests, hepatic blood flow is often altered in ACHD, therefore impairing hepatic extraction of benzodiazepines. Midazolam with a high extraction ratio is more effective by insufficient hepatic perfusion as compared to lorazepam which has a much lower extraction ratio [104]. Another adverse effect of lorazepam with prolonged administration is the risk for metabolic acidosis due to its solvent propylene glycol [105]. Key adverse effect of any benzodiazepine is the risk for prolonged sedation and the need for mechanical ventilation. Risk factors for prolonged sedation are older age, obesity, and hepatic and renal impairment [106]. Even though benzodiazepines are not recommended as primary sedative anymore, there are specific indications where benzodiazepines may have some benefits. With its minimal side effects on blood pressure and heart rate, they may be the drugs of choice to achieve deeper level of sedation in significantly hemodynamically unstable patients. Especially in young patients and patients with a history of drug and alcohol abuse, this may be advantageous. Patients who are chronically taking benzodiazepines can benefit from its use by avoiding symptoms of withdrawal. Due to their strong anticonvulsive properties, benzodiazepine infusions are often used in patients with seizure activity in the neuro-ICU setting.

ACHD patients often suffer psychological trauma from multiple previous hospitalization at a young age. Prior exposure to sedatives leads to drug tolerance, and the use of benzodiazepines may be a good choice in this subset of patients. However, given the high risk for cognitive impairment and delirium in ICU and ACHD patients, benzodiazepines should not be the primary choice of sedation regimen but rather used as a backup should other agents such as propofol or dexmedetomidine fail.

8.4.3 Propofol

Originating from the use for induction and maintenance of general anesthesia, propofol has become one of the main ICU sedatives worldwide. Similar to benzodiazepines, its main effect is mediated through the central GABA receptor system. Propofol causes variable depression of consciousness from sedation to hypnosis, as well as anxiolysis and amnesia. Additionally, antiemetic and anticonvulsant attributes can be beneficial when used in the ICU. With an onset and half-life shorter than benzodiazepines or dexmedetomidine, it provides excellent ability to titrate to an optimal effect. Propofol is partially metabolized by the liver, but the majority of the drug is directly excreted by the kidneys. Therefore, hepatic or renal impairment does not cause accumulation or prolongation of the drug [107]. Propofol causes dose-dependent central respiratory depression, but no direct analgesia or muscle relaxation. Among sedatives, propofol exhibits the most potent hemodynamic effects causing hypotension. The etiology is mostly due to systemic vasodilation and sympathectomy rather than a decrease in cardiac output. Myocardial depression is not seen in dose ranges used for ICU sedation. A rare but life-threatening complication of propofol use in high doses is propofol infusion syndrome (PRIS). Due to impaired fatty acid metabolism, it presents with hypertriglyceridemia, worsening metabolic acidosis, hypotension, rhabdomyolysis with acute kidney injury, and malignant arrhythmias [108]. It is usually associated with prolonged and high-dose propofol sedation, and specific risk factors to develop PRIS are unknown. Even though PRIS in ACHD has not been described to our knowledge, coexisting inborn errors of metabolism manifesting as abnormalities of fatty acid break down warrants the avoidance of propofol use.

Propofol-induced hypotension can worsen overall hemodynamic instability and increase the risk of myocardial ischemia, and represents the greatest disadvantage of this drug. Given the otherwise benign side-effect profile and great benefits of controlled sedation management, propofol is the primary choice for sedation in ACHD as in most other critically ill patients.

8.4.4 Dexmedetomidine

Dexmedetomidine is an alpha-2 receptor agonist with sedative, anxiolytic, analgesic, and significant sympatholytic properties. Unlike with benzodiazepines or propofol, patients sedated with dexmedetomidine are much easier to arouse, and no intrinsic respiratory depression is seen while still providing notable anxiolysis and analgesia. Analgesic effects are partly through intrinsic mechanisms on spinal cord receptors, but the main pain relief with dexmedetomidine results from its ability to augment the analgesic effects of other drugs. These key characteristics make dexmedetomidine an almost ideal drug for the use in ICU patients, and with rapidly rising experience and decreasing drug costs, it is replacing propofol in many situations. Other attributes making this drug attractive for the ICU setting are its association with decreased incidence of delirium and tachyarrhythmias [31, 80]. Even though it is well tolerated by a majority of patients including the cardiac and ACHD patient population [109, 110], non-responders to the sedative effects of dexmedetomidine are described in up to 50% [111, 112]. Common side effects seen are bradycardia and hypotension induced by indirect sympatholysis resulting in decreased norepinephrine release. When initiating the drug in high doses or as a bolus, profound bradycardia and hypertension can occur. For this reason, many clinicians in the ICU start continuous infusions directly rather than use initial boluses. Metabolism of dexmedetomidine occurs in the liver, and its dose may need to be adjusted in patients with liver failure to avoid prolonged drug effect [113, 114]. Dexmedetomidine fulfills many characteristics beneficial for sedation in the ACHD population. The main concern for its use in ACHD patients is prevalence of profound bradycardia.

8.4.5 Ketamine

The use of ketamine in the past has been mainly for general anesthesia, procedural purposes in the ICU and the emergency department, and as adjunctive analgesic in the multimodal approach to patients with chronic pain or increased tolerance to pain medications. Due to its hemodynamic stability, its use has been particularly common in pediatric CHD and cardiac anesthesia field. Ketamine is a potent analgesic, sedative, and hypnotic without amnestic effects. Its main mechanism of action is through antagonism of the *N*-methyl-D-aspartic acid (NMDA) receptor, and metabolism occurs via enzymatic pathways by the liver. Similar to propofol, it has a rapid onset and short half-life and distinguishes itself from other sedatives by its hemodynamic stability. While all other sedatives cause vasodilation and sympathectomy, ketamine results in increase in systemic vascular resistance (SVR), HR, and pulmonary vasodilation. Ketamine as a potential sedative in the critically ill possesses a narrow safety profile in patients with multi-organ impairment, and some of the major adverse effects are increase in oxygen consumption, significant mental status alterations with risk of hallucinations, cognitive impairment, and significant secretion production [115]. Theoretically benefits of routine ketamine use for prolonged

ICU sedation only apply to a narrow, and not yet defined, patient population [116, 117]. Despite its potential hemodynamic benefits, the main indication for ketamine in the ICU remains procedural or as analgesic adjunct.

8.5 Current Management Recommendations

The approach to sedation of ACHD patients in the ICU should follow modern concepts of adult ICU sedation and incorporate management of pain, agitation, and delirium. Current guidelines for adult patients can be applied to ACHD with some modifications keeping specific pathophysiologic aspects in mind.

Frequent preexisting cognitive impairment and susceptibility for stroke and seizures warrant to keep sedation as light as possible and with regular awakening trials to maintain close monitoring of the neurological status. With a high incidence of anxiety and tolerance to sedatives, sedation and analgesia should be adjusted to individual needs. Caution ought to be taken of possible drug interactions with the patients' home medications.

Marginal pulmonary function in ACHD requires vigilance in balancing adequate sedation and analgesia while avoiding impairment of respiratory drive and mechanics. Minimizing time of sedation, mechanical ventilation, and immobilization is pertinent in these patients with poor physical reserve. Acid-base abnormalities need to be avoided as these can have significant effect on the pulmonary vascular bed as well as interfere with pacemaker function in extreme cases.

Most concerning cardiovascular abnormalities are pHTN and RV dysfunction, arrhythmias, and marginal global myocardial function. Sedation-induced sympathectomy in any of these settings can be detrimental as ACHD patients are often dependent on HR to maintain cardiac output. Systemic hypotension can lead to myocardial ischemia, especially in patients with abnormal coronary anatomy or RV hypertrophy, quickly resulting in decompensation of hemodynamics.

Patients with liver or renal dysfunction need to be closely monitored for prolongation of sedation or other adverse effects. Benzodiazepines have the highest risk for prolonged sedation, while Propofol can be used safely. Sedation-associated hypotension can lead to acute organ dysfunction in preexisting hepatic or renal impairment and should be avoided.

ACHD-associated musculoskeletal deconditioning and decreased exercise tolerance should prompt light sedation regimens, early liberation from mechanical ventilation, and avoidance of immobilization.

Choosing the optimal sedation agent by adjusting to each individual ACHD lesion and its comorbidities is the safest way to approach sedation for ACHD in the ICU. Unless specifically indicated, benzodiazepines should be avoided, and propofol or dexmedetomidine should be utilized in addition to appropriate analgesia. Given its beneficial side-effect profile with lack of respiratory depression and decrease in arrhythmias and delirium, dexmedetomidine may be considered as the superior sedative in the future. When used, caution is required in patients who are dependent on their HR for cardiac output.

References

1. Barr J, Fraser GL, Puntillo K, Ely EW. Clinical practice guidelines for the management of pain, agitation, and delirium in adult patients in the intensive care unit. Crit Care. 2013;41:263–306.
2. Fraser GL, Riker RR, Prato S. The frequency and cost of patient-initiated device removal in the ICU. Pharmacotherapy. 2001;21:1–6.
3. Atkins PM, Mion LC, Mendelson W, Palmer RM. Characteristics and outcomes of patients who self-extubate from ventilatory support: a case-control study. Chest. 1997;112:1317–23.
4. Conti J, Smith D. Haemodynamic responses to extubation after cardiac surgery with and without continued sedation. Br J Anaesth. 1998;80:834–6.
5. Reade MC, Finfer S. Sedation and delirium in the intensive care unit. N Engl J Med. 2014;370:444–54.
6. Jakob SM, Ruokonen E, Grounds RM, Sarapohja T. Dexmedetomidine for long-term sedation investigators: dexmedetomidine vs midazolam or propofol for sedation during prolonged mechanical ventilation: two randomized controlled trials. JAMA. 2012;307:1151–60.
7. Fraser GL, Devlin JW, Worby CP, Alhazzani W, Barr J, Dasta JF, et al. Benzodiazepine versus nonbenzodiazepine-based sedation for mechanically ventilated, critically ill adults: a systematic review and meta-analysis of randomized trials. Crit Care Med. 2013;41(9 Suppl 1):S30–8.
8. Sessler CN, Gosnell MS, Grap MJ, Brophy GM, O'Neal PV, Keane KA, et al. The Richmond agitation-sedation scale: validity and reliability in adult intensive care unit patients. Am J Respir Crit Care Med. 2002;166(10):1338–44.
9. Ely EW, Truman B, Shintani A, Thomason JWW, Wheeler AP, Gordon S, et al. Monitoring sedation status over time in ICU patients: reliability and validity of the Richmond agitation-sedation scale (RASS). JAMA. 2003;289(22):2983–91.
10. Riker RR, Picard JT, Fraser GL. Prospective evaluation of the sedation-agitation scale for adult critically ill patients. Crit Care Med. 1999;27:1325–9.
11. Ely EW, Inouye SK, Bernard GR, Gordon S, Francis J, May L, et al. Delirium in mechanically ventilated patients: validity and reliability of the confusion assessment method for the intensive care unit (CAM-ICU). JAMA. 2001;286(21):2703–10.
12. Brummel NE, Vasilevskis EE, Han JH. Implementing delirium screening in the intensive care unit: secrets to success. Crit Care. 2013;41:2196–208.
13. Brook AD, Ahrens TS, Schaiff R, Prentice D, Sherman G, Shannon W, et al. Effect of a nursing-implemented sedation protocol on the duration of mechanical ventilation. Crit Care Med. 1999;27(12):2609–15.
14. Shehabi Y, Bellomo R, Reade MC, Bailey M, Bass F, Howe B, et al. Early goal-directed sedation versus standard sedation in mechanically ventilated critically ill patients: a pilot study. Crit Care Med. 2013;41(8):1983–91.
15. Kress JP, Pohlman AS, O'Connor MF, Hall JB. Daily interruption of sedative infusions in critically ill patients undergoing mechanical ventilation. N Engl J Med. 2000;342(20):1471–7.
16. Girard TD, Kress JP, Fuchs BD, Thomason J. Efficacy and safety of a paired sedation and ventilator weaning protocol for mechanically ventilated patients in intensive care (awakening and breathing controlled trial): a randomised controlled trial. Lancet. 2008;371(9607):126–34.
17. Morris PE. Moving our critically ill patients: mobility barriers and benefits. Crit Care Clin. 2007;23(1):1–20.
18. Hermans G, Van Mechelen H, Clerckx B, Vanhullebusch T, Mesotten D, Wilmer A, et al. Acute outcomes and 1-year mortality of intensive care unit-acquired weakness. A cohort study and propensity-matched analysis. Am J Respir Crit Care Med. 2014;190(4):410–20.
19. Kress JP, Hall JB. ICU-acquired weakness and recovery from critical illness. N Engl J Med. 2014;370(17):1626–35.
20. Schweickert WD, Pohlman MC, Pohlman AS, Nigos C, Pawlik AJ, Esbrook CL, et al. Early physical and occupational therapy in mechanically ventilated, critically ill patients: a randomised controlled trial. Lancet. 2009;373(9678):1874–82.

21. Marra A, Ely EW, Pandharipande PP, Patel MB. The ABCDEF bundle in critical care. Crit Care Clin. 2017;33:225–43.
22. Lin S-M, Liu C-Y, Wang C-H, Lin H-C, Huang C-D, Huang P-Y, et al. The impact of delirium on the survival of mechanically ventilated patients. Crit Care Med. 2004;32(11):2254–9.
23. Salluh JIF, Wang H, Schneider EB, Nagaraja N, Yenokyan G, Damluji A, et al. Outcome of delirium in critically ill patients: systematic review and meta-analysis. BMJ. 2015;350:h2538.
24. Ely EW, Shintani A, Truman B, Speroff T, Gordon SM. Delirium as a predictor of mortality in mechanically ventilated patients in the intensive care unit. JAMA. 2004;291:1753–62.
25. Pandharipande PP, Girard TD. Long-term cognitive impairment after critical illness. N Engl J Med. 2013;369:1306–16.
26. Pandharipande P, Shintani A. Lorazepam is an independent risk factor for transitioning to delirium in intensive care unit patients. Anesthesiology. 2006;104:21–6.
27. Pandharipande P, Girard TD, Sanders RD. Comparison of sedation with dexmedetomidine versus lorazepam in septic ICU patients. Crit Care. 2008;12:P275.
28. Riker RR, Shehabi Y, Bokesch PM, Ceraso D, SEDCOM (Safety and Efficacy of Dexmedetomidine Compared with Midazolam) Study Group. Dexmedetomidine vs midazolam for sedation of critically ill patients: a randomized trial. JAMA. 2009;301:489–99.
29. Maldonado JR, Wysong A, van der Starre PJA, Block T, Miller C, Reitz BA. Dexmedetomidine and the reduction of postoperative delirium after cardiac surgery. Psychosomatics. 2009;50(3):206–17.
30. Mo Y, Zimmermann AE. Role of dexmedetomidine for the prevention and treatment of delirium in intensive care unit patients. Ann Pharmacother. 2013;47:869–76.
31. Djaiani G, Silverton N, Fedorko L. Dexmedetomidine versus Propofol sedation reduces delirium after cardiac surgery: a randomized controlled trial. Anesthesiology. 2016;124:362.
32. Su X, Meng Z-T, Wu X-H, Cui F, Li H-L, Wang D-X, et al. Dexmedetomidine for prevention of delirium in elderly patients after non-cardiac surgery: a randomised, double-blind, placebo-controlled trial. Lancet. 2016;388(10054):1893–902.
33. Devlin JW, Roberts R, Fong JJ. Efficacy and safety of quetiapine for delirium in the ICU: a randomized, double-blind, placebo-controlled pilot study. Crit Care Med. 2010;38:419–27.
34. Devlin JW, Fraser GL, Ely EW, Kress JP. Pharmacological management of sedation and delirium in mechanically ventilated ICU patients: remaining evidence gaps and controversies. Semin Respir Crit Care Med. 2013;34:201–15.
35. Trogrlić Z, van der Jagt M, Bakker J, Balas MC, Ely EW, van der Voort PHJ, et al. A systematic review of implementation strategies for assessment, prevention, and management of ICU delirium and their effect on clinical outcomes. Crit Care. 2015;19(1):157.
36. Ehlenbach WJ, Hough CL, Crane PK, Haneuse S. Association between acute care and critical illness hospitalization and cognitive function in older adults. JAMA. 2010;303:763–70.
37. Jackson JC, Pandharipande PP, Girard TD. Depression, post-traumatic stress disorder, and functional disability in survivors of critical illness in the BRAIN-ICU study: a longitudinal cohort study. Lancet Respir Med. 2014;2:369–79.
38. Patel MB, Jackson JC, Morandi A, Girard TD, Hughes CG, Thompson JL, et al. Incidence and risk factors for intensive care unit-related post-traumatic stress disorder in veterans and civilians. Am J Respir Crit Care Med. 2016;193(12):1373–81.
39. Girard TD, Shintani AK, Jackson JC, Gordon SM, Pun BT, Henderson MS, et al. Risk factors for post-traumatic stress disorder symptoms following critical illness requiring mechanical ventilation: a prospective cohort study. Crit Care. 2007;11(1):R28.
40. Ramnarain D, Gnirrip I, Schapendonk W. Post-traumatic stress disorder after ICU discharge: results of a post-ICU aftercare program. Crit Care. 2015;19:P553.
41. Svenningsen H. Associations between sedation, delirium and post-traumatic stress disorder and their impact on quality of life and memories following discharge from an intensive care unit. Dan Med J. 2013;60(4):B4630.
42. Hohlfelder B, Szumita PM, Lagambina S, Weinhouse G, Degrado JR. Safety of Propofol for oxygenator exchange in extracorporeal membrane oxygenation. ASAIO J. 2017;63(2):179–84.
43. Shekar K, Roberts JA, Mullany DV, Corley A, Fisquet S, Bull TN, et al. Increased sedation requirements in patients receiving extracorporeal membrane oxygenation for respiratory and cardiorespiratory failure. Anaesth Intensive Care. 2012;40(4):648–55.

44. Lemaitre F, Hasni N, Leprince P, Corvol E. Propofol, midazolam, vancomycin and cyclosporine therapeutic drug monitoring in extracorporeal membrane oxygenation circuits primed with whole human blood. Crit Care. 2015;19:40.
45. Dzierba AL, Abrams D, Brodie D. Medicating patients during extracorporeal membrane oxygenation: the evidence is building. Crit Care. 2017;21:66.
46. Williams RG, Pearson GD, Barst RJ, Child JS, del Nido P, Gersony WM, et al. Report of the National Heart, Lung, and Blood Institute Working Group on research in adult congenital heart disease. J Am Coll Cardiol. 2006;47:701–7.
47. Price S, Jaggar SI, Jordan S, Trenfield S, Khan M, Sethia B, et al. Adult congenital heart disease: intensive care management and outcome prediction. Intensive Care Med. 2007;33(4):652–9.
48. Allan CK. Intensive care of the adult patient with congenital heart disease. Prog Cardiovasc Dis. 2011;53:274–80.
49. Cohen SB, Ginde S, Bartz PJ. Extracardiac complications in adults with congenital heart disease. Congenital Heart Dis. 2013;8:370–80.
50. Jerrell JM, Shuler CO, Tripathi A, Black GB, Park Y-MM. Long-term neurodevelopmental outcomes in children and adolescents with congenital heart disease. Prim Care Companion CNS Disord. 2015;17(5). https://doi.org/10.4088/PCC.15m01842.
51. Marino BS, Lipkin PH, Newburger JW, Peacock G, Gerdes M, Gaynor JW, et al. Neurodevelopmental outcomes in children with congenital heart disease: evaluation and management: a scientific statement from the American Heart Association. Circulation. 2012;126:1143–72.
52. Bromberg JI, Beasley PJ, D'Angelo EJ, Landzberg M, DeMaso DR. Depression and anxiety in adults with congenital heart disease: a pilot study. Heart Lung. 2003;32(2):105–10.
53. Kovacs AH, Saidi AS, Kuhl EA, Sears SF, Silversides C, Harrison JL, et al. Depression and anxiety in adult congenital heart disease: predictors and prevalence. Int J Cardiol. 2009;137(2):158–64.
54. Bhatt AB, Foster E, Kuehl K, Alpert J, Brabeck S. Congenital heart disease in the older adult. Circulation. 2015;131:1884–931.
55. Jackowski AP, Rando K, Maria de Araújo C, Del Cole CG, Silva I, Tavares de Lacerda AL. Brain abnormalities in Williams syndrome: a review of structural and functional magnetic resonance imaging findings. Eur J Paediatr Neurol. 2009;13(4):305–16.
56. Gaeta SA, Ward C, Krasuski RA. Extra-cardiac manifestations of adult congenital heart disease. Trends Cardiovasc Med. 2016;26(7):627–36.
57. Jensen AS, Idorn L, Thomsen C, Recke von der P, Mortensen J, Sørensen KE, et al. Prevalence of cerebral and pulmonary thrombosis in patients with cyanotic congenital heart disease. Br Heart J. 2015;101(19):1540–6.
58. Leisner MZ, Madsen NL, Ostergaard JR, Woo JG, Marino BS, Olsen MS. Congenital heart defects and risk of epilepsy: a population-based cohort study. Circulation. 2016;134(21):1689–91.
59. Padula MA, Ades AM. Neurodevelopmental implications of congenital heart disease. NeoReviews. 2006;7:e363.
60. Martinez-Biarge M, Jowett VC, Cowan FM. Neurodevelopmental outcome in children with congenital heart disease. Semin Fetal Neonatal Med. 2013;18:279–85.
61. Bellinger DC, Jonas RA, Rappaport LA, Wypij D, Wernovsky G, Kuban KC, et al. Developmental and neurologic status of children after heart surgery with hypothermic circulatory arrest or low-flow cardiopulmonary bypass. N Engl J Med. 1995;332(9):549–55.
62. Healy F, Hanna BD, Zinman R. Pulmonary complications of congenital heart disease. Paediatr Respir Rev. 2012;13:10–5.
63. Alonso-Gonzalez R, Borgia F, Diller G-P, Inuzuka R, Kempny A, Martinez-Naharro A, et al. Abnormal lung function in adults with congenital heart disease: prevalence, relation to cardiac anatomy, and association with survival. Circulation. 2013;127(8):882–90.
64. Sun XG, Hansen JE, Oudiz RJ, Wasserman K. Exercise pathophysiology in patients with primary pulmonary hypertension. Circulation. 2001;104:429–35.

65. Ingle L, Sloan R, Carroll S, Goode K, Cleland JG, Clark AL. Abnormalities of the ventilatory equivalent for carbon dioxide in patients with chronic heart failure. Pulm Med. 2012;2012(12):589164–6.
66. Sietsema KE, Cooper DM, Perloff JK, Rosove MH, Child JS, Canobbio MM, et al. Dynamics of oxygen uptake during exercise in adults with cyanotic congenital heart disease. Circulation. 1986;73(6):1137–44.
67. Dimopoulos K, Okonko DO, Diller G-P, Broberg CS, Salukhe TV, Babu-Narayan SV, et al. Abnormal ventilatory response to exercise in adults with congenital heart disease relates to cyanosis and predicts survival. Circulation. 2006;113(24):2796–802.
68. Khan AM, Paridon SM, Kim YY. Cardiopulmonary exercise testing in adults with congenital heart disease. Expert Rev Cardiovasc Ther. 2014;12(7):863–72.
69. Fahed AC, Roberts AE, Mital S, Lakdawala NK. Heart failure in congenital heart disease: a confluence of acquired and congenital. Heart Fail Clin. 2014;10(1):219–27.
70. Diller G-P, Kempny A, Alonso-Gonzalez R, Swan L, Uebing A, Li W, et al. Survival prospects and circumstances of death in contemporary adult congenital heart disease patients under follow-up at a large tertiary Centre. Circulation. 2015;132(22):2118–25.
71. Engelings CC, Helm PC, Abdul-Khaliq H, Asfour B, Bauer UMM, Baumgartner H, et al. Cause of death in adults with congenital heart disease—an analysis of the German National Register for congenital heart defects. Int J Cardiol. 2016;211:31–6.
72. Moussa NB, Karsenty C, Pontnau F, Malekzadeh-Milani S, Boudjemline Y, Legendre A, et al. Characteristics and outcomes of heart failure-related hospitalization in adults with congenital heart disease. Arch Cardiovasc Dis. 2017;110:283–91.
73. Triedman JK. Arrhythmias in adults with congenital heart disease. Heart. 2002;87:383–9.
74. Walsh EP, Cecchin F. Arrhythmias in adult patients with congenital heart disease. Circulation. 2007;115:534–45.
75. Norozi K, Wessel A, Alpers V, Arnhold JO, Binder L, Geyer S, et al. Chronotropic incompetence in adolescents and adults with congenital heart disease after cardiac surgery. J Card Fail. 2007;13(4):263–8.
76. Diller GP, Dimopoulos K, Okonko D, Uebing A. Heart rate response during exercise predicts survival in adults with congenital heart disease. J Am Coll Cardiol. 2006;48:1250–6.
77. Witte KK, Clark AL. Chronotropic incompetence in heart failure. J Am Coll Cardiol. 2006;48:595.
78. LeRiger M, Naguib A, Gallantowicz M, Tobias JD. Dexmedetomidine controls junctional ectopic tachycardia during tetralogy of Fallot repair in an infant. Ann Card Anaesth. 2012;15(3):224–8.
79. Geng J, Qian J, Cheng H, Ji F, Liu H. The influence of perioperative dexmedetomidine on patients undergoing cardiac surgery: a meta-analysis. PLoS One. 2016;11(4):e0152829.
80. Liu X, Zhang K, Wang W, Xie G, Fang X. Dexmedetomidine sedation reduces atrial fibrillation after cardiac surgery compared to propofol: a randomized controlled trial. Crit Care. 2016;20(1):298.
81. Asrani SK, Asrani NS, Freese DK, Phillips SD. Congenital heart disease and the liver. Hepatology. 2012;56:1160–9.
82. Hilscher M, Sanchez W. Congestive hepatopathy. Clin Liver Dis. 2016;8:68.
83. Kiesewetter CH, Sheron N, Vettukattill JJ, Hacking N, Stedman B, Millward-Sadler H, et al. Hepatic changes in the failing Fontan circulation. Br Heart J. 2007;93(5):579–84.
84. Wu FM, Ukomadu C, Odze RD. Liver disease in the patient with Fontan circulation. Congenit Heart Dis. 2011;6:190–201.
85. Harbrecht BG, Zenati MS, Doyle HR, McMichael J, Townsend RN, Clancy KD, et al. Hepatic dysfunction increases length of stay and risk of death after injury. J Trauma. 2002;53(3):517–23.
86. Kramer L, Jordan B, Druml W, Bauer P. Incidence and prognosis of early hepatic dysfunction in critically ill patients—a prospective multicenter study. Crit Care. 2007;35:1099–104.
87. Dimopoulos K, Diller G-P, Koltsida E, Pijuan-Domenech A, Papadopoulou SA, Babu-Narayan SV, et al. Prevalence, predictors, and prognostic value of renal dysfunction in adults with congenital heart disease. Circulation. 2008;117(18):2320–8.

88. Norozi K, Oechslin E. Renal dysfunction in adults with congenital heart defects. Prog Pediatr Cardiol. 2016;41:51–7.
89. Bock JS, Gottlieb SS. Cardiorenal syndrome. Circulation. 2010;121:2592–600.
90. Giallourakis CC, Rosenberg PM, Friedman LS. The liver in heart failure. Clin Liver Dis. 2002;6:947–67.
91. Rodighiero V. Effects of liver disease on pharmacokinetics. An update. Clin Pharmacokinet. 1999;37(5):399–431.
92. Verbeeck RK. Pharmacokinetics and dosage adjustment in patients with hepatic dysfunction. Eur J Clin Pharmacol. 2008;64(12):1147–61.
93. Carrero JJ, Chmielewski M, Axelsson J, Snaedal S, Heimbürger O, Bárány P, et al. Muscle atrophy, inflammation and clinical outcome in incident and prevalent dialysis patients. Clin Nutr. 2008;27(4):557–64.
94. Rehn TA, Munkvik M, Lunde PK, Sjaastad I, Sejersted OM. Intrinsic skeletal muscle alterations in chronic heart failure patients: a disease-specific myopathy or a result of deconditioning? Heart Fail Rev. 2012;17(3):421–36.
95. Gea J, Casadevall C, Pascual S. Clinical management of chronic obstructive pulmonary disease patients with muscle dysfunction. J Thorac Dis. 2016;8:3379–400.
96. Greutmann M, Le TL, Tobler D, Biaggi P, Oechslin EN, Silversides CK, et al. Generalised muscle weakness in young adults with congenital heart disease. Br Heart J. 2011;97(14):1164–8.
97. Haehling v S, Ebner N, Santos Dos MR, Springer J, Anker SD. Muscle wasting and cachexia in heart failure: mechanisms and therapies. Nat Rev Cardiol. 2017;11:177.
98. Cordina R, O'Meagher S, Gould H, Rae C, Kemp G, Pasco JA, et al. Skeletal muscle abnormalities and exercise capacity in adults with a Fontan circulation. Br Heart J. 2013;99(20):1530–4.
99. Young-McCaughan S, Miaskowski C. Definition of and mechanism for opioid-induced sedation. Pain Manag Nurs. 2001;2(3):84–97.
100. Muellejans B, López A, Cross MH. Remifentanil versus fentanyl for analgesia based sedation to provide patient comfort in the intensive care unit: a randomized, double-blind controlled trial [ISRCTN43755713]. Crit Care. 2004;8:R1–R11.
101. Wilhelm W, Kreuer S. The place for short-acting opioids: special emphasis on remifentanil. Crit Care. 2008;12(Suppl 3):S5.
102. Barr J, Zomorodi K. A double-blind, randomized comparison of iv lorazepam versus midazolam for sedation of ICU patients via a pharmacologic model. Anesthesiology. 2001;95:286–98.
103. Bauer TM, Ritz R, Haberthür C, Haefeli WE. Prolonged sedation due to accumulation of conjugated metabolites of midazolam. Lancet. 1995;346:145–7.
104. Swart EL, Zuideveld KP, De Jongh J. Comparative population pharmacokinetics of lorazepam and midazolam during long-term continuous infusion in critically ill patients. Br J Clin Pharmacol. 2004;57:135–45.
105. Arroliga AC, Shehab N, McCarthy K, Gonzales JP. Relationship of continuous infusion lorazepam to serum propylene glycol concentration in critically ill adults. Crit Care Med. 2004;32(8):1709–14.
106. Greenblatt DJ, Abernethy DR, Locniskar A, Harmatz JS, Limjuco RA, Shader RI. Effect of age, gender, and obesity on midazolam kinetics. Anesthesiology. 1984;61(1):27–35.
107. Kanto J, Gepts E. Pharmacokinetic implications for the clinical use of propofol. Clin Pharmacokinet. 1989;17(5):308–26.
108. Krajčová A, Waldauf P, Anděl M, Duška F. Propofol infusion syndrome: a structured review of experimental studies and 153 published case reports. Crit Care. 2015;19(1):398.
109. Ji F, Li Z, Nguyen H, Young N, Shi P, Fleming N, et al. Perioperative dexmedetomidine improves outcomes of cardiac surgery. Circulation. 2013;127(15):1576–84.
110. Goyal R, Singh S, Bangi A, Singh SK. Case series: dexmedetomidine and ketamine for anesthesia in patients with uncorrected congenital cyanotic heart disease presenting for noncardiac surgery. J Anaesthesiol Clin Pharmacol. 2013;29(4):543–6.
111. Holliday SF, Kane-Gill SL, Empey PE, Buckley MS, Smithburger PL. Interpatient variability in dexmedetomidine response: a survey of the literature. ScientificWorldJournal. 2014;2014(1):805013–2.

112. Smithburger PL, Smith RB, Kane-Gill SL. Identification of patient predictors for dexmedetomidine effectiveness for ICU sedation. Am J Crit Care. 2014;23:160–5.
113. Gertler R, Brown HC, Mitchell DH. Dexmedetomidine: a novel sedative-analgesic agent. Proc (Bayl Univ Med Cent). 2001;14(1):13–21.
114. Anand VG. Sedation in intensive care unit: is dexmedetomidine the best choice? Int J Crit Illn Inj Sci. 2012;2(1):3–5.
115. Kurdi MS, Theerth KA, Deva RS. Ketamine: current applications in anesthesia, pain, and critical care. Anesth Essays Res. 2014;8(3):283–90.
116. Benken ST, Goncharenko A. The future of intensive care unit sedation: a report of continuous infusion ketamine as an alternative sedative agent. J Pharm Pract. 2017;30:576–81.
117. Umunna B-P, Tekwani K, Barounis D, Kettaneh N, Kulstad E. Ketamine for continuous sedation of mechanically ventilated patients. J Emerg Trauma Shock. 2015;8(1):11–5.

Part II

Advanced Management of the Critically-Ill Adult with Congenital Heart Disease

Cardiopulmonary Interactions in Adults with Congenital Heart Disease

9

Ronald A. Bronicki and Andrew N. Redington

9.1 Introduction

The population of adults with CHD has increased dramatically over the past few decades, with the number of adults with CHD now surpassing the pediatric population. These adult survivors reflect the results of decades of evolution of treatment for CHD, some of which have stood the test of time, others of which have been long since abandoned, but all of which require specific expertise to fully understand their implications. It is no overstatement to suggest that some of the procedures, for example, the Fontan operation for "single ventricle" patients, result in unique cardiopulmonary physiology that has never before been encountered in human biology. Even in biventricular hearts, the nature of the resulting hemodynamic load, for example, chronic pulmonary valve incompetence, results in completely novel cardiovascular responses for which there is no precedent in those with acquired heart disease. That is not to discount the additional effects of acquired heart and lung disease however. These comorbidities further complicate an already complex hemodynamic milieu, and while much has been learned over the past three to four decades, there is much still to learn. Indeed, specific data regarding cardiopulmonary interactions in adults with CHD are sparse. Nonetheless, in this review we describe the physiologic underpinnings of the interaction between the respiratory

R. A. Bronicki (✉)
Sections of Critical Care Medicine and Cardiology, Baylor College of Medicine, Texas Children's Hospital, Houston, TX, USA
e-mail: Bronicki@BCM.edu; rxbronic@texaschildrens.org

A. N. Redington
Cincinnati College of Medicine, Cincinnati Children's Hospital Medical Center, Cincinnati, OH, USA
e-mail: Andrew.Redington@cchmc.org

E. da Cruz et al. (eds.), *Intensive Care of the Adult with Congenital Heart Disease*, Congenital Heart Disease in Adolescents and Adults,
https://doi.org/10.1007/978-3-319-94171-4_9

and cardiovascular systems and their potential clinical impact in adults with CHD. Specifically, we will review the physiologic underpinnings of cardiopulmonary interactions and the effects of respiration on cardiovascular function, the impact of respiration on cardiovascular function in adult patients with congenital and acquired heart disease, the effects of respiratory disease on cardiovascular function, and the impact of cardiovascular disease on respiratory function.

9.2 Volume—Pressure and Pressure—Flow Relationships

The physiologic underpinnings of cardiopulmonary interactions are largely based on the general laws of hydrodynamics applied to a distensible or compressible structure. The extent to which a structure undergoes deformation in response to a force depends on its compliance and the magnitude and direction of the pressure exerted across its wall or its transmural pressure (Ptm). A positive Ptm distends the structure and may result from an increase in the internal pressure and/or from a fall in the surrounding pressure. A negative Ptm causes the structure to decrease in size and may result from a decrease in the internal pressure and/or from an increase in the surrounding pressure. Compliance describes the pressure–volume relationship for a distensible structure such that for a given Ptm, a more compliant structure undergoes greater deformation than a less compliant structure.

The physical properties that govern the flow of fluids (liquid or air) through conducting passages, such as vessels and airways, whether rigid or collapsible, are based on the general laws of hydrodynamics. The behavior of flow (*Q*) through a collapsible structure depends on the inflow pressure (Pi), the outflow pressure (Po), the surrounding pressure (Ps), the Ptm, and the compliance of the structure (Fig. 9.1). When the Ptm throughout the structure is positive, the tube is widely patent and *Q* is proportional to the pressure gradient Pi–Po (also known as zone III conditions).

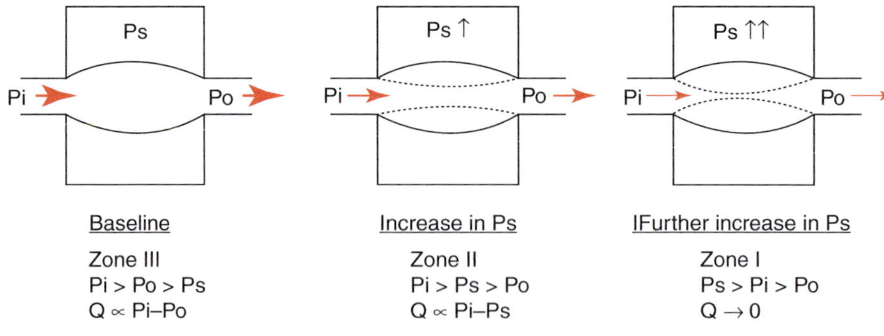

Fig. 9.1 Pi, Po, and Ps represent inlet, outlet, and surrounding pressure, respectively. At low Ps, the magnitude of flow through the tube is principally governed by the difference between Pi and Po (zone III conditions). If Ps is increased above Po, resistance to flow has increased, and flow is governed by the difference between Pi and Ps (zone II conditions). Further increases in Ps to levels greater than Pi result in cessation of flow

With a constant Pi and Po, as the Ps increases, the Ptm decreases. As a result, the volume of the structure decreases, the pressure within increases, and as a result volume is translocated from this compartment to the next. Resistance to flow has increased, and flow is now proportional to the pressure gradient Pi–Ps (zone II conditions). With a greater increase in the Ps, the Ptm decreases further, and as the Ptm becomes negative, the structure collapses and Ps > Pi and flow ceases (zone I conditions). The physiologic significance of these principles is that many structures within the pulmonary and cardiovascular systems behave analogously as intrathoracic, intra-abdominal, and intravascular pressures and volumes vary.

9.3 The Effects of Respiration on Cardiovascular Function

9.3.1 The Effects of Respiration on Right Ventricular Preload

Respiration has a significant impact on systemic venous return; thus a review of the determinants of systemic venous return is germane to any discussion of cardiopulmonary interactions. The force responsible for driving systemic venous return from the periphery to the central venous structures is the pressure gradient that exists between the systemic venous reservoirs and the right atrium [1]. Based on this conceptual framework, the systemic arterial portion of the circulation affects systemic venous return only insofar as it is responsible for filling the venous reservoirs (Fig. 9.2) [1–5]. The resistance to venous return remains remarkably constant under

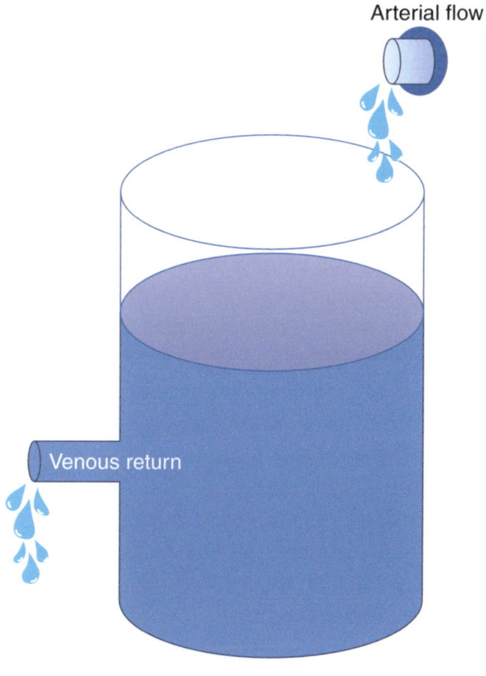

Fig. 9.2 Tub analogy for systemic venous return. Water in a tub represents blood within the systemic venous reservoirs. The inflow tap is arterial flow. The water leaves the tub (systemic venous return) at a rate that depends on the diameter of the hole (resistance to venous return) and the height of the water above the hole. Venoconstriction is represented by a downward displacement of the hole, or an increase in the height of the water above the hole, and venodilation by an upward displacement of the hole, or a decrease in the height of the water above the hole

a number of conditions, including large adrenergic stimulation [6–10]. The resistance to venous return changes appreciably with extremes in viscosity and arterial venous fistulae and with collapse of the vena cava due to the generation of a negative Ptm at the thoracic inlet (zone I conditions) (to be discussed below) [1, 6–10].

The pressure within the systemic venous reservoirs is equal to the mean systemic pressure (Pms) [11, 12]. The Pms may be measured by arresting the circulation, allowing blood to redistribute and for pressures throughout the entire circulation to equilibrate prior to activation of compensatory circulatory reflexes. Guyton and colleagues found the Pms to be 7 mmHg in dogs, and the normal mean right atrial pressure is 2 mmHg, producing a driving pressure for systemic venous return under normal conditions of 5 mmHg [1].

The Pms is a function of intravascular volume and vascular capacitance, the vast majority of which reside within and with the systemic venous reservoirs [11, 12]. These venous reservoirs, the most important of which are located within the splanchnic, splenic, and hepatic circulations, have 18 times greater capacitance than the systemic arterial resistance vessels and thus contain the majority of intravascular volume (upward of 70% of total). The Pms increases as intravascular volume expands, which occurs over hours with activation of neurohormonal pathways or acutely with the administration of volume. Intravascular volume expansion produces a linear increase in the Pms [12–14]. An immediate compensatory increase in the Pms occurs with vasoconstriction of the venous capacitance vessels. An increase in venomotor tone reduces the capacity of the venous reservoirs, increasing the pressure within [12–14]. Studies have demonstrated that venoconstriction increases the Pms and then plateaus, with the most pronounced increase in vasomotor tone occurring with the Cushing reflex [12–14]. Endogenous catecholamines, angiotensin, and vasopressin are the primary mediators of this acute compensatory circulatory mechanism for maintaining systemic venous return. Pharmacologic agents such as furosemide, nitric oxide donors (nitroprusside and nitroglycerin), and combined inodilators such as milrinone and dobutamine vasodilate venous reservoirs, increasing their capacitance and decreasing the Pms and systemic venous return. A systemic inflammatory response syndrome, as is seen in severe sepsis and which may be seen following cardiopulmonary bypass, induces vasomotor paresis increasing venous capacitance while decreasing intravascular volume as a result of an increase in microvascular permeability and the generation of interstitial fluid. The net effect is a marked reduction in the Pms and systemic venous return.

The downstream pressure for systemic venous return is the right atrial pressure, which is affected by a number of factors, specifically cardiac function and the cardiac cycle (so-called cardiac suction factors) [15, 16], and respiration. During spontaneous respiration intrathoracic pressure (ITP) decreases, the Ptm for the right atrium increases, and as a result the right atrium distends and the pressure within falls, driving systemic venous return. Contributing to the pressure gradient for systemic venous return is diaphragmatic descent, which increases intra-abdominal pressure, causing the Ptm and the capacity of the intra-abdominal venous reservoirs to decrease and the pressure within to rise [17–20]. This creates a longitudinal pressure gradient for systemic venous return from the largest of venous reservoirs. In other words, during inspiration, systemic venous return from the abdominal compartment results from phasic decreases in right atrial pressure and increases in the Pms within the abdominal venous reservoirs. This is in contrast to venous return from the head and neck vessels, which are exposed to atmospheric pressure.

During spontaneous respiration venous return increases as right atrial pressure decreases and then plateaus. The negative ITP is transmitted to the right atrium and to the vena cava as they enter the thorax. When the vascular Ptm becomes negative at the thoracic inlet, as what may occur with marked inspiratory effort, the vena cava collapses as they enter the chest limiting venous return (zone I conditions are created). Further decreases in right atrial pressure have no effect on systemic venous return because flow is now a function of the difference between Pms and atmospheric pressure (for the superior vena cava) or abdominal pressure (for the inferior vena cava) [21]. When the Po or downstream pressure is elevated, as in heart failure, the propensity for the Ptm of the vena cava at the thoracic inlet to become negative decreases.

With positive pressure ventilation (PPV), the opposite occurs. During PPV, the ITP throughout the respiratory cycle is above atmospheric pressure, which decreases the Ptm for the right atrium thereby increasing right atrial pressure. For a given Pms, an increase of only 1 mmHg in right atrial pressure decreases systemic venous return by 14%. As the right atrial pressure approaches Pms, systemic venous return ceases unless circulatory reflexes compensate by increasing Pms [13, 14, 22, 23]. As described above this is accomplished acutely with adrenergic stimulation and over time with an increase in intravascular volume [13, 14, 22, 23].

It is important to appreciate that the increase in right atrial pressure that occurs during PPV results from an increase in ITP and decrease in the right atrial Ptm and not from an increase in systemic venous return and right atrial filling. It may seem counterintuitive that an increase in right atrial pressure may be associated with a decrease in systemic venous return and ultimately right ventricular end-diastolic volume because right atrial pressure is used as an indicator of right ventricular preload. However, the increase in right atrial pressure is due to a decrease in its effective compliance as a result of an increase in the Ps. Pinsky and colleagues demonstrated that it is the effect of interventions such as changes in ITP or intravascular volume on the right atrial Ptm and not the right atrial pressure per se that correlates with right ventricular preload and stroke volume [24].

In addition to the adequacy of compensatory circulatory reflexes to maintain an adequate Pms with an elevated right atrial pressure, the extent to which PPV affects systemic venous return, stroke volume, and cardiac output depends on where the right ventricle (RV) resides on its pressure stroke volume curve and on the degree to which alveolar pressure is transmitted to the cardiac fossa. A congested ventricle will tolerate a decrease in systemic venous return (i.e., stroke volume will be unchanged) so long as it remains operating on the flat portion of its pressure stroke volume curve. In addition, it is the magnitude of the rise in airway pressure and respiratory mechanics (airway resistance and lung compliance) that determine the extent to which airway pressure is transmitted to intrathoracic structures and sensed, for example, on the pericardium and in the pleural space [25, 26].

In addition to inducing changes in systemic venous return, respiration alters the effective compliance of the RV and left ventricle (LV) [27–29]. The determinant of ventricle filling is the diastolic Ptm. A noncompliant ventricle or one surrounded by positive pressure requires a proportionally elevated Ptm (in this case driven by an increase in the internal pressure) to generate an adequate end-diastolic volume. The importance of this relationship cannot be overstated as ventricular compliance is often impaired and the surrounding pressure may be elevated, confounding the use of an atrial pressure or ventricular end-diastolic pressure as an indicator of ventricular preload [24].

9.3.2 The Effects of Respiration on Right Ventricular Afterload

Respiration affects pulmonary vascular resistance (PVR) by altering blood pH, alveolar oxygen tension, and lung volumes. Respiratory and metabolic alkalosis induces pulmonary vasodilation, whereas acidosis causes vasoconstriction.

Respiration also affects PVR by altering lung volumes. This cardiopulmonary interaction is not mediated by changes in ITP per se but rather is a function of the alveolar Ptm or transpulmonary pressure (regardless of the mode of ventilation) and lung compliance. Alveolar vessels lie within the septa, which separate adjacent alveoli. Alveolar pressure is the Ps for these vessels. Extra-alveolar vessels are located in the interstitium and are exposed to intrapleural pressure. Because alveolar and extra-alveolar vessels are in series, the resistance provided by each are additive. Functional residual capacity (FRC) is the lung volume from which normal tidal volume breathing occurs. PVR is lowest near the FRC and increases at both high- and low-lung volumes.

At low-lung volumes, the radial traction provided by the pulmonary interstitium diminishes, leading to a decrease in the cross-sectional area of the extra-alveolar vessel. In addition, at low end-expiratory lung volumes, alveoli collapse and hypoxic pulmonary vasoconstriction ensues, and the resistance of extra-alveolar vessels increases further. However, the Ptm of alveolar vessels increases at low-lung volumes because the alveolar Ptm falls. Nonetheless, the net effect is for PVR to increase with lung volumes well below FRC.

As lung volumes rise above FRC, PVR increases. Large tidal volumes or tidal volumes superimposed on an elevated FRC significantly increase PVR. With large lung volumes, distended alveoli compress interalveolar vessels, decreasing the Ptm for the interalveolar vessel (creating zone I and II conditions) and increasing PVR. With PPV the interstitial pressure is positive, decreasing the Ptm for the extra-alveolar vessels as well, contributing to PPV-induced increases in PVR. In other words, during PPV alveolar and intrapleural pressures are positive during inspiration and expiration, and resistance is elevated in both alveolar and extra-alveolar vessels throughout the respiratory cycle. This is in contrast to an increase in lung volume due to negative pressure ventilation where interstitial pressure is negative. This is an important consideration when using PPV, particularly in patients with a normal pulmonary venous pressure and underlying pulmonary vascular disease and/or right heart dysfunction (to be discussed below).

The extent to which lung volume affects PVR also depends on pulmonary vascular hydrostatic pressures, which can be appreciated by applying the general laws of hydrodynamics to the pulmonary vasculature. In the lung, pulmonary arterial pressure is the Pi, pulmonary venous pressure is the Po or downstream pressure, and alveolar pressure is the Ps. In addition, there is a vertical hydrostatic pressure gradient from the most dependent to the most superior portions of the lung. Because the weight of air is negligible, there is no measurable vertical gradient for alveolar pressure. In the gravity-dependent portions of the lung, Pi and Po are greater than Ps, and the Ptm for the alveolar vessel is positive throughout (zone III conditions) (Fig. 9.1). With progression to the non-gravity-dependent regions of the lung, PVR begins to increase as Ps becomes greater than Pv but remains less than Pi (zone II conditions) (Fig. 9.1). In the event that Ps becomes greater than Pi and the Ptm for the alveolar vessel becomes negative, the vessel collapses and flow ceases (zone I conditions) (Fig. 9.1). In the absence of cardiopulmonary disease, zone I conditions do not exist. However, the proportion of lung units under zone I and II conditions increases in a variety of clinical settings. The use of PPV in patients with a normal Po (pulmonary venous pressure) increases the proportion of lung units under zone I and II conditions. Conversely, left heart failure with its attendant pulmonary venous hypertension will increase the proportion of lung units under zone III conditions, rendering the pulmonary vasculature less susceptible to large lung volume-induced increases in PVR.

The interaction between lung volumes and PVR is compounded by the impact of this interplay on gas exchange. Large lung volumes create high ventilation to perfusion ratios (*V*/*Q* ratios), which leads to wasted ventilation and is characterized by an elevated arterial to end-tidal carbon dioxide (CO_2) gradient. Increasing ventilatory support may seem intuitive as the arterial PCO_2 is elevated; however, this may exacerbate the inefficiency in gas exchange if lung volumes (afterload related) and/or ITP are increased (preload related) because ventricular loading conditions will be adversely affected, causing right ventricular stroke volume to decrease further. Large *V*/*Q* ratios do not directly cause pulmonary venous admixture. However, a worsening of oxygenation may occur due to the creation of zone I conditions. This occurs if blood flow is shunted from overdistended lung units to normally or underventilated lung units, which creates lung units with low *V*/*Q* ratios and causes pulmonary venous admixture.

9.3.3 The Effect of Respiration on Left Ventricular Preload

As discussed above, respiration impacts left ventricular preload by altering right ventricular loading conditions and output as well as the effective compliance of each ventricle. The *response* of the RV to alterations in loading conditions and ventricular interdependence also impact left ventricular preload.

As a thin-walled structure that functions as a bellow during shortening, the unprepared RV has much less contractile reserve than the LV and is therefore much more sensitive to increases in and less able to maintain stroke volume with increases in afterload [30]. In addition enlargement of the RV adversely affects left ventricular filling through ventricular interdependence. The ventricles have an intimate anatomical relationship as both ventricles are bound together by spiraling muscle bundles and share a common septum and all chambers are contained within and constrained by the pericardial membrane and surrounding structures. This intimate anatomical relationship sets up a continuous physiologic interplay between the chambers of the heart throughout the cardiac cycle, leading to diastolic and systolic ventricular interdependence. These interactions describe how the change in the volumes and pressures of one ventricle affects the volumes and pressures of the other [30].

Right ventricular enlargement is associated with an increase in right ventricular diastolic pressure, which decreases the normal transseptal pressure gradient. Under normal conditions, left ventricular diastolic pressure is greater than right causing the interventricular septum to bow into the RV. With an elevated right ventricular diastolic pressure, the interventricular septum occupies a more neutral position between the two ventricles. If the right ventricular diastolic pressure were to rise above left, the septum would bow into the LV. In either case, the LV becomes restrained not only by right ventricular pressure and the deviated septum, but also its free wall becomes constrained by the pericardium and lung. These factors decrease the effective compliance of the LV. Even though the left ventricular filling pressure is elevated, intrapericardial pressure has risen to a greater extent, and the net effect is reduced left ventricular diastolic Ptm, end-diastolic volume, and output. This phenomenon is known as *diastolic ventricular interdependence*. This also occurs in the normal circulation albeit to a lesser extent. Spontaneous inspiration increases systemic venous return and right ventricular filling and diastolic pressure, altering the position of the interventricular septum. This mechanism is the diastolic component of pulsus paradoxus, the decrease in systolic arterial blood pressure that occurs during spontaneous inspiration [31].

As left ventricular end-diastolic volume decreases, the pressure-generating capability of the LV is diminished. Further, right ventricular enlargement alters left ventricular geometry adversely affecting the mechanical efficiency of left ventricular systolic contraction [32–34]. The significance of all this as it relates to the patient with increased right ventricular afterload is that the LV is responsible for generating upward of 40% of right ventricular systolic pressure [35]. This decrease in left ventricular assistance to right ventricular ejection leads to further increases in right ventricular volume and pressure, which further impairs left ventricular filling and pressure-generating capabilities. This phenomenon is known as *systolic ventricular interdependence* and plays a central role in the pathophysiology of right ventricular failure due to pulmonary hypertension [30].

Manipulating left ventricular afterload may be a strategy by which to acutely manage isolated right ventricular failure and right ventricular failure due to pulmonary hypertension [36–39]. In patients with intact left ventricular systolic function, increases in left ventricular afterload alter septal configuration as left ventricular diastolic volume and pressure increase. Further, an increase in left ventricular afterload increases the inotropic state of the LV through homeo- and heterometric autoregulation [36, 38, 39], which in conjunction with an increase in left ventricular end-diastolic volume increase left ventricular systolic pressure and stroke volume, and left ventricular assistance to right ventricular ejection [40].

9.3.4 The Effects of Respiration on Left Ventricular Afterload

Respiration may have a profound impact on left ventricular output. Changes in ITP modulate not only the pressure gradient for systemic venous return but also the pressure gradient responsible for propelling blood from the thoracic cavity. While the right atrium and vena cava are much more compliant than the systemic arterial vessels, it is the compliance and Ptm for the thoracic arterial vessels that determine the extent to which changes in ITP create a pressure gradient for driving blood from the chest and therefore to the extent that changes in ITP affect left ventricular afterload [41–43].

During spontaneous inspiration, the fall in ITP increases the Ptm and therefore volume for the thoracic arterial system. As a result, the pressure within the thoracic arterial system decreases relative to the extrathoracic arterial system, and left ventricular afterload increases [41–43]. According to Laplace's law, the effect of a decrease in ITP on left ventricular afterload is physiologically the same as a rise in the systemic arterial blood pressure (Fig. 9.3).

If the fall in ITP occurs during ventricular diastole, antegrade flow runoff decreases, resulting in an increase in thoracic arterial blood volume and an increase in the inertial forces opposing ejection during the following systole [41–44]. A fall in ITP during ventricular systole decreases the egress of blood from the thorax as well as left ventricular ejection and stroke volume [41–44]. The distension of the thoracic arterial vessels and decrease in left ventricular output are responsible for

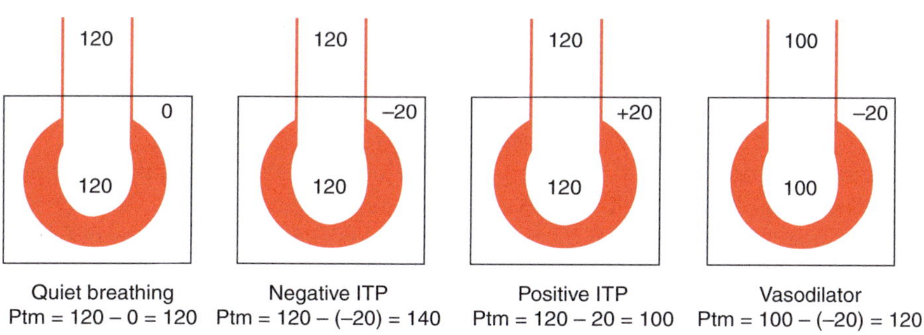

Fig. 9.3 During periods of quiet breathing in which intrathoracic pressure (ITP) is 0, the left ventricular (LV) transmural pressure (Ptm) is equal to LV systolic pressure (120 mmHg) (left-hand panel). When ITP is negative the LV distending pressure is increased and wall stress within the ventricle is elevated (the LV Ptm rises to 140 mmHg). The opposite occurs when positive pressure ventilation eliminates exaggerated negative ITP, as may be seen in cardiogenic pulmonary edema (the Ptm is reduced by 30% to 100 mmHg). The LV Ptm may also be lowered pharmacologically (right-hand panel)

the decrease in blood pressure during systole that occurs with spontaneous inspiration and is the mechanism responsible for the systolic component of pulsus paradoxus [41]. As left ventricular systolic function wanes or as ITP becomes more negative, the adverse impact of respiration on left ventricular afterload increases. Further, during exaggerated negative pressure breathing, the sympathetic nervous system is stimulated, which leads to an increase in endogenous catecholamine release, systemic vascular resistance (SVR), and arterial blood pressure, contributing to further increases in left ventricular afterload, and a vicious cycle ensues.

With PPV, the decrease in Ptm for the thoracic arterial vessels increases the pressure within creating a waterfall-like effect, driving blood into the extrathoracic arterial vessels. If the increase in ITP is confined to diastole, the LV ejects into a relatively depleted thoracic aorta with reduced inertial forces opposing ejection, while a selective increase in ITP during ventricular systole augments left ventricular ejection without compromising the gradient for systemic venous return [43, 44]. An increase in ITP therefore unloads the LV while increasing aortic diastolic and systolic pressures, creating a so-called reverse pulsus paradoxus [45, 46]. Even though aortic pressures increase, the left ventricular Ptm has decreased, as ITP has risen to a greater extent than left ventricular and thoracic arterial pressures.

Understanding the physiologic principles that govern the interplay between cardiovascular and respiratory systems is essential to optimizing the care of critically ill patients. Consideration must be given to intravascular volume status and the function of the venous capacitance vessels, whether right and/or left ventricular dysfunction is present and to what extent the primary problem is ventricular filling or emptying, and whether right and/or left ventricular afterload is affected and to what extent ventricular interdependence plays in the pathophysiologic process.

9.4 The Impact of Respiration on Cardiovascular Function in Patients with Congenital and Acquired Cardiac Disease

9.4.1 Left Ventricular Systolic Dysfunction

The most common cause of impaired left ventricular systolic function is ischemic heart disease [47, 48]. While this is relatively uncommon in adults with CHD, it may become more prevalent as the population ages [48]. Progression to heart failure in adults with CHD usually results from the hemodynamic burden of their primary defect and/or residual lesions. Nonetheless, for the most part, these patients obey the "rules" of acquired heart failure (at least acutely) and can usually be treated in a similar way.

In patients with primarily left ventricular systolic dysfunction, stroke volume and cardiac output are low despite elevated ventricular end-diastolic volume and pressure. Because pulmonary venous pressure is elevated, the impact of PPV and lung volumes on the pulmonary vasculature and right ventricular afterload is much less as a disproportionate number of lung units are in zone III conditions. If systemic venous return is reduced (preload effect), so long as the ventricles remain on the flat portion of their pressure stroke volume curve, the reduction in systemic venous return will not reduce stroke volume. Thus, the predominant effect of PPV is on reducing left ventricular afterload.

Studies have demonstrated in patients with LV systolic heart failure that stroke volume/cardiac output increases significantly so long as an adequate albeit elevated left ventricular filling pressure is present at baseline [49–54]. In patients with normal and impaired left ventricular systolic function and normal filling pressures, stroke volume will not increase and may decrease depending on the factors discussed previously [49–54].

In addition to improving cardiac output, increases in ITP and mechanical ventilation improve the myocardial and respiratory, and therefore global, oxygen supply–demand relationship by reducing myocardial and respiratory muscle oxygen consumption. In accordance with Laplace's law, by decreasing the ventricular diastolic and systolic Ptm, PPV reduces myocardial oxygen demand. In patients with cardiogenic pulmonary edema and exaggerated negative pressure breathing, the PPV-induced reduction in left ventricular systolic Ptm is profound (Fig. 9.3). In addition, by unloading the respiratory muscles, mechanical ventilation reduces respiratory muscle oxygen demand and in doing so allows for a redistribution of a limited cardiac output from the respiratory pump to other vital organs (to be discussed further below). The unloading of the respiratory pump and cardiovascular system during PPV also leads to a partial withdrawing of sympathetic nervous system activity, contributing to a reduction in SVR and left ventricular afterload (Fig. 9.3) [53, 55].

The importance of these principles has been demonstrated in several studies and in different lines of investigation. Rasanen and colleagues found that progressing from PPV to spontaneous respiration adversely affected the myocardial oxygen supply–demand relationship in patients with acute myocardial infarction complicated by respiratory failure, resulting in myocardial ischemia and significant elevations in the left ventricular filling pressure [56]. Scharf and colleagues demonstrated acute left ventricular regional akinesis in patients with preexisting left ventricular dysfunction during performance of the Mueller maneuver [57]. Jubran and colleagues demonstrated in adult patients with underlying cardiopulmonary disease receiving PPV that patients who failed a spontaneous breathing trial were unable to increase their cardiac output in order to meet the metabolic demand of the respiratory muscles, which was reflected in the progressive increase in their oxygen extraction ratios, and developed a 2.5-fold increase in left ventricular filling pressures. In contrast those patients who tolerated the spontaneous breathing trial demonstrated a significant compensatory increase in cardiac output and maintained a normal oxygen extraction ratio and left ventricular filling pressure [58].

Continuous positive airway pressure (CPAP) or PPV may be delivered noninvasively so long as the patient is cooperative. In adult patients with decompensated left ventricular systolic heart failure and pulmonary edema, meta-analyses have shown a significant reduction in the need for intubation and early mortality with noninvasive positive airway pressure [59, 60]. The long-term benefits of noninvasive positive airway pressure have also been demonstrated in adult patients with chronic heart failure. Haruki and colleagues found that the prolonged use of noninvasive PPV delivered for at least 4 h per day for 6 months led to ventricular remodeling and significantly improved left ventricular diastolic and systolic function [61].

9.4.2 Ventricular Diastolic Dysfunction

The impact of respiration in patients with ventricular diastolic dysfunction/failure has been clearly demonstrated in infants immediately following repair of tetralogy of Fallot. In these patients biventricular systolic function is usually normal; however, varying degrees of right ventricular diastolic dysfunction are common [62]. In a subset of these patients, right ventricular diastolic function is significantly impaired, and restrictive ventricular physiology is present, which is characterized by atrial systole causing ventricular diastolic pressure to rise above pulmonary artery diastolic pressure, producing diastolic pulmonary arterial flow [62–64]. Shekerdemian and colleagues demonstrated a significant increase in stroke volume and cardiac output when patients were converted from PPV to negative pressure ventilation using a cuirass (mimicking "normal" breathing), with a greater response found in those patients with restrictive ventricular physiology [64].

Restrictive and hypertrophic cardiomyopathies have varying degrees of diastolic dysfunction. Systolic function is preserved in most cases. Ventricular end-diastolic volumes may be normal or decreased, while ventricular end-diastolic pressures, and therefore pulmonary vascular pressures, are elevated [65–68]. One would expect the predominant effect of PPV to be on systemic venous return and ventricular filling. In hypertrophic cardiomyopathies, if the substrate for an obstruction to left ventricular outflow is present, by decreasing left ventricular preload and afterload, PPV may create or will exacerbate an obstruction to left ventricular outflow by reducing left ventricular systolic volumes [69, 70]. In adult patients with CHD, progression of an outflow tract obstruction will lead to compensatory concentric hypertrophy and varying degrees of diastolic dysfunction; thus one would expect the predominant effect of PPV to be on ventricular filling.

9.4.3 Specific Congenital Heart Lesions

9.4.3.1 The Fontan Circulation

Following the Fontan procedure, as in the normal circulation, the Pms is the upstream pressure for driving systemic venous return, while the pressure within the confluence of the venae cavae and pulmonary artery is the downstream pressure [71, 72]. However, because the Fontan circulation lacks a subpulmonic pumping chamber, the Pms is the upstream pressure for driving systemic venous return not only to the central confluence of the venae cavae and pulmonary artery but also the pressure responsible for driving blood across the pulmonary circulation to the common atrium [71, 72]. Over time changes within the circulation occur that serve to maintain an elevated Pms, including activation of neurohormonal pathways, leading to venoconstriction (reducing venous capacitance) and an increase in intravascular volume, as well as adaptations within the microvasculature that elevate the filtration threshold [72–74].

Spontaneous inspiration by decreasing ITP enhances systemic venous return to vena cava–pulmonary artery confluence; however, no pressure gradient is generated during respiration between the confluence and the common atrium. In addition, as ITP falls, the effective compliance of the ventricle increases, as discussed previously. Finally, a decrease in the common atrial pressure during the cardiac cycle contributes to the pressure gradient for driving pulmonary venous return [75, 76].

Because the Fontan circulation lacks a subpulmonic pumping chamber, it is particularly sensitive to increases in PVR. Further compounding this limitation is the common presence of varying degrees of diastolic dysfunction, although end-diastolic pressure is usually not elevated, and elevated ventricular afterload [77–80]. As a result of these factors, there is diminished capacity to deliver an adequate systemic venous return and in turn to generate an adequate end-diastolic pressure and volume to overcome diastolic dysfunction and elevated ventricular afterload [79–81]. For these reasons the creation of a fenestration between the vena cava and heart significantly increases cardiac output (in those with or without elevated PVR), and it is why hemi-diaphragmatic paralysis has a particularly adverse impact on inferior vena cava flow in the Fontan circulation [82–85].

Acutely following the Fontan procedure, systolic function is generally normal, while there are varying degrees of ventricular diastolic dysfunction. For these reasons, the effects of changes in ITP on systemic venous return and the ventricular diastolic Ptm predominate over its effects on afterload of the systemic ventricle. Shekerdemian and colleagues demonstrated a marked increase in pulmonary blood flow and cardiac output when patients were transitioned from PPV to negative pressure ventilation using a cuirass immediately following the Fontan procedure [86]. In those patients studied during elective cardiac catheterization remote from the time of surgery, converting from PPV to negative pressure ventilation also resulted in a significant increase in cardiac output [86].

Remote from the Fontan procedure, systolic and/or diastolic dysfunction is common [87, 88]. In those patients that develop heart failure with intact systolic function, so-called failing Fontan physiology, one would expect PPV to adversely affect stroke volume and cardiac output.

9.4.3.2 Ebstein's Anomaly

The most common presentation of symptomatic adult patients with Ebstein's anomaly is severe right ventricular dysfunction/failure and right heart enlargement resulting from long-standing tricuspid regurgitation, which may be compounded by an underlying right ventricular myopathy [89, 90]. The RV is usually very thin walled and vulnerable to progressive dilation and dysfunction due to tricuspid regurgitation. All of this will amplify the adverse effects of PPV on right heart hemodynamics. Consequently, if high airway pressures are required and lung volumes become significantly elevated, as may occur despite the judicious use of airway pressure in parenchymal lung disease (to be discussed), right ventricular stroke volume and output will fall to a greater extent than in those with relatively preserved right ventricular function. Contributing to a decrease in systemic output would be a worsening of adverse diastolic ventricular interaction and altered left ventricular geometry and systolic function. When PPV is used postoperatively, the hemodynamic milieu is usually substantially more favorable. Nonetheless, efforts should be made to minimize PVR. The use of systemic arterial vasodilators should be avoided or used judiciously, as hypotension will have an adverse effect on ventricular interdependence, while the acutely failing RV may be supported by the use of systemic vasoconstrictors, as discussed previously.

9.4.3.3 Tetralogy of Fallot

While a small percentage of patients can have persistent restrictive right ventricular physiology in the long term, most adult patients with a history of tetralogy of Fallot have right ventricular dysfunction and enlargement due to long-standing pulmonary insufficiency [89]. These patients often undergo pulmonary valve replacement, and significant complications or postoperative hemodynamic problems are rare. Nonetheless, the effects of PPV and the role of ventricular interactions on the circulation in these patients would be similar to those seen in patients with Ebstein's anomaly, and similar therapeutic strategies may be considered to improve cardiac output.

9.5 The Effects of Respiratory Disease on Cardiovascular Function

9.5.1 Sleep-Disordered Breathing

Sleep-disordered breathing (SDB) occurs in 5–10% of the general population. In patients with cardiovascular disease, the incidence increases significantly ranging between 47% and 83%, depending on the specific disorder surveyed [91]. Obstructive SDB (OSDB) like other diseases of the respiratory system primarily affects cardiovascular function by altering ITP. OSDB is characterized by repetitive episodes of inspiratory flow limitation or cessation of inspiratory flow and occurs when sleep-related withdrawal of respiratory drive to the upper airway dilator muscles is superimposed on an upper airway with underlying structural and/or functional abnormalities, leading to the generation of exaggerated negative ITP. Upper airway obstruction also causes hypoxia and acidosis, increasing pulmonary vascular resistance. The increase in the work of breathing also activates the sympathetic nervous system and renin–angiotensin–aldosterone systems, contributing to increases in biventricular afterload [92]. Exaggerated negative pressure breathing also leads to an increase in system venous return and diastolic ventricular interaction, contributing to a decrease in left ventricular output.

The impact of exaggerated negative pressure breathing and an increase in biventricular afterload on cardiovascular function is greatest in subjects with underlying left ventricular systolic dysfunction. Contributing to the spectrum of sleep-disordered breathing seen in patients with heart failure is the relatively common finding of central sleep apnea, which is manifested as Cheyne–Stokes respiration, a form of periodic breathing with a crescendo–decrescendo pattern of breathing [91]. Stimulation of pulmonary vagal irritant receptors by pulmonary edema augments the respiratory drive causing hyperventilation and a decrease in the $PaCO_2$, which falls below the apnea threshold, leading to a loss of central drive. Ventilation returns as carbon dioxide production increases the $PaCO_2$ to levels above the apnea threshold, stimulating hyperventilation, which in turn causes the $PaCO_2$ to fall below the apnea threshold. Bradley and colleagues demonstrated that central events alone did not cause stroke volume to decrease, while isolated obstructive events caused a significant decrease in stroke volume in adult patients with heart failure [93].

The net effect of obstructive and central sleep apnea in patients with a limited cardiac output is a disturbance in the oxygen supply–demand relationship for all viscera, including the brain and myocardium, leading to repeated episodes of ischemia reperfusion injury [91]. The adverse impact of these effects on the myocardium is exemplified in the findings by Kuniyoshi and colleagues who evaluated the relationship between the day and night variation of presentation for acute myocardial infarction [94]. The odds of having OSDB in those patients whose acute myocardial infarction occurred during sleeping hours was sixfold higher than in those having an acute myocardial infarction during the remainder of the day, and of all the patients having an acute myocardial infarction between midnight and 6 a.m., 91% had OSDB.

The cumulative effects of sleep-disordered breathing on cardiovascular function can precipitate or contribute to the development of ventricular remodeling and right and left ventricular diastolic and systolic disease [91, 95–98]. Noninvasive continuous positive airway pressure has been shown to reverse ventricular remodeling and improve biventricular diastolic and systolic function while chronically lowering systemic blood pressure [95, 99].

9.5.2 The Acute Respiratory Distress Syndrome and Cardiovascular Function

The use of PPV in patients with the acute respiratory distress syndrome (ARDS) may induce significant cardiopulmonary interactions that adversely impact gas exchange, cardiac output, and ultimately systemic oxygen delivery. Jardin and colleagues evaluated patients receiving PPV for ARDS and found a significant decrease in right ventricular shortening and increase in right ventricular systolic dimensions consistent with an increase in right ventricular impedance, which was temporally related to the inspiratory phase of PPV [100, 101]. Right ventricular end-diastolic dimensions remained unchanged consistent with a limitation of systemic venous return, since an increase in right ventricular afterload should lead to an increase in right ventricular end-diastolic volume. The extent to which alveolar overdistension occurs during PPV decreases with the use of a volume-protective strategy. Nonetheless, due to the nonhomogeneous distribution of disease in ARDS, even the judicious use of positive airway pressure does not preclude the development of alveolar overdistension [102, 103]. The creation of zone I conditions in the lungs in addition to the underlying pathophysiology of ARDS including hypoxic pulmonary vasoconstriction due to atelectasis, pulmonary endothelial injury and dysfunction, and microvascular occlusion due to dysregulated coagulation contributes to increases in PVR, which may not be tolerated in patients with underlying right ventricular dysfunction [104, 105].

An additional related interaction between the cardiovascular and pulmonary systems that is seen in patients receiving PPV for ARDS is the not uncommon occurrence of a patent foramen ovale, which allows for right to left atrial shunting [106]. The presence of right to left shunting in patients with a patent foramen ovale has been shown to be associated with significantly greater pulmonary arterial pressures and RV dimensions than seen in patients with a patent foramen ovale and no cardiac shunting [106]. It is important to consider not only the impact of continuous positive airway pressure and PPV on oxygenation in patients with hypoxic respiratory failure but also to consider the impact of these therapies on cardiac output and ultimately systemic oxygen delivery.

9.6 The Impact of Cardiovascular Disease on Respiratory Function

9.6.1 Heart Failure and Respiratory Function

Under normal conditions, the diaphragm consumes less than 3% of global oxygen consumption and receives less than 5% of cardiac output. However, with an increase in respiratory load, diaphragmatic oxygen consumption may increase to values over 50% of total oxygen consumption [107, 108]. The increase in respiratory muscle oxygen consumption correlates with an increase in minute ventilation and increases further with impairment of respiratory mechanics. Because the baseline arteriovenous oxygen content difference for the diaphragm is high, diaphragmatic blood flow must increase to meet the increase in oxygen demand, which if cardiac output is limited occurs at the expense of other vital organs [107, 108].

Studies using animal models of cardiogenic and septic shock have evaluated the distribution of cardiac output during spontaneous and mechanical ventilation [109, 110]. Viires and colleagues as well as Hussain and colleagues demonstrated that respiratory muscle blood flow increases significantly in animal models of shock. Both studies demonstrated that in animals receiving mechanical ventilation, respiratory muscle blood flow is significantly less and perfusion to other vital organs, including the brain, is significantly greater than that seen in the spontaneously breathing animals. These studies demonstrate that diaphragmatic blood flow is protected to an equal or even greater extent than is cerebral blood flow when cardiac output is limited and that by unloading the respiratory pump, mechanical ventilation allows for a redistribution of a limited cardiac output to other vital organs. Separate from PPV-induced increases in ITP and decreases in ventricular afterload, mechanical ventilation represents an additional tool in the armamentarium to treat low cardiac output states.

There is also a competition for blood flow among vital viscera in patients with heart failure and a limited cardiac output. In subjects without underlying cardiac disease undergoing strenuous exercise, perfusion of the brain as well as muscles of locomotion becomes relatively limited, as manifested by changes in near-infrared spectroscopy (NIRS)-derived oxygenation indices [111, 112]. In patients at rest with compensated heart failure, cerebral oxygenation may be significantly depressed [113–115]. In patients with compensated heart failure undergoing exercise, oxygenation of the cerebrum decreases further as muscles of respiration and locomotion become loaded [116–118]. Further, with therapies that improve cardiac output such as cardiac transplantation, cardiac resynchronization therapy, and afterload reduction, cerebral blood flow increases significantly [115, 119, 120]. Not only may cerebral blood flow be limited and contribute to impaired cognition in patients with chronic heart failure [121–123], but in patients with decompensated heart failure, cerebral oxygenation may become more depressed and approach if not exceed the anaerobic threshold for the brain in the absence of hypotension. The discussion of competition for a limited cardiac output in spontaneously breathing subjects is germane to a review of cardiopulmonary interaction because it highlights an important and unique interplay between the two systems that plays a key role in the acute management of heart failure and shock.

Conclusion

Under normal conditions, the interplay between the respiratory and cardiovascular systems is inconsequential. However, in the presence of underlying cardiopulmonary disease, the importance of the interaction between these two organ systems cannot be overstated. A thorough understanding and the clinical application of cardiopulmonary interactions are essential to management of patients with congenital and acquired cardiovascular disease.

References

1. Guyton AC, Jones CE, Coleman TG. Peripheral vascular contribution to cardiac output regulation—the concept of "venous return". In: Guyton AC, Jones CE, Coleman TG, editors. Circulatory physiology: cardiac output and its regulation. 2nd ed. Philadelphia, PA: WB Saunders; 1973. p. 173–87.
2. Funk DJ, Jacobsohn E, Kumar A. The role of venous return in critical illness and shock—part I: physiology. Crit Care Med. 2013;41:255–62.
3. Gelman S. Venous function and central venous pressure. Anesthesiology. 2008;108:735–48.
4. Herndon CW, Sagawa K. Combined effects of aortic and right atrial pressures on aortic flow. Am J Phys. 1969;217:65–72.
5. Landis EM, Hortenstine JC. Functional significance of venous blood pressure. Am Physiol Soc. 1950;30:1–32.
6. Hatanakah T, Potts JT. Invariance of the resistance to venous return to carotid sinus baroreflex control. Am J Phys. 1996;271(3 Pt 2):H1022–30.
7. Caldini P, Permutt S, Waddell JA, et al. Effect of epinephrine on pressure, flow, and volume relationships in the systemic circulation in dogs. Circ Res. 1974;34:606–23.

8. Greene AS, Shoukas AA. Changes in canine cardiac function and venous return curves by the carotid baroreflex. Am J Phys. 1986;251:H288–96.
9. Guyton AC, Lindsey AW, Abernathy B, et al. Mechanism of the increased venous return and cardiac output caused by epinephrine. Am J Phys. 1958;192:126–30.
10. Guyton AC, Richardson TQ. Effect of hematocrit on venous return. Circ Res. 1961;9:157–64.
11. Rothe CF. Mean circulatory filling pressure: its meaning and measurement. J Appl Physiol. 1993;74:499–509.
12. Guyton AC, Jones CE, Coleman TG. Mean circulatory pressure, mean systemic pressure, and mean pulmonary pressure and their effects on venous return. In: Guyton AC, Jones CE, Coleman TG, editors. Circulatory physiology: cardiac output and its regulation. 2nd ed. Philadelphia, PA: WB Saunders; 1973. p. 205–21.
13. Drees JA, Rothe CF. Reflex venoconstriction and capacity vessel pressure-volume relationships in dogs. Circ Res. 1974;XXXIV:360–73.
14. O'Brien LJ. Negative diastolic pressure in the isolated hypothermic dog heart. Circ Res. 1960;10:188–96.
15. Nakatani S, Beppu S, Nagata S, et al. Diastolic suction in the human ventricle: observation during balloon mitral valvuloplasty with a single balloon. Am Heart J. 1994;127:143–7.
16. Yellin EL, Hori M, Yoran H, et al. Left ventricular relaxation in the filling and nonfilling intact canine heart. Am J Phys. 1986;250:H620–9.
17. Takata M, Wise RA, Robotham JL. Effects of abdominal pressure on venous return: abdominal vascular zone conditions. J Appl Physiol. 1990;69:1961–72.
18. Takata M, Robotham JL. Effects of inspiratory diaphragmatic descent on inferior vena caval venous return. J Appl Physiol. 1992;72:597–607.
19. Lloyd TC Jr. Effect of inspiration on inferior vena caval blood flow in dogs. J Appl Phyisol. 1983;55:1701–8.
20. Karim F, Hainsworth R. Responses of abdominal vascular capacitance to stimulation of splanchnic nerves. Am J Phys. 1976;231:434–40.
21. Guyton AC, Adkins LH. Quantitative aspects of the collapse factor in relation to venous return. Am J Phys. 1954;177:523–7.
22. Bark H, LeRoith D, Myska M, et al. Elevations in plasma ADH levels during PEEP ventilation in the dog: mechanisms involved. Am J Phys. 1980;239:E474–80.
23. Scharf SM, Ingram RH Jr. Influence of abdominal pressure and sympathetic vasoconstriction on the cardiovascular response to positive end-expiratory pressure. Am Rev Respir Dis. 1977;116:661–70.
24. Pinsky M. Determinants of pulmonary arterial flow variation during respiration. J Appl Physiol. 1984;56:1237–45.
25. Cabrera MR, Nakamura GE, Montague DA, et al. Effect of airway pressure on pericardial pressure. Am Rev Respir Dis. 1989;140:659 667.
26. Novak R, Matuschak GM, Pinsky MR. Effect of positive-pressure ventilatory frequency on regional pleural pressure. J Appl Physiol. 1988;65:1314–23.
27. Fewell JE, Abendschein DR, Carlson J, et al. Mechanism of decreased right and left ventricular end-diastolic volumes during continuous positive-pressure ventilation in dogs. Circ Res. 1980;47:467–72.
28. O'Quin R, Marini JJ. Pulmonary artery occlusion pressure: clinical physiology, measurement, and interpretation. Am Rev Respir Dis. 1983;128:319–26.
29. Takata M, Robotham JL. Ventricular external constraint by the lung and pericardium during positive end-expiratory pressure. Am Rev Respir Dis. 1991;143:872–5.
30. Bronicki RA, Baden HP. Pathophysiology of right ventricular failure in pulmonary hypertension. Pediatr Crit Care Med. 2010;11(Suppl):S15–22.
31. Peters J, Kindred MK, Robotham JL. Transient analysis of cardiopulmonary interactions. I. Diastolic events. J Appl Physiol. 1988;64:1506–17.
32. Buckberg G, Hoffman JIE, Nanda NC. Ventricular torsion and untwisting: further insights into mechanics and timing interdependence: a viewpoint. Echocardiography. 2011;28:782–804.
33. van Dalen BM, Kauer F, Vletter WB, et al. Influence of cardiac shape on left ventricular twist. J Appl Physiol. 2010;108:146–51.

34. Brookes C, Ravn H, White P, et al. Acute right ventricular dilatation in response to ischemia significantly impairs left ventricular systolic performance. Circulation. 1999;100:761–7.
35. Santamore WP, Gray L. Significant left ventricular contributions to right ventricular systolic function. Chest. 1995;107:1134–45.
36. Belenkie I, Horne SG, Dani R, et al. Effects of aortic constriction during experimental acute right ventricular pressure loading. Circulation. 1995;92:546–54.
37. Ricciardi MJ, Bossone E, Bach DS, et al. Echocardiographic predictors of an adverse response to a nifedipine trial in primary pulmonary hypertension: diminished left ventricular size and leftward ventricular septal bowing. Chest. 1999;116:1218–23.
38. Apitz C, Honjo O, Humpl T, et al. Biventricular structural and functional responses to aortic constriction in a rabbit model of chronic right ventricular pressure overload. J Thorac Cardiovasc Surg. 2012;144:1494–501.
39. Apitz C, Honjo O, Friedberg MK, et al. Beneficial effects of vasopressors on right ventricular function in experimental acute right ventricular failure in a rabbit model. Thorac Cardiovasc Surg. 2012;60:17–25.
40. Page RD, Harringer W, Hodakowski GT, et al. Determinants of maximal right ventricular function. J Heart Lung Transplant. 1992;11:90–8.
41. Peters J, Kindred MK, Robotham JL. Transient analysis of cardiopulmonary interaction. II. Systolic events. J Appl Physiol. 1988;64:1518–26.
42. Fessler HE, Brower RG, Wise RA, et al. Mechanism of reduced LV afterload by systolic and diastolic positive pleural pressure. J Appl Physiol. 1988;65:1244–50.
43. Pinsky MR, Matuschak GM, Bernardi L, et al. Hemodynamic effects of cardiac cycle-specific increases in intrathoracic pressure. J Appl Physiol. 1986;60:604–12.
44. Pinsky MR, Marquez J, Martin D, et al. Ventricular assist by cardiac cycle-specific increases in intrathoracic pressure. Chest. 1987;91:709–15.
45. Viellard-Baron A, Chergui K, Augarde R, et al. Cyclic changes in arterial pulse during respiratory support revisited by Doppler echocardiography. Am J Respir Crit Care Med. 2003;168:671–6.
46. Massumi RA, Mason DT, Vera Z, et al. Reversed pulsus paradoxus. New Engl J Med. 1973;289:1272–5.
47. He J, Ogden LG, Bazzano LA, et al. Risk factors for congestive heart failure in US men and women: NHANES I epidemiologic follow-up study. Arch Intern Med. 2001;161:996–1002.
48. Giannakoulas G, Dimopoulos K, Engel R, et al. Burden of coronary artery disease in adults with congenital heart disease and its relation to congenital and traditional heart risk factors. Am J Cardiol. 2009;103:1445–50.
49. Grace MP, Greenbaum DM. Cardiac performance in response to PEEP in patients with cardiac dysfunction. Crit Care Med. 1982;10:358–60.
50. Bradley TD, Holloway RM, McLauglin PR, et al. Cardiac output response to continuous positive airway pressure in congestive heart failure. Am Rev Respir Dis. 1982;145:377–82.
51. Scharf SM. Ventilatory support in cardiac failure. Curr Opin Crit Care. 1997;3:71–7.
52. Rasanen J, Vaisanen IT, Heikkila J, et al. Acute myocardial infarction complicated by left ventricular dysfunction and respiratory failure. The effects of continuous positive airway pressure. Chest. 1985;87:158–62.
53. Scharf SM, Chen L, Rao PS. Effects of continuous positive airway pressure on cardiac output and plasma norepinephrine in sedated pigs. J Crit Care. 1996;11:57–64.
54. Genovese J, Moskowitz M, Tarasiuk A, et al. Effects of continuous positive airway pressure on cardiac output in normal and hypervolemic unanesthetized pigs. Am J Respir Crit Care Med. 1994;150:752–8.
55. Kennedy SK, Weintraub RM, Skillman JJ. Cardiorespiratory and sympathoadrenal responses during weaning from controlled ventilation. Surgery. 1977;82:233–40.
56. Rasanen J, Nikki P, Heikkila J. Acute myocardial infarction complicated by respiratory failure. Chest. 1984;85:21–8.
57. Scharf SM, Bianco JA, Tow DE, et al. The effects of large negative intrathoracic pressure on left ventricular function in patients with coronary artery disease. Circulation. 1981;63:871–5.

58. Jubran A, Mathru M, Dries D, et al. Continuous recordings of mixed venous oxygen saturation during weaning from mechanical ventilation and the ramifications thereof. Am J Respir Crit Care Med. 1998;158:1763–9.
59. Winck J, Azevedo LF, Costa-Pereira A, et al. Efficacy and safety of non-invasive ventilation in the treatment of acute cardiogenic pulmonary edema—a systematic review and meta-analysis. Crit Care. 2006;10:1–18.
60. Massip J, Roque M, Sanchez B, et al. Noninvasive ventilation in acute cardiogenic pulmonary edema. JAMA. 2005;294:3124–30.
61. Haruki N, Takeuchi M, Kaku K, et al. Comparison of acute and chronic impact of adaptive servo-ventilation on left chamber geometry and function in patients with chronic heart failure. Eur J Heart Fail. 2011;10:1140–6.
62. Cullen S, Shore D, Redington A. Characterization of right ventricular diastolic performance after complete repair of tetralogy of Fallot. Circulation. 1995;91:1782–9.
63. Appleton CP, Hatle LK, Popp RL. Demonstration of restrictive ventricular physiology by Doppler echocardiography. J Am Coll Cardiol. 1988;11:757–68.
64. Shekerdemian LS, Bush A, Shore DF, et al. Cardiorespiratory responses to negative pressure ventilation after tetralogy of Fallot repair: a hemodynamic tool for patients with a low-output state. J Am Coll Cardiol. 1999;33:549–55.
65. Kushwaha SS, Fallon JT, Fuster V. Restrictive cardiomyopathy. N Engl J Med. 1997;336:267–76.
66. Fifer MA, Vlahakes GJ. Management of symptoms in hypertrophic cardiomyopathy. Circulation. 2008;117:429–39.
67. Gotsman MS, Lewis BS. Left ventricular volumes and compliance in hypertrophic cardiomyopathy. Chest. 1974;66:498–505.
68. Thomson HL, Morris-Thurgood J, Atherton J, et al. Reflex responses of venous capacitance vessels in patients with hypertrophic cardiomyopathy. Clin Sci. 1998;94:339–46.
69. Braunwald E, Oldham H Jr, Ross J, et al. The circulatory response of patients with idiopathic hypertrophic subaortic stenosis to nitroglycerin and to the Valsalva maneuver. Circulation. 1964;29:422–31.
70. Braunwald E, Ebert PA. Hemodynamic alterations in idiopathic hypertrophic subaortic stenosis induced by sympathomimetic drugs. Am J Cardiol. 1962;10:489–95.
71. Mace L, Dervanian P, Bourriez A, et al. Changes in venous return parameters associated with univentricular Fontan circulations. Am J Physiol Heart Circ Physiol. 2000;279:H2335–43.
72. Myers CD, Ballman K, Riegle LE, et al. Mechanisms of systemic adaptation to univentricular Fontan conversion. J Thorac Cardiovasc Surg. 2010;140:850–6.
73. Kelley JR, Mack GW, Fahey JT. Diminished venous vascular capacitance in patients with univentricular hearts after the Fontan operation. Am J Cardiol. 1995;76:158–63.
74. Krishnan US, Taneja I, Gewitz M, et al. Peripheral vascular adaptation and orthostatic tolerance in Fontan physiology. Circulation. 2009;120:1775–83.
75. Fogel MA, Weinberg PM, Hoydu A, et al. The nature of low in the systemic venous pathway measured by magnetic resonance blood tagging in patients having the Fontan operation. J Thorac Cardiovasc Surg. 1997;114:1032–41.
76. Qureshi S, Richheimer R, McKay R, et al. Doppler echocardiographic evaluation of pulmonary artery flow after modified Fontan operation: importance of atrial contractions. Br Heart J. 1990;64:272–6.
77. Penny DJ, Rigby ML, Redington AN. Abnormal patterns of intraventricular flow and diastolic filling after the Fontan operation: evidence for incoordinate ventricular wall motion. Br Heart J. 1991;66:375–8.
78. Cheung YF, Penny DJ, Redington AN. Serial assessment of left ventricular diastolic function after Fontan procedure. Heart. 2000;83:420–4.
79. Rychik J, Goldberg DJ. Late consequences of the Fontan operation. Circulation. 2014;130:1525–8.
80. Gewillig M, Brown SC. The Fontan circulation after 45 years: update in physiology. Heart. 2016;102:1081–6.

81. Anderson PAW, Sleeper LA, Mahony L, et al. Contemporary outcomes after the Fontan procedure: a pediatric heart network multicenter study. J Am Coll Cardiol. 2008;52:85–98.
82. Lloyd TR, Rydberg A, Ludomirsky A, et al. Late fenestration closure in the hypoplastic left heart syndrome: comparison of hemodynamic changes. Am Heart J. 1998;136:302–6.
83. Grosse-Wortmann L, Dragulescu A, Drolet C, et al. Determinants and clinical significance of flow via the fenestration in the Fontan pathway: a multimodality study. Int J Cardiol. 2013;168:811–7.
84. Kuhn MA, Jarmakani JM, Laks H, et al. Effect of late postoperative atrial septal defect closure on hemodynamic function in patients with a lateral tunnel Fontan procedure. J Am Coll Cardiol. 1995;26:259–65.
85. Hsia T-Y, Khambadkone S, Redington AN, et al. Effects of respiration and gravity on infradiaphragmatic venous flow in normal and Fontan patients. Circulation. 2000;102(Suppl III):III-148–53.
86. Shekerdemian LS, Bush A, Shore DF, et al. Cardiopulmonary interactions after the Fontan operation. Augmentation of cardiac output using negative pressure ventilation. Circulation. 1997;96:3934–42.
87. Jayakumar KA, Addonizio LJ, Kichuk-Chrisant MR, et al. Cardiac transplantation after the Fontan or Glenn procedure. J Am Coll Cardiol. 2004;44:2065–72.
88. Griffiths ER, Kaza AK, Wyler von Ballmoos MC, et al. Evaluating failing Fontans for heart transplantation: predictors of mortality. Ann Thorac Surg. 2009;88:558–64.
89. Warnes CA. Adult congenital heart disease. J Am Coll Cardiol. 2009;54:1903–10.
90. Anderson KR, Lie JT. The right ventricular myocardium in Ebstein's anomaly: a morphometric histopathologic study. Mayo Clin Proc. 1979;54:181–4.
91. Kasai T, Floras JS, Bradley TD. Sleep apnea and cardiovascular disease: a bidirectional relationship. Circulation. 2012;126:1495–510.
92. Somers VK, Dyken ME, Abboud FM. Sympathetic neural mechanisms in obstructive sleep apnea. J Clin Invest. 1995;96:1897–904.
93. Yumino D, Kasai T, Kimmerly D, et al. Differing effects of obstructive and central sleep apneas on stroke volume in patients with heart failure. Am J Respir Crit Care Med. 2013;187:433–8.
94. Kuniyoshi F, Garcia-Touchard A, Gami AS, et al. Day-night variation of acute myocardial infarction in obstructive sleep apnea. J Am Coll Cardiol. 2008;52:343–6.
95. Arias MA, Garcia-Rio F, Alonso-Fernandez A, et al. Obstructive sleep apnea syndrome affects left ventricular diastolic function: effects of nasal continuous positive airway pressure in men. Circulation. 2005;112:375–83.
96. Sofer S, Weinhouse E, Tal A, et al. Cor pulmonale due to adenoid or tonsillar hypertrophy or both in children. Chest. 1988;93:119–22.
97. Amin RS, Kimball TR, Bean JA, et al. Left ventricular hypertrophy and abnormal ventricular geometry in children and adolescent with obstructive sleep apnea. Am J Crit Care Respir Med. 2002;165:1395–9.
98. Shivalkar B, Van De Heyning C, Kerremans M, et al. Obstructive sleep apnea syndrome. More insights on structural and functional cardiac alterations, and the effects of treatment with continuous positive airway pressure. J Am Coll Cardiol. 2006;47:1433–9.
99. Kaneko Y, Floras JS, Usui K, et al. Cardiovascular effects of continuous positive airway pressure in patients with heart failure and obstructive sleep apnea. N Engl J Med. 2003;348:1233–41.
100. Vieillard-Baron A, Loubieres Y, Schmitt J-M, et al. Cyclic changes in right ventricular output impedance during mechanical ventilation. J Appl Physiol. 1999;87:1644–50.
101. Jardin F, Viellard-Baron A. Right ventricular function and positive pressure ventilation in clinical practice: from hemodynamic subsets to respirator settings. Intensive Care Med. 2003;29:1426–34.
102. Bone R. The ARDS lung: new insights from computed tomography. JAMA. 1993;269:2134–5.
103. Gattinoni L, Marini JJ, Pesenti A, et al. The "baby lung" became an adult. Intensive Care Med. 2016;42:663–73.

104. Price LC, McAuley DF, Marino PS, et al. Pathophysiology of pulmonary hypertension in acute lung injury. Am J Physiol Lung Cell Mol Physiol. 2010;302:L803–15.
105. Hill NS, Roberts K, Preston I. Editorial. Pulmonary vasculopathy in acute respiratory distress syndrome. Something new, something old…. Am J Respir Crit Care Med. 2010;182:1093–7.
106. Dessap AM, Boissier F, Leon R, et al. Prevalence and prognosis shunting across patent foramen ovale during acute respiratory distress syndrome. Crit Care Med. 2010;38:1786–92.
107. Roussos C, Macklem PT. The respiratory muscles. N Engl J Med. 1982;307:786–97.
108. Rochester DF, Bettini G. Diaphragmatic blood flow and energy expenditure in the dog. Effects of inspiratory airflow resistance and hypercapnia. J Clin Invest. 1976;57:661–72.
109. Viires N, Aubier SM, Rassidakis A, et al. Regional blood flow distribution in dog during induced hypotension and low cardiac output. J Clin Invest. 1983;72:935–47.
110. Hussain SNA, Roussos C. Distribution of respiratory muscle and organ blood flow during endotoxic shock in dogs. J Appl Physiol. 1985;59:1802–8.
111. Thomas R, Stephane P. Prefrontal cortex oxygenation and neuromuscular responses to exhaustive exercise. Eur J Appl Physiol. 2008;102:153–63.
112. Rooks CR, Thom NJ, McCully KK, et al. Effects of incremental exercise on cerebral oxygenation measured by near-infrared spectroscopy: a systematic review. Prog Neurobiol. 2010;92:134–50.
113. Madsen PL, Nielsen HB, Christiansen P. Well-being and cerebral oxygen saturation during acute heart failure in humans. Clin Physiol. 2000;20:158–64.
114. Choi B-R, Kim JS, Yang YJ, et al. Factors associated with decreased cerebral blood flow in congestive heart failure secondary to idiopathic dilated cardiomyopathy. Am J Cardiol. 2006;97:1365–9.
115. Gruhn N, Larsen FS, Boesgaard S, et al. Cerebral flood flow in patients with chronic heart failure before and after heart transplantation. Stroke. 2001;32:2530–3.
116. Fu T-C, Wang C-H, Hsu C-C, et al. Suppression of cerebral hemodynamics is associated with reduced functional capacity in patients with heart failure. Am J Physiol Heart Circ Physiol. 2011;300:H1545–55.
117. Koike A, Hoshimoto M, Tajima A, et al. Critical level of cerebral oxygenation during exercise in patients with left ventricular dysfunction. Circ J. 2006;70:1457–61.
118. Koike A, Hoshimoto M, Nagayama O, et al. Cerebral oxygenation during exercise and exercise recovery in patients with idiopathic dilated cardiomyopathy. Am J Cardiol. 2004;94:821–4.
119. Van Bommel RJ, Marsan NA, Koppen H, et al. Effect of cardiac resynchronization therapy on cerebral blood flow. Am J Cardiol. 2010;106:73–7.
120. Rajagopalan B, Raine AEG, Cooper R, et al. Changes in cerebral blood flow in patients with severe congestive cardiac failure before and after captopril treatment. Am J Med. 1984;76:86–90.
121. Luijckx G-J, van den Berg MP. Heart failure and the brain, a wake-up call. Eur J Heart Fail. 2011;13:597–8.
122. Vogels RL, Oosterman JM, Laman DM, et al. Transcranial Doppler blood flow assessment in patients with mild heart failure: correlates with neuroimaging and cognitive performance. Congest Heart Fail. 2008;14:61–5.
123. Lee CW, Lee J-H, Kim J-J, et al. Cerebral metabolic abnormalities in congestive heart failure detected by proton magnetic resonance spectroscopy. J Am Coll Cardiol. 1999;33:1196–202.

Critical Care Management of the Adult with Tetralogy of Fallot

10

Giuseppe Isgro, Marco Ranucci, and Massimo Chessa

10.1 Introduction

Tetralogy of Fallot (ToF) in adulthood is one of the most frequent cardiac anomalies that need surgery for different reasons, of which replacement of severely regurgitant pulmonary valve and correction of residual defects following previous surgeries (i.e., residual ventricular septal defect (VSD) or right ventricle outflow tract (RVOT) obstruction) are the most frequent [1].

Complete correction of ToF in natural history is uncommon in developed countries but can be more frequent in developing countries or for patients coming from environments where a congenital cardiac surgery program is not available.

Surgery involving the RV in the adult ToF patient is always a challenge for anesthesiologists and intensivists who take care of these complex patients.

The expertise required for the appropriate treatment of these patients belongs to the congenital heart domain, and physicians used to treat pediatric congenital heart patients are probably better poised to be in charge of the perioperative management of these patients. However, the expertise that characterizes clinicians and surgeons trained with adult patients is also needed; hence, the ideal hospital setting is that of a cardiac surgical program that treats both adult and pediatric patients. Moreover, adults with congenital heart disease (ACHD) experience long-term modifications of cardiovascular physiology that affect multiple organ systems and may relatively

G. Isgro (✉)
Congenital Cardiac Intensive Care Unit, IRCCS Policlinico San Donato, Milan, Italy

M. Ranucci
Department of Cardiothoracic and Vascular Anesthesia and Intensive Care, IRCCS Policlinico San Donato, Milan, Italy

M. Chessa
Pediatric and Adult Congenital Heart Center, IRCCS Policlinico San Donato, Milan, Italy
e-mail: Massimo.Chessa@grupposandonato.it

E. da Cruz et al. (eds.), *Intensive Care of the Adult with Congenital Heart Disease*, Congenital Heart Disease in Adolescents and Adults,
https://doi.org/10.1007/978-3-319-94171-4_10

increase the risk of failure in the postoperative period, and this is the most important reason to involve a multidisciplinary team with specific training in ACHD care before and after surgery.

This chapter deals with perioperative problems in adult ToF, focusing on the different models of RV perioperative pathophysiology, pharmacological treatment of the failing RV, hemodynamic monitoring, and mechanical circulatory support of refractory RV failure.

10.2 Pathophysiological Aspects of the RV in Adult Tetralogy of Fallot

Adult ToF patients may present to the operating room with different pathophysiologic conditions of the RV function. Basically, patients scheduled for late corrective surgery of a ToF have a chronic RV pressure overload that, after correction, may be converted into an acute volume overload. Conversely, patients who undergo surgery for severe pulmonary regurgitation after a previous ToF correction have a pattern of chronic volume overload. Patients requiring correction of a residual RVOT obstruction may have a mixed pattern of chronic pressure and volume overload. Finally, when the operation is required for correction of residual VSD, the hemodynamic pattern depends on the extent of the left-to-right shunt and consequent degree of pulmonary hypertension, the severity of pulmonary regurgitation, and the presence of residual RVOT obstruction. In the setting of ACHD patients, acute right ventricular systolic dysfunction is relatively uncommon. Indeed, maladaptive right ventricular systolic dysfunction, with RV dilatation and reduced ejection fraction, is rather a common manifestation of end-stage congenital heart disease. The congenitally malformed RV is not immune to coronary ischemia (e.g., after surgery involving the right coronary artery) and can be more directly adversely affected by specific congenital heart operations (e.g., surgery for pulmonary valve replacement). Since the RV is so dependent on a low afterload for optimal function, all efforts should be made to minimize afterload. For these reasons, ventilation support, cardiovascular drugs, and correct fluid replacement avoiding fluid overload have a significant influence on early postoperative outcome. Generally, the right ventricle is considered a volume-loaded ventricle rather than a pressure-loaded ventricle; this entails that it tolerates better volume overload than pressure overload, especially in congenital heart disease conditions. In normal individuals, the pulmonary circulation is a low resistance, high capacitance system capable of accommodating a three- to fourfold increase in RV stroke volume without significantly raising pulmonary pressures. In pathological conditions, alteration of the geometry of the RV makes the chamber poorly tolerant to acute elevations in afterload mainly because it can cause acute RV dilation, with resultant RV failure. Right ventricular systolic function is also dependent on RV preload. Elevations in RV preload most commonly occur secondary to an elevation in intravascular volume or tricuspid regurgitation. With progressive RV dilation, the RV works on the descending part of the Frank-Starling curve,

Table 10.1 Clinical manifestation of RV dysfunction

• Hypotension
• Tachycardia
• Elevated right atrial pressure
• Oliguria
• Anuria
• Acute kidney injury
• Oxygen desaturation
• Liver dysfunction
• Ascites
• Pleural effusion
• Right jugular vein distension
• Coagulation dysfunction

causing cardiac output reduction. The most important clinical manifestations of RV dysfunction soon after congenital cardiac surgery procedures are listed in Table 10.1.

10.3 Tetralogy of Fallot: Natural History or After Palliation

Unoperated ToF patients surviving the natural history, or those who were submitted to shunt palliation during infancy, suffer for different and severe degrees of RV chronic pressure overload that induce RV hypertrophy. This pattern is always accompanied by a RV diastolic dysfunction, with elevation of the right ventricular end-diastolic pressure (RVEDP), whereas the systolic function may be normal or decreased. It has been demonstrated that previous palliation more frequently determines an impaired systolic function of the RV. In a retrospective series of 52 adult patients who underwent total repair of ToF, Attenhofer Jost and coworkers [2] found that patients with previous palliation had a significantly higher rate of decreased RV ejection fraction before the operation (70% vs. 4% in non-palliated patients), increased central venous pressure (CVP), and signs of caval stasis, with impaired venous return mainly at the level of the inferior vena cava and visceral organs. Both chronic cyanosis and increased RVEDP are risk factors for kidney injury in the postoperative course of any surgery for adult ToF. Echocardiography is the first line method for the assessment of the RV function (Fig. 10.1), routinely performed in the early follow-up of patient after correction of ToF.

Quantification of the RV diastolic dysfunction is based on echocardiographic measurements that are derived from those developed for the left ventricle. The trans-tricuspid diastolic flow pattern may be explored using the same relative changes in E- and A-wave velocities, E/A ratios, and deceleration time as for trans-mitral diastolic flow in left ventricle relaxation analysis [3]. Tissue Doppler evaluation of the tricuspid valve motion may partially overcome the loading-dependent changes in trans-tricuspid valve diastolic flow. Additional information may be obtained by the analysis of the hepatic flow pattern with transesophageal echocardiography (TEE) and by analogy to the pulmonary vein flow for the left ventricle [4]. Finally, restrictive RV filling may be diagnosed in the presence of a late

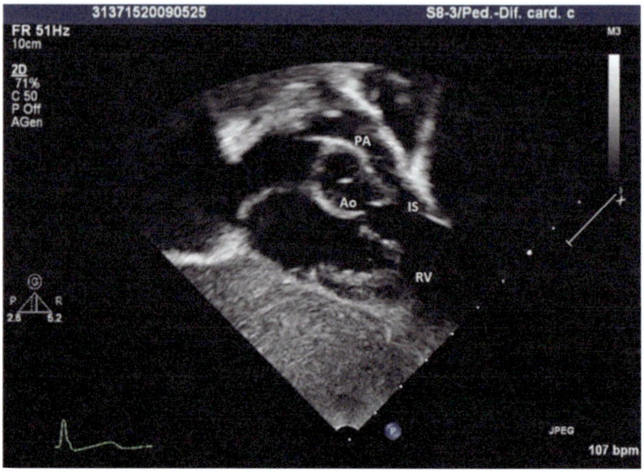

Fig. 10.1 Tetralogy of Fallot (natural history): echocardiography (*Ao* aorta, *PA* stenotic pulmonary artery and branches, *IS* infundibular stenosis, *RV* right ventricle)

diastolic forward flow in the pulmonary artery [5]. The hemodynamic changes after correction of ToF greatly depend on the type of correction applied to the RVOT and pulmonary valve. In the past, different types of corrections have been applied: (1) transannular outflow patch, (2) RVOT patch with sparing of the native valve, and (3) replacement of the native pulmonary valve with or without the use of conduits. Various series have now highlighted that adult ToF patients referred for surgical correction do not tolerate transannular patch repair well, resulting in consequent severe pulmonary regurgitation. Acute and severe pulmonary regurgitation may be easily detected immediately after the repair using TEE color-flow Doppler and continuous wave (CW) Doppler. The presence of an acute pulmonary regurgitation causes a further deterioration of diastolic RV function. Diastolic filling of the RV is already impaired by the hypertrophic myocardial condition, and the retrograde diastolic filling of the RV due to the pulmonary regurgitation further impairs the ability of the RV to recruit volume through the pulmonary circulation into the systemic circulation. Patients with this pattern often experience a postoperative low cardiac output syndrome (LCOS) and are more prone to subsequent operations (pulmonary valve replacement) [6, 7].

10.4 Reoperation of Adult Tetralogy of Fallot Patients with Severe Pulmonary Regurgitation: The Chronic Volume Overload

Pulmonary valve regurgitation (PVR) is the most common indication for late reoperation in adult patients submitted to correction of ToF during infancy. Besides PVR, RV dilation and dysfunction, aneurysm of the RVOT, and tricuspid regurgitation (TR) secondary to RV dilatation are commonly associated as clinical manifestation of progressive disease (Fig. 10.2).

The chronic volume overload determines a deterioration of the systolic function of the RV [8]. By transthoracic echocardiography (TTE) or transesophageal

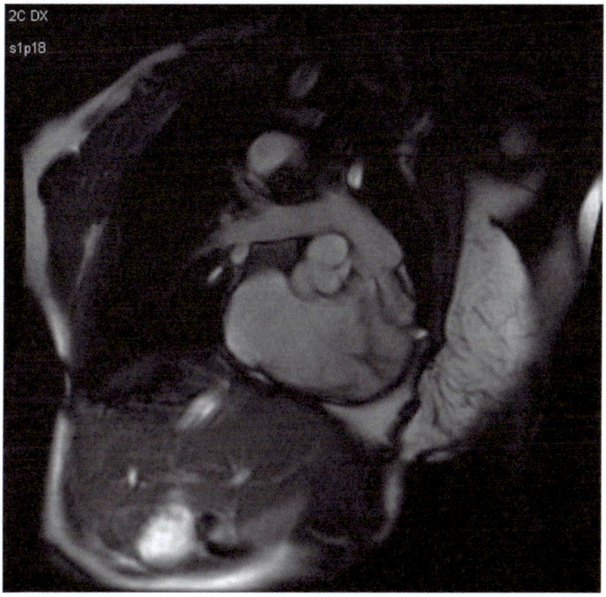

Fig. 10.2 MRI depicting a pulmonary regurgitation and right ventricular dilatation in tetralogy of Fallot

echocardiogram (TEE), the systolic function of the RV can be addressed with techniques that differ from the assessment of left ventricular function. Due to its elliptical shape that cannot be easily translated into a solid geometrical volume, the RV ejection fraction is rarely used. Tricuspid annular plane systolic excursion (TAPSE) quantifies the movement of the lateral tricuspid valve annulus toward the RV apex during systole. This measurement overcomes the problems related to the difficult geometry of the RV and correlates well with the angiographically determined RV ejection fraction. Normal values of TAPSE are around 25 mm, and severe RV systolic function may be diagnosed when TAPSE is less than 12–14 mm. Since the RV contractility greatly depends on the free wall movement, a M-mode study of the free wall excursion may be done with either TTE or TEE (in the inflow-outflow view). Other more complex assessments of the systolic RV function include the total ejection isovolume (TEI) index and tissue velocity, strain, and strain rate with tissue Doppler. Patients previously operated for ToF may demonstrate systolic dysfunction of the left ventricle, which appears not to be related to the severity of pulmonary regurgitation. Conversely, systolic RV dysfunction appears significantly associated with systolic left ventricular dysfunction. Both pressure and volume overload of the RV have deleterious reflections on left ventricular systolic function: the mechanical interaction of the two ventricles is even enhanced by the presence of the septal defect patch. Other mechanisms that link the RV and left ventricular function are electrical dyssynchrony and neurohormonal coupling. Tricuspid regurgitation makes the RV end-diastolic volume and ejection fraction calculations unreliable. Pulmonary artery catheter (PAC) is not the first-choice monitoring tool, due to the anatomical difficulties that make the insertion sometimes impossible and to the surgical manipulations that can dislocate the catheter. Finally, the use of patches,

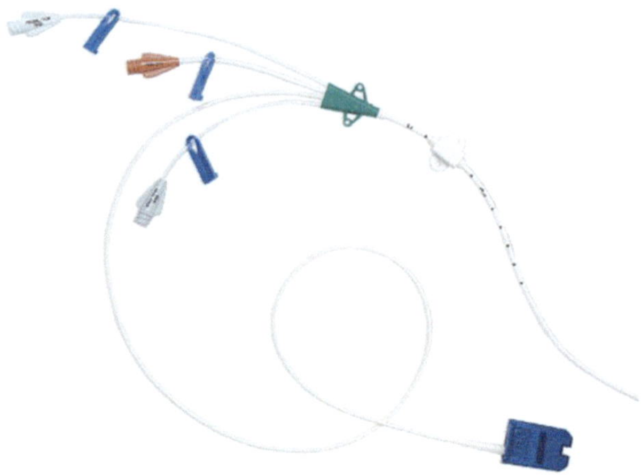

Fig. 10.3 Oximeter catheter (PreSep, courtesy of Edwards Lifesciences)

conduits, and prosthetic valves on right heart chambers makes a long-permanence PAC a threat for infections. As an adjunct to the standard CVC, it is reasonable to use oximetric catheters (Fig. 10.3) that can provide a continuous measurement of the central mixed venous oxygen saturation (SvO_2).

SvO_2 provides reliable information about the adequacy of the cardiac output with respect to the metabolic needs and may guide diagnosis and treatment in case of perioperative RV failure. A central role in the hemodynamic monitoring of the adult ToF patient is played by the TEE. The RV and its hemodynamic measurements may be studied using four standard TEE views. The mid-esophageal, four-chamber view allows detection of the border of the RV and its relationship with the left ventricle. The hypertrophic RV appears as a structure with a greatly enhanced myocardial wall, whereas the dilated RV loses its natural elliptic shape and occupies the apex of the heart. The subaortic ventricular septal defect or the defective patch may be appreciated in this view. From this position, by simply shifting to a 45 °C view, the RV inflow-outflow view is obtained. This image is of paramount importance, because it includes many of the typical findings of ToF. The RV is visible as a structure that embraces the aortic valve (in short axis in the middle of the screen), with the tricuspid valve on the left side (inflow) and the pulmonary valve and artery on the right side (outflow) of the screen. The RV free wall (at the bottom of the screen) may be appreciated for its movement and excursion using a M-mode analysis. The tricuspid valve can be explored for TAPSE in this view and in the presence of tricuspid valve regurgitation. This is one of the best views to obtain a parallelism with the regurgitant flow and therefore measuring the systolic pulmonary pressure with a CW Doppler. Finally, this is the best view to appreciate the extent and position of the RVOT obstruction. The anatomy of the pulmonary valve and artery may be evaluated using an upper esophageal aortic arch short axis view. In this image the final part of the aortic arch is located at the top of the screen, with the left subclavian artery visible, and on the left side of the screen, there is the long axis view of the pulmonary artery and valve. In this position, it is very easy to obtain a perfect parallelism and to assess the degree of the transpulmonary gradient and pulmonary regurgitation using a color Doppler and a CW Doppler study. Finally, inserting the probe into the stomach, the trans-gastric view is obtained. In this incidence, the left ventricle is on the right side of the screen, and the right ventricle is on the left. The ratio between the two ventricles' volume may be assessed, and it is possible to obtain again a good parallel with the transpulmonary flow, measuring the systolic gradient and the diastolic regurgitant flow.

Other hemodynamic monitoring tools may be useful in case of perioperative RV failure. Arterial waveform pulse contour analysis systems may be used for obtaining an estimate of the cardiac output and of the left ventricular filling status (derived from the systolic pressure variation). Near-infrared spectroscopy can provide a continuous indirect estimate of the regional (cerebral and somatic) SvO_2, and serial blood lactate determination may provide information related to the adequacy of the cardiac output with respect to the metabolic needs [9–11].

10.5 The Failing Right Ventricle

Adult patients receiving complete ToF correction or additional procedures after a previous complete correction may experience acute right ventricular failure after the operation. This pattern may appear immediately after completion of the operation in the operating room or during the first postoperative hours in the intensive care unit. The basic pathophysiological mechanisms recognize the preoperative diastolic and/or systolic dysfunction, which may deteriorate due to the ischemia-reperfusion insult during the operation. The hypertrophic right ventricle may be difficult to protect during the ischemic time of the aortic cross-clamping, despite the use of adequate cardioplegic solutions. The hemodynamic marker of the RV failure is its inability to recruit volume into the systemic circulation. Under these conditions, the clinical pattern is quite specific: the left ventricle appears unloaded, with all the dynamic fluid responsiveness indicators (pulse pressure variation, systolic pressure variation) suggestive of a hypovolemic condition. Actually, this condition is a relative rather than absolute hypovolemia of the systemic circulation, with a large amount of unrecruitable fluids placed in the venous bed. As a result, the CVP is high (>15 mmHg) and the inferior vena cava and hepatic veins are overloaded. The right ventricle may appear dilated in case of systolic dysfunction with pulmonary regurgitation or hypertrophic with a reduced end-diastolic volume in the restrictive diastolic pattern. The global cardiac output is inadequate, with reduced systemic arterial pressure, urine output, SvO_2 (<68%), and increased arterial serum lactates (>3 mMol/L). The end-tidal CO_2 is typically reduced, as an expression of a reduced pulmonary blood flow, and a large venous-arterial CO_2 gradient may appear [12].

10.6 Pharmacological Strategies for the Treatment of Acute RV Failure

Different drugs may be used for the treatment of the failing RV, and many therapeutic algorithms greatly depend on the physician's preference. However, there is a general agreement on the use of the phosphodiesterase inhibitor milrinone (0.375–0.75 μg/kg/min). This drug may be particularly useful for the treatment of systolic dysfunction, without deteriorating the diastolic function due to its action which is independent of the adrenoreceptor activity. Milrinone seems to improve myocardial relaxation and induces a limited increase in myocardial oxygen demands. Its role in the treatment of acute heart failure following pediatric cardiac surgery is well established. However, it must be considered that milrinone induces a considerable systemic vasodilation, and its effects should be considered within a comprehensive strategy of RV preload preservation. In this respect, the patients with RV diastolic dysfunction and no left ventricular dysfunction may benefit from a moderate systemic vasoconstriction (e.g., with norepinephrine, 0.05–0.2 μg/kg/min). When milrinone alone is insufficient, direct adrenoreceptor agents like dopamine (3–8 μg/kg/min) or epinephrine (0.02–0.2 μg/kg/min) may be added. Both of these agents increase the heart rate and may be responsible for arrhythmias. Levosimendan, a new calcium-sensitizer inodilator drug, is currently used in the treatment of acute heart failure in adult non-congenital patients after cardiac surgery and looks promising in reducing low cardiac output syndrome (LCOS); notwithstanding this fact, recent articles show no difference in reducing 30-day mortality in patient with left ventricle dysfunction after elective cardiac surgery.

The role of both milrinone and levosimendan in reducing afterload of the failing right ventricle and improving simultaneously lusitropic effect is interesting [13–15].

10.7 Non-pharmacological Strategies for the Treatment of Acute RV Failure

The failing RV needs an appropriate preload to recruit blood from the venous system toward the systemic circulation. Therefore, CVP values in the range of 12–15 mmHg are not unusual and may be required. Diastolic filling should be facilitated by ensuring adequate atrioventricular conduction and a normal heart rate. Tachycardia decreases the diastolic filling time, and junctional rhythm or any pattern of atrioventricular block excludes the atrial contribution to the diastolic filling. Therefore, the use of atrioventricular pacing is mandatory in the absence of a spontaneous normal conduction and heart rate. The cardiopulmonary interaction under mechanical ventilation is of particular importance in the setting of an impaired blood flow through the pulmonary vascular bed. Positive pressure ventilation decreases venous return, RV preload, and cardiac output, especially when a positive end-respiratory pressure is applied. At the same time, pulmonary vessel compression during positive pressure ventilation increases the RV afterload. Mechanical ventilation should therefore be settled at the lowest possible positive pressure regimen, however avoiding the occurrence of hypoxia and/or hypercapnia, which determines pulmonary vasoconstriction. Inhaled nitric oxide (iNO) is a powerful pulmonary arterial vasodilator. Its role in congenital heart surgery is limited to the treatment of pulmonary hypertension and is of course absent in the treatment of the ToF. However, some patients who received a Blalock–Taussig palliation may have areas of inhomogeneous pulmonary blood flow after correction, and anecdotal reports of the use of iNO in the treatment of RV failure exist.

RV failure refractory to pharmacological treatment may require additional measures, ranging from the need for leaving an open sternum to mechanical circulatory support. Even if the primary culprit for the low cardiac output state is RV failure, isolated RV assistance is difficult to perform, due to the need for pulmonary artery cannulation and the presence of different degrees of residual pulmonary regurgitation. Therefore, mechanical assistance of the failing RV in the adult ToF is based on the placement of an extracorporeal membrane oxygenation (ECMO) system [16]. This includes a venous and arterial cannulation, a centrifugal pump, an oxygenator, and a heat exchanger. Depending on the situation, the cannulas can be directly inserted into the right atrium and the ascending aorta when the chest is open or through the groin (femoral vein and artery) once it is closed. Extracorporeal life support (ECLS) strategies in refractory RV failure after cardiac operations in adult ToF patients should be considered a bridge to recovery or a bridge to transplant, depending on the clinical characteristics and risk factors of the patient.

10.8 Renal Function and Renal Protection

Renal function in ToF patient may be impaired chronically due to many reasons: elevated RVEDP, venous congestion, or chronic cyanosis. In CHD patients, impaired renal function may lead to kidney failure in the postoperative period, increasing the risk of mortality threefold for those patients who have moderately to severely impaired glomerular filtration rate (GFR). Preexisting renal insufficiency in adult ToF patients should be recognized prior to surgery in order to start proactive measures to protect renal perfusion and kidney function during and after surgery, in the ICU setting. Cardiopulmonary bypass (CPB), associated to various changes in physiology (decreased renal blood flow, changes in renin-angiotensin-aldosterone production, fluid retention, excessive hemodilution with low hematocrit), may exacerbate underlying renal dysfunction, complicated in the postoperative course by RV failure with increased RVEDP and filling pressures, rise in intra-abdominal pressure due to ascites, or low cardiac output syndrome (LOS), leading to acute kidney injury (AKI) with the necessity to treat the patient with continuous venous-venous hemofiltration (CVVH). Continuous dialysis should promptly begin according to AKI definitions and recommended treatment and patient clinical conditions. Maintaining good mean arterial pressure, reducing central venous pressure, avoiding nephrotoxic drugs, and reducing use and dosage of vasoactive drugs are essential steps toward renal protection. Pharmacologic strategies may also be useful to optimize renal perfusion. Many different drugs have been studied in non-CHD adult patient demonstrating reduction in renal insufficiency. Fenoldopam, a dopamine 1 receptor-specific agonist that causes arterial and arteriolar vasodilation, has been studied in the general adult cardiac populations as a renal protective agent on the basis of its ability to increase renal blood flow in the setting of cardiac surgery. A meta-analysis of 13 randomized and case-matched studies of fenoldopam administration during cardiopulmonary bypass in a standard (non-CHD) adult population demonstrated reduced need for renal replacement therapy, decreased in-hospital death, and shorter duration of ICU stay. For this reason many intensivists suggest the use of fenoldopam as a prophylactic treatment for those patients with preoperative renal impairment, although no specific data exist in the setting of ACHD. Adult ToF patients, especially survivors of natural history or palliated during infancy, are more prone to develop postoperative AKI [17].

10.9 Hematological Changes in Adult Tetralogy of Fallot

ToF patients are at increased risk of both bleeding and clotting in the postoperative course due to hematological changes, in particular for those unoperated or palliated patients with longstanding cyanosis. Cyanosis itself induces erythrocytosis that exposes to high risk of thrombosis, while bleeding is generally related to iron deficiency and alteration in number and function of platelets, particularly in patients with underlying liver disease as a consequence of right ventricular failure or increased RVEDP. Hepatic synthetic function leading to prolonged prothrombin times and bleeding risk should be recognized and treated during and after interventions take place, according to careful monitoring of coagulation status. Use of point-of-care tests (i.e., thromboelastography and platelet function tests) provides crucial information about the comprehensive coagulation profile to treat post-CPB coagulopathy with blood products and prothrombin complex concentrates or exogenous fibrinogen [18, 19].

10.10 Arrhythmias

Arrhythmias are a significant cause of morbidity and mortality in adults with CHD and occur with increasing frequency with age. Arrhythmias are the most important risk factor for sudden cardiac death (SCD) among ACHD patients. Arrhythmias can also complicate the postoperative course increasing morbidity and mortality on operated adult ToF patients. Atrial re-entrant tachycardia is the most common form of arrhythmia in adult ToF patients, while high-grade ventricular arrhythmias account to about 10% of patients. Close collaboration with electrophysiologists is required for adult ToF patients to plan a consistent and efficient approach to decrease postoperative arrhythmias, including preoperative electrophysiological studies and eventual ablation and surgical arrhythmia treatment during the forthcoming surgery. In a study from the Toronto Group, 12 of 41 ToF reoperated patients had supraventricular tachycardia prior to the reoperation; the 7.5-year freedom from arrhythmia recurrence was 75% for the intraoperatively ablated patients and 34% for those without ablation. ToF patients often have chronic atrial fibrillation (AF) correlated with longstanding chronic pulmonary valve regurgitation resulting in right ventricular failure, functional tricuspid regurgitation, and arrhythmia [20, 21].

10.11 Myocardial Infarction

TOF patients may have anomalous coronary origin or abnormal coronary tract crossing the RVOT in between 2% and 10% of cases. Preoperative coronary artery imaging studies are mandatory to identify those patients who can be injured during surgery and to minimize the correlated risk of myocardial ischemia and infarction particularly in redo patients.

Postoperative myocardial ischemia should be suspected when 12-lead electrocardiogram (ECG) shows ST tract alterations or other ischemic signs coupled with TTE ventricular abnormalities and rise in plasma troponin I level. When myocardial ischemia is detected, the underlying mechanisms should be clarified as soon as possible in order to expedite intervention to solve the occlusive problem. It is unequivocal that the coronary pattern needs to be well identified preoperatively, to warrant a safe surgical correction especially for patients in need for a RVOT operation [15, 22].

10.12 Pulmonary Function

Patients with tetralogy of Fallot may have compromised pulmonary function related to many different conditions: chronic hypoxemia, restrictive lung disease, chronic obstructive pulmonary disease (COPD), smoking history, scoliosis or other orthopedic illnesses, or diaphragmatic paralysis secondary to prior phrenic nerve injury. Diminished pulmonary reserve with forced expiratory volume (FEV_1) reduction increases the risk of postoperative pulmonary lung failure and will be further compromised in patients who are significantly desaturated at baseline. In the postoperative course, good respiratory support is mandatory to counteract the negative effect of mechanical ventilation on hemodynamic parameters, mainly with those patients affected by right ventricular dysfunction. High-positive end-expiratory pressure during positive pressure ventilation can be significantly deleterious in patients with right ventricular dysfunction. Under- or overdistension of the lungs will cause an increase in pulmonary vascular resistance, effectively increasing right ventricular afterload and potentially diminishing pulmonary blood flow, decreasing left ventricular filling and leading to low cardiac output (LCO). Early extubation and avoidance of high levels of positive end-expiratory pressures, according to good clinical status, are recommended to reduce the negative impact on cardiac output. If pulmonary function worsens despite appropriate ventilation strategies, respiratory support ECMO may be useful to prevent LCO and consequently the risk of multiorgan failure (MOF) with the subsequent high risk of mortality [15, 18].

References

1. Sadiq A, Shyamkrishnan KG, Theodore S, Gopalakrishnan S, Tarakan JM, Karunakan J. Long-term functional assessment after correction of tetralogy of Fallot in adulthood. Ann Thorac Surg. 2007;83(5):1790–5.
2. Attenhofer Jost CH, Connolly HM, Burkhart HM, et al. Tetralogy of Fallot repair in patients 40 years or older. Mayo Clin Proc. 2010;85:1090–4.
3. Spencer KT, Weinert L, Lang RM. Effect of age, heart rate and tricuspid regurgitation on the Doppler echocardiography evaluation of right ventricular diastolic function. Cardiology. 1999;92:59–64. PubMed CrossRef.
4. Cicala S, Galderisi M, Caso P, et al. Right ventricular diastolic dysfunction in arterial systemic hypertension: analysis by pulsed tissue Doppler. Eur J Echocardiogr. 2002;3:135–42. PubMed CrossRef.
5. Nomura T, Lebowitz L, Koide Y, et al. Evaluation of hepatic venous flow using transesophageal echocardiography in coronary artery bypass surgery: an index of right ventricular function. J Cardiothorac Vasc Anesth. 1995;9:9–17. PubMed CrossRef.
6. Gatzoulis MA, Clark AL, Cullen S, et al. Right ventricular diastolic function 15 to 35 years after repair of tetralogy of Fallot: restrictive physiology predicts superior exercise performance. Circulation. 1995;91:1775–81. PubMed CrossRef.
7. Bacha EA, Scheule AM, Zurakowski D, et al. Long-term results after early primary repair of tetralogy of Fallot. J Thorac Cardiovasc Surg. 2001;122:154–61.
8. Apitz C, Webb GD, Redington AN. Tetralogy of Fallot. Lancet. 2009;374:1462–71.
9. Friedberg MK, Redington AN. Right versus left ventricular failure differences, similarities, and interactions. Circulation. 2014;129:1033–44.
10. Alonso-González R, Dimopoulos K, Ho SY, Oliver JM, Gatzoulis MA. The right heart in adults with congenital heart disease. Rev Esp Cardiol. 2010;63(9):1070–86.
11. Lucy Roche S, Redington AN. The failing right ventricle in congenital heart disease. Can J Cardiol. 2013;29:768–78.
12. Villafañe J, et al. Hot topics in Tetralogy of Fallot. J Am Coll Cardiol. 2013;62(23):2155–66.
13. Mehta RH, et al. Levosimendan in patients with left ventricular dysfunction undergoing cardiac surgery. New Engl J Med. 2017;376:2032–42. https://doi.org/10.1056/NEJMoa1616218.
14. Landoni G, et al. Levosimendan for hemodynamic support after cardiac surgery. New Engl J Med. 2017;376:2021–31. https://doi.org/10.1056/NEJMoa1616325.
15. Dos L, et al. Pulmonary valve replacement in repaired Tetralogy of Fallot: determinants of early postoperative adverse outcomes. J Thorac Cardiovasc Surg. 2009;138:553–9.
16. Acheampong B, et al. Postcardiotomy ECMO support after high-risk operations in adult congenital heart disease. Congenit Heart Dis. 2016;11:751–5.
17. Morgan C, et al. Chronic kidney disease in congenital heart disease patients: a narrative review of evidence. Can J Kidney Health Dis. 2015;2:27.
18. Allan CK. Intensive care of the adult patient with congenital heart disease. Prog Cardiovasc Dis. 2011;53:274–80.
19. Ranucci M. Outcome measures and quality markers for perioperative blood loss and transfusion in cardiac surgery. Can J Anaesth. 2016;63(2):169–75.
20. Page RL, et al. 2015 ACC/AHA/HRS guideline for the management of adult patients with supraventricular tachycardia. A report of the American College Cardiology/American Heart Association Task Force on Clinical Practice Guidelines and the Heart Rhythm Society. Circulation. 2016;133:e506–74.
21. Giamberti A, et al. Surgery for supraventricular tachycardia and congenital heart defects: long-term efficacy of the combined approach in adult patients. Europace. 2016;19:1542–8.
22. Warnes CA, et al. ACC/AHA 2008 guidelines for the management of adults with congenital heart disease. J Am Coll Cardiol. 2008;52(23):e143–263.

Critical Care Management of the Adult with Aortic Coarctation

11

Barry A. Love

11.1 Introduction

Coarctation of the aorta is defined as a narrowing of the aorta distal to the transverse aortic arch. With an incidence of 4 in 10,000 live births [1], it is one of the more common congenital heart lesions. While most patients are identified in infancy or childhood, a small number of patients with coarctation are identified for the first time in adulthood.

Coarctation is often found in association with bicuspid aortic valve (40%). This association is especially important in the adult as the aortopathy with ascending aortic dilation may coexist with coarctation making management decisions more complex. Other congenital associations are frequently associated and are typically left-sided obstructive lesions, including ventricular septal defect (28%), aortic stenosis (6%), subaortic membrane (26%), and mitral valve abnormalities (25%) [2].

Coarctation of the aorta may also be seen in association with other more complex forms of congenital heart disease mainly transposition of the great arteries (12%) [2].

A genetic basis for coarctation has not been identified in most cases. The main genetic syndrome where coarctation is seen is Turner's syndrome (X,O karyotype) where the incidence of coarctation is about 15% [3].

B. A. Love
Pediatrics and Medicine, Icahn School of Medicine, Mount Sinai Medical Center, New York, NY, USA
e-mail: barry.love@mssm.edu

E. da Cruz et al. (eds.), *Intensive Care of the Adult with Congenital Heart Disease*, Congenital Heart Disease in Adolescents and Adults,
https://doi.org/10.1007/978-3-319-94171-4_11

11.2 Presentations

The adult patient with coarctation of the aorta may be admitted to the intensive care unit (ICU) as a result of intervention for the coarctation, as a complication of operated or unoperated coarctation, or this may be an associated diagnosis for a patient admitted for another reason to the ICU. The pregnant patient with repaired or unrepaired coarctation presents special ICU challenges.

11.3 Natural History

Coarctation was firstly described in the pathology literature in 1791 [4]. In the 1920s [5] and then in the 1940s [6], postmortem series of coarctation were published. The median age of death in these series was 31 years, and 76% of deaths were attributable to a complication of coarctation. The most common causes of death in these early series were heart failure (26%) and occurred at a mean age of 37 years. Other causes of death included aortic rupture (21%), bacterial endocarditis (18%) and intracranial hemorrhage (12%). Of the patients with intracranial hemorrhage, 1/3 had ruptured cerebral aneurysms.

In these early presurgical era series, coronary artery disease was not a significant cause of death. This is also in keeping with the low incidence of coronary artery disease in the general population prior to the 1950s. However, a recent cohort of patient has shown atherosclerotic coronary and cerebrovascular events to now be the leading cause of late death in coarctation patients after repair [7]. A population study from Quebec demonstrated than coarctation was not a risk factor for coronary artery disease independent of hypertension [8]. Unfortunately, at least half of patients with repaired coarctation will have hypertension [9] and that, along with other common risk factors (smoking, hyperlipidemia, diabetes), puts these patients at higher risk for coronary artery disease.

11.4 Indications for Intervention

The most common ICU admission for a patient with coarctation is for postoperative or post-procedural management after intervention for coarctation or recoarctation of the aorta. The majority will be to address narrowing of the aorta. Most consensus documents advocate for intervention for a peak-to-peak gradient of 20 mmHg or more as an indication for intervention [10, 11], but lower gradients are often intervened on in the presence of significant anatomic narrowing with significant collaterals. The presence of hypertension, an exaggerated blood pressure response with exercise, or left ventricular hypertrophy or dysfunction are factors that may influence a decision to move forward with intervention for gradients less than 20 mmHg if there is a suitable anatomic target.

Other operative or procedural indications for intervention besides narrowing would include aneurysm formation at the site of prior surgical repair or aneurysm or pseudoaneurysm at the site of a prior balloon dilation or stenting.

11.5 Preoperative Management

Prior to intervention for coarctation of the aorta, a full assessment needs to be undertaken. A complete history, physical examination, and appropriate testing are mandatory to plan the correct intervention, anticipate issues, and avoid surprises.

11.6 History

Past history of prior cardiac surgeries and current cardiac symptoms including angina, claudication, shortness of breath, and orthopnea should be elicited. It is ideal to obtain prior surgical records; however, with widespread adoption of the electronic medical record, it is becoming increasingly difficult to obtain older archived records.

11.7 Physical Examination

Four limb blood pressures are important to assess the degree of obstruction at the site of coarctation. In the absence of other issues, the right arm to leg blood pressure systolic difference is a reasonable correlate to a peak-to-peak gradient across the coarctation measures in the catheterization laboratory. However, in some patients the right subclavian artery is aberrant arising distal to the coarctation site, so knowing this is important. In addition, many adult patients with coarctation had arterial catheterization from the femoral approach in childhood. This may have led to narrowing or occlusion of the femoral artery especially if a cut-down approach was used. Typically, vascular narrowing in the femoral artery that occurred early in life is asymptomatic because of collateral formation, but femoral arterial stenosis can exaggerate an arm-leg blood pressure difference making that leg an unreliable site for assessing coarctation gradient.

Many adult patients will have scars over their radial and femoral arteries as a result of prior cut-down approaches in infancy and childhood. This can make accessing these sites for monitoring or intervention difficult or impossible.

The neurologic exam prior to coarctation repair is important as a baseline. Because interventions on the aorta may lead to paraplegia, stroke, and recurrent laryngeal nerve injury, assessing these neurologic parameters prior to intervention is of clinical and medicolegal importance.

11.8 Testing

11.8.1 Transthoracic Echocardiogram

A transthoracic echocardiogram will be able to assess other cardiac anatomic abnormalities that may coexist including bicuspid aortic valve or aortic stenosis, a dilated ascending aorta, mitral valve abnormalities, subaortic stenosis, and left ventricular function. The coarctation area can frequently be visualized by transthoracic echocardiogram and a Doppler gradient obtained, but these gradients often overestimate the true peak-to-peak gradient found at catheterization, and visualization of the area is often limited. Transesophageal echocardiogram is usually not performed as there are better diagnostic tests available.

Imaging of the aorta is important for preoperative planning and can be best done with contrast CT or MRI. CT or MRI will show the degree of narrowing and the anatomic location, the presence of ascending aortic dilation especially with a bicuspid aortic valve, and any aneurysm formation at the coarctation site. In addition, these tests can show the degree of collateral formation. The proximity of the coarctation to the left subclavian artery is an especially important consideration for transcatheter stent placement. Transverse arch hypoplasia is another important consideration for intervention.

In addition to anatomic information, MRI can predict coarctation severity and predict peak-to-peak gradients of less than or greater than 20 mmHg found at catheterization using a combination of anatomic and flow parameters [12, 13]. In patients with prior stenting of the coarctation, CT is superior to MRI because of metal artifact.

In addition to the aorta, both contrast CT and MRI can be used to assess for the presence of cerebral aneurysms which are present in 3–10% of patients with coarctation [14] compared with 2–3% in the general population. The 2008 American College of Cardiology/American Heart Association guidelines recommend that every patient with coarctation of the aorta receive at least one MRI or CT to evaluate the thoracic aorta and intracranial vessels (level of evidence B) [10].

11.8.2 Cardiac Catheterization

Noninvasive CT and/or MRI has now replaced angiography as the best imaging for coarctation. However, peak-to-peak pressure gradient measured across the coarctation remains the "gold standard" for planning intervention. It is best to obtain the gradient in an adult patient under minimal sedation. In addition, simultaneous pressure measurement above and below the coarctation is the most accurate method for assessment. This can be accomplished in a variety of ways. A 6-French double-lumen pigtail catheter (Langston, Vascular Solutions, Inc., Minneapolis, MN) that has multiple side holes near the tip and another set further back on the shaft is commonly employed. Although the "magic" number of 20 mmHg is oft-used as the threshold for intervention, the gradient is the result of both the narrowing and the flow. If the cardiac output is reduced or there is significant runoff around the coarctation by collateral vessels, the gradient will be less even in the presence of important narrowing. Other hemodynamic parameters that are important in the pre-procedure assessment of coarctation include the left ventricle end-diastolic pressure as well as the pulmonary capillary wedge pressure as an indication of LV diastolic compliance.

Coronary angiography in patients over 40 years of age is an important consideration because of the earlier incidence of coronary artery disease in those patients with coarctation and concomitant hypertension. Coronary assessment by CT scanning is another alternative.

Cardiac catheterization may then be extended to perform intervention for coarctation or may be used as a preoperative planning modality.

11.9 Indications for Intervention

Patients with significant coarctation or recoarctation of the aorta should undergo intervention to relieve the obstruction. Most consensus documents agree on a peak-to-peak gradient of 20 mmHg or more as an indication for intervention [10, 11]. In addition, lesser gradients should also be considered for intervention in the presence of significant anatomic narrowing with significant collaterals. In patients with borderline gradients, the presence of hypertension, an exaggerated blood pressure response with exercise, or left ventricular hypertrophy or dysfunction would be additional factors to weigh in clinical decision-making. The presence of aneurysm at the coarctation site is another indication for intervention.

11.10 Treatment

Treatment for the adult with primary coarctation or recoarctation can be surgical or transcatheter.

11.10.1 Surgical Approaches

11.10.1.1 End-to-End

The first reported repair for coarctation of the aorta was performed in 1944 on a 12-year-old boy in Sweden using an end-to-end technique [15]. The end-to-end repair is performed from a left thoracotomy. The aorta is clamped proximal and distal to the narrowed segment. The narrowed segment is excised, and the distal aorta is mobilized. The two ends are then anastomosed together. There was initially a high incidence (20–86%) incidence of recurrent narrowing at the site of repair [16, 17]. This was thought to be due to circumferential scar formation and growth issues. Other surgical techniques were developed in an attempt to overcome this problem. With experience (and suboptimal results with other techniques), the end-to-end anastomosis again became the preferred method of repair—especially in children. The method to avoid recoarctation in the end-to-end repair appears to be largely dependent on the ability of the surgeon to create a tension-free anastomosis. This is critically dependent on mobilization of the distal aorta to approximate it to the proximal segment. In the modern era, the end-to-end anastomosis has the lowest rate of recoarctation compared to other methods (8% versus up to 35%) [18]. In the adult, it is more difficult to mobilize the aorta, and so the end-to-end technique is used in short, discrete coarctation where the amount of mobilization required will be minimal. The adult patient also has the option of a tube graft to bridge a longer resected segment without the need for mobilization of the aorta and without the concerns for growth that are present in the young child.

11.10.1.2 Patch-Plasty

The patch-plasty repair is also performed from a left thoracotomy. The aorta is cross-clamped above and below the narrowed segment. In this repair method, the posterior wall of the aorta is opened and enlarged with a patch. Gore-Tex, Dacron, and Hemashield materials as well as others have been used as patch material. There is a significantly higher residual coarctation rate in this type of repair. A significant rate of aneurysm formation opposite the patch was also encountered. This method is rarely used in the current era, but there is a substantial group of adult patients with coarctation who had this type of repair in childhood and may need residual issues addressed.

11.10.1.3 Left Subclavian Flap

Because of the initial finding of a significant incidence of recoarctation following end-to-end repair of coarctation in children, other methods of repair were developed in an attempt to address this issue. The left subclavian flap repair was thought to be a potentially superior method as it did not leave a circumferential scar and used autologous tissue rather than synthetic material for the patch. This method, first described in 1966, involves cross-clamping the aorta proximal to the left subclavian artery and distal to the coarctation. The left subclavian artery is then divided proximal to the vertebral origin. The posterior wall of the proximal left subclavian artery is then incised along its length carrying the incision down the back wall of the aorta opposite to the coarctation segment. The edges are then anastomosed together such that the proximal left subclavian artery is used as patch to augment the narrowed segment. This method was popular in the 1970s and 1980s, but the long-term results showed that there continued to be a significant residual coarctation rate [19, 20]. In addition, the left subclavian artery was ligated leaving the vertebral artery to perfuse the left arm retrograde through the circle of Willis. While rarely clinically apparent, it can lead to a vertebral artery "steal" phenomenon with exercise of the left arm causing the blood to be diverted from the cerebral circulation to the left arm.

11.10.1.4 Interposition Graft

In the adult with a longer segment of coarctation, excision of the narrowed segment and replacement with a synthetic tube of matching diameter to the normal segment is a good option. For patients with postsurgical aneurysm at the site of prior repair, it is the surgical method of choice, though this problem can usually be addressed using endovascular techniques. If a mycotic aneurysm is present, excision of the infected segment and replacement with a synthetic tube is usually the best option. The interposition graft is avoided in growing children as they run the risk of outgrowing the graft leading to a fixed stenosis at the site.

11.10.1.5 Arch Augmentation

If the transverse arch is hypoplastic, then simply addressing the coarctation site will lead to residual stenosis proximal to the repair. In the infant and young child, this problem is usually managed with arch augmentation—a technique performed on cardiopulmonary bypass with hypothermia (sometimes with circulatory arrest) from a median sternotomy approach where the aortic arch is transected and augmented with patch material. The coarctation segment is usually excised in the repair. This repair is possible in the infant and young child because of the relative ease of mobilizing the arch and aorta but much more difficult in the adult patient. Even in the young patient, while good anatomic augmentation of the arch is usually achieved, there is a significant residual risk of narrowing at the coarctation site.

11.10.1.6 Ascending–Descending Conduit

The ascending to descending aortic conduit repair [21] is a good option in the adult patient for complex arch narrowing or when other concomitant cardiac surgery is required, for example, an ascending aortic aneurysm repair or coronary artery bypass grafting. A tube graft is anastomosed to the right side of the ascending aorta and then brought down to the right of the heart to the level of the diaphragm where it can be anastomosed to the side of the descending aorta. The repair is performed on cardiopulmonary bypass because of the significant manipulation of the heart that needs to occur in order to achieve the distal anastomosis.

11.10.2 Complications of Surgical Repair

Complications of surgical repair of coarctation can be divided into those that occur early postoperatively and those that occur later in follow-up (Tables 11.1 and 11.2).

11.10.2.1 Early

Spinal Cord Ischemia

Spinal cord ischemia with lower limb paraplegia is the most feared complication of surgical repair of coarctation of the aorta. The incidence in large early series of repair was between 0.9% and 2.4% of cases. Improved surgical techniques and protection strategies have lowered, but not eliminated this risk. Spinal cord ischemia may result from prolonged cross-clamping of the aorta, ligation of the arterial supply to the spinal cord. The arterial supply to the spinal cord arises from a number of vessels from the posterior aspect of the descending aorta. While there is redundancy

Table 11.1 Interventional management for native and recurrent aortic coarctation

	Native coarctation	Recurrent coarctation
Surgery		
Resection and end-to-end anastomosis	Appropriate for short-segment coarctation only Adequate mobilization of descending aorta is critical	Rarely performed to relieve recurrent coarctation
Subclavian flap	Rarely performed in the adult because of risk of aneurysm formation and loss of pulsatile flow to left arm	Rarely performed for recurrent coarctation
Interposition tube graft	Good technique for longer-segment coarctation Aorta should be at or near full growth	Often used is aneurysm present—resect abnormal tissue with placement of interposition graft
Patch angioplasty	Rarely performed now as risk of aneurysm formation	May be used if difficulty exposing aorta circumferentially. Less risk of aneurysm in recurrent coarctation because of prior scar tissue formation
Ascending-descending bypass	Excellent option for patient who needs concomitant cardiac procedure on bypass (e.g., aortic valve replacement) or for those with small transverse arch	Excellent option for patients with complex arch anatomy or for those who need other cardiac surgery
Interventional catheterization		
Balloon angioplasty alone	Has been shown to be higher risk with poorer outcomes than stenting or surgery	Reasonable choice in patients where stent placement would be problematic (cover carotid or subclavian origin) Recoil leads to suboptimal gradient relief
Bare-metal stent	Results comparable to those of surgery with respect to gradient relief Usually needs a staged approach with subsequent balloon dilation to achieve desired final stent diameter	Procedure of choice in most instances for adult with recurrent coarctation
Covered stent	Covering may decrease risk of dissection and rupture	May prevent aneurysm formation and can be used to treat aortic wall injury after bare-metal stenting

Table 11.2 Early complications after surgical coarctation repair

Complication	Treatment
Bleeding	Medical management, surgical reintervention
Pseudoaneurysm	Surgical reintervention or transcatheter covered stent
Recurrent laryngeal nerve palsy	Conservative
Chylothorax	Chest tube drainage, parental nutrition, octreotide, surgical ligation of the thoracic duct
Spinal cord ischemia	Avoidance. Steroids no longer recommended
Post-coarctectomy syndrome	NPO, IV antihypertensives to achieve high-normal blood pressure range
Hypertension	IV antihypertensives to achieve high-normal blood pressure range

of the arterial supply, ligation of many in close proximity puts the spinal cord at risk. Mobilizing the aorta to approximate the edges of an end-to-end repair necessitates surgical division of these vessels. For this reason, the end-to-end anastomosis for primary repair of coarctation in the adult should be limited to those patients where only a short segment needs to be excised and mobilization is minimized.

The typical cross-clamp time of the aorta for coarctation surgery is between 20 and 30 min. In the adult patient with significant primary coarctation, extensive collateral vessels will usually provide significant flow back into the aorta. However if the duration of cross-clamping is expected to be longer or if the collateral circulation appears underdeveloped, spinal cord protection techniques may be employed.

Spinal cord protection strategies are variable. There is no good data or consensus as to the best strategy [22]. Intraoperatively, spinal cord function may be assessed with somatosensory evoked response that evaluates the brain's reception of signals from the spinal cord in response to a stimulus. While this assesses the sensory pathways, it does not appraise the motor pathways that run in a different part of the cord.

Although there was enthusiasm for early steroid administration as a treatment strategy for spinal cord injury (usually traumatic), this has fallen out of favor with more data suggesting higher likelihood of harm [23]. If spinal cord injury is suspected early postoperatively, there was once enthusiasm to use steroids based on the recommendations for traumatic spinal cord injury, but this too has fallen out of favor.

Left Heart Bypass

Left heart bypass is used to perfuse distal to the cross-clamped aorta. The left atrium is cannulated from the same left thoracotomy incision used for the repair and is connected to a centrifugal pump. The outflow cannula is placed in the aorta distal to the cross-clamp to provide flow to the lower body. A heat exchanger can also be introduced in the circuit to provide modest hypothermia (30–34 °C) and decrease tissue oxygen demand. With left heart bypass, the lower body including the kidneys and distal spinal arteries are perfused during cross-clamping allowing for a longer period of occlusion and a potentially safer operation. This technique is typically considered when cross-clamping of more than 30 min is anticipated. It can also be instituted mid-procedure if difficulties are encountered that prolong the cross-clamp time.

Epidural Cooling

One method to potentially decrease spinal cord injury is to decrease oxygen demand. Infusing cooled 4 °C saline into the epidural space can potentially achieve this goal. The infusion catheter is typically placed at the T10–11 level and a drainage catheter in the lumbar epidural space. There are no studies demonstrating efficacy of this treatment. It must be instituted prior to surgical incision.

11.10.2.2 Bleeding, Blood Loss, and Transfusion

The suture line at the repair site must be meticulous to avoid postoperative bleeding and pseudoaneurysm formation. Postoperative blood pressure control is important to avoid disruption of the suture line. In adult patients with coarctation, collateral vessels increase the risk of intra- and postoperative bleeding and need to be meticulously controlled. Extensive chest tube output that does not respond to correction of coagulation factors or a large increase in chest tube output mandates a return to the operating room for re-exploration and control of surgical bleeding.

For most adult patients undergoing coarctation repair, administration of blood products is not required; however in the presence of complications, patients may need significant blood replacement, and protocols for autotransfusion and large volume donor transfusion need to be in place.

11.10.2.3 Chylothorax

The lymphatic system collects lymph from the lower extremities where it meets the lymphatic channels draining the intestines at the cisterna chyli. From there, the thoracic duct ascends typically to the right of the spine. In the thorax at about the T5 level, the thoracic duct crosses to the left of the midline and enters the innominate vein. The course of the thoracic duct is very variable and practically invisible to the surgeon in the fasting state when the lymph is clear. In thoracic surgery for repair of coarctation, the thoracic duct may be disrupted leading to chylothorax. This manifests as prolonged chylous drainage from the chest tube or accumulation of fluid in the left thoracic cavity if the chest tube has been removed. Testing of the fluid reveals a high lymphocyte count. In the fed state, the fluid will appear milky white and will have a high triglyceride level. Most patients with chylothorax are managed conservatively with chest tube drainage and fasting with parenteral nutrition or low-fat diet for several days or weeks. Intravenous octreotide may be used in some refractory cases. Pleurodesis can be used in refractory cases as can reoperation and surgical ligation or embolization of the thoracic duct ligation is required [24].

11.10.2.4 Recurrent Laryngeal Nerve Injury

The nerve supply to the vocal cords is the recurrent laryngeal nerve. This nerve descends from the neck and loops under the last remaining aortic arch. On the right, this is the subclavian artery. On the left side, it is the ductus arteriosus (which becomes the ligamentum arteriosus postnatally) before ascending to supply the ipsilateral vocal cord. In coarctation surgery, the ligamentum arteriosus is divided in order to excise the coarctation segment. The surgeon must take care not to put traction or divide the recurrent laryngeal nerve during manipulation in this area. Even traction on the nerve can lead to temporary or permanent damage to the nerve that can result in hoarseness. Because the paretic vocal cord position is closed, aspiration is rarely seen.

11.10.2.5 Post-coarctectomy Syndrome and Postoperative Hypertension

In patients with coarctation of the aorta undergoing surgical repair, a number will develop paradoxical increase in systemic blood pressure in the first week after repair even in the absence of residual obstruction. The phenomenon is usually the worst in the first 48 h after surgery [24]. The phenomenon is thought to be due to stimulation of sympathetic nerve fibers between the media and adventitia of the aortic isthmus stimulating the release of plasma norepinephrine as well as a spinal reflex that stimulates renin release [25]. The renin release is thought to constrict mesenteric vessels that can lead to abdominal pain and intestinal ischemia if left untreated. Interestingly, this finding is rarely observed in patients who have coarctation treated percutaneously with balloon dilation [26] and/or stenting. The incidence of post-coarctectomy syndrome was reported to be as high as 56% in surgical series with the syndrome more commonly seen in patients after adolescence [26]. Pretreatment with a nonselective beta-blocker (propranolol) was found to diminish the paradoxical hypertensive response and also blunt the rise in plasma renin levels [27].

Although adult patients undergoing surgical coarctation repair should ideally be pretreated with a nonselective beta-blocker prior to surgery, there has been less focus on the need for this pretreatment in the current era. This is likely because the postoperative medications to treat hypertension in the intensive care unit are much better than they were in the 1970s and 1980s when treatment of postoperative hypertension was more difficult.

Good control of blood pressure following surgical repair of coarctation of the aorta is of utmost importance. The suture lines after repair are subject to significantly increased stress in the presence of hypertension and are at risk for tearing with uncontrolled hypertension. On the other hand, hypotension could risk cerebral hypoperfusion and watershed infarction with a cerebral vasculature that had been accommodating chronic hypertension. For this reason, rapid, short-acting antihypertensives are usually the treatment of choice in the adult intensive care unit. Intravenous nicardipine has proven to be a popular choice for acute blood pressure management as it has a rapid onset and offset and can be titrated to achieve the desired blood pressure [28]. Other choices include intravenous sodium nitroprusside, esmolol, enalaprilat, and labetalol [28]. It is critical to have reliable, continuous arterial blood pressure monitoring in the postoperative period for these patients. Equally important is to avoid arterial monitoring in an extremity that does not reflect the central blood pressure. For instance, the left radial artery would be a poor choice for an arterial line in a patient with a left subclavian flap repair where the left arm blood pressure is typically 20 or 30 mmHg less than the opposite arm.

11.10.3 Late Complications

While it would seem that repair of simple coarctation should be a definitive procedure, the results of late follow-up tell a different story. A series from the Mayo Clinic published in 1989 examined patients operated on there from 1946 to 1981 [29]. They found that those patients operated on after age 14 had much worse outcomes than those operated on at a younger age. The mean survival for those operated on after age 14 was only 38 years. The most common causes of death were coronary artery disease (37%), sudden death (13%), heart failure (9%), stroke (7%), and ruptured aortic aneurysm (7%). The Mayo study showed that hypertension was an important residual sequelae with older age at repair predicting persistent hypertension even in the absence of residual narrowing. For patients operated on at age 9 years or later, 25% had persistent hypertension, whereas only 6% had hypertension if they had their operation before age 9. Other studies have confirmed the correlation between later age of repair and persistent hypertension [30].

Recoarctation can be seen in up to 25% of patients with surgical repair of coarctation with 10% of patients having significant narrowing by one MRI study [31]. Significant recoarctation is usually treated with transcatheter stenting but is also sometimes addressed surgically. Aneurysmal dilation of the aorta can be seen at the repair site as well as the ascending aorta in those with a bicuspid aortic valve. The recommendation is for all adult patients with repaired coarctation of the aorta to have contrast CT or MRI imaging of the aorta at least once to exclude this condition [10].

In addition to recoarctation, patients may develop aneurysm at the repair site. This is reported in 13% of patients in one study [31] but is also seen in native coarctation without repair and can be fatal as described in the early pathology series [5, 6].

Between 7% and 28% of adult patients with childhood coarctation repair will require reintervention at the coarctation site [29].

As described in the paper from Mayo, many patients following coarctation repair will have heart failure that may even be fatal. The biggest risk factor is late repair and also recurrent coarctation. These patients develop both systolic and diastolic heart failure. The mechanism is likely increased afterload on the left ventricle with increased wall stress. The treatment of heart failure is similar to those patients without congenital disease; however if residual coarctation is present, it should be eliminated, usually with transcatheter stenting, to reduce as much as possible the ongoing elevated afterload on the left ventricle. Pharmacologic reduction of afterload is also very important along with diuretics, beta-blockers, and other contemporary heart failure medical management. Pharmacologic afterload reduction in the presence of significant residual coarctation is unlikely to be helpful and is probably harmful.

The incidence of sudden and non-sudden death in patients following coarctation repair was evaluated in a population-based study from Oregon between 1958 and 1996 [32]. The incidence of non-sudden death was 0.25%/year, and the incidence of sudden death was 0.13%/year. This is not much different that the incidence of sudden death in the repaired tetralogy of Fallot population in this study where the incidence of sudden death was found to be 0.15%/year. This incidence of sudden death makes consideration of an implantable defibrillator in those with reduced ejection fraction all the more compelling.

11.11 Transcatheter Treatment for Adults with Coarctation of the Aorta

Transcatheter stenting has become the first-line approach for adults with recurrent coarctation of the aorta (Table 11.3). For those patients with aneurysm formation at the coarctation site, covered endografts are the preferred approach. For adults with unrepaired coarctation, primary stenting or covered stenting is an option. Balloon dilation alone in the adult with primary or recurrent coarctation appears to have a high risk of incomplete gradient relief and recurrent coarctation (44%) as well as a high risk of aneurysm formation (7.5%) [3, 34], and so this has mostly fallen out of favor.

Table 11.3 Early complications following transcatheter repair for coarctation

Complication	Treatment
Femoral pseudoaneurysm	Thrombin injection, sometimes surgery
Retroperitoneal hematoma	Conservative, sometimes surgery
Femoral arterial occlusion	Vascular surgery consult, surgery
Aortic tear	Placement covered stent, sometimes surgery
Occlusion of left subclavian artery with a covered stent	Carotid to left subclavian artery anastomosis
Stroke	Conservative
Hypertension	IV antihypertensive to achieve high-normal blood pressure

11.12 Bare-Metal Stenting

Balloon-expandable stenting of coarctation of the aorta offers advantages over balloon dilation alone in that the stent prevents recoil of the vessel so the balloon does not need to be expanded beyond the normal vessel diameter, thus improving the final vessel diameter and decreasing the risk of aneurysm formation. Several stents can be used. The NuMED Cheatham-Platinum (CP) stent is the only stent to have received FDA approval for the indication of aortic stenting, though others are also commonly used for this indication. Self-expanding stents are rarely used as they do not have sufficient radial strength to offer much in the way of prevention of recoil.

Because the adult aorta is very noncompliant, if there is a tight narrowing especially for primary coarctation, it is inadvisable to expand the balloon to the nominal diameter of the normal aorta as this risks aortic wall tearing. Typically, the stent is deployed to expand the aortic lumen several millimeters with the plan to re-dilate the stent at a second and even third setting, months apart, up to the fully desired diameter of close to the normal diameter of the proximal aortic segment. Care must be taken not to use the distal aortic diameter as the reference measurement as there is usually post-stenotic dilation of this segment.

Results of stenting for native coarctation of the aorta in the adult are quite good. Recent experience suggests the risk of aortic dissection or aneurysm with staged stenting procedures is about 1% in the current era with other risks including femoral arterial injury and stent malposition about 0.5–2% [35]. Gradient relief appears to be very good with acute success 96% and long-term gradient relief and freedom from unplanned intervention 77% at 18–60 months.

The COAST trial (Coarctation of the Aorta Stent Trial) looked at the effectiveness of the CP stent for treatment of coarctation in 105 children and adults up to age 60 years [36]. There was good immediate and late gradient relief. There was a 6% incidence of aortic wall injury with pseudoaneurysm formation that required treatment with a covered stent. In addition, there was an increasing number of stent wire fractures noted with 2 at 1 year, 11 at 2 years, and 24 after 2 years. The wire fractures have not appeared to be clinically significant to date. After 2 years, 19 patients required reintervention to treat pseudoaneurysm or re-dilate the initially placed stent.

Patients who have undergone stenting for primary coarctation continue to have a significant incidence of residual hypertension [35] with one study showing 23% of patients with ongoing hypertension and 32% of patients on antihypertensive medications in long-term follow-up.

Patients who are not good candidates for stenting include those with aortic arch hypoplasia, or tortuous anatomy. In addition, it is important to note that the aorta becomes much less compliant with age. Older age becomes a risk for aortic wall tearing, rupture, and pseudoaneurysm.

11.13 Covered Stent

In order to prevent and also treat aortic wall injury associated with bare-metal stenting, covered stents were developed. There are a number of case reports and small case series describing self-made polytetrafluorethylene (PTFE) coverings for bare-metal stents, albeit the only commercially available covered stent to have received FDA approval is the NuMED Covered Cheatham-Platinum stent (NuMED, Hopkinton, NY). This stent has been available outside the USA for several years and was recently FDA approved on the data of the COAST II trial [37]. This trial enrolled 158 patients with a mean age of 19 years. Eighty-three patients had preexisting aortic wall injury, and the remaining covered stents were placed in patients that were felt to be at high risk of aortic wall injury. There was good gradient relief in the group as 93% of patients had the aortic wall injury completely covered by a single covered stent. There were no reinterventions in the short term. Four patients had important vascular injury including two with iliac artery dissection, one with femoral pseudoaneurysm, and one with femoral arterial occlusion related to suture closure of the vascular access site. The risk of vascular injury appears to be higher with the covered stents because of the larger sheath required for implantation of these stents. The lower rate of reintervention compared with bare-metal stents is related to the shorter-term follow-up of these patients but also the requirement for a covered stent that the proximal and distal ends of the stent be well-approximated to the vessel edge. If a significant part of the stent is not against the vessel wall, the leading edge risks folding into the stent lumen causing obstruction. For this reason and also because the stent is covered, the final diameter may and must be larger than it would be for initial placement of a bare-metal stent.

11.14 Surgery or Stent?

A non-randomized observational study from the Congenital Cardiovascular Interventional Study Consortium (CCISC) looked at 350 patients from 36 institutions of children and adults treated for native coarctation [33]. Patients were treated with either surgical repair by a variety of methods, bare-metal stenting, or balloon dilation alone. The findings of the study were that stented patients had the lowest overall incidence of complications (2.3%) though they had a 20% incidence of planned or unplanned intervention. Patients who underwent surgery or stenting had equally high rates of complete gradient relief (81% and 85%, respectively). Balloon dilation alone fared poorly with a complete gradient relief achieved in only 68%. Finally, balloon dilation patients were more likely to have aortic injury (dissection or aneurysm) (21%) than surgery (11.5%) or stent (3.1%). This data supports stenting or surgery as reasonable options for treatment of primary coarctation in the adult.

A randomized study comparing covered with non-covered CP stents for treatment of native coarctation in 120 adolescents and adults showed good results with both approaches [38]. There were two pseudoaneurysms seen in follow-up at the stent site, interestingly, both in the covered stent group. These were treated with implantation of a second covered stent to cover the leak.

For patients with recurrent coarctation after surgical repair, consensus statements [10, 11] recommend transcatheter intervention. A recent paper by the Mayo Clinic reviewed their experience comparing patients who underwent surgery for recoarctation compared to those who underwent stenting. They found both had low risk, but the surgical approach had a 96% freedom from reintervention at 5 years, whereas the transcatheter stenting group had only a 72% freedom from reintervention. Both surgery and stenting decreased the number of patients with hypertension (57% compared with 74% pre-intervention) and reduced the need for antihypertensive medication from a median of two prior to intervention to a median of one post-intervention [39].

11.15 Special Considerations

11.15.1 Pregnancy

Patients who have repaired coarctation of the aorta with no significant residual gradient, no aortic wall aneurysm, and good baseline blood pressure control generally tolerate pregnancy well [40]. There is some increased risk of pregnancy-induced hypertension in these patients that should be managed in the usual way by the obstetrical service. These patients do not generally require Cesarean delivery for maternal cardiac indications.

For patients with repaired coarctation who have residual hypertension managed medically without significant anatomic obstruction, they should not be on angiotensin-converting enzyme (ACE) inhibitors or angiotensin receptor blockers (ARBs) if they are contemplating pregnancy because of the potential teratogenic effect on the fetal kidney. The absolute risk of these medications is not high, however, and more of an issue in the second trimester. If a woman discovers she is pregnant while on an ACE or ARB, stopping the medication and following the fetus is usually all that is required. These patients with hypertension are at an even higher risk for pregnancy-induced hypertension, and close maternal follow-up is mandatory during pregnancy.

Patients with unrepaired coarctation or repaired coarctation with residual obstruction should not become pregnant; however the scenario does present where expectant mothers with unrepaired coarctation are only first diagnosed during pregnancy. Depending on the severity of the coarctation, blood pressure, the status of the left ventricular function, and symptoms, consideration for termination versus continuing the pregnancy can be made. In this instance, the risk of pregnancy-induced hypertension is elevated, and assisted second-stage delivery or Cesarean delivery should be considered.

Both repaired and unrepaired patients with coarctation should have imaging of the aorta to exclude aneurysm prior to pregnancy. If not performed prior to the pregnancy, then cardiac MRI without gadolinium would be test of choice in the expectant mother. Aneurysm of the aorta is worrisome during pregnancy because of the risk of rupture. In addition to the increased cardiac output and increase in blood pressure with labor and delivery, estrogen is known to weaken the arterial wall. If an aneurysm is found, then consideration should be given to termination or intervention during pregnancy which may include a covered stent. Delivery should avoid pushing and is probably best accomplished with a Cesarean section [40].

The risk of left-sided obstructive lesions in the fetus of mothers with coarctation of the aorta may be as high as 10%. This includes everything from an isolated bicuspid aortic valve all the way to most severe hypoplastic left heart syndrome [41]. There is no specific genetic test available to ascertain who is most at risk. Early fetal ultrasound at 14–16 weeks and follow-up scans may be needed to exclude serious congenital heart disease. This can be very important in the management of the fetus but also in decision-making for the mother.

11.16 Other Non-cardiac Surgeries

For patients with unrepaired coarctation or repaired coarctation with residual stenosis, ICU management perioperatively for non-cardiac surgery may arise. Again, knowing which limbs reflect the central blood pressure is important. These patients may need their upper extremity blood pressure managed to reflect "what they are used to" rather than normotension as the kidneys will still see the blunted lower pressure beyond the coarctation. Creating normotension in the upper body will lead to relative hypotension in the lower body potentially compromising renal and splanchnic flow.

References

1. Bjornard K, Riehle-Colarusso T, Gilboa SM, Correa A. Patterns in the prevalence of congenital heart defects, metropolitan Atlanta, 1978 to 2005. Birth Defects Res Part A: Clin Mol Teratol. 2013;97:87–94.
2. Becker AE, Becker MJ, Edwards JE. Anomalies associated with coarctation of the aorta. Particular reference to infancy. Circulation. 1970;41:1067–75.
3. Sybert VP. Cardiovascular malformations and complications in Turner Syndrome. Pediatrics. 1998;101(1):E11.
4. Paris M. Retrecissement considerable de l'aorta pectorale observe a l'Hotel Dieu de Paris. Jour de Chirurgie de Desault. 1791;ii:107.

5. Abbott ME. Statistical study and historical retrospect of 200 recorded cases, with autopsy, of stenosis or obliteration of the descending arch in subjects above the age of two years. Am Heart J. 1928;3:392–421. 574–618
6. Reifenstein GH, Levine SA, Gross RE. Coarctation of the aorta: a review of 104 autopsied cases of the "adult-type", 2 years of age or older. Am Heart J. 1947;33:146–68.
7. Bambul Heck P, Pabst von Ohain J, Kaemmerer H, et al. Survival and cardiovascular events after coarctation repair in long-term follow-up (COAFU): predictive value of clinical variables. Int J Cardiol. 2017;228:347–51.
8. Roifman I, Therrien J, Ionescu-Ittu R, Pilote L, Guo L, Kotowycz MA, Martucci G, Marelli AJ. Coarctation of the aorta and coronary artery disease: fact or fiction? Circulation. 2012;126(1):16–21.
9. Rinnstrom D, Dellborg M, Thilen U, et al. Hypertension in adults with repaired coarctation of the aorta. Am Heart J. 2016;181:10–5.
10. Warnes CA, Williams RG, Bashore TM, Child JS. ACC/AHA 2008 Guidelines for the management of adults with congenital heart disease. J Am Coll Cardiol. 2008;52:e143–263.
11. Silversides CK, Kiess M, Beauchesne L, Bradley T, Connelly M, Niwa K, Mulder B, Webb G, Colman J, Therrien J. Canadian Cardiovascular Society 2009 Consensus Conference on the management of adults with congenital heart disease: outflow tract obstruction, coarctation of the aorta, tetralogy of fallot, Ebstein anomaly and Marfan's syndrome. Can J Cardiol. 2010;26(3):e80–97.
12. Nielsen JC, Powell AJ, Gavreau K, Marcus EN, Prakash A, Geva T. Magnetic resonance imaging predictors of coarctation severity. Circulation. 2005;111(5):622–8.
13. Muzzarelli S, Meadows AK, Ordovas KG, et al. Prediction of hemodynamic severity of coarctation by magnetic resonance imaging. Am J Cardiol. 2011;108:1335–40.
14. Connolly HM, Huston J III, Brown RD Jr, Warnes CA, Ammash NM, Tajik AJ. Intracranial aneurysms in patients with coarctation of the aorta: a prospective magnetic resonance angiographic study of 100 patients. Mayo Clin Proc. 2003;78:1491–9.
15. Crafoord C, Nylin G. Congenital coarctation of the aorta and its surgical treatment. J Thorac Surg. 1945;14:347–61.
16. Williams WG, Shindo G, Trusler GA, Dische MR, Olley PM. Results of repair of coarctation of the aorta during infancy. J Thorac Cardiovasc Surg. 1980;79:603–8.
17. Kappetein AP, Zwinderman AH, Bogers AJJC, Rohmer J, Huysmns HA. More than thirty five years of coarctation repair: an unexpected high relapse rate. J Thorac Cardiovasc Surg. 1994;107:87–95.
18. Presbitero P, Demarie D, Villani M, Perinetto EA, Rivera G, Orzan F, Bobbio M, Morea M, Brusca A. Long term results (15–30 years) of surgical repair of aortic coarctation. Br Heart J. 1987;57:462–7.
19. Sanchez GR, Balsara RK, Dunn JM, Mehta AV, O'Riordan AC. Recurrent obstruction after subclavian flap repair of coarctation of the aorta in infants. J Thorac Cardiovasc Surg. 1986;91:738–46.
20. Cobanoglu A, Teply JF, Grunkeimier GL, Sunderland CO, Starr A. Coarctation of the aorta in patients younger than three months: a critique of the subclavian flap operation. J Thorac Cardiovasc Surg. 1985;89:128–35.
21. Connolly HM, Schaff HV, Izhar U, Dearani JA, Warnes CA, Orszulak TA. Posterior pericardial ascending-to-descending aortic bypass: an alternative surgical approach for complex coarctation of the aorta. Circulation. 2001;104:133–7.
22. Hadley MN, Walters BC, Aarabi B, et al. Guidelines for the management of acute cervical spine and spinal cord injuries. Neurosurgery. 2013;72:1–259.
23. Tawes RL Jr, Bull JC, Roe BB. Hypertension and abdominal pain after resection of aortic coarctation. Ann Surg. 1970;171:409–12.
24. McGrath EE, Blades Z, Anderson PB. Chylothorax: aetiology, diagnosis and therapeutic options. Respir Med. 2010;104(1):1–8.
25. Fox S, Pierce W, Waldhausen JA. Pathogenesis of paradoxical hypertension after coarctation repair. Ann Thorac Surg. 1978;29(2):135–41.

26. Choy M, Rocchini AP, Beekman RH, Rosenthal A, Dick M, Crowley D, Behrendt D, Snider AR. Paradoxical hypertension after repair of coarctation of the aorta in children: balloon angioplasty versus surgical repair. Circulation. 1987;75:1186–91.
27. Gidding SS, Rochchini AP, Beekman R, Szpunar CA, Moorehead C, Behrendt D, Rosenthal A. Therapeutic effect of propranolol on paradoxical hypertension after repair of coarctation of the aorta. N Engl J Med. 1985;312(19):1224–8.
28. Salgado DR, Silva E, Vincent JL. Control of hypertension in the critically ill: a pathophysiological approach. Ann Intensive Care. 2013;3:17.
29. Cohen M, Fuster V, Steele PM, Driscoll D, McGoon DC. Coarctation of the aorta. Long-term follow-up and prediction of outcome after surgical correction. Circulation. 1989;80:840–5.
30. Brouwer RMHJ, Erasmus ME, Ebels T, Aijgelaar A. Influence of age on survival, late hypertension and recoarctation in elective aortic coarctation repair. J Thorac Cardiovasc Surg. 1994;108:525–31.
31. Chen SS, Dimopoulos K, Alonso-Gonzalez R, et al. Prevalence and prognostic implication of restenosis or dilation at the aortic coarctation repair site assessed by cardiovascular MRI adult patients late after coarctation repair. Int J Cardiol. 2014;173:209–15.
32. Silka MJ, Hardy BG, Menashe VD, Morris CD. A population-based prospective evaluation of risk of sudden cardiac death after operation for common congenital heart defects. J Am Coll Cardiol. 1998;32(1):245–51.
33. Forbes TJ, Kim DW, Wei D, et al. Comparison of surgical, stent, and balloon angioplasty treatment of native coarctation of the aorta. J Am Coll Cardiol. 2011;58:2664–74.
34. Hassan W, Awad M, Fawzy ME, et al. Long-term effects of balloon angioplasty on left ventricular hypertrophy in adolescent and adult patients with native coarctation of the aorta. Up to 18 years follow-up results. Catheter Cardiovasc Interv. 2007;70:881–6.
35. Holzer R, Qureshi S, Ghasemi A, et al. Stenting of aortic coarctation: acute, intermediate and long-term results of a prospective, multiinstitutional registry—Congenital Cardiovascular Interventional Study Consortium (CCISC). Catheter Cardiovasc Interv. 2010;76:553–63.
36. Meadows J, Minahan M, DB ME, et al. Intermediate outcomes in the prospective, multicenter coarctation of the aorta stents trial (COAST). Circulation. 2015;131(19):1656–64.
37. Taggart NW, Minahan M, Cabalka AK, et al. Immediate outcomes of covered stent placement for treatment or prevention of aortic wall injury associated with coarctation of the aorta (COAST II). JACC Cardiovasc Interv. 2016;9(5):484–93.
38. Sohrabi B, Jamshidi P, Yaghoubi A, et al. Comparison between covered and bare Cheatham-Platinum stents for endovascular treatment of patients with native post-ductal aortic coarctation: immediate and intermediate results. JACC Cardiovasc Interv. 2014;4:416–23.
39. Brown ML, Bukhart HM, Connolly HM, Dearani JA, Hagler DJ, Schaff HV. Late outcomes of reintervention on the descending aorta after repair of aortic coarctation. Circulation. 2010;122(suppl 1):s81–4.
40. Swan L, Lupton M, Anthony J, Yentis SM, Steer PJ, Gatzoulis MA. Controversies in pregnancy and congenital heart disease. Congenit Heart Dis. 2006;1(1–2):27–34.
41. Cripe L, Andelfinger G, Martin LJ, et al. Bicuspid aortic valve is heritable. J Am Coll Cardiol. 2004;44:138–43.

Critical Care Management of the Adult with the Univentricular Heart

12

Mina Hafzalah, John M. Costello, Carl L. Backer, R. Andrew de Freitas, and Constantine Mavroudis

M. Hafzalah (✉)
Division of Pediatric Critical Care Medicine, Children's Hospital of Illinois/UICOMP, Peoria, IL, USA
e-mail: mhafza@uic.edu

J. M. Costello
Department of Pediatrics, Medical University of South Carolina, Charleston, SC, USA

Department of Pediatric Cardiology, Medical University of South Carolina Children's Hospital, Charleston, SC, USA
e-mail: costello@musc.edu

C. L. Backer
Department of Surgery, Northwestern University Feinberg School of Medicine, Chicago, IL, USA

Cardiovascular-Thoracic Surgery, Ann & Robert H. Lurie Children's Hospital of Chicago, Chicago, IL, USA
e-mail: cbacker@luriechildrens.org

R. Andrew de Freitas
Department of Pediatrics, Medical University of South Carolina, Charleston, SC, USA

Adult Congenital Heart Disease Service, Ann & Robert H. Lurie Children's Hospital of Chicago, Chicago, IL, USA

Bluhm Cardiovascular Institute, Northwestern Memorial Hospital, Chicago, IL, USA

C. Mavroudis
Department of Surgery, Johns Hopkins University School of Medicine, Baltimore, MD, USA

Johns Hopkins Children's Heart Surgery, Florida Hospital for Children, Orlando, FL, USA

E. da Cruz et al. (eds.), *Intensive Care of the Adult with Congenital Heart Disease*, Congenital Heart Disease in Adolescents and Adults,
https://doi.org/10.1007/978-3-319-94171-4_12

12.1 Introduction

The functionally univentricular heart includes a broad category of congenital cardiac malformations characterized by both atria related entirely or almost entirely to one functionally single ventricular chamber [1]. Although often referred to as having a "single ventricle," in most cases, a second rudimentary or hypoplastic ventricle is present. Functionally univentricular hearts account for approximately 15% of all congenital cardiac defects. Common types include hypoplastic left heart syndrome (HLHS), tricuspid atresia, unbalanced atrioventricular septal defects, double inlet left ventricle, and pulmonary atresia with intact ventricular septum.

Improvements in surgical palliation, perioperative care, and outpatient management in recent decades have allowed more patients with functionally univentricular heart defects to survive to adulthood [2]. Given the unique cardiovascular anatomy, physiology, and non-cardiac comorbidities present in this patient population, an in-depth understanding of the esoteric nuances in the diagnostic evaluation and critical care management is necessary to achieve optimal outcomes. Access to multiple clinicians with expertise in adult congenital heart disease is often needed, and when feasible, intensive care for this patient population should be provided in a regional adult congenital heart disease center [3].

In this chapter, we review the cardiac surgical approach to the patient with a functionally univentricular heart. We then summarize the primary principles for evaluation and management, focusing on issues most relevant to the underlying cardiac anatomy and cardiovascular physiology.

12.2 Surgical Palliation for Functionally Univentricular Hearts

The ultimate goal of surgical palliation for functionally univentricular hearts is to convert the circulation from a "complete mixing" circulation, in which systemic and pulmonary venous return mix in the single ventricle before being actively pumped to both the pulmonary and systemic vascular beds, to a series circulation in which the single ventricle provides systemic blood flow and pulmonary blood flow is dependent on passive systemic venous return. Each operation is performed with the goal of optimizing anticipated Fontan physiology [4]. Efforts are made to limit volume and pressure loading on the systemic ventricle, thereby limiting myocardial hypertrophy. Preservation of atrioventricular and semilunar valve function and avoidance of systemic outflow tract obstruction are important. Minimizing resistance in the pulmonary vascular circuit is also essential. Prolonged periods of excessive pulmonary blood flow or obstructed pulmonary venous return, both of which may increase pulmonary vascular resistance, are avoided. The cross-sectional area of the pulmonary vascular bed must be preserved and proximal pulmonary artery distortion minimized. Maintenance of atrioventricular synchrony optimizes cardiac efficiency.

12.2.1 Neonatal Palliation

The initial operation is typically performed in the neonatal period. The guiding principles for this first operation are to provide balanced pulmonary and systemic perfusion while optimizing the performance of each circuit. These principles are accomplished by providing an unobstructed pathway from the single ventricle to the systemic circulation, a regulated, temporary source of pulmonary blood flow, and unobstructed systemic and pulmonary venous return [5]. In patients with severe pulmonary stenosis or atresia, the regulated source of pulmonary blood flow is provided by a systemic to pulmonary shunt (Fig. 12.1), whereas those with excessive pulmonary blood flow may undergo placement of a pulmonary artery band (Fig. 12.2). The Norwood procedure, which is commonly used for initial palliation of neonates with HLHS, embodies these guiding principles [6]. An unobstructed systemic outflow tract is created by reconstructing the aortic arch and amalgamating the diminutive native aorta with the pulmonary artery. The distal pulmonary artery is oversewn, and regulated pulmonary blood flow is provided by a modified Blalock–Taussig shunt or right ventricular to pulmonary artery conduit (i.e., "Sano shunt") [7]. An atrial septectomy is performed to allow unobstructed egress of pulmonary venous return from the left atrium.

12.2.2 Superior Cavopulmonary Connection

Historically, patients with functionally univentricular hearts who outgrew their initial source of pulmonary blood flow were palliated with additional systemic to pulmonary shunts prior to the Fontan operation. While acutely effective in alleviating hypoxemia, this approach led to additional volume loading of the single ventricle and potential distortion of the pulmonary arteries. Since the 1990s, the second-stage operation has typically entailed the creation of a superior cavopulmonary connection (i.e., a bidirectional Glenn or hemi-Fontan) at 4–6 months of age [8]. During the bidirectional Glenn procedure, the superior vena cava is routed directly to the pulmonary arteries, and any previously placed systemic to pulmonary shunts are taken down (Fig. 12.3). The creation of a superior cavopulmonary connection serves to improve systemic oxygen saturation and reduce the volume load on the single ventricle, with the intent of optimizing ventricular function in anticipation of eventual Fontan physiology [9].

12.2.3 Fontan Operation

The Fontan operation connects systemic venous return directly to the pulmonary artery circulation, thereby bypassing the underdeveloped right or left heart. The resulting circulation relies on passive, nonpulsatile flow through the lungs. The original Fontan operation, first reported in 1971 in patients with tricuspid atresia,

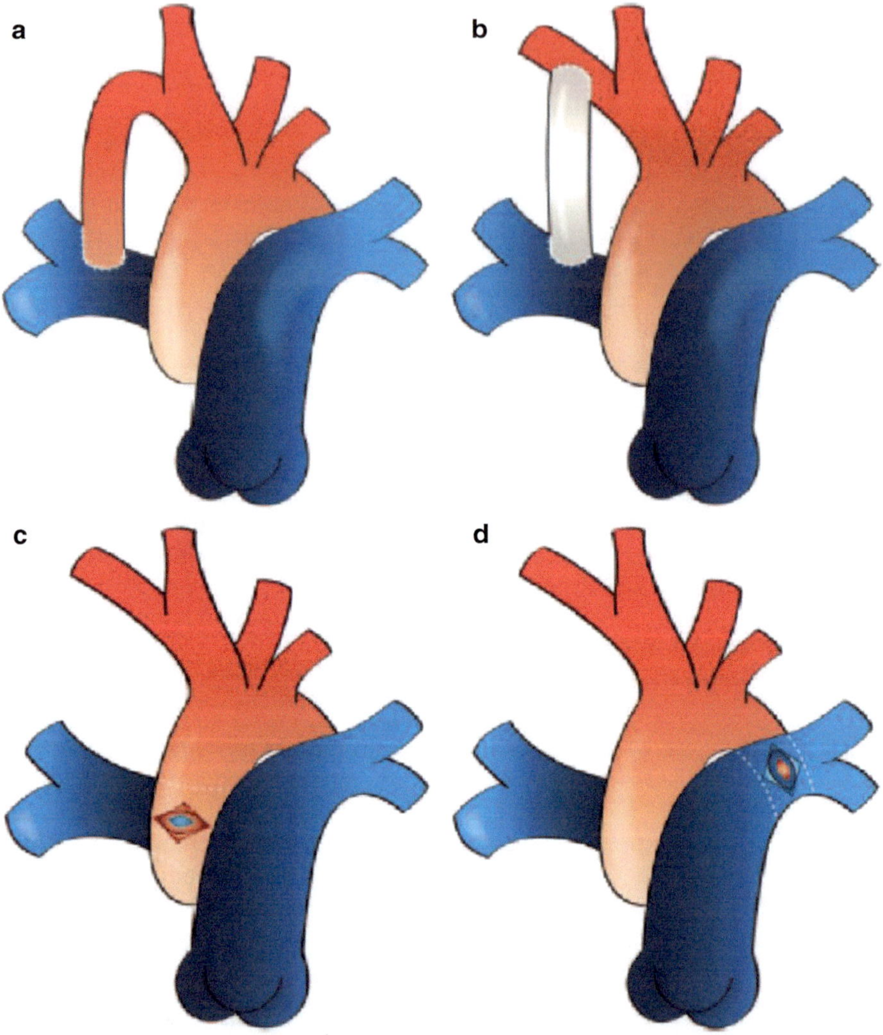

Fig. 12.1 Aortopulmonary shunts. (**a**) The classic Blalock–Taussig shunt consists of an end-to-side anastomosis of the subclavian artery and pulmonary artery. (**b**) The modified Blalock–Taussig shunt consists of an interposition tube graft that connects the subclavian artery to the ipsilateral pulmonary artery. (**c**) A Waterston shunt consists of a connection between the ascending aorta and pulmonary artery. (**d**) A Potts shunt involves a communication between the descending aorta and ipsilateral pulmonary artery. In the current era, modified Blalock–Taussig shunts, aortopulmonary shunts (figure not shown), and right ventricular to pulmonary conduits (i.e., "Sano" shunt, figure not shown) are the most common type of systemic to pulmonary shunts. Reprinted from Khairy et al., Circulation 2007;115:800–12, with permission

included a direct anastomosis of the right atrium to the main pulmonary artery and a separate connection of the superior vena cava to the right pulmonary artery [10]. Conceptually, the pulsatile right atrium was thought to optimize flow to the pulmonary arteries. However, many such "classic" Fontan patients developed atrial

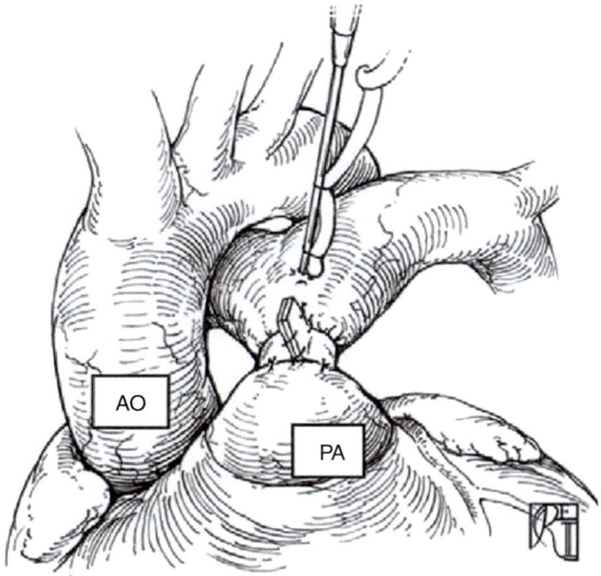

Fig. 12.2 Pulmonary artery band. Reprinted from Backer CL. W Journal Pediatr Cong Heart Surg 2012;3;165–70, with permission

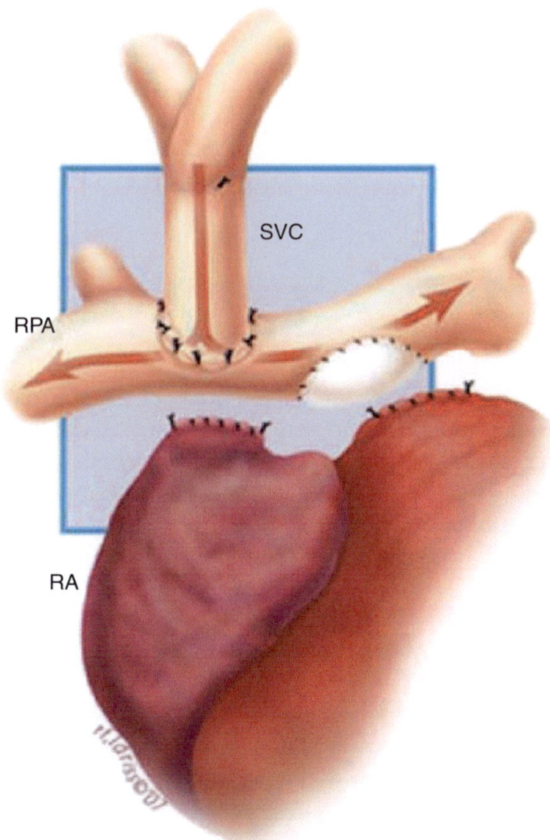

Fig. 12.3 Illustration of a completed bidirectional cavopulmonary anastomosis (i.e., bidirectional Glenn operation). Reprinted from MacIver RH. Cardiol Young 2008;18:147–52, with permission

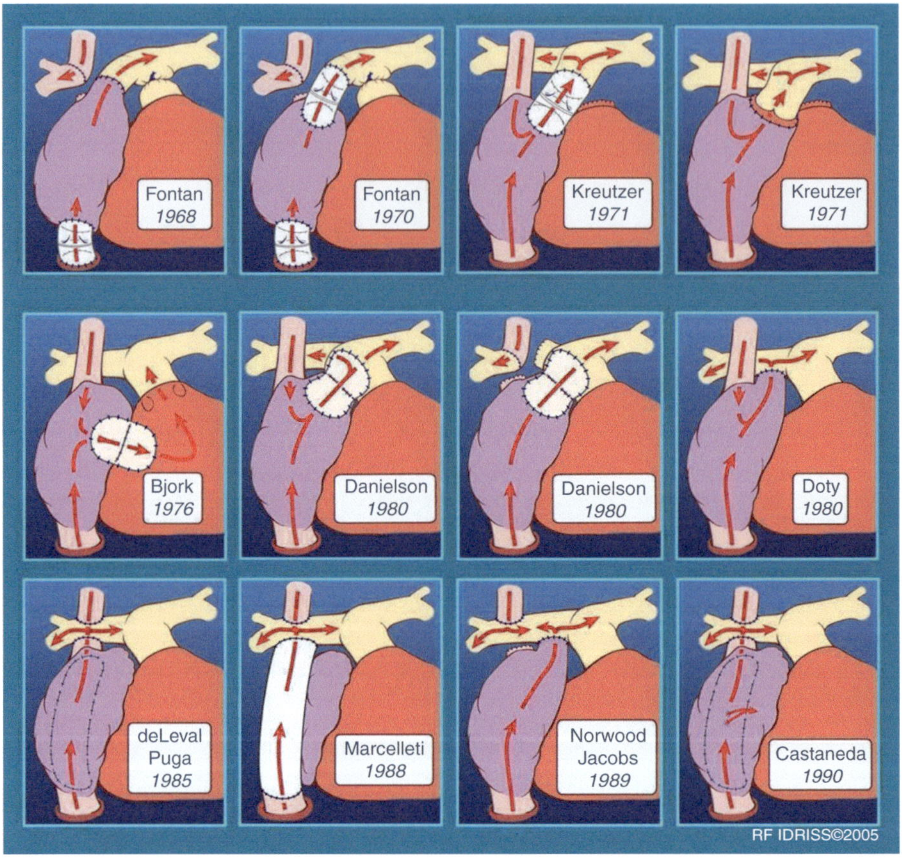

Fig. 12.4 Illustrations depicting the evolution of the Fontan procedure

dilation with resultant energy loss, arrhythmias, and thromboemboli. Over the years, a number of modifications have been made to the Fontan operation (Fig. 12.4). In the current era, at 2–4 years of age, an extracardiac conduit or intra-atrial lateral tunnel is used to reroute inferior vena cava flow to the pulmonary arteries [11, 12]. A fenestration may be created in the Fontan pathway to allow right-to-left shunting at the atrial level, which serves to lower the Fontan pathway pressure and maintain preload to the systemic ventricle at the expense of mild cyanosis [13, 14].

12.2.4 Fontan Conversion

Following the Fontan operation, patients may undergo one or more unplanned cardiac reinterventions for a variety of indications. Ablation procedures may be attempted for atrial arrhythmias. A permanent pacemaker may be placed to treat sinus node dysfunction and atrioventricular block or to facilitate treatment of atrial tachyarrhythmias. Atrioventricular or semilunar valve dysfunction, compromised Fontan pathway, systemic ventricular outflow tract obstruction, and aortopulmonary or veno-venous collateral vessels may warrant reintervention by surgery and/or by cardiac catheterization.

The "Fontan conversion" operation may be undertaken in selected Fontan patients, typically those with an atriopulmonary connection who suffer from right atrial dilation with refractory atrial arrhythmias and energy loss [15]. This operation typically involves takedown of the atriopulmonary connection with conversion to an extracardiac Fontan, atrial reduction, atrial arrhythmia surgery (e.g., right-sided maze or Cox Maze III), and placement of a permanent pacemaker. Other residual lesions (e.g., atrioventricular valve regurgitation, pulmonary artery stenosis) are addressed as needed. Operative mortality for the Fontan conversion operation as reported in the Society of Thoracic Surgeons Congenital Heart Surgery Database (July 2012–June 2016) is 5.7%. In the largest reported single-center experience with this operation, operative mortality occurred in 2 of 140 cases (1.4%), and freedom from cardiac death or transplant was 84% at 10 years [16].

12.2.5 Unoperated Functionally Univentricular Heart

The natural history of patients with functionally univentricular hearts who do not undergo surgical intervention is poor, with the vast majority dying in infancy or childhood [17]. Occasionally patients survive to adult age with an unoperated single ventricle heart defect. Such patients typically have a morphological left ventricle with either pulmonary stenosis (resulting in a "balanced" circulation) or Eisenmenger's syndrome [18]. Such patients may be admitted to an ICU for arrhythmias, thromboembolism, complications of hyperviscosity, and eventual heart failure. Although typically not good candidates for Fontan palliation or cardiac transplantation, survival to the sixth and seventh decade of life has been reported in a small number of patients.

Carefully selected adults with unoperated single ventricles may be considered for creation of a bidirectional Glenn operation [19]. Similarly, occasionally a late-presenting patient may undergo Fontan completion for the first time as an adult. Recent data indicate that operative mortality and intermediate-term Fontan failure rates for such patient are quite high relative to patients who underwent Fontan operation in early childhood [20].

12.3 Critical Care Issues

12.3.1 Intensive Care Unit Admission Epidemiology

Data from the National Inpatient Sample indicate that rates of hospitalization for adults with functionally univentricular hearts are increasing [21]. Admissions for cardiothoracic surgical procedures, cardiac catheterization, and electrophysiology

Table 12.1 Common indications for ICU admission in adults with functionally univentricular hearts

Indication	Examples
Postoperative care following cardiac surgery	• Fontan conversion • Valve repair/replacement • Pacemaker placement/revision
Postoperative care following non-cardiac cardiac surgery	• Wide variety
Post-procedural monitoring	• Cardiac catheterization • Invasive electrophysiology procedure
Acutely decompensated heart failure	• Ventricular failure • Endocarditis • Atrioventricular valve regurgitation
Arrhythmia	• Atrial reentrant tachycardia • Atrial flutter • Advanced heart block • Permanent pacemaker malfunction
Cardiac arrest	• Arrhythmia • Peri-procedural
Non-cardiac acute medical condition	• Stroke • Central nervous system hemorrhage • Gastrointestinal bleeding • Hepatic or renal insufficiency • Infection/sepsis

procedures are common. Admitted patients commonly have comorbid medical conditions, including congestive heart failure, arrhythmia, cyanosis, valvar disease, pulmonary vascular conditions, and thrombus within the cardiovascular system [21, 22]. Other common non-cardiac ICU admission diagnoses for adults with functionally univentricular hearts include acute kidney injury, urosepsis, pneumonia, asthma, esophageal reflux, hypothyroidism, liver cirrhosis, obstructive sleep apnea, and neurologic symptoms that raise concern for stroke [23]. Common indications for ICU admission for adults with functionally univentricular hearts are summarized in Table 12.1. Regardless of the anticipated need for postoperative intensive care, elective procedures in adults with functionally univentricular hearts should be performed in a regional adult congenital heart disease center [24]. The threshold for ICU admission for young adults with functionally univentricular hearts is likely lower than that used for young adults without heart disease who are admitted for similar conditions.

12.3.2 Intake to the Intensive Care Unit

Optimal evaluation and management of adults with functionally univentricular hearts may be achieved by understanding the anatomic and physiologic details of each case. In addition to receiving a detailed handoff from the clinicians providing care for the patient immediately prior to ICU admission (e.g., emergency room clinicians, surgeon, interventional cardiologist), it is important to review relevant medical records (e.g., most recent clinic letter) and communicate with the adult congenital heart disease physician who is providing outpatient care for the patient. Note that neurodevelopmental issues are common in patients with complex congenital heart disease, which may compromise the accuracy and level of detail of histories provided by some patients.

It is essential for ICU clinicians to understand the details of the cardiopulmonary anatomy. This includes knowledge of the primary cardiac defect, any surgeries or transcatheter interventions, and the presence of any hemodynamic lesions, either fixed or dynamic. Additionally, an understanding is needed of baseline physiology, including hemoglobin, blood pressure, systemic oxygen saturation, and heart rate and rhythm. An appreciation is needed of the impact that any interventions (e.g., oxygen, vasoactive infusions, positive pressure ventilation) may have on this physiology. Limited vascular access (e.g., prior occlusion, anatomic variants), noncardiac comorbidities, and advanced directives may influence decision-making in the ICU. Early during the ICU stay, collaboration with congenital heart surgeons, heart failure specialists, and electrophysiologists may be beneficial.

12.3.3 Low Cardiac Output

12.3.3.1 Etiologies of Low Cardiac Output

In adults with functionally univentricular hearts, a low cardiac output syndrome may be present upon ICU admission or may develop during the ICU stay. Even in the best of circumstances, many patients with functionally univentricular hearts exist in a state of chronic heart failure, particularly by the time they reach adulthood [25]. Myriad factors contribute to this chronic low cardiac output state (Table 12.2). An acute on chronic heart failure state may develop for a wide variety of reasons, most commonly including worsening myocardial failure, arrhythmias, and postoperative ischemia-reperfusion injury. Factors that compromise systemic venous return may be poorly tolerated in patients with cavopulmonary connections (i.e., Glenn or Fontan). For example, general anesthesia and the use of positive pressure ventilation during operative or transcatheter procedures may compromise pulmonary blood flow, leading to inadequate ventricular preload and low cardiac output. The pneumoperitoneum created to facilitate laparoscopic abdominal surgery may decrease systemic venous return and increase systemic vascular resistance, both of which may decrease cardiac output.

Arrhythmias may lead to a low cardiac output state in adults with functionally univentricular hearts. Atrial tachyarrhythmias (especial atrial reentrant tachycardia and atrial fibrillation) are particularly common due to the high prevalence of atrial dilation, suture lines, atrioventricular valve dilation, and poor ventricular compliance. Atrial systole contributes to approximately 20% of ventricular preload and cardiac output, and thus the loss of atrioventricular synchrony may result in rapid hemodynamic deterioration. Incessant atrial tachyarrhythmias may result in a "tachycardia mediated cardiomyopathy" that may be reversible with restoration of sinus rhythm.

Table 12.2 Factors contributing to chronic heart failure in adults with functionally univentricular hearts

Pathophysiology	Key contributing factors	Comments
Ventricular dysfunction	• Chronic volume/pressure overload (e.g., parallel circulation, valvar regurgitation, aortopulmonary collaterals) • Cyanosis • Ischemia-reperfusion injury	• Single right ventricle not morphologically designed to support systemic circulation
Incessant atrial arrhythmias	• Atrial dilation • Suture lines	• 50% of patients with Fontan physiology will experience supraventricular tachycardia • 10 years post Fontan the risk of SVT is 20% and 50% for patients with atriopulmonary classic Fontan
Atrioventricular valve regurgitation	• Chronic volume/pressure overload	• Tricuspid valve not morphologically designed to withstand systemic pressure
Fontan pathway obstruction	• Pulmonary artery stenosis • Obstruction of extracardiac conduit anastomosis	• Obstruction may be present despite low pressure gradients (e.g., 1–2 mmHg)
Elevated pulmonary vascular resistance	• Thromboembolism • Longstanding ↑ pulmonary blood flow	• Thromboembolism caused by antithrombin III deficiency, venous congestion, atrial dilation, stagnant blood flow
Systemic venous hypertension	• Fontan physiology • ↑ Pulmonary artery pressure	• Manifests with gastrointestinal symptoms, hepatic congestion, ascites
Chronic cyanosis	• Fontan fenestration • Fontan baffle leak • Veno-venous collaterals • Pulmonary arteriovenous malformations	• SvO_2 must be interpreted in the context of baseline SaO_2
Systemic ventricular outflow obstruction	• Residual aortic arch obstruction • Restrictive bulboventricular foramen	• Minimal gradients (e.g., ~10 mmHg) may be important in functionally univentricular hearts

SaO_2 systemic arterial oxygen saturation, *SvO_2* systemic venous oxygen saturation

12.3.3.2 Evaluation of Low Cardiac Output

Although many principles regarding the evaluation of low cardiac output in patients with structurally normal hearts may be applied to those with functionally univentricular hearts (e.g., assessment of heart rate/rhythm, ventricular function, loading conditions, etc.), several important nuances warrant comment. For example, assessment of ventricular function by echocardiogram may be difficult as the ventricular geometry may be distorted, making calculation of ejection fraction by conventional techniques unreliable. The baseline electrocardiogram appearance is highly variable in adults with functionally univentricular hearts which may confound the assessment of rhythm or ischemia. For example, patients with heterotaxy syndrome and right atrial isomerism may have two sinus nodes, whereas those with left atrial isomerism often have none. The atrioventricular node may be displaced in patients with atrioventricular discordance or atrioventricular septal defects. Patients with double inlet left ventricles may have Q waves in over the right precordial and inferior limb leads. Additionally, the proper interpretation of chest computed tomography angiogram (CTA) scan images may be difficult due to distorted systemic venous flow patterns and issues related to the timing of contrast injection.

Monitoring for low cardiac output should be undertaken with an appreciation for the underlying cardiac anatomy and physiology. Hemodynamic monitoring lines should be placed with prior knowledge of vascular anatomy and potentially occluded vessels. For example, in a patient with a prior classic Blalock–Taussig shunt, blood pressure measurements in the ipsilateral arm may be falsely low, and an arterial line should not be placed in that extremity. In patients with a bidirectional Glenn operation, pressure measured through an internal jugular line will reflect the pulmonary artery pressure, which is often 5–10 mmHg higher than the right atrial pressure. Evaluation of systemic venous oxygen saturation measurements must be made in the context of systemic arterial oxygen saturation values, which may be abnormal at baseline in patients with functionally univentricular hearts (Table 12.3).

Table 12.3 Causes of hypoxemia in patients with functionally univentricular hearts

Physiology	Examples	Initial evaluation	Comments
Pulmonary venous/left atrial desaturation	*Acute:* • Pneumothorax • Pleural effusion • Pulmonary edema • Pneumonia • Atelectasis • Aspiration *Chronic:* • Veno-venous collaterals • Pulmonary arteriovenous malformations • Fontan baffle leak • Fontan fenestration	• CXR for acute pulmonary issues • ECHO for baffle leak, fenestration	• Consider catheterization to diagnose veno-venous collaterals • Consider bubble study or catheterization to diagnose pulmonary arteriovenous malformations
Systemic venous desaturation	*Acute:* • ↑ VO_2 *Acute or Chronic:* • ↓ Cardiac output • Anemia	• Hemoglobin • Temperature • ECG, ECHO, SvO_2	• Any cause of systemic venous desaturation will cause systemic desaturation in patients with right to left shunts or intracardiac mixing
Decreased pulmonary blood flow	*Acute:* • ↓ SVR in patient with S-P shunt • Pulmonary embolus *Chronic:* • Pulmonary artery obstruction • Pulmonary vein obstruction • Small systemic to pulmonary shunt • ↑ PVR	• Exclusion of pulmonary and systemic venous desaturation • Arterial blood gas • Echo to assess shunt, pulmonary artery anatomy (echo windows often limited in adults)	• Consider CT angiography or catheterization to evaluate anatomic issues, PE • Consider catheterization to evaluate anatomy, PVR

CXR chest radiograph, *CT* computed tomography, *ECHO* echocardiogram, *ECG* electrocardiogram, *PE* pulmonary embolism, *PVR* pulmonary vascular resistance, *S-P* systemic to pulmonary, *SVR* systemic vascular resistance, SvO_2 systemic venous oxygen saturation, VO_2 oxygen consumption

Table 12.4 Hemodynamic changes seen in common causes of low cardiac output with Fontan physiology

Fontan [59] pressure	Common (left) atrial pressure	Common etiologies
Low	Low	Hypovolemia: • Bleeding • Inadequate preload
High	Low	• Fontan pathway or pulmonary artery obstruction (e.g., anatomic, clot) • Elevated pulmonary vascular resistance • Clotted fenestration
High	High	• Ventricular failure • Arrhythmia • Atrioventricular valve stenosis or regurgitation • Ventricular outflow tract obstruction • Tamponade

Hemodynamic changes seen in Fontan patients with various causes of low cardiac output are summarized in Table 12.4. Of note, caution is needed to minimize the chances of a paradoxical air embolism related to central venous catheters.

In adults with functionally univentricular hearts, consideration must be given to iatrogenic causes of low cardiac output and hypotension caused by delayed clearance of medications commonly used in the ICU. Many of these patients have chronic hepatic and renal insufficiency due to chronic cyanosis, elevated venous pressure, chronic low cardiac output, and prior exposure to nephrotoxic medications and cardiopulmonary bypass. Delayed metabolism and clearance of many drugs, such as milrinone, benzodiazepines, and narcotics, may contribute to sustained hypotension.

12.3.3.3 Management of Low Cardiac Output

The management of low cardiac output syndrome in patients with functionally univentricular hearts can be particularly challenging. Similar to patients with structurally normal hearts, general strategies are focused on optimizing systemic oxygen delivery while minimizing oxygen consumption [26]. However, a number of important nuances exist in the management of adults with functionally univentricular heart defects. Attention to factors that influence stroke volume (i.e., preload, contractility, and afterload) is important. Patients with Fontan physiology are preload dependent. A reasonable target Fontan (i.e., CVP) pressure in a critically ill adult is 14–16 mmHg, although occasionally slightly higher pressures (e.g., 18–22 mmHg) are needed to maintain cardiac output, particularly in patients receiving positive pressure ventilation. If available, a reasonable common ("left") atrial pressure target range is ~6–10 mmHg. Patients with hypertrophy of the single ventricle may benefit from slightly higher filling pressures due to the inherent restrictive physiology.

Maintaining adequate oxygen carrying capacity (e.g., hemoglobin) is obviously important when managing a low cardiac output state. Patients with functionally univentricular hearts who are cyanotic often have compensatory erythrocytosis.

Transfusing packed red blood cells to keep hemoglobin levels near the patient's baseline may be useful to augment systemic oxygen delivery.

Factors that increase oxygen consumption, such as fever or agitation, should be addressed promptly. In a critically ill Fontan patient with low cardiac output, a high fever may be caused by cutaneous vasoconstriction and a resultant failure to dissipate heat. This scenario is a medical emergency that warrants immediate attention with the initiation of rapid cooling, judicious fluid resuscitation, and consideration for inodilator infusions.

Once preload and oxygen carrying capacity have been optimized, some patients with functionally univentricular hearts who are in a low cardiac output state may benefit from judicious administration of a vasoactive infusion. Low-dose catecholamine infusions may be helpful, particularly in patients with marginal systemic blood pressure, provided that arrhythmias are not triggered or exacerbated. Similar to other adults with long-standing heart failure, those with functionally univentricular hearts (particularly Fontan patients) often develop systemic vasoplegia early after cardiac surgery. In this scenario, low-dose infusions of vasopressin or phenylephrine are often well tolerated and serve to normalize blood pressure without causing tachycardia or arrhythmias.

Milrinone may have a role in some patients given its inotropic and lusitropic effects and systemic and pulmonary vasodilatory properties. However, because milrinone has a relatively long half-life (2–3 h) and clearance is dependent on renal function, this inodilator must be used cautiously, particularly in patients with Fontan physiology. Patients with an adequate or high blood pressure may benefit from a pure vasodilator. A randomized double-blind placebo-controlled trial of empiric milrinone and nesiritide infusions in children recovering from the Fontan operation failed to show benefit of either drug [27]. Data regarding the use of these drugs in adults with functionally univentricular heart defects are lacking. Of note, inadequate analgesia may increase SVR, which may be poorly tolerated by the single ventricle.

Maintenance of an adequate renal perfusion pressure is of particular importance in critically ill adults with functionally univentricular heart defects. Renal perfusion pressure is calculated by subtracting the Fontan pressure from the mean systemic arterial pressure. Critically ill adult Fontan patients may have a CVP as high as 18–24 mmHg. Thus in order to maintain a renal perfusion pressure of 60–70 mmHg, a mean arterial pressure of 80–90 mmHg is needed. Significant ascites may compromise renal venous drainage and when present in significant amounts warrant consideration for therapeutic paracentesis. Patients with evolving acute renal failure despite the optimization of critical care therapies noted above may benefit from the early initiation of continuous renal replacement therapy (CRRT) with the specific intent of lowering the CVP. Of note, caution is warranted with the use of citrate anticoagulation during CRRT in Fontan patients with significant hepatic insufficiency.

Management of hemodynamically significant arrhythmias in critically ill adults with functionally univentricular heart defects may be challenging for several reasons. The positioning of pad placement for cardioversion or defibrillation may need to be modified based on the underlying cardiac and chest wall anatomy (e.g., dextrocardia; scoliosis) so that the shock vector traverses the intended myocardium.

Transvenous access to the atrium for temporary pacing is not feasible in patients with an extracardiac non-fenestrated Fontan. Underlying hepatic and renal function may influence the metabolism of antiarrhythmic agents. Consultation with an electrophysiologist with specific expertise in the management of adult congenital heart disease patients is prudent.

A thorough understanding of cardiopulmonary interactions is needed to optimize ICU outcomes for adult patients with functionally univentricular hearts [28]. Spontaneous ventilation has been shown to increase pulmonary blood flow in patients with cavopulmonary connections (i.e., Glenn and Fontan physiology). Furthermore, negative pressure cuirass ventilation has been shown to increase stroke volume and cardiac output in patients with Fontan physiology, but this ventilator strategy is not available in most ICU settings [29]. Conversely, positive pressure ventilation may impede pulmonary blood flow and thereby limit cardiac output in patients with passive pulmonary blood flow (i.e., Glenn or Fontan physiology).

Given the above cardiopulmonary interactions, in patients with a cavopulmonary connection who are receiving positive pressure ventilation, the following principles may be useful. Ventilator settings are chosen to achieve the lowest mean airway pressure that still prevents atelectasis. MAP is calculated using the following formula:

$$\mathrm{MAP} = \left(\mathrm{PIP}^{*}\%\mathrm{IT}\right) + \left(\mathrm{PEEP}^{*}\%\mathrm{ET}\right),$$

where *PIP* is the peak inspiratory pressure, *IT* the inspiratory time, *PEEP* the positive end expiratory pressure, and *ET* the expiratory time.

A PEEP of 4–5 mmHg is often used to prevent atelectasis. Maximum peak inspiratory pressures less than 20–25 mmHg, low inspiratory time, and low respiratory rate are used to minimize mean airway pressure [30]. Hypoxemia, hypercarbia, and overdistension of the lungs may elevate pulmonary vascular resistance and should be avoided. Parenchymal lung processes (e.g., pneumonia, atelectasis) and extrapleural collections (e.g., hemothorax, pneumothorax, pleural effusion, chylothorax) may increase pulmonary vascular resistance, increase cavopulmonary pressures, and impede pulmonary blood flow and thus should be promptly and aggressively treated. In patients with a superior cavopulmonary connection (i.e., Glenn), hyperventilation may impair oxygenation as the resultant hypocarbia increases cerebral vascular resistance and lowers cerebral blood flow, thereby diminishing SVC return and lowering PBF [31]. Patients with a Glenn shunt who are hypoxemic often have improved systemic oxygenation with mild hypoventilation [32]. In all patients with a cavopulmonary connection, early extubation with resumption of spontaneous ventilation (when feasible) reliably increases pulmonary blood flow and cardiac output.

12.3.4 Other Intensive Care Issues

12.3.4.1 Cyanosis

Adults with functionally univentricular hearts may be admitted to the ICU with unexplained cyanosis or may develop cyanosis during the course of an ICU stay. Common causes of hypoxemia and initial evaluation in patients with functionally univentricular hearts are summarized in Table 12.3. Of note, patients with systemic to pulmonary shunts (Fig. 12.1) may have "pressure-dependent pulmonary blood flow." Baseline cyanosis may worsen with an acute illness that results in decreased systemic vascular resistance (e.g., sepsis). The use of vasopressors may be beneficial in this scenario to increase systemic blood pressure and thus pulmonary blood flow.

12.3.4.2 Hemoptysis

Adults with functionally univentricular hearts occasionally develop hemoptysis [33]. Potential etiologies of particular interest in this patient population include pulmonary embolism or rupture of aortopulmonary collateral vessels into the proximal or distal bronchi. An underlying bleeding diathesis or use of antiplatelet or anticoagulation may exacerbate the problem. Bronchoscopy and aortic angiography may be useful to localize the site of bleeding and assess for collateral vessels.

12.3.4.3 Plastic Bronchitis

Plastic bronchitis occurs in 2–4% of Fontan patients and has also been reported in those with superior cavopulmonary connections [34]. The pathophysiology of bronchial cast formation in Fontan patients is unknown but has been proposed to be related to some combination of chronic low cardiac output, elevated CVP, mucous hypersecretion, heparin sulfate mutations, and inflammation [35]. Patients may present to the ICU with acute respiratory distress, wheezing, and hypoxemia. The bronchial casts may also cause life-threatening upper airway obstruction. Some patients may expectorate the casts making the diagnosis evident, although others may present with recurring episodes of respiratory distress with shifting infiltrates on chest radiograph.

Acute management of plastic bronchitis includes the provision of supplemental oxygen if hypoxemia is present. Inhaled steroids, bronchodilators, recombinant DNAse, and N-acetyl cysteine have all been used with variable degrees of success [36]. Inhaled tissue plasminogen activator may be used to facilitate breakdown of the fibrin component of the casts [37, 38]. Bronchoscopy may be considered to establish a diagnosis and facilitate cast removal. Hypercarbia and severe hypoxemia may be present in advanced cases of plastic bronchitis and is often particularly poorly tolerated by patients with cavopulmonary connections. Positive pressure ventilation may be helpful, with care to select ventilator settings that will minimize mean airway pressure in the context of passive pulmonary blood flow. Thoracic duct ligation or selective lymphatic embolization have been reported to be efficacious in small number of patients [39–41]. Cardiac transplantation is often efficacious in refractory cases [42].

12.3.4.4 Protein-Losing Enteropathy

Protein-losing enteropathy (PLE) develops in 3–18% of patients after the Fontan operation, with typical onset in childhood or adolescence [34]. The underlying pathophysiology is likely a combination of chronic venous hypertension and low cardiac output with resultant reduced overall gut perfusion and impaired mucosal and enterocyte function. Furthermore, as the thoracic duct drains into the innominate vein, elevated Fontan pressures result in backpressure to the lymphatic circulation. Intestinal protein loss leads to hypoalbuminemia, lymphopenia, and hypogammaglobulinemia. The diagnosis is made by a combination of presenting signs and symptoms and the documentation of decreased serum albumin and elevated fecal alpha-1-antitrypsin levels.

The diarrhea and dependent edema associated with PLE may typically be managed in the outpatient setting. A variety of therapies have been employed, including increased protein and decreased fat intake, diuretics, albumin and IVIG infusions, pulmonary vasodilators, corticosteroids, heparin infusions, and Fontan fenestration [43]. Intensive care may be needed for management of pleural or pericardial effusions, significant ascites, worsening heart failure, arrhythmias, thromboembolism, or sepsis. Following the diagnosis of PLE, the generally accepted 5-year survival rate is approximately 50%, although with comprehensive evaluation and management strategies, 5-year survival of 88% has been reported [43–45]. PLE resolves in the vast majority of patients who undergo cardiac transplantation [46].

12.3.4.5 Hepatic Dysfunction

Adults with a Fontan circulation are at risk for developing chronic hepatic disease; this entity has been described as Fontan-associated liver disease or FALD [47]. The combination of a chronic low cardiac output state and long-standing elevated Fontan pathway (i.e., CVP) pressure leads to hepatic congestion with associated fibrosis, cirrhosis, portal hypertension, ascites, and, in some patients, hepatocellular carcinoma [48]. Hepatic insufficiency including coagulopathy, hyperammonemia, and encephalopathy may complicate the management of critically ill patients with a Fontan palliation. Such patients may also have esophageal and gastric varices predisposing them to gastrointestinal bleeding that may require interventional endoscopy for management. Afflicted patients may require intensive care primarily for treatment of acute complications of underlying hepatic disease. Acute on chronic liver injury may also occur following cardiac surgery or other acute illnesses.

12.3.4.6 Thromboembolism and Stroke

Adults with functionally univentricular hearts are at risk for thromboembolic events for several reasons [49]. These may include low flow states, erythrocytosis, iron deficiency anemia, intracardiac prosthetic devices, decreased hepatic production of protein C, protein S, and antithrombin III, among others. The incidence of venous thromboemboli may be as high a 33% on patients with Fontan physiology [34, 50]. Pulmonary embolism occasionally occurs in Fontan patients and has been reported as the most common cause of out-of-hospital sudden death [50]. A thromboembolism to a coronary artery may cause an acute myocardial infarction or sudden death.

Cyanosis in adult Fontan patients commonly reflects right-to-left shunting through either veno-venous collaterals or pulmonary arteriovenous malformations. This right-to-left shunt places them at risk for paradoxical embolization if embolic material is administered intravenously. These patients therefore require meticulous attention to "deairing" of intravenous lines ("right-to-left shunt precautions"), something that is often not routine in adult critical care settings, and thus warrants emphasis. Embolic strokes, cerebral abscess, and intracranial hemorrhage may also occur.

Adults with cavopulmonary connections may have an abnormal cerebral circulation that may predispose to the development of acute cerebral ischemia. The chronically elevated cerebral venous pressure in patients with a cavopulmonary connection may compromise cerebral perfusion pressure. Carotid arteries and jugular veins may have been sacrificed during ECMO support. Additionally, the vertebral arteries that normally arise from the subclavian arteries may have been compromised during the creation of systemic to pulmonary shunts. Such patients are predisposed to brainstem ischemia, and afflicted patients may benefit from the maintenance of higher cerebral perfusion pressures during anesthesia or critical illness [51].

12.3.5 Cardiac Arrest

Many of the principles and guidelines for prevention and management of cardiac arrest in adults may be extrapolated to those with functionally univentricular hearts [52]. However, a number of issues warrant specific comment [53].

In adult patients with functionally univentricular heart defects who have undergone cavopulmonary connections (i.e., Glenn, Fontan), achieving a good outcome after resuscitation is particularly challenging for a number of reasons. In patients with cavopulmonary connections, the high cerebral venous pressure and atrioventricular valve regurgitation that typically exist at the onset of the arrest make it difficult to achieve adequate cerebral perfusion pressure with chest compressions.

In the peri-arrest period, avoiding over ventilation in patients with cavopulmonary connections is paramount for several reasons. Hypocarbia may worsen cerebral perfusion in the face of reduced cerebral blood flow. Additionally, high intrathoracic pressure may reduce Glenn or Fontan blood flow.

In a refractory cardiac arrest, the initiation of extracorporeal membrane oxygenation (ECMO) could be considered in carefully selected adult patients with functionally univentricular hearts. Barriers to success for E-CPR in this patient population may include limited vascular access for ECMO cannula placement, difficulties achieving adequate ECMO flows, end-organ injury that may ensue in the context of high CVP (Fontan pressure), and prolonged CPR needed while placing the patient on ECMO [54].

12.3.6 Mechanical Circulatory Support and Cardiac Transplantation

Mechanical circulatory support is an option for selected adult patients with functionally univentricular heart defects who develop refractory low cardiac output. Venoarterial ECMO may be useful for short-term support in patients with coexistent acute lung disease.

Carefully selected adults with functionally univentricular hearts defects who have refractory heart failure may be considered for placement of a ventricular assist device, typically as a bridge to cardiac transplantation. In a recent report from the Interagency Registry for Mechanically Assisted Circulatory Support (INTERMAX), of 16,182 adult patients, only 17 (0.1%) had a functionally univentricular heart defect. However, survival for these 17 patients (~70% at 12 months) was similar to adult congenital heart patients with two ventricles and with that of adults without CHD [55].

Cardiac transplantation may be considered for carefully selected adult patients with functionally univentricular hearts defects [46, 56]. Particular attention during transplant evaluation should be paid to antibody sensitization. Those with important hepatic or renal dysfunction may warrant consideration for dual-organ transplantation [57, 58]. Additional surgical procedures may be needed at the time of transplant, including pulmonary artery reconstruction or rerouting of abnormal systemic venous return. Operative mortality following heart transplant for failing Fontan patients is somewhat higher than that reported for many other indications [46, 56].

References

1. Khairy P, Poirier N, Mercier LA. Univentricular heart. Circulation. 2007;115(6):800–12.
2. Marelli AJ, Mackie AS, Ionescu-Ittu R, Rahme E, Pilote L. Congenital heart disease in the general population: changing prevalence and age distribution. Circulation. 2007;115(2):163–72.
3. Webb G, Mulder BJ, Aboulhosn J, Daniels CJ, Elizari MA, Hong G, et al. The care of adults with congenital heart disease across the globe: current assessment and future perspective: a position statement from the International Society for Adult Congenital Heart Disease (ISACHD). Int J Cardiol. 2015;195:326–33.
4. Prakash A, Khan MA, Hardy R, Torres AJ, Chen JM, Gersony WM. A new diagnostic algorithm for assessment of patients with single ventricle before a Fontan operation. J Thorac Cardiovasc Surg. 2009;138(4):917–23.
5. Ohye RG, Schranz D, D'Udekem Y. Current therapy for hypoplastic left heart syndrome and related single ventricle lesions. Circulation. 2016;134(17):1265–79.
6. Norwood WI, Lang P, Hansen DD. Physiologic repair of aortic atresia-hypoplastic left heart syndrome. N Engl J Med. 1983;308(1):23–6.
7. Sano S, Ishino K, Kawada M, Arai S, Kasahara S, Asai T, et al. Right ventricle-pulmonary artery shunt in first-stage palliation of hypoplastic left heart syndrome. J Thorac Cardiovasc Surg. 2003;126:504–10.
8. Forbess JM, Cook N, Serraf A, Burke RP, Mayer JE Jr, Jonas RA. An institutional experience with second- and third-stage palliative procedures for hypoplastic left heart syndrome: the impact of the bidirectional cavopulmonary shunt. J Am Coll Cardiol. 1997;29(3):665–70.
9. Tanoue Y, Sese A, Ueno Y, Joh K, Hijii T. Bidirectional Glenn procedure improves the mechanical efficiency of a total cavopulmonary connection in high-risk Fontan candidates. Circulation. 2001;103(17):2176–80.
10. Fontan F, Baudet E. Surgical repair of tricuspid atresia. Thorax. 1971;26(3):240–8.
11. Kumar SP, Rubinstein CS, Simsic JM, Taylor AB, Saul JP, Bradley SM. Lateral tunnel versus extracardiac conduit Fontan procedure: a concurrent comparison. Ann Thorac Surg. 2003;76(5):1389–96.
12. Iyengar AJ, Winlaw DS, Galati JC, Wheaton GR, Gentles TL, Grigg LE, et al. The extracardiac conduit Fontan procedure in Australia and New Zealand: hypoplastic left heart syndrome predicts worse early and late outcomes. Eur J Cardiothorac Surg. 2014;46(3):465–73.

13. Bridges ND, Mayer JE Jr, Lock JE, Jonas RA, Hanley FL, Keane JF, et al. Effect of baffle fenestration on outcome of the modified Fontan operation. Circulation. 1992;86(6):1762–9.
14. Lemler MS, Scott WA, Leonard SR, Stromberg D, Ramaciotti C. Fenestration improves clinical outcome of the fontan procedure: a prospective, randomized study. Circulation. 2002;105(2):207–12.
15. Mavroudis C, Deal BJ. Fontan conversion: literature review and lessons learned over 20 years. World J Pediatr Cong Heart Surg. 2016;7(2):192–8.
16. Deal BJ, Costello JM, Webster G, Tsao S, Backer CL, Mavroudis C. Intermediate-term outcome of 140 consecutive Fontan conversions with arrhythmia operations. Ann Thorac Surg. 2016;101(2):717–24.
17. Moodie DS, Ritter DG, Tajik AJ, O'Fallon WM. Long-term follow-up in the unoperated univentricular heart. Am J Cardiol. 1984;53(8):1124–8.
18. Poterucha JT, Anavekar NS, Egbe AC, Julsrud PR, Connolly HM, Ammash NM, et al. Survival and outcomes of patients with unoperated single ventricle. Heart. 2016;102(3):216–22.
19. Abdelbar A, Mahadevan VS, Austin C, Hoschtitzky JA. Late bidirectional Glenn anastomosis in a 54-year-old patient with unoperated functionally univentricular heart. World J Pediatr Cong Heart Surg. 2013;4(4):444–6.
20. Forsdick V, Iyengar AJ, Carins T, Gentles TL, Weintraub RG, Celermajer DS, et al. Unsatisfactory early and late outcomes after Fontan surgery delayed to adolescence and adulthood. Semin Thorac Cardiovasc Surg. 2015;27(2):168–74.
21. Collins RT 2nd, Doshi P, Onukwube J, Fram RY, Robbins JM. Risk factors for increased hospital resource utilization and in-hospital mortality in adults with single ventricle congenital heart disease. Am J Cardiol. 2016;118(3):453–62.
22. Cedars A, Benjamin L, Vyhmeister R, Harris K, Bradley EA, Wadia S, et al. Contemporary hospitalization rate among adults with complex congenital heart disease. World J Pediatr Cong Heart Surg. 2016;7(3):334–43.
23. Seckeler MD, Moe TG, Thomas ID, Meziab O, Andrews J, Heller E, et al. Hospital resource utilization for common noncardiac diagnoses in adult survivors of single cardiac ventricle. Am J Cardiol. 2015;116(11):1756–61.
24. Warnes CA, Williams RG, Bashore TM, Child JS, Connolly HM, Dearani JA, et al. ACC/AHA 2008 guidelines for the management of adults with congenital heart disease: a report of the American College of Cardiology/American Heart Association Task Force on Practice Guidelines. Circulation. 2008;118(23):e714–833.
25. Atz AM, Zak V, Mahony L, Uzark K, D'Agincourt N, Goldberg DJ, et al. Longitudinal outcomes of patients with single ventricle after the Fontan procedure. J Am Coll Cardiol. 2017;69(22):2735–44.
26. Costello JM, Mazwi ML, McBride ME, Gambetta KE, Eltayeb O, Epting CL. Critical care for paediatric patients with heart failure. Cardiol Young. 2015;25(Suppl 2):74–86.
27. Costello JM, Dunbar-Masterson C, Allan CK, Gauvreau K, Newburger JW, McGowan FX Jr, et al. Impact of empiric nesiritide or milrinone infusion on early postoperative recovery after Fontan surgery: a randomized, double-blind, placebo-controlled trial. Circ Heart Fail. 2014;7(4):596–604.
28. Bronicki RA, Anas NG. Cardiopulmonary interaction. Pediatr Crit Care Med. 2009;10(3):313–22.
29. Shekerdemian LS, Bush A, Shore DF, Lincoln C, Redington AN. Cardiopulmonary interactions after Fontan operations: augmentation of cardiac output using negative pressure ventilation. Circulation. 1997;96(11):3934–42.
30. Mossad EB, Motta P, Vener DF. Anesthetic considerations for adults undergoing Fontan conversion surgery. Anesthesiol Clin. 2013;31(2):405–19.
31. Bradley SM, Simsic JM, Mulvihill DM. Hyperventilation impairs oxygenation after bidirectional superior cavopulmonary connection. Circulation. 1998;98(19 Suppl):II372–6.
32. Bradley SM, Simsic JM, Mulvihill DM. Hypoventilation improves oxygenation after bidirectional superior cavopulmonary connection. J Thorac Cardiovasc Surg. 2003;126:1033–9.

33. Ohuchi H, Yasuda K, Miyazaki A, Ono S, Hayama Y, Negishi J, et al. Prevalence and predictors of haemostatic complications in 412 Fontan patients: their relation to anticoagulation and haemodynamics. Eur J Cardiothorac Surg. 2015;47(3):511–9.
34. Allen KY, Downing TE, Glatz AC, Rogers LS, Ravishankar C, Rychik J, et al. Effect of Fontan-associated morbidities on survival with intact Fontan circulation. Am J Cardiol. 2017;119(11):1866–71.
35. Larue M, Gossett JG, Stewart RD, Backer CL, Mavroudis C, Jacobs ML. Plastic bronchitis in patients with Fontan physiology: review of the literature and preliminary experience with fontan conversion and cardiac transplantation. World J Pediatr Cong Heart Surg. 2012;3(3):364–72.
36. Singhi AK, Vinoth B, Kuruvilla S, Sivakumar K. Plastic bronchitis. Ann Pediatr Cardiol. 2015;8(3):246–8.
37. Costello JM, Steinhorn D, McColley S, Gerber ME, Kumar SP. Treatment of plastic bronchitis in a Fontan patient with tissue plasminogen activator: a case report and review of the literature. Pediatrics. 2002;109(4):e67.
38. Avitabile CM, Goldberg DJ, Dodds K, Dori Y, Ravishankar C, Rychik J. A multifaceted approach to the management of plastic bronchitis after cavopulmonary palliation. Ann Thorac Surg. 2014;98(2):634–40.
39. Shah SS, Drinkwater DC, Christian KG. Plastic bronchitis: is thoracic duct ligation a real surgical option? Ann Thorac Surg. 2006;81(6):2281–3.
40. Itkin M. Lymphatic intervention techniques: look beyond thoracic duct embolization. J Vasc Interv Radiol. 2016;27(8):1187–8.
41. Dori Y, Keller MS, Rome JJ, Gillespie MJ, Glatz AC, Dodds K, et al. Percutaneous lymphatic embolization of abnormal pulmonary lymphatic flow as treatment of plastic bronchitis in patients with congenital heart disease. Circulation. 2016;133(12):1160–70.
42. Gossett JG, Almond CS, Kirk R, Zangwill S, Richmond ME, Kantor PF, et al. Outcomes of cardiac transplantation in single-ventricle patients with plastic bronchitis: a multicenter study. J Am Coll Cardiol. 2013;61(9):985–6.
43. John AS, Johnson JA, Khan M, Driscoll DJ, Warnes CA, Cetta F. Clinical outcomes and improved survival in patients with protein-losing enteropathy after the Fontan operation. J Am Coll Cardiol. 2014;64(1):54–62.
44. Binotto MA, Maeda NY, Lopes AA. Altered endothelial function following the Fontan procedure. Cardiol Young. 2008;18(1):70–4.
45. Silvilairat S, Cabalka AK, Cetta F, Grogan M, Hagler DJ, O'Leary PW. Protein-losing enteropathy after the Fontan operation: associations and predictors of clinical outcome. Congenit Heart Dis. 2008;3(4):262–8.
46. Backer CL, Russell HM, Pahl E, Monge MC, Gambetta K, Kindel SJ, et al. Heart transplantation for the failing Fontan. Ann Thorac Surg. 2013;96(4):1413–9.
47. Wu FM, Kogon B, Earing MG, Aboulhosn JA, Broberg CS, John AS, et al. Liver health in adults with Fontan circulation: a multicenter cross-sectional study. J Thorac Cardiovasc Surg. 2017;153(3):656–64.
48. Goldberg DJ, Surrey LF, Glatz AC, Dodds K, O'Byrne ML, Lin HC, et al. Hepatic fibrosis is universal following Fontan operation, and severity is associated with time from surgery: a liver biopsy and hemodynamic study. J Am Heart Assoc. 2017;6(5):e004809.
49. Egbe AC, Connolly HM, Niaz T, Yogeswaran V, Taggart NW, Qureshi MY, et al. Prevalence and outcome of thrombotic and embolic complications in adults after Fontan operation. Am Heart J. 2017;183:10–7.
50. Gewillig M. The Fontan circulation. Heart. 2005;91(6):839–46.
51. Broomall E, McBride ME, Deal BJ, Ducharme-Crevier L, Shaw A, Mazwi M, et al. Posterior circulation ischemia or occlusion in five adults with failing Fontan circulation. Ann Thorac Surg. 2016;101(6):2315–20.
52. Neumar RW, Shuster M, Callaway CW, Gent LM, Atkins DL, Bhanji F, et al. Part 1: executive summary: 2015 American Heart Association guidelines update for cardiopulmonary resuscitation and emergency cardiovascular care. Circulation. 2015;132(18 Suppl 2):S315–67.

53. Marino BS, Tibby SM, Hoffman GM. Resuscitation of the patient with the functionally univentricular heart. Curr Pediatr Rev. 2013;9(2):148–57.
54. Booth KL, Roth SJ, Thiagarajan RR, Almodovar MC, del Nido PJ, Laussen PC. Extracorporeal membrane oxygenation support of the Fontan and bidirectional Glenn circulations. Ann Thorac Surg. 2004;77(4):1341–8.
55. Arnaoutakis GJ, Blitzer D, Fuller S, Eckhauser AW, Montenegro LM, Rossano JW, et al. Mechanical circulatory support as bridge to transplantation for the failing single ventricle. Ann Thorac Surg. 2017;103(1):193–7.
56. Matsuda H, Fukushima N, Ichikawa H, Sawa Y. Orthotropic heart transplantation for adult congenital heart disease: a case with heterotaxy and dextrocardia. Gen Thorac Cardiovasc Surg. 2017;65(1):47–51.
57. Hill AL, Maeda K, Bonham CA, Concepcion W. Pediatric combined heart-liver transplantation performed en bloc: a single-center experience. Pediatr Transplant. 2012;16(4):392–7.
58. Hollander SA, Reinhartz O, Maeda K, Hurwitz M, D NR, Bernstein D. Intermediate-term outcomes after combined heart-liver transplantation in children with a univentricular heart. J Heart Lung Transplant. 2013;32(3):368–70.
59. Kelley JR, Mack GW, Fahey JT. Diminished venous vascular capacitance in patients with univentricular hearts after the Fontan operation. Am J Cardiol. 1995;76(3):158–63.

Critical Care Management of the ACHD Patient with Aortopathies

13

David Briston and Curt Daniels

13.1 Introduction

The aorta is the main artery of the body, which connects to a systemic ventricle and supplies oxygenated blood to tissues. The aorta is composed of multiple segments, and variations at different levels require different treatments, which are discussed within this chapter (Fig. 13.1). Aortopathies discussed herein are related to the thoracic aorta. Figure 13.2 nicely shows where measurements are made using multidetector computed tomography. Usually connected to a left ventricle but in rare circumstances to a right ventricle, the aorta emanates from its superior aspect and is separated from the myocardium by the aortic valve. In most adults, just above the aortic valve, the aorta measures approximately 3 cm. In this region just superior to the aortic valve called the aortic root, there are aortic ostia from which coronary arteries take off and supply blood to the myocardium. This region may dilate and require intervention. As the aortic root tapers down at the sinotubular junction, the ascending aorta continues to move superiorly as it twists in counterclockwise fashion with the pulmonary artery anterior to the aorta. The ascending aorta moves posteriorly and then commonly to the left as it arches over the left main stem bronchus although less commonly it can arch rightward. The aortic arch comes next and gives off arterial branches supplying the head, neck, and arms. The aortic isthmus, where the ductus arteriosus inserts and typically just distal to the takeoff of the subclavian artery ipsilateral to the arch sidedness, comes last and is sometimes a site of narrowing in certain congenital defects discussed later. The descending thoracic aorta is the next segment of the aorta as it descends toward the diaphragm typically on the left side of the vertebral column in a posterior location. The aorta descends

D. Briston · C. Daniels (✉)
Nationwide Children's Hospital, The Ohio State University, Columbus, OH, USA
e-mail: David.Briston@nationwidechildrens.org; curt.daniels@nationwidechildrens.org

E. da Cruz et al. (eds.), *Intensive Care of the Adult with Congenital Heart Disease*, Congenital Heart Disease in Adolescents and Adults,
https://doi.org/10.1007/978-3-319-94171-4_13

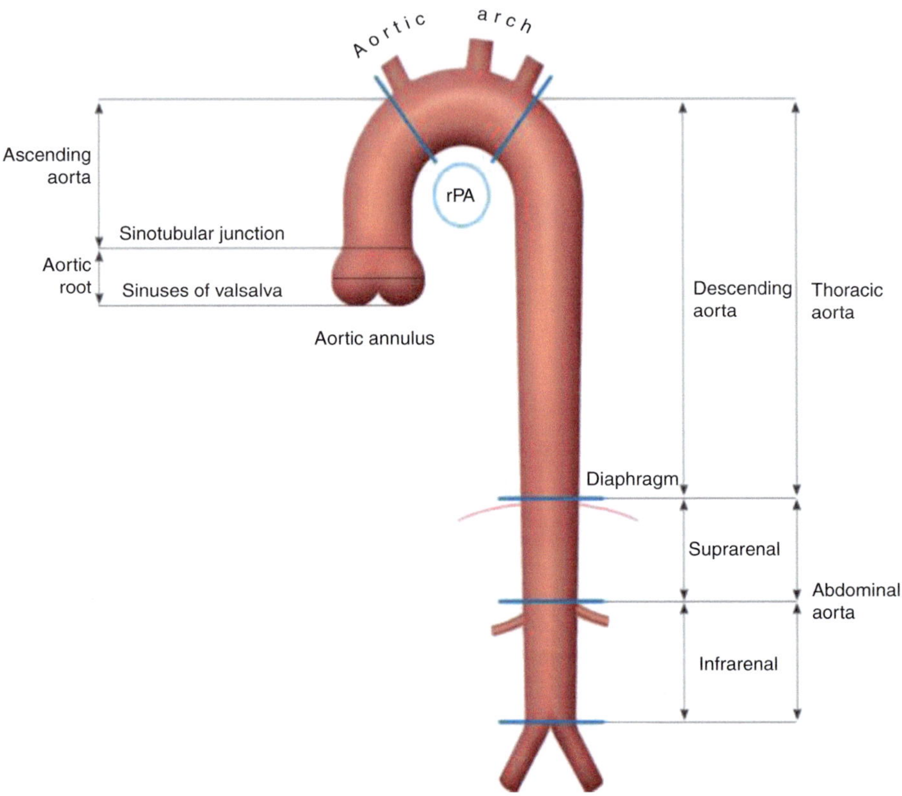

Fig. 13.1 The multiple levels of the aorta in the thorax and abdomen are depicted. From: 2014 ESC Guidelines on the diagnosis and treatment of aortic diseases: document covering acute and chronic aortic diseases of the thoracic and abdominal aorta of the adult. The Task Force for the Diagnosis and Treatment of Aortic Diseases of the European Society of Cardiology (ESC). Erbel R, Aboyans V, Boileau C, Bossone E, Bartolomeo RD, Eggebrecht H, Evangelista A, Falk V, Frank H, Gaemperli O, Grabenwöger M, Haverich A, Iung B, Manolis AJ, Meijboom F, Nienaber CA, Roffi M, Rousseau H, Sechtem U, Sirnes PA, Allmen RS, Vrints CJ; ESC Committee for Practice Guidelines. Eur Heart J. 2014; 35(41): 2873–926

through the diaphragm at the aortic hiatus and supplies blood to the abdomen before bifurcating in the pelvis into the bilateral iliac arteries.

Arteries have three layers, listed from internal to external: the tunica intima (mostly endothelial cells), the tunica media (mostly smooth muscle cells and elastic fibers), and the tunica adventitia (mostly connective tissue). The aortic tunica media contains smooth muscle cells and extracellular matrix, which is composed of ground substance. This is essentially elastic fibers and collagen in a hydrated gel layer. This architecture permits for significant elasticity, which is important as the aorta transmits the systemic blood pressure from the ventricle.

The aorta has multiple roles. It is most commonly thought of as the main hub in the arterial system that connects the oxygenated blood from the lungs and heart and

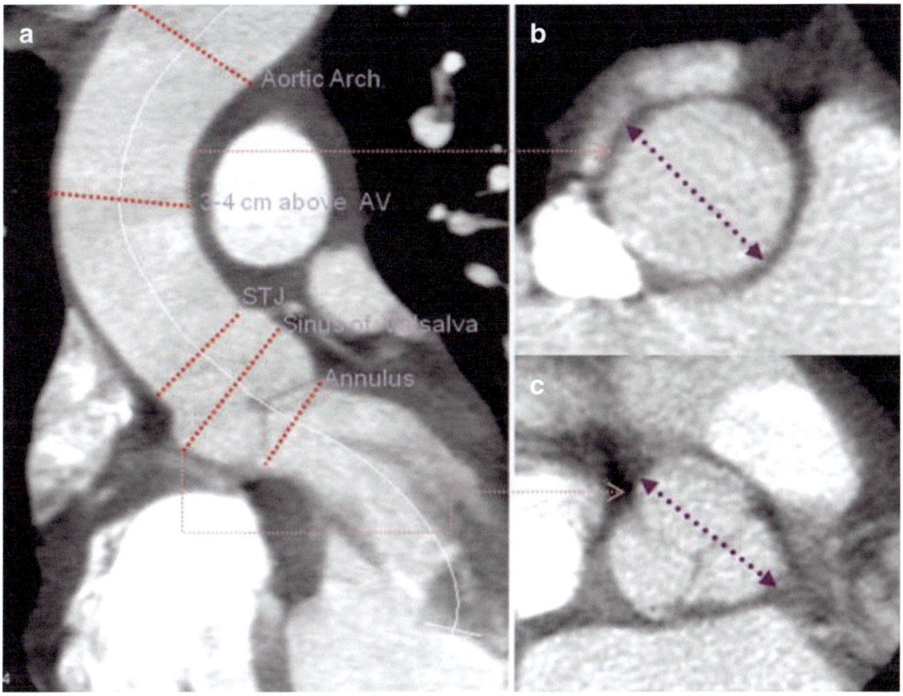

Fig. 13.2 Aortic dimensions by multi-detector computed tomography. (**a**) Depicts a view of the aorta emanating from the left ventricle and rising into the aortic arch. (**b**) Demonstrates the cross-sectional measurement of the ascending aorta with correlation to (**a**). (**c**) Demonstrates the cross-sectional measurement location of the aortic sinuses with correlation to (**a**). From: Aortic dimensions by multi-detector computed tomography versus echocardiography. Blondheim DS, Vassilenko L, Glick Y, Asif A, Nachtigal A, Meisel SR, Shochat M, Shotan A, Zeina AR. J Cardiol. 2016; 67 (4): 365–70

sends it to the body. Another role of the aorta relates to its elastic properties. Distention and recoiling with each ventricular contraction augment pulsatile blood flow. This reduces the afterload against which the ventricle must pump and improves diastolic coronary filling.

Understanding normal aortic anatomy and physiology as well as the nature and types of aortic disease is important prior to distinguishing aspects of their care in the ICU.

13.2 Aortic Disease

Aortic diseases are complex and disparate in nature. Bicommissural, often termed bicuspid, aortic valve (BAV) is a relatively common occurrence seen in about 1.5–2% of the population [1] (Fig. 13.3). It is the most common valvular defect and tends to affect males more than females. It is seen in about 70% of patients who

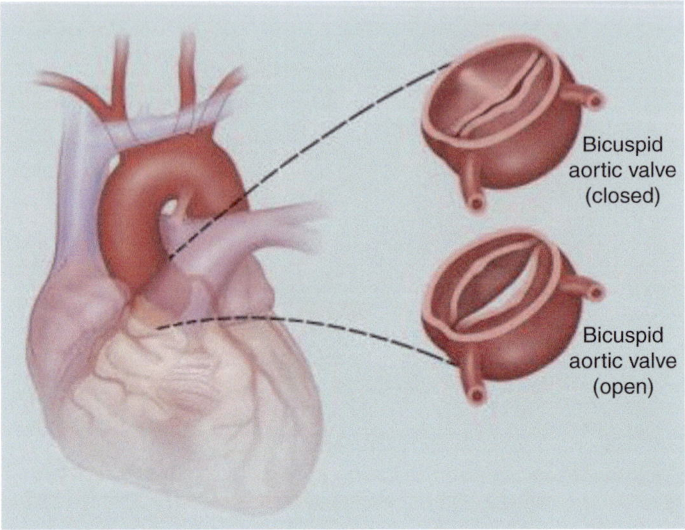

Fig. 13.3 Pictorial demonstration of a bicuspid aortic valve in the open and closed positions. From: Bicupsid Aortic Valve Disease. Siu SC, Silversides CK. J Am Coll Cardiol. 2010; 55 (25): 2789–800

have coarctation of the aorta (CoA), which is another relatively common congenital heart defect (CHD). Occurring alone, with BAV, or in concert with other lesions, CoA is reported to occur in about 0.04% of live births in isolation, but this number is likely an underestimate since many cases are not detected until adolescence or adulthood [2]. Also, CoA may be underreported when coexisting with other lesions. The reduced detection rate is related to the difficulty in identifying this lesion on neonatal echocardiography, while the ductus arteriosus remains open and also because inconsistences regarding palpating femoral pulses hinder diagnosis. Having recognized this, neonatal screening is performed in most centers in the USA to aid in diagnosis early in life [3]. Should a neonate not undergo screening or have been born before such practices went into place, manifestations such as claudication with activity, hypertension, heart failure, and cold lower extremities will become evident later in life. Distinct from the valvular disease associated with BAV, CoA even in the repaired form has been associated with hypertension, recoarctation after repair, pseudoaneurysms, aneurysms, cerebrovascular disease, early coronary artery disease, aortic dissection, and sudden cardiac death. There is an increased rate of BAV and CoA in families suggesting a heritable component to its transmission. Genetic studies have shown an increased rate of 22q11 microdeletion syndrome in these patients [4]. While not acutely necessary, genetic testing might affect clinical management and family planning. Not only single genes but also copy number variants and single nucleotide polymorphisms may predispose to aortopathy by modifying the genetic sequence and altering protein production. Future discoveries may allow different types of genetic sequence testing that identify BAV phenotypes associated with the need for early intervention. Testing can be performed in consultation with aortopathy patients' primary cardiologist on an outpatient basis.

Interrupted aortic arch is the other significant form of aortopathy. It is considered by many to be a severe form of CoA, so caring for patients with this includes mindfulness for aspects of care seen in CoA patients. It exists when there is complete luminal discontinuity between the aortic arch and the descending aorta, sometimes with the gap spanned by fibrous tissue. It is categorized by the location of discontinuity relative to the head and neck vessels. The ductus arteriosus must remain patent to provide pulsatile blood flow to the infradiaphragmatic areas, and most cases are identified and corrected surgically early in life. If not, robust collateralization is necessary for prolonged survival. Care in the ICU is not different from that of CoA regarding how to set up equipment and monitoring, but procedures to alleviate this obstruction are adaptations on CoA repairs but technically can be more challenging.

Aortopathies coexist in association with other CHD lesions [5]. Conotruncal defects such as tetralogy of Fallot, transposition of the great arteries, pulmonary atresia, and double outlet right ventricle can be associated with an enlarged aorta and aortopathy. However, reports of dissection are rare [6, 7]. Surgical replacement is commonly unnecessary, and a few case reports describe such patients [8, 9]. Few guidelines for intervention on CHD patients with aortopathy exist [10, 11].

The aorta also plays an important role in atherosclerotic disease. Plaque buildup can obstruct flow or embolize. Disruptions in the normal vascular wall architecture can hasten platelet and red blood cell aggregation, which can augment plaque or embolic phenomena.

13.3 Bicuspid Aortic Valve

The details of BAV are important to understand when considering care for these patients. BAV is the primary indication for surgical intervention on isolated aortic valve disease [10]. Also, there is a strong association between BAV and aortic dilation as is discussed later. For these reasons, BAV patients are commonly seen in the ICU in a postoperative setting; however, these patients may be in the ICU setting for other reasons or because of sequela of undetected or underappreciated valve disease. There is a male predilection with 2:1 male: female ratio [12]. While CoA is associated with BAV as well, only a minority of patients with BAV exhibit this CHD [1]. Many patients with BAV are identified incidentally on echocardiograms. Figure 13.4 (from Siu Silversides 2005 JACC paper (Fig. 2)) depicts echocardiographic views of BAV, which are used to make this diagnosis, as well as a cardiac magnetic resonance image showing an associated aortopathy in one such patient.

There are multiple subtypes of BAV with fusions of different commissures, which always lead to an aortic valve with leaflets of unequal size. Flow dynamics relate to the subtlety of differences in geometry of the BAV. Previous studies have suggested that fusion of the right and left coronary cusps is associated with more rapid aortic dilation in adults [13]. Fusion of the left or right coronary cusp

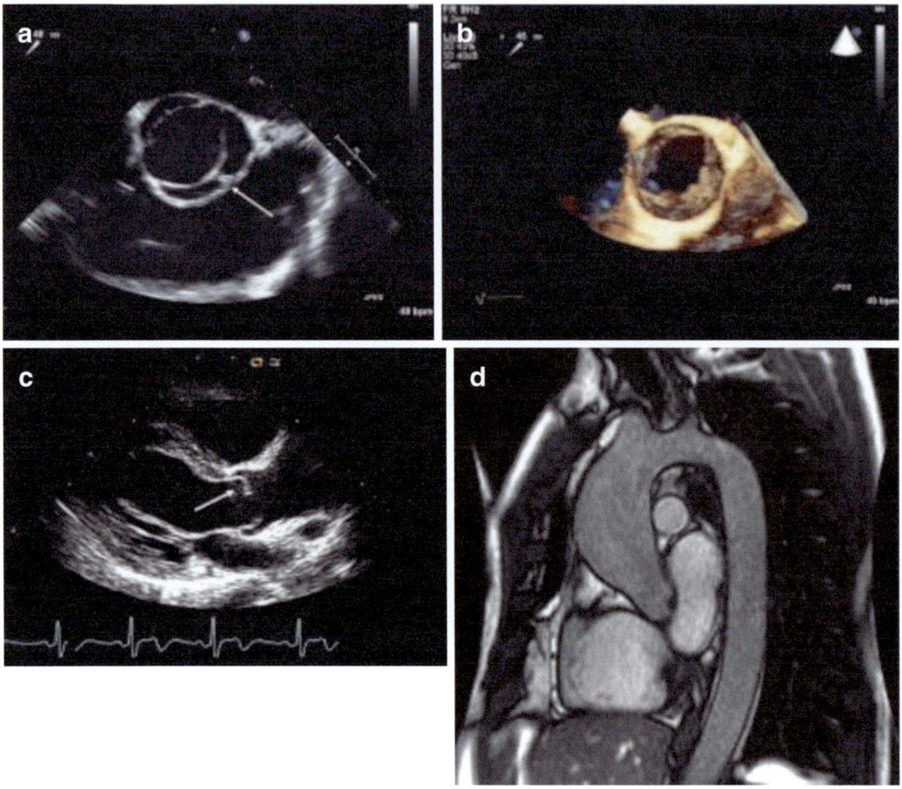

Fig. 13.4 Echocardiography of a bicuspid aortic valve. (**a–c**) Demonstrate echocardiographic pictures of a bicuspid aortic valve. (**d**) Demonstrates an MRI of the same patient, which demonstrates an enlarged aorta. From: Bicuspid Aortic Valve Disease. Siu SC, Silversides CK. J Am Coll Cardiol. 2010; 55 (25): 2789–800

with the noncoronary cusp was associated with more significant valve dysfunction in children [14]. When looking at the same anatomical cohorts, another study identified no such valvular dysfunction but noted ascending aortic dilation in adults [15]. Wall stress and flow velocity may be different in BAV patients as compared to those without [16] (Figs. 13.5, 13.6, and 13.7). The BAV morphology subtype leads to different locations of wall shear stress, and this potentially offers a physiologic explanation as to how different BAV phenotypes lead to dissimilar aortopathies.

The pathophysiology of BAV and its associated aortopathy is noted on the histologic level. Cystic medial necrosis results from abnormal signaling within the vascular smooth muscle cells within the media layer of the aortic wall. Irregularities in cell signaling lead to increased matrix metalloproteinases and tissue inhibitors. These changes are thought to adversely affect the structural

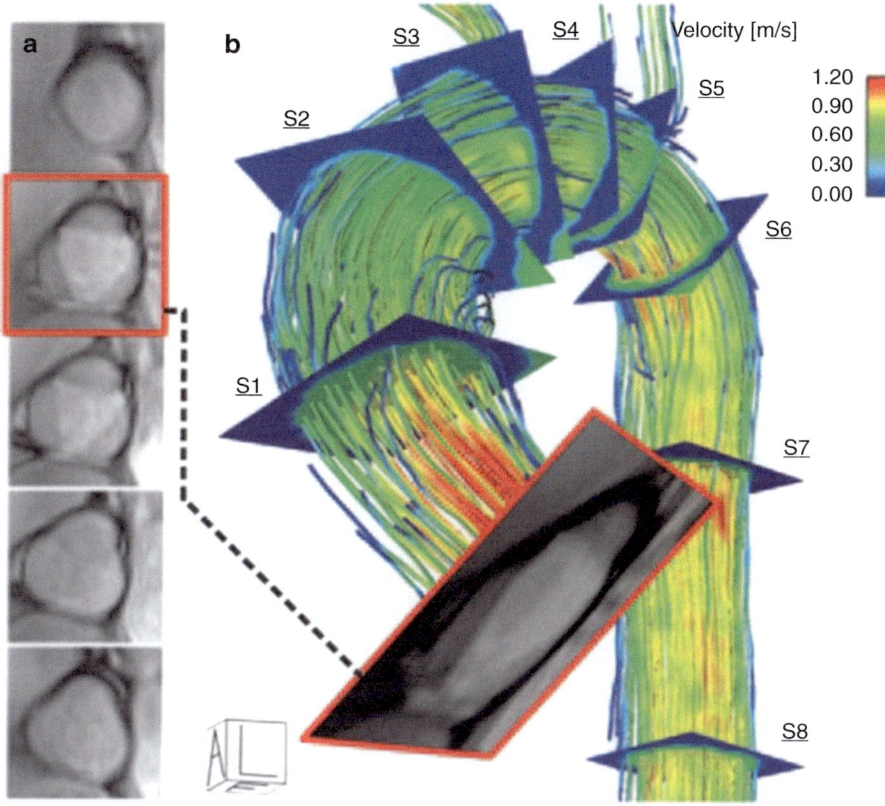

Fig. 13.5 Ascending aorta wall shear stress with a bicuspid aortic valve. (**a**) Demonstrates aortic valve images during stages ventricular contraction starting with contraction for a trileaflet aortic valve. (**b**) Demonstrates four-dimensional flow data for this valve. S1–S8 indicates the standardized positions chosen for flow and wall shear stress quantification. From: Barker AJ, Markl M, Bürk J, Lorenz R, Bock J, Bauer S, Schulz-Menger J, von Knobelsdorff-Brenkenhoff F. Bicuspid aortic valve is associated with altered wall shear stress in the ascending aorta. Circ Cardiovasc Imaging. 2012; 5 (4): 457–66

integrity and elasticity of the aorta. Recently published data suggest that MRI has identified abnormal transvalvular-flow patterns across the aortic valve, which further supports this theory [17].

Regardless of the underlying anatomic variation within the scope of BAV, the physiologic consequences are upon what clinical care decisions depend. If the aortic valve is regurgitant, then considerations must be given to a dilated and hypertrophied left ventricle that may or may not be providing adequate systemic output and coronary perfusion. Whether or not this is the primary reason that a patient is in the ICU, care must be given to avoid agents that markedly increase systemic vascular

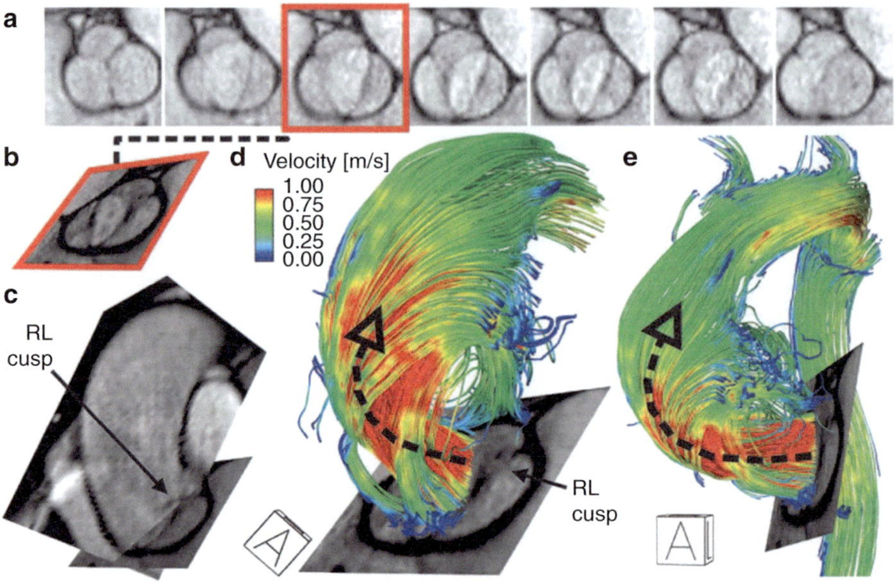

Fig. 13.6 Flow patterns and wall shear stress with a bicuspid aortic valve. (**a–c**) Shows steady-state free precession images that provide anatomic landmarks, which are used to locate the direction and propagation of a systolic flow jet. There is fusion of the right and left leaflets of the aortic valve. (**d**, **e**) Demonstrate the eccentric jet of ejected blood with arrows demonstrating its impact with the right-anterior aorta wall in a right-handed helical direction. From: Barker AJ, Markl M, Bürk J, Lorenz R, Bock J, Bauer S, Schulz-Menger J, von Knobelsdorff-Brenkenhoff F. Bicuspid aortic valve is associated with altered wall shear stress in the ascending aorta. Circ Cardiovasc Imaging. 2012; 5 (4): 457–66

resistance or further reduce coronary perfusion. Guidelines for the timing of intervention are previously reported based on the degree of regurgitation and patient symptoms [10]. On the other extreme of the spectrum is BAV associated with stenosis. Similar to other causes of aortic stenosis, strict guidelines are in place to guide management strategies based on the degree of stenosis and symptomatology [10]. Aortic stenosis has multiple treatment options including surgery, transcatheter aortic valve replacement (TAVR), and other catheterization procedures. These patients often have low systemic blood pressure and benefit from increased ventricular filling time. Within the ICU, monitoring for signs of poor coronary and systemic perfusion as well as valvular deterioration is important.

Among BAV patients in the ICU who are not in the postoperative setting, many factors influence their care. Invasive lines should be checked and ensured to be accurate given that the systemic blood pressure can be reduced in many of these patients. Afterload-reducing agents may be necessary if a regurgitant BAV has worsened and is related to the cause of ICU admission. All standard monitoring practices for non-BAV patients also should be employed as it is not protective against other problems. Special vigilance should be offered to those patients with BAV who display fever or unexplained tachycardia in the ICU. There is an increased

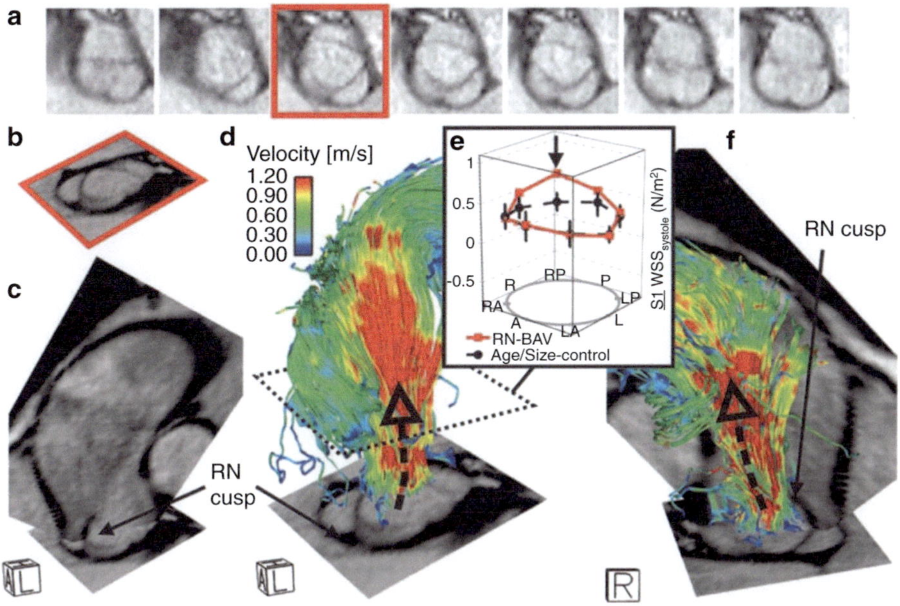

Fig. 13.7 Ascending aorta wall shear stress with a right-noncoronary cusp fusion of the bicuspid aortic valve. (**a**–**d**) Demonstrate right-noncoronary cusp fusion of the bicuspid aortic valve. The jet pattern shows interaction with the posterior wall of the aorta on the opposite side from the fused right and noncoronary cusps. (**e**) Demonstrates that the peak wall shear stress occurs at the right posterior portion of the aorta wall as shown by the arrow. (**f**) Demonstrates that the fusion of leaflets causes incomplete opening of the fused cusp and influences the direction of the velocity jet as is seen in the black open arrow. From: Barker AJ, Markl M, Bürk J, Lorenz R, Bock J, Bauer S, Schulz-Menger J, von Knobelsdorff-Brenkenhoff F. Bicuspid aortic valve is associated with altered wall shear stress in the ascending aorta. Circ Cardiovasc Imaging. 2012; 5 (4): 457–66

risk of infective endocarditis in this cohort as is thought to be related to the unusual aortic valve architecture.

BAV is commonly associated with aortopathy, and sometimes surgical intervention is undertaken wherein the aortic valve and aortic root are replaced or aortic valve sparing aortic root replacement. Studies have associated BAV with dilated aortic sinuses and ascending aorta [18]. It has been demonstrated that BAV patients have a larger ascending aorta, which increases in size at a rate faster than those patients with trileaflet aortic valve [19]. While the wall shear theory suggests an explanation as to why this occurs, the aortic phenotype associated with various types of BAV provides another explanation, and these types have been standardized [17]. Type 1 is the most common form wherein the ascending aorta is tubular in shape and is associated with varying amounts of aortic root dilatation. This type of ascending aorta is associated with older age at diagnosis and aortic stenosis and is associated with the most common bicuspid aortic valve architecture, fusion of the right and left coronary cusps. Type 2 arches include a tubular shape of the ascending aorta without aortic root dilation. Sometimes the tubular shape may extend distally to the transverse aorta. This is thought to occur more commonly with fusion of the right and noncoronary cusps. Type 3 is the least common phenotype and is associated with a young age of diagnosis and isolated aortic root dilation without significant effects on the ascending aorta.

Caring for BAV with associated aortopathy patients in the ICU in the postoperative period after having had the mechanical aortic valve replacement and aortic root replacement is similar to caring for those patients who have had either of these procedures, regardless of the congenital cause. Special care must be given to ensure that no postsurgical issues such as bleeding or hemolysis are occurring. Monitoring ventilatory status and determining the optimal time for extubation are critical while also simultaneously providing sufficient analgesia. Ensuring adequate coronary blood flow through the reimplanted coronary arteries also must be screened for. If mechanical aortic valve replacement was undertaken, anticoagulation guidelines exist and should be followed [20]. Close monitoring of vital signs as significant fluid shifts occur is necessary to identify problems early, similar to other surgical procedures.

13.4 Coarctation of the Aorta

Coarctation of the aorta (CoA) is present in 5–10% of patients with CHD and has multiple associations leading to a relatively high morbidity and mortality and the need for lifelong follow-up. The majority of patients with CoA also have BAV. Unlike BAV wherein many patients do not require intervention until later in life, CoA patients often have had at least one prior procedure. Details of any prior procedures are critical to understanding physiology and management. Through the different surgical eras, multiple techniques with varying degrees of success and morbidity have been utilized. More recently, catheterization procedures have been used to address CoA detected later after childhood. While rare that patients present with undiagnosed CoA to the hospital setting, it certainly is not unheard of. Oftentimes, echocardiography or chest imaging is performed for other reasons, and the CoA is incidentally found such as when performing workup for renal dysfunction.

Surgical treatments utilized in the past have included end-to-end anastomosis, subclavian artery patch aortoplasty ("subclavian flap" technique), and interposition graft placement (Fig. 13.8). Other approaches such as the patch aortoplasty technique and bypass "jump" graft procedure have also been utilized in certain patients. The end-to-end anastomosis is commonly utilized nowadays in the modern surgical era given evidence that pseudoaneurysms and recoarctation are thought to be less likely in the decades subsequent to repair. When performing a subclavian artery patch aortoplasty, the limb (commonly left arm) blood pressure may be markedly reduced. This reduced blood pressure does not reflect the true systemic blood pressure, and special care must be taken to avoid the use of this limb for medical monitoring and blood draws if possible given that its vascular supply is not directly emanating from the aortic arch. Interposition graft placement is sometimes necessary due to anatomic considerations. It is more susceptible to long-term complications than the

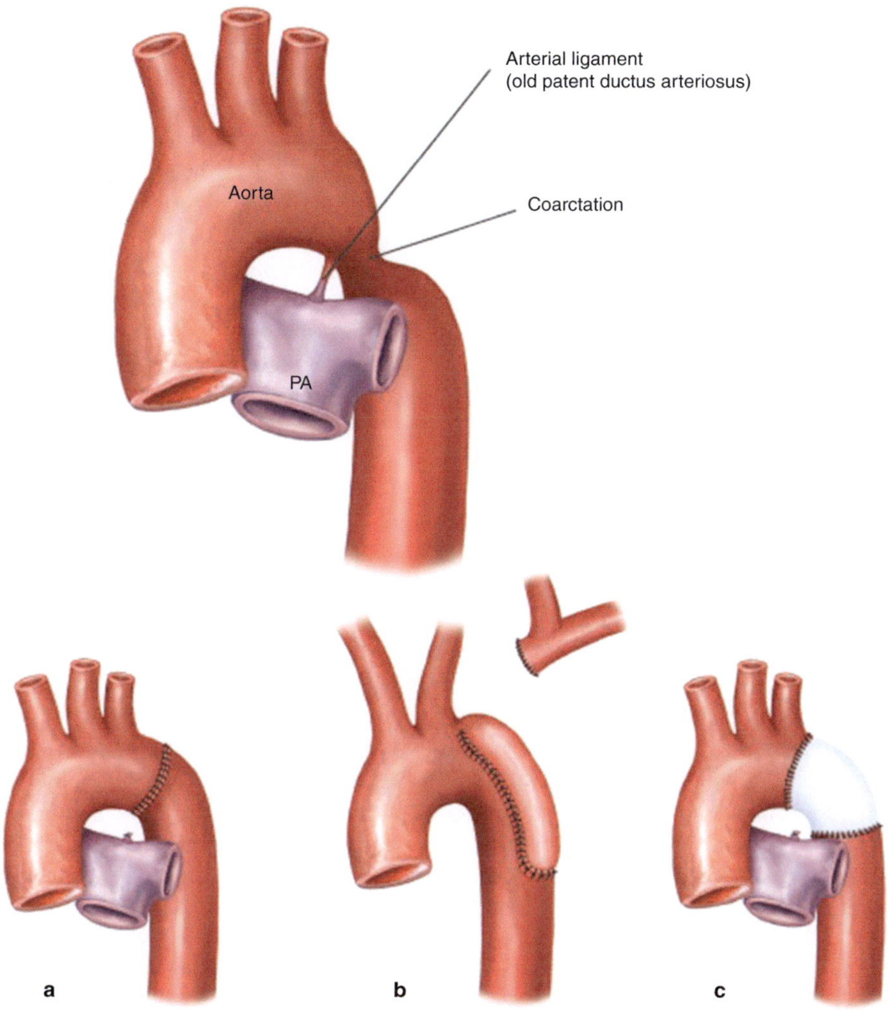

Fig. 13.8 Surgical techniques to repair coarctation of the aorta. There are multiple surgical techniques available to repair CoA. Image A demonstrates the commonly utilized end-to-end anastomosis repair. Image B demonstrates the subclavian flap repair. Image C demonstrates the interposition graft technique

end-to-end anastomosis and therefore is not typically chosen when options exist. The patch aortoplasty technique is susceptible to pseudoaneurysm formation, which when detected can be treated in the catheterization lab often but sometimes may require surgical intervention. If a bypass graft was placed from the ascending aorta to the descending aorta, then blood pressures in the arms may not reflect those in the legs given that obstructions may develop acutely because of the procedure or chronically because of it. Details regarding what type of intervention was performed and when are crucial to providing proper care of the CoA patient in the ICU.

Covered stent technology has been widely used to care for CoA patients especially among those who are adults at the time of diagnosis. It has been shown to be a safe procedure with comparable results to surgery. Inpatient hospitalization time is shorter although more planned re-interventions are noted as compared to surgery [21]. The rates of pseudoaneurysm formation are thought to be lower, but the relatively young age of the technology limits long-term data acquisition. The technical aspects of a transcatheter stenting procedure to expand CoA are elsewhere described but depend on careful measurements and appropriate sizing [22].

Within the ICU, adult patients with CoA must be monitored in different ways than other patients. Hypertension is known to be present in patients with CoA with several proposed mechanism [23, 24]. Close monitoring of blood pressure is critical. Prevention of hypertension-related end-organ damage is primary among ICU care goals. There is an increased association with cerebral aneurysms, and rupture is associated with hypertension. Also, at the repair site, prosthetic material and native tissue are subjected to increased wall stress when the heart rate and blood pressure are elevated. Infrequently discussed is a recent study, which showed that CoA is the third highest frequency lesion associated with sudden cardiac death as well as death or transplantation even when no evidence of coronary artery disease is present [25]. While it is unclear if sudden death is during times of stress or is a random event, patients should remain on telemetry monitoring, and close arrhythmia surveillance is recommended.

Not all CoA patients are alike, and details regarding additional CHD lesions are imperative to providing appropriate care. The presence of a patent ductus arteriosus is unlikely in an adult patient, but it must be ruled out. Robust collateral arteries exist to circumvent the CoA in adults who have not been repaired. In those patients who do not have a patent ductus arteriosus but have a coarctation of the aorta, significant differences in blood pressure can be appreciated with relatively increased pre-ductal as compared to post-ductal values. In those with unrepaired lesions and a patent ductus arteriosus, differences in oxygen saturation will be appreciated as well. Clubbing and cyanosis may be seen in such adult patients in tissues supplied by the descending thoracic aorta, with the brain and coronary arteries receiving fully oxygenated blood as indicated by a pulse oximetry monitor on the limb on the pre-ductal side of the body. As it relates to care, having invasive or noninvasive blood pressure monitoring is necessary and is achieved with blood pressure cuffs in the pre-ductal region and post-ductal limbs. The pre-ductal region is usually opposite to the side of the aortic arch, so knowing this detail of aortic anatomy is also crucial although anomalous subclavian arteries may confound such diagnostic monitoring. Placing a blood pressure cuff on the right arm in the setting of a left aortic arch provides accurate pre-ductal BP. Blood pressure cuffs on either leg (best placed on the lower thigh) will monitor post-ductal pressure. In higher acuity settings, invasive lines may be placed. Commonly, a right radial arterial line provides pre-ductal blood pressure, while a femoral artery line delivers post-ductal blood pressure data. As noted above, arterial lines should be placed carefully, and in the femoral artery, they should be distinct from where prior catheterization procedures were performed due to complications of femoral artery irregularities such as aneurysms, pseudoaneurysms, and stenoses. If a catheter intervention was performed, checking cuff blood pressures in the contralateral leg from arterial access is advisable for true post-ductal blood pressure monitoring. Also, in the setting of those patients with patent ductus arteriosus, monitoring saturations in a similar fashion also provides important information.

In the first few months post-procedure (surgery or catheter-based) when endothelialization has not yet occurred, an indwelling line could potentially disrupt the aortic wall especially if a pseudoaneurysm exists. Even many months or years after repair, entrance into a pseudoaneurysm could be associated with rupture.

Lastly, for patients who have coarctation of the aorta, the current guidelines in adults recommend intervention when there is ≥20 mmHg blood pressure gradient [26]. Many patients may have a lower blood pressure in their legs than pre-ductal but not meet criteria for intervention. In CoA patients with reduced blood pressure in the legs, medications that lead to decreased splanchnic blood flow should be avoided if possible. For example, in an adult with an upper gastrointestinal bleed octreotide decreases splanchnic blood flow and could possibly exacerbate suboptimal mesenteric blood flow. Vasopressin is sometimes used as adjunctive therapy for septic shock, but its vasoconstrictive effects are widespread, and for patients with already diminished blood flow, vasopressin could lead to mesenteric ischemia.

Once appropriate monitoring lines are in place, the ICU must ensure adequate cardiac output is maintained without any deleterious effects. Peri-procedurally, hypertension may be present and is related to increased sympathetic tone in the form of circulating catecholamines [27]. For this reason, beta-blockers are often utilized during or after a procedure is performed. Some data suggest that catheter interventions are associated with a less catecholamine release and a lesser hypertensive response [28]. Selective beta-blockers are commonly utilized because of their negative chronotropic and inotropic effects while also having a lesser contribution to mesenteric constriction. Calcium channel blockers are also commonly utilized and may be preferred with significant reactive airway disease. Intravenous nicardipine may be titrated to achieve adequate heart rate and blood pressure control. In the subsequent days, the primary driver of hypertension shifts away from catecholamines and becomes more centered around the renin-angiotensin-aldosterone system [27]. Medications such as angiotensin-converting enzyme inhibitors and aldosterone receptor blockers may be more beneficial in the more prolonged phase of hypertension. In addition to blood pressure management, regardless of the type of repair, careful monitoring for evidence of acute recoarctation, aneurysm formation, and femoral artery complications should be undertaken.

In the modern surgical era, surgical complications are less common than in the past. Most centers with surgeons who have congenital heart disease training perform end-to-end anastomoses when able to do so, and this technique has lower complication rates [29, 30]. Despite medical advances, complications related to surgical technique remain. An appropriate sign out should be received from the operating room personnel regarding what procedure was performed and the degree of collateralization. Nerve damage is relatively common and may be chronic. Left recurrent laryngeal nerve palsy may be seen in patients and associated with vocal cord dysfunction, which can hinder extubation. Phrenic nerve injury may occur, and diaphragmatic paresis can result. This is commonly identified on chest X-ray with flattening of the diaphragm. Similar to phrenic nerve injury, a conservative extubation strategy should be employed, and if needed, diaphragmatic plication to optimize lung volumes should be pursued. Chylothorax may occur if lymphatic vessels are damaged. If chest tube output becomes cloudy, then triglyceride levels should be checked. Modification of diet and prolonged courses of diuretic therapy have been advocated to bridge patients while collateralization occurs. Subclavian steal phenomena may become evident in the setting of subclavian flap repairs. Flow into the affected limb will come retrograde from the ipsilateral vertebral artery. Symptoms of poor flow into the posterior cerebral circulation or fatigue in the affected limb with activity may be present. Though uncommon, vascular flow issues related to small vessels that emanate at the site of surgical repair can cause significant morbidity [30]. Small vertebral arteries often take off from the descending aorta near to the left subclavian artery, and downstream ischemia in these vessels has been associated with paraplegia, so performance of neurologic examination is warranted to rule out this rare complication.

While complications for patients who have undergone catheterization procedures are less common, they remain important. In an observational study, patients who underwent stent procedures for CoA had lower acute complications but required repeat interventions [21]. Patients who underwent balloon angioplasty for CoA had poorer short- and intermediate-term hemodynamic and radiologic outcomes [21]. Balloon angioplasty requires damage to the intimal layer of the aortic wall in order to achieve results, and therefore in the ICU, one must be vigilant for acute aortic aneurysm rupture. In the current era, covered stents are placed rather than balloon angioplasty or bare-metal stents for many adult patients. Fewer morbidities and shorter hospitalization make it a desirable treatment alternative to surgical procedures. The COAST I trial was performed in the last decade and showed that 105 children (mean age 16 years) had stent implantation to native or recurrent coarctation with 99% success rate [31]. All patients had reduced blood pressure gradient without significant morbidity, and 19 patients required reintervention (planned or unplanned) in the first 2 years post-procedure. The use of covered stents as opposed to bare-metal stents is thought to reduce the rate of aneurysms.

Conclusion

Patients with aortopathies have multiple medical comorbidities as well as CHD that may lead to ICU admission. While in many ways similar to other patients, special considerations must be undertaken to ensure that accurate information is garnered. The placement of lines and pulse oximeters is important to achieving accurate data regarding blood perfusing the heart and brain as well as to the extremities. While guidelines and checklists are important to optimal outcomes in the ICU, caregivers must also be cognizant of congenital anatomy and physiology. Having a healthcare team knowledgeable about what to do and how to do it will provide the ideal care environment for patients with aortopathies.

References

1. Hoffman JI, Kaplan S. The incidence of congenital heart disease. J Am Coll Cardiol. 2002;39(12):1890–900.
2. Bjornard K, Riehle-Colarusso T, Gilboa SM, Correa A. Patterns in the prevalence of congenital heart defects, metropolitan Atlanta, 1978 to 2005. Birth Defects Res Part A: Clin Mol Teratol. 2013;97:87–94.
3. Glidewell J, Olney RS, Hinton C, Pawelski J, Sontag M, Wood T, Kucik JE, Daskalov R, Hudson J. Centers for Disease and Control and Prevention (CDC). State Legislation, Regulations, and Hospital Guidelines for Newborn Screening for Critical Congenital Heart Defects—United States, 2011–2014. MMWR Morb Mortal Wkly Rep. 2015;64(23):625–30.
4. Lee MY, Won HS, Baek JW, Cho JH, Shim JY, Lee PR, Kim A. Variety of prenatally diagnosed congenital heart disease in 22q11.2 deletion syndrome. Obstet Gynecol Sci. 2014;57(1):11–6.
5. Francois K. Aortopathy associated with congenital heart disease: a current literature review. Ann Pediatr Cardiol. 2015;8(1):25–36.
6. Yetman AT, Graham T. The dilated aorta in patients with congenital cardiac defects. J Am Coll Cardiol. 2009;53(6):461–7.
7. Crestanello JA, Cook S, Daniels C, Hitchcock CL, Sai-Sudhakar C. Medial necrosis in aortic root aneurysm after repair of tetralogy of Fallot. J Card Surg. 2010;25(2):230–2.
8. Rathi VK, Doyle M, Williams RB, Yamrozik J, Shannon RP, Biederman RWW. Massive aortic aneurysm and dissection in repaired tetralogy of Fallot; diagnosis by cardiovascular magnetic resonance imaging. Int J Cardiol. 2005;101:169–70.
9. Bradley EA, Zaidi AN, Goldsmith P, Sisk T, Colombo D, Roble S, Bradley D, Daniels C. Major adverse maternal cardiovascular-related events in those with aortopathies. What should we expect? Int J Cardiol. 2014;177(1):229–34.
10. Nishimura RA, Otto CM, Bonow RO, Carabello BA, Erwin JP 3rd, Guyton RA, O'Gara PT, Ruiz CE, Skubas NJ, Sorajja P, Sundt TM 3rd, Thomas JD, American College of Cardiology/American Heart Association Task Force on Practice Guidelines. 2014 AHA/ACC guideline for the management of patients with valvular heart disease: a report of the American College of Cardiology/American Heart Association Task Force on Practice Guidelines. Circulation. 2014;63(22):e57–185.
11. Baumgartner H, Bonhoeffer P, De Groot NM, de Haan F, Deanfield JE, Galie N, Gatzoulis MA, Gohlke-Baerwolf C, Kaemmerer H, Kilner P, Meijboom F, Mulder BJ, Oechslin E, Oliver JM, Serraf A, Szatmari A, Thaulow E, Vouhe PR, Walma E, Task Force on the Management of Grown-up Congenital Heart Disease of the European Society of Cardiology (ESC), Association for European Paediatric Cardiology (AEPC), ESC Committee for Practice Guidelines (CPG). ESC Guidelines for the management of grown-up congenital heart disease (new version 2010). Eur Heart J. 2010;31(23):2915–57.
12. Roberts WC, Ko JM. Frequency by decades of unicuspid, bicuspid, and tricuspid aortic valves in adults having isolated aortic valve replacement for aortic stenosis, with or without associated aortic regurgitation. Circulation. 2005;111(7):920–5.
13. Thanassoulis G, Yip JW, Filion K, Jamorski M, Webb G, Siu SC, Therrien J. Retrospective study to identify predictors of the presence and rapid progression of aortic dilatation in patients with bicuspid aortic valves. Nat Clin Pract Cardiovasc Med. 2008;5(12):821–8.
14. Fernández B, Durán AC, Fernández-Gallego T, Fernández MC, Such M, Arqué JM, Sans-Coma V. Bicuspid aortic valves with different spatial orientations of the leaflets are distinct etiological entities. J Am Coll Cardiol. 2009;54(24):2312–8.
15. Schaefer BM, Lewin MB, Stout KK, Gill E, Prueitt A, Byers PH, Otto CM. The bicuspid aortic valve: an integrated phenotypic classification of leaflet morphology and aortic root shape. Heart. 2008;94(12):1634–8.
16. Barker AJ, Markl M, Bürk J, Lorenz R, Bock J, Bauer S, Schulz-Menger J, von Knobelsdorff-Brenkenhoff F. Bicuspid aortic valve is associated with altered wall shear stress in the ascending aorta. Circ Cardiovasc Imaging. 2012;5(4):457–66.

17. Verma S, Siu SC. Aortic dilation in patients with bicuspid aortic valve. N Engl J Med. 2014;370(20):1920–9.
18. Michelena HI, Khanna AD, Mahoney D, Margaryan E, Topilsky Y, Suri RM, Eidem B, Edwards WD, Sundt TM 3rd, Enriquez-Sarano M. Incidence of aortic complications in patients with bicuspid aortic valves. JAMA. 2011;306(10):1104–12.
19. Siu SC, Silversides CK. Bicuspid aortic valve disease. J Am Coll Cardiol. 2010; 55(25):2789–800.
20. Whitlock RP, Sun JC, Fremes SE, Rubens FD, Teoh KH. Antithrombotic and thrombolytic therapy for valvular disease: Antithrombotic Therapy and Prevention of Thrombosis, 9th ed: American College of Chest Physicians Evidence-Based Clinical Practice Guidelines. Chest. 2012;141(2 Suppl):e576S–600S.
21. Forbes TJ, Kim DW, Du W, Turner DR, Holzer R, Amin Z, Hijazi Z, Ghasemi A, Rome JJ, Nykanen D, Zahn E, Cowley C, Hoyer M, Waight D, Gruenstein D, Javois A, Foerster S, Kreutzer J, Sullivan N, Khan A, Owada C, Hagler D, Lim S, Canter J, Zellers T, CCISC Investigators. Comparison of surgical, stent, and balloon angioplasty treatment of native coarctation of the aorta: an observational study by the CCISC (Congenital Cardiovascular Interventional Study Consortium). J Am Coll Cardiol. 2011;58(25):2664–74.
22. Kische S, D'Ancona G, Stoeckicht Y, Ortak J, Elsässer A, Ince H. Percutaneous treatment of adult isthmic aortic coarctation: acute and long-term clinical and imaging outcome with a self-expandable uncovered nitinol stent. Circ Cardiovasc Interv. 2015;8:e001799.
23. Cohen M, Fuster V, Steele PM, Driscoll D, McGoon DC. Coarctation of the aorta. Long-term follow-up and prediction of outcome after surgical correction. Circulation. 1989;80(4):840–5.
24. Daniels SR. Repair of coarctation of the aorta and hypertension: does age matter. Lancet. 2001;358:89.
25. Gallego P, Gonzalez AE, Sanchez-Recalde A, Peinado R, Polo L, Gomez-Rubin C, Lopez-Sendon JL, Oliver JM. Incidence and predictors of sudden cardiac arrest in adults with congenital heart defects repaired before adult life. Am J Cardiol. 2012;110(1):109–17.
26. Warnes CA, Williams RG, Bashore TM, Child JS, Connolly HM, Dearani JAACC. AHA 2008 Guidelines for the Management of Adults with Congenital Heart Disease: a report of the American College of Cardiology/American Heart Association Task Force on Practice Guidelines (writing committee to develop guidelines on the management of adults with congenital heart disease). Circulation. 2008;118:714–833.
27. Rocchini AP, Rosenthal A, Barger AC, Castaneda AR, Nadas AS. Pathogenesis of paradoxical hypertension after coarctation resection. Circulation. 1976;54(3):382–7.
28. Choy M, Rocchini AP, Beekman RH, Rosenthal A, Dick M, Crowley D, Behrendt D, Snider AR. Paradoxical hypertension after repair of coarctation of the aorta in children: balloon angioplasty versus surgical repair. Circulation. 1987;76(6):1186–91.
29. Vergales JE, Gangemi JJ, Rhueban KS, Lim DS. Coarctation of the aorta—the current state of surgical and transcatheter therapies. Curr Cardiol Rev. 2013;9(3):211–9.
30. Hershberger R, Cho JS. Neurologic complications of aortic diseases and aortic surgery. Handb Clin Neurol. 2014;119:223–38.
31. Meadows J, Minahan M, McElhinney DB, McEnaney K, Ringel R, Investigators COAST. Intermediate outcomes in the prospective, multicenter coarctation of the aorta stent trial (COAST). Circulation. 2015;131(19):1656–64.

Critical Care Management of the ACHD Patient with Heart Failure

14

Leigh Christopher Reardon, Eugene Depasquale, and Weiyi Tan

14.1 Introduction

The progression of surgical techniques and improvement of diagnosis and medical management of patients with congenital heart defects has altered the natural history of many previously fatal cardiac conditions. As a result, more and more patients with CHD are living into adulthood, and studies suggest that there are now more adults living with CHD (ACHD) than there are children with CHD [1, 2]. Between 2000 and 2010, the proportion of adults to children with CHD changed from 49% to 66%, and when extrapolated to the US population, there are approximately 1.5 million adults with CHD [1].

L. C. Reardon (✉)
Department of Medicine and Pediatric Cardiology, Ronald Reagan UCLA Medical Center, Los Angeles, CA, USA

Department of Medicine and Cardiology, Ronald Reagan UCLA Medical Center, Los Angeles, CA, USA
e-mail: lreardon@mednet.ucla.edu

E. Depasquale
Division of Cardiology, Department of Medicine, Ahmanson/UCLA Cardiomyopathy Center, David Geffen School of Medicine, Los Angeles, CA, USA
e-mail: EDepasquale@mednet.ucla.edu

W. Tan
Department of Medicine and Cardiology, Ronald Reagan UCLA Medical Center, Los Angeles, CA, USA
e-mail: WeiyiTan@mednet.ucla.edu

E. da Cruz et al. (eds.), *Intensive Care of the Adult with Congenital Heart Disease*, Congenital Heart Disease in Adolescents and Adults,
https://doi.org/10.1007/978-3-319-94171-4_14

Adults with CHD are at increased risk of late complications, including heart failure, arrhythmias, and sudden death. Despite advances in the field, death rates in the ACHD population can be two to seven times higher than for the general population [3]. There are over 13,500 admissions for heart failure annually according to one study out of the 24,800 admissions for ACHD every year [4]. With the annual increase of number of adults with congenital heart disease, this problem will only become greater in the future.

The 2008 ACC/AHA (American College of Cardiology/American Heart Association) guidelines for adults with CHD and the 2010 ESC (European Society of Cardiology) guidelines for the management of grown-up congenital heart disease provide some guidance about the management of heart failure in the adult population [5, 6]. Some of the guidelines highlighted in the ACC/AHA 2009 update about the management of adult patients with heart failure can be extrapolated to adults with congenital heart disease, but many of the recommendations are based on studies that excluded these types of patients, and thus applying these recommendations to patients with CHD is fraught with assumptions [7]. We focus on synthesizing and summarizing the evidence available to date in order to describe the critical care management of adult patients with CHD who present to the hospital with heart failure.

14.2 Types of Heart Failure

There are many definitions of heart failure, but we define it similarly to how the American Heart Association (AHA) and the Heart Failure Society of America guidelines define heart failure (HF): "In physiologic terms, HF is a syndrome characterized by either or both pulmonary and systemic venous congestion and/or inadequate peripheral oxygen delivery, at rest or during stress, caused by cardiac dysfunction." [8]. Adult patients with CHD can present with varied symptoms of heart failure, ranging from classic symptoms of fatigue, dyspnea, and exercise intolerance, but may also have more subtle findings like malnutrition, cachexia, or growth failure [8]. Many patients fail to even report symptoms despite objective evidence of exercise intolerance [9]. When applying the ACC/AHA guidelines on staging heart failure, most adults with CHD fall into at least stage B (structural heart disease but without signs of HF), but we focus on patients admitted to the hospital with at least stage C or stage D heart failure (structural heart disease with prior or current symptoms of HF and refractory HF requiring specialized interventions, respectively) [8].

14.3 Types of ACHD Patients

When an adult patient with CHD is admitted to the hospital, understanding their underlying anatomy and history of prior interventions and/or surgeries is paramount, as patients can be surgically repaired, palliated, or unrepaired. Surgical procedures early in life for a patient with CHD are generally life prolonging, and thus survival for patients with CHD has increased. Many of these procedures, however, are not curative, and consequently the adult patient with CHD will often times have residua of their initial congenital cardiac diagnosis and sequelae of their prior interventions. These patients may commonly face a lifetime of repeated interventions and long-term effects of structural abnormalities that will eventually lead to heart failure [10]. There are aspects of HF management that are universally applicable to adults with and without CHD, but many patients will have unique anatomic and physiological constraints that will make management individualized. It is useful to think of patients with CHD as those with a systemic left ventricle, those with a systemic right ventricle, or those with a single ventricle physiology (either left or right ventricular morphology). Furthermore, it is useful to understand that depending on the surgical technique available at the time of their birth and at the particular center performing the palliation, patients will have varying historical surgical repairs. For example, a patient with a Fontan palliation may have a classic atriopulmonary connection, an intracardiac lateral tunnel conduit, or an extracardiac cavopulmonary connection. To summarize, adults with congenital heart disease should be treated in accordance with their specific anatomy and not uniformly like typical adults with congestive heart failure.

14.4 Epidemiology

As stated earlier, there are more adults with congenital heart disease than there are children with the condition [1]. The number of hospital admissions is increasing, and one study demonstrated an increase of 102% from 1998 to 2005 [4]. Twenty percent of hospital admissions for patients with ACHD are for heart failure [3]. One recent study noted that patients with pulmonary arterial hypertension, a history of HF, and atrial arrhythmias are at the highest risk for HF admissions [11]. Heart failure is the leading cause of death for patients with ACHD [12]. While the prevalence of heart failure in adults with CHD is unknown, some reports suggest that nearly 50% of patients after a Fontan procedure will develop HF [8, 13] (Fig. 14.1).

With advances in surgery and medical therapy, children with congenital heart disease are living longer. One study showed that median age at death increased by

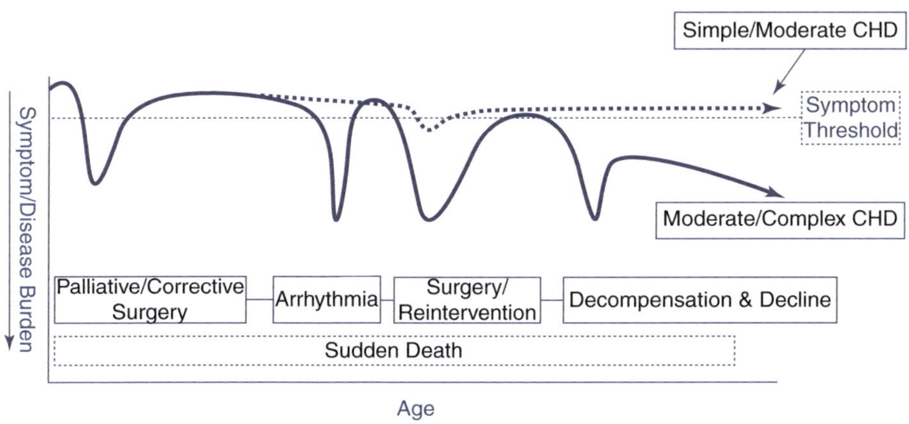

Fig. 14.1 Cited from [12]

15 years from 1987 to 2005 [14]. Another study shows that for patients with CHD, the cause of late death after pediatric cardiac surgery was heart failure in 43% of cases in their study cohort [15]. The cost of these hospitalizations has been estimated to be $3.16 billion per year [4]. Per the 2008 guidelines for adults with congenital heart disease, certain patients may be at higher risk for developing heart failure, including those with left-sided valvular defects, unoperated atrial septal defect (ASD), congenitally corrected transposition of the great arteries (ccTGA), D-transposition of the great arteries (dTGA) after a Mustard or Senning procedure, single ventricle physiology, tetralogy of Fallot (TOF) with early-era surgery or long-standing shunt, and Fontan surgery [5]. Compared to those with a systemic left ventricle and biventricular physiology, patients with a systemic RV or single right ventricles are at high risk of heart failure and associated mortality [13].

14.5 Etiology and Pathophysiology

Clinical heart failure in patients with CHD is due to a multitude of factors, some of which may be lesion specific. In traditional patients with acquired HF, the most common cause of heart failure is systemic ventricular dysfunction from ischemia, which is uncommon in ACHD patients [8]. According to the AHA statement on chronic heart failure in ACHD patients, abnormal myocardial architecture, abnormal myocardial perfusion due to cyanotic lesions, neurohormonal activation, myocardial fibrosis and adverse remodeling, surgical complications, and an underlying geometric and anatomic disadvantage from poor ventricular-ventricular dependence and ventriculo-arterial coupling all contribute to clinical HF in this population [8].

For example, the patient with repaired tetralogy of Fallot may not necessarily suffer from systolic left ventricular dysfunction due to ischemia from blocked coronary arteries. Heart failure may occur due to myocardial damage from shunts, multiple cardiac surgeries, or inadequate myocardial protection from the original surgery. Chronic volume and pressure overload from an insufficient pulmonary valve may contribute to right ventricular dysfunction and signs of right-sided heart failure. Impaired electrical conduction systems from the multiple surgeries and ventricular septal defect patches may prevent efficient ventricular function as well as sudden cardiac death episodes. Finally, some patients may also have anomalous coronary arteries that may lead to ischemia [10]. In patients with atrial level switches for D-transposition of the great arteries, pulmonary venous obstruction can cause heart failure. In a Fontan patient, the single ventricle has to pump against three resistance beds in a series (the systemic vascular bed, the cavopulmonary connection, and the pulmonary vascular bed) [16], which can lead to chronic heart failure. Nevertheless, as adults with CHD get older, they may also be susceptible to traditional risk factors for developing ischemia, such as hypertension, hyperlipidemia, and diabetes [3].

The neurohormonal aspects of heart failure are well documented, but it is unclear what standard therapies are beneficial in adults with congenital heart disease. There is evidence to suggest that patients with adult congenital heart disease do have

Table 14.1 Causes of heart failure in patients with congenital heart disease

Volume overload from left-to-right shunts and valvular regurgitation
Pressure overload from stenotic valves and other obstructive lesions
Intrinsic myocardial dysfunction, genetic syndromes
Pulmonary hypertension caused by congenital heart disease lesions, or from comorbidities like obstructive sleep apnea
Systemic arterial hypertension from coarctation of the aorta, renal disease, or essential hypertension
Coronary artery disease
Cyanosis
Tachycardia induced cardiomyopathy from recurrent atrial arrhythmias

similar increases in activation of neurohormonal pathways [17]. Studies have confirmed that an elevation in BNP is predictive of mortality and worsening functional status [18, 19].

Pulmonary hypertension is also a risk factor for heart failure. One study out of Canada showed that the prevalence of pulmonary hypertension in patients with congenital heart disease was around 5.8% [20]. This finding increased the risk of mortality and heart failure in these patients, by more than two times and three times, respectively, when compared to a matched cohort of CHD patients without pulmonary hypertension.

In addition to acquired etiologies of heart failure, adults with congenital heart disease may also have complex genetic pathways that contribute to their myocardial dysfunction. Certain genetic syndromes, such as Noonan, DiGeorge, or Williams-Beuren syndrome, all present with cardiomyopathy, and the ACHD population may have a unique interaction between genetic and acquired factors that may make treatment of heart failure more difficult [21]. There are currently few studies highlighting the effect of genetic variation in the ACHD population on adverse ventricular remodeling, but as these studies emerge, the future of "personalized" medicine will become more of a reality [22] (Table 14.1).

14.6 Management

14.6.1 General Principles of Heart Failure Management

Increasing numbers of adults with congenital heart disease will be admitted to the hospital for cardiac procedures, pregnancy, or other non-cardiac conditions. Nevertheless, proper management of ACHD patients with clinical and subclinical heart failure will be a priority in all these settings. If there is a patient with CHD who has critical care needs, they should ideally be in a center that has experience with treatment of ACHD patients [5, 6].

When discussing patients with CHD and CHF, many of the general principles highlighted in the ESC and ACC/AHA guidelines will remain the same. For example, the ESC guidelines espouse a method of parallel assessments when working up a patient with acute heart failure, including assessing for heart failure or other causes of their symptoms, identifying the trigger for the heart failure episode, and managing any life-threatening conditions like hypoxemia or hypotension [23]. Nevertheless, some differences exist; for example, the ubiquitous use of oxygen for hypoxic patients may not be applicable, especially in patients with intracardiac shunts.

In patients with pulmonary hypertension or persistent intracardiac or extracardiac shunts, the balance between pulmonary and systemic vascular resistance must be maintained. Any therapy that increases PVR will reduce cardiac output, and patients with shunts will have increased right-to-left shunting with therapies that decrease systemic vascular resistance [24].

Assessment and management of traditional risk factors should occur. Existing guidelines for tobacco cessation and screening for traditional risk factors should be applied [8]. The prevalence of hypertension, diabetes, and dyslipidemia closely mirrors, if not exceeds, the rates of these risk factors in the general population [25]. Early detection and treatment should be then applied for these traditional cardiovascular risk factors, understanding that certain patients may have variable response to treatment depending on their cardiac anatomy. Patients should be vaccinated with an annual influenza vaccine and the pneumococcal vaccine as well [6].

Medical management of ACHD patients with heart failure should focus on optimizing their preload, afterload, and cardiac contractility. In terms of preload, the use of diuretics is accepted to improve symptoms in a fluid-overloaded patient. The detection of fluid overload may be difficult in certain patients with CHD; for example, patients with a Fontan or a Glenn procedure will not have an interpretable jugular venous waveform to guide therapy [5]. Afterload reduction agents, such as ACE inhibitors (ACE-I) and angiotensin receptor blockers (ARB), are the cornerstone of heart failure therapy for those with acquired heart disease, but caregivers should extrapolate cautiously from heart failure trials as these studies enrolled very few patients with ACHD [5]. Some of the few studies involving ACHD patients did not show as robust of a clinical benefit when using these traditional agents. For example, the appropriate trial did not show a difference between groups that received ramipril or placebo in terms of right ventricular ejection fraction as measured by cardiac MRI [26]. When discussing contractility, the role of pacemaker therapy and multisite pacing (or cardiac resynchronization therapy) is also being investigated. There is no evidence to support the use of cardiac resynchronization therapy (CRT) in patients with a single ventricle morphology, but the traditional criteria for CRT implantation still apply (two-ventricle morphology and HF symptoms with a QRS duration ≥120 ms with a left bundle-branch block morphology in the setting of sinus rhythm) [5].

Many patients will have comorbidities that may make management of heart failure difficult, such as anemia, renal insufficiency, pulmonary hypertension, and hepatic dysfunction. Renal insufficiency has been associated with worse outcomes in adults with CHD [27]. Patients with single ventricle physiology, such as those with the Fontan circuit, are susceptible to external changes that will affect passive filling of the pulmonary bed. Thus, ascites, positive-pressure ventilation, and decreased diaphragmatic excursion will lead to increased Fontan or right-sided pressures and decreased pulmonary venous return [28]. Pulmonary hypertension (PH) is also a difficult situation to manage, especially in patients with Eisenmenger syndrome. The use of advanced therapies for pulmonary hypertension will be discussed in other chapters, but some studies demonstrate a mortality benefit in these patients [29]. Nonetheless, more studies are needed to investigate the use of PH-targeted therapy in adults with CHD. Hepatic dysfunction and right heart failure are also concerns in ACHD patients. Cardiac cirrhosis, especially in patients with a Fontan circulation, is quite common. Consider the use of bladder pressure monitors to avoid intra-abdominal hypertension from ascites and decreased renal perfusion. The use of inotropes, aggressive diuresis and the use of dialysis, and drainage of ascites may be required for optimization [30].

Specific therapeutic strategies tailored to different forms of CHD will be highlighted in future sections.

14.6.2 Diagnosis and Risk Prediction

Heart failure occurs when the heart cannot meet the metabolic demands of the body. In older patients, classic symptoms may manifest, but younger patients with CHD may maintain blood pressure and urine output due to autoregulation and may underreport symptoms given their lifetime of chronic heart disease [9, 31]. Conversely, for example, in cyanotic patients, dyspnea may occur within the first 30 seconds of initiating exercise due to hypoxemic and acidotic blood arriving at central receptors, and thus their symptom of dyspnea on exertion is not due to pulmonary congestion from heart failure [5]. When patients with ACHD are admitted to the hospital, there are no specific tools to identify the ones at highest risk for heart failure and morbidity/mortality from their cardiac conditions, and relying on just physical exam findings may be misleading. One study demonstrated that use of the Seattle HF model can be applied to a population of adults with CHD, and those that have a 5-year predicted survival of <70% can be classified as high risk of having a cardiovascular event [32]. A high index of suspicion should be maintained when treating patients with high risk for late heart failure, such as those with bicuspid valves, subvalvular or supravalvular pathology, severe aortic stenosis and/or regurgitation, unoperated ASD or partial AVSD, ccTGA, atrial-level switch with dTGA, tetralogy of Fallot with early-era surgery, a long-standing shunt, pulmonary regurgitation, pulmonary hypertension, single ventricle physiology, and a history of a Fontan/Glenn operation [5]. On top of their underlying high-risk lesions, patients with ACHD may have sequelae from their disease or reparative surgeries, such as prolonged cyanosis, pressure and volume overload, ventricular scars, residual LVOT or RVOT obstructions or shunts, arrhythmias, and obesity, that could contribute to the development of heart failure. Finally, unrelated conditions may also cause an "imbalance" between the heart's ability to provide for the metabolic demands of the body and manifest as heart failure, such as pregnancy, endocarditis, illicit drug use, hyperthyroidism, or obstructive sleep apnea [5].

14.7 Laboratory Analysis and Studies

At the onset of worsening symptoms, the ACHD patient and suspected HF should undergo right-sided and left-sided anatomic and hemodynamic evaluation with a variety of studies best suited for their condition. In addition to basic laboratory studies (chemistry panel, liver function studies, and complete blood count), a measurement of the serum BNP level may also be useful in helping risk-stratify patients [18, 19]. The 2008 ACC/AHA guidelines for management of ACHD and the 2010 guidelines for the management of grown-up congenital heart disease both also recommend an electrocardiogram, chest X-ray, pulse oximetry, and echocardiogram for most patients being evaluated in an acute setting [5, 6]. If patients are stable enough, data from a cardiopulmonary exercise testing may be helpful for quantitative assessment of cardiac function. Advanced imaging, such as cardiac MRI, is playing an increased role in the initial evaluation, especially in patients with systemic right ventricles and single ventricles, and may even be considered the reference standard for RV volume quantification, outflow tract obstruction, pulmonary valve function, and assessment of the great arteries [33, 34]. Cardiac computed tomography is also another option for an imaging modality if MRI is not feasible or available. More invasive procedures, such as cardiac catheterization, may be necessary for a comprehensive evaluation for an adult patient with CHD in clinical HF [8] (Table 14.2).

14.7.1 Echocardiogram

Echocardiography remains as a first-line investigative tool. Echocardiography can provide a wealth of information, such as assessment of volume overload, pressure overload, and detailed data about structure and function of the ventricle. Echocardiograms establish segmental anatomy and can provide measures of and follow-up assessments of valves. Echocardiography also provides crucial hemodynamic data through measurement of gradients across obstructions, conduits, and valves, as well as flow calculations. Doppler images allow for identifying arterial and venous vascular anomalies and shunts.

Transthoracic echocardiography is complemented by transesophageal echocardiography (TEE) and other specialized techniques, such as contrast imaging, strain imaging, real-time three-dimensional and four-dimensional imaging, and stress echocardiography with or without Doppler [3]. Of note, certain echocardiographic variables are subject to changes with age, such as diastolic flow parameters (E- and A-wave peak velocities) and pulmonary pressure cutoffs for pulmonary hypertension [3].

Nevertheless, when assessing an adult patient with CHD, advanced training is required to properly acquire and interpret the echocardiographic images, since many of these patients have complicated surgical history and complex anatomy that makes for unorthodox or unconventional image views [6, 35].

Echocardiographic parameters, besides the Simpson method, are required for measuring RV function. Strain imaging is shown to be helpful, in addition to FAC

Table 14.2 Imaging modalities used for diagnosis and management of adult congenital heart disease

Modality	Widely available	Scan time	Advanced equipment required	Cost	Radiation (in millisieverts)	Contrast	Comments
Echocardiography	Yes	Slow	No	$$	None	None	Workhorse imaging modality, requires expert readers dedicated to ACHD
Non-contrast CT	Yes	Fast	No	$	3–7	None	Limited to calcification assessments
ECG-gated cardiac CT/CTA	No	Fast	Yes	$$$	8–12	Yes	Excellent spatial resolution. Preferred method for evaluating coronary artery patency and anatomy
MRI/MRA	No	Slow	Yes	$$$	None	Yes for late gadolinium enhancement	Good for tissue characterization and anatomy. Can also evaluate real-time cardiac function and be used for flow quantification

(fractional area change) and tissue Doppler [34]. Non-geometric techniques for assessing ventricular function are also useful in patients with CHD, and include the rate of pressure rise (dP/dt), the Tei (myocardial performance) index, and tissue Doppler imaging, strain imaging, and tricuspid annular plane systolic excursion (TAPSE) [34].

Strain imaging is a new technique that can identify ventricular dysfunction in patients with traditional systemic left ventricles, as well as systemic RVs or single ventricles. The commercial software available for analyzing myocardial strain is designed for the morphologic left ventricle, and thus may not be as useful for the right ventricle. Furthermore, the strain measurement varies widely depending on the type of machine and software being used, so serial measurements must be performed with the same device and software package [34]. Nevertheless, multiple studies have shown that myocardial strain is predictive of myocardial dysfunction and can have prognostic value in patients with a systemic right ventricle in dTGA after an atrial switch and in patients with repaired tetralogy of Fallot [36, 37].

Contrast echocardiography is useful in opacifying heart chambers in patients with a large body habitus or with difficult acoustic windows. While not approved by the FDA for use in patients with right-to-left or bidirectional shunts, the use of agitated saline is a useful tool in patients with ACHD. These techniques are used to detect residual shunts, baffle leaks, or anatomic anomalies like a persistent left-sided super vena cava [3].

Stress echocardiography can be used to screen for coronary ischemia, assess the physiologic response to severe AV valve regurgitation, and evaluate for subaortic stenosis, aortic coarctation, or aortic valve disease in the presence of low ejection fraction [34].

Transesophageal echocardiography (TEE) is an important adjunctive modality to transthoracic studies. Similar to adults without CHD, it is useful when the patient has poor acoustic transthoracic windows. TEE is effective at assessing the intrathoracic aorta, native and prosthetic valves, ventricular function, atrial-level shunts, baffle function, detecting endocarditis, and other cardiac sources of emboli. TEE is also a useful technique during procedures and surgeries [3]. One methodology of TEE includes the use of a miniature TEE probe to evaluate real-time hemodynamic data, including LV function, in critically ill patients [38]. Another study also found that a TEE-derived cardiac output calculation correlated well with a thermodilution method in critically ill ICU patients, and thus TEE has been demonstrated to be useful in patients who may be too unstable for transport to receive other imaging modalities or invasive procedures [39].

14.7.2 Cardiac Magnetic Resonance Imaging (CMR)

CMR is useful as an alternative to echocardiography, as a second method when echocardiography is not adequate, or as a superior imaging modality to echocardiography in certain situations, such as quantifying RV volumes, tissue characterization, and evaluation of the great vessels [6, 40]. This imaging modality enables excellent three-dimensional anatomical reconstruction that is not restricted by body size or acoustic windows, unless the patient has a pacemaker or dense calcification. CMR has limitless angles of acquisition [3]. It is the reference standard for assessing the right ventricle for structure and function [34]. CMR allows for detailed pre-procedural planning, such as prior to a percutaneous valve replacement, an electrophysiology study and ablation, or a surgery with redo sternotomy in the setting of complex conotruncal anatomy or anomalous coronary arteries [3]. The ability for CMR to provide tissue characterization, specifically identifying patients with scar and fibrosis (through late gadolinium enhancement), can have important prognostic value, as there have been studies highlighting associations between scar and arrhythmias, ventricular dysfunction, and poor clinical outcomes in patients with CHD [34]. Another promising CMR technique is fibrosis imaging using extracellular volume (ECV) fraction via T1 mapping, which has been associated with surrogate markers of myocardial dysfunction, including higher BNP and longer QRS duration [34]. Patients with implanted pacemakers or defibrillators may not be able to be imaged with CMR, and thus cardiac CT is a possible alternative. Furthermore, the relatively long acquisition times and requirement for repeated breath holds in a setting that promotes claustrophobia may make it a prohibitive study for some ACHD patients [3].

CMR also allows for accurate calculations of shunt fractions and regurgitation volumes using two-dimensional phase contrast imaging. In fact, CMR is considered the reference standard for assessing the severity of pulmonary regurgitation [34]. Four-dimensional magnetic resonance velocity mapping (4D flow) also encodes blood flow in a 3D volume set over time, which may provide future insight into the ventriculo-arterial coupling relationship in complex CHD patients, such as in the Fontan circuit [34].

14.7.3 Cardiac Computed Tomography (CT)

CT has excellent spatial resolution and has a much more rapid acquisition time than CMR, which makes it attractive in acute settings, but lacks the ability of CMR for tissue characterization. Furthermore, CT imaging systems are more widely available, and thus it is a more practical imaging option as well. CT delineates epicardial coronary arteries and collateral arteries with accurate detail. CT is also useful in ruling out complications like intracardiac thrombus, baffle obstruction, and prosthetic valve dysfunction [34]. Ionizing radiation is required for CT, which is a drawback for using this modality for serial studies [6].

CT angiography is useful for pre-procedure planning prior to a percutaneous catheter-based intervention or a redo sternotomy when assessing for the structural relationship of the great vessels, coronary arteries, and sternum. Inexperienced interpreters, however, may misdiagnose abnormalities in pulmonary vascular blood flow in the setting of known shunt lesions or palliative circulations, such as making an incorrect diagnosis of pulmonary embolism in a patient with a Fontan surgery [3].

14.7.4 Exercise Testing with CPET

Cardiopulmonary testing is valuable in predicting morbidity and mortality. The entire cohort of ACHD patients has reduced exercise tolerance when compared to an age-matched control, and even asymptomatic patients have reduced VO_2 consumption [9]. CPET, especially peak VO_2 and heart rate reserve, may provide prognostic information in ACHD [41], but this study modality may be too strenuous for patients who are critically ill in heart failure.

14.8 Procedures

14.8.1 Invasive Hemodynamic Monitoring

The ESCAPE trial did not show much benefit in using Swan-Ganz catheters routinely [42]. Furthermore, many adults with CHD will have limited vascular access, and using a Swan-Ganz catheter in patients with intracardiac shunts and Fontan physiology may not give accurate information that can be used for clinical decision-making.

14.8.2 Arterial Line

If placing an arterial line, caregivers need to make sure it is in an artery that has adequate blood flow; patients with previous BT shunts may not have a reliable waveform, and achieving access may be impossible.

14.8.3 Peripheral IV with Bubble Filters

If a patient with ACHD has a right-to-left shunt, there is always a risk of paradoxical air or thromboembolism traveling to the brain. Thus all intravenous lines, including peripheral IVs, should have 23 micron bubble filters attached [24].

14.8.4 Implantable Hemodynamic Monitors

Newer technologies, including the use of implantable hemodynamic monitors, such as the CardioMEMS™ device, have demonstrated that they can reduce the incidence of heart failure hospitalizations [43]. While it has not been approved for use in the ACHD population, one study did show that implantation of this device was possible in a patient with a Fontan procedure, and thus the utilization of this device in the ACHD population will most likely be increased in the future [44]. Risk of clot in a low-flow circulation is a reason to use judicious caution in placing such devices in higher-risk patients.

14.8.5 Cardiac Catheterization

With the advent and development of advanced imaging techniques, cardiac catheterization is an invasive procedure that is reserved to resolve specific anatomic or physiological questions or for interventional treatment. For example, cardiac catheterization procedures can assess for pulmonary hypertension, measure pressure gradients, be used for closure of aortopulmonary, arteriovenous, or venovenous collaterals, and shunt calculations. Catheterization procedures in ACHD patients can be more complex due to vascular access issues and abnormal anatomy that limits appropriate entry to desired chambers of the heart. Usually, a team of operators is needed, one with expertise in CHD lesions and evaluation of intracardiac shunts and one with experience in coronary artery angiography and intervention of left-sided heart disease [3].

14.9 Therapies

14.9.1 Medications

The role of neurohormonal agents like ACE inhibitors, angiotensin receptor blockers, and beta-blockers for patients with reduced systolic function is not as established for patients with ACHD. Yet, some guidelines state that without specifically tailored evidence, caregivers have to carefully extrapolate evidence and apply them to patients with CHD [8, 45]. These therapies may be helpful in patients with two-ventricle circulations and a dysfunctional systemic LV but may be less helpful with diastolic dysfunction, systemic RV, Eisenmenger syndrome, or single ventricle patients. Standard heart failure therapies may even have worse adverse effects [8]. In one trial, losartan was given to patients with a systemic RV and it did not improve exercise tolerance or reduce BNP levels [46]. Another study did not demonstrate a benefit of beta-blockers in patients with systemic right ventricles [47]. Nevertheless, the medical therapies for each set of congenital lesions will be described here.

14.9.1.1 Systemic LV

If patients have left-sided pressure overload lesions, they will need intervention for the coarctation or stenosis. For patients with systolic failure of the left ventricle, many guidelines suggest that evidence for traditional medications used for adults with HF can extrapolated to adults with CHD and HF [8, 24]. Thus, beta-blockers, ACE inhibitors or angiotensin receptor blockers, aldosterone inhibitors, and diuretics can all be used in these patients.

14.9.1.2 Systemic RV

The systemic RV will eventually fail. No data exist about when a systemic RV with impaired ejection fraction should warrant treatment. If the patient is asymptomatic, it is difficult to ascertain when the appropriate time is to initiate treatment. Some studies (using arbitrary measures) state that heart failure occurs in 22% of dTGA with Mustard and 32% of patients with ccTGA [13]. Diagnosis with the use of a BNP and echocardiography is helpful. Cardiac MRI provides detailed RV imaging and can be useful in diagnosing RV dysfunction as well. In patients with a Mustard or Senning procedure, vasodilators may reduce preload and reduce cardiac output due to a concomitant baffle obstruction. Beta-blockers may have some beneficial effects in these patients in terms of AV valve regurgitation and RV remodeling [47], but a lot of these patients have conduction abnormalities that may be exacerbated by the use of an AV nodal blocking agent. Studies investigating the use of neuromodulators of the renin-angiotensin-aldosterone system (RAAS) system did not show a benefit in patients with HF and a systemic RV [46, 48]. Despite inconsistent evidence and lack of data supporting improved clinical outcomes, the use of ACE-I/ARB is common for patients with a systemic RV [8]. If the patient is suffering from symptomatic HF, many physicians will start neurohormonal therapy empirically [49, 50].

14.9.1.3 Systolic Failure of the Morphologic Sub-pulmonary RV

These patients usually have Ebstein's anomaly of the tricuspid valve or repaired TOF with pulmonary regurgitation. Long-term sequelae of these conditions lead to volume overload, dilation, myocardial dysfunction and clinical HF. RV dysfunction and enlargement can lead to LV dysfunction due to ventricular interdependence. Poor RV output also leads to low LV preload. As both ventricles share myocardial fibers, fibrosis can affect both ventricles and neurohormonal activation will also lead to long-term structural changes in both chambers [8]. The use of beta-blockers and ACE inhibitors in these patients is common, but evidence does not suggest robust outcomes [26, 51]. There are no randomized controlled trials for medical therapies for this group of patients. Even the traditional guidelines have few recommendations about therapies in this group of adults without CHD. Diuretics are the main treatment option for symptomatic patients. If pulmonary hypertension is thought to be the primary cause of RV failure, then advanced therapy may play a role, although the data for these drugs do not include many ACHD patients [24]. That being said, there have been some studies showing that advanced therapies (mainly bosentan) do have a favorable effect on exercise capacity and hemodynamics in Eisenmenger patients [52].

14.9.1.4 Systolic Failure of the Single Ventricle

These patients do not have the benefit of a sub-pulmonary pumping chamber and thus have to rely on passive filling of the pulmonary vasculature. This results in improved oxygenation, but at the sacrifice of elevated CVP. These patients are dependent on respiratory mechanics, the diastolic function of the ventricle, and the pulmonary vascular resistance [8]. Low velocity flow through an atriopulmonary or cavopulmonary connection can increase the risk of thrombosis, which can lead to an increase in the pulmonary vascular resistance. The high CVP in a Fontan circuit can lead to hepatic congestion and dysfunction. Right-to-left shunting through a fenestration in the Fontan can also lead to cyanosis. Thus, CHF findings of cyanosis, hepatic dysfunction, and increased pulmonary vascular resistance may arise in the setting of preserved myocardial function. When managing a Fontan patient in HF, clinicians must search for potentially reversible causes of HF, such as arrhythmias, obstruction of the Fontan pathway, and residual shunting [8]. In Fontan patients, where increased pulmonary vascular resistance can impair ventricular filling, the use of phosphodiesterase inhibitors may improve exercise performance and myocardial performance [29, 53]. The use of spironolactone may also improve endothelial function and reduce the incidence of PLE [54, 55]. One study did not show beneficial effects with RAAS inhibition in Fontan patients, so their use is uncertain in this group [56]. Use of diuretics and digoxin is also popular, but without evidence. Carvedilol has been shown to improve HF signs and symptoms in Fontan patients [57], so reducing pulmonary vascular resistance and afterload may have the best benefits, while diuretics should be used judiciously as it may induce cardiorenal syndrome from reduced preload.

14.9.1.5 Heart Failure with Preserved Ejection Fraction (HFpEF)

There are no good evidence-based treatments that reduce morbidity or mortality in adults with heart failure with preserved ejection fraction [7, 23]. Diuretics are mainly used for symptomatic relief (Fig. 14.2).

Of note, there are no studies looking at the newer treatments, including ivabradine [58] and the neprilysin inhibitors [59] in patients with CHD. Nevertheless, the data can be extrapolated to patients with systolic dysfunction and systemic left ventricles. For ACHD patients with systemic RVs or single ventricle physiology, use of

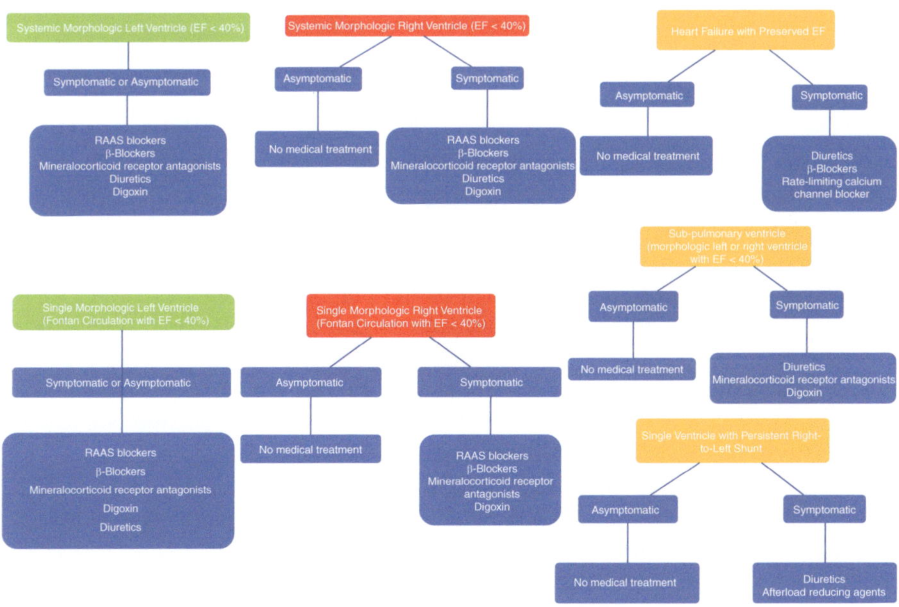

Fig. 14.2 Medical treatment for heart failure related to intrinsic myocardial dysfunction

these newer treatments cannot be recommended at this time. Iron deficiency anemia is an important comorbidity that should be addressed in patients with CHD and heart failure, especially in those who are chronically hypoxic [60].

14.10 Pulmonary HTN and Eisenmenger Physiology

Management of these patients will be discussed in another chapter. Nevertheless, these patients often present with failing right or sub-pulmonic ventricles. Patients with Eisenmenger physiology are recommended to avoid pregnancy, dehydration, severe strenuous exercise, exposure to excessive heat, high altitudes, and iron deficiency. The 2008 ACC/AHA guidelines also encourage prompt treatment of arrhythmia [5]. Treatment with advanced therapies, such as endothelin antagonists, showed improved mortality in retrospective studies [61], and some patients may even need long-term dual vasodilator therapy for improved outcomes [62].

14.11 Drips, Inotropes, and Vasopressors

There are no robust studies with the use of inotropes and vasopressors in critically ill patients with CHD in heart failure. Right ventricular failure manifests as an increase in jugular venous pressure and renal and hepatic dysfunction. Management includes inotropic support of the RV with phosphodiesterase inhibitors like milrinone, adrenaline, aggressive management of pulmonary hypertension (inhaled NO, prostacyclins), and systemic blood pressure support [30]. Use of such drugs must be aimed at optimizing blood pressure and cardiac output understanding that ACHD patients are acutely sensitive to changes to SVR and PVR, especially if they have intracardiac shunts.

14.12 Percutaneous Interventions

Percutaneous techniques and interventions may be helpful in certain patients. For one example, percutaneous replacement of the pulmonary valve for severe PR in repaired TOF patients may lead to improved outcomes [10]. Percutaneous closure of shunts like ASDs and VSDs and coiling of AP (aortopulmonary) collaterals are now commonplace [3] and carry a lower morbidity than with surgical interventions [63]. Percutaneous clips to treat severe mitral regurgitation are becoming more popular [64], and while the use of this new technology has not been studied on a wide scale, there are reports of the use of the MitraClip™ in the tricuspid position [65]. Other technologies, such as the Mitralign™, TriCinch™, and even percutaneous tricuspid valve replacements are being tested and studied currently and will provide a wealth of options for interventional cardiologists aiming to treat severe valvular dysfunction in the future [66]. As adults with CHD often have right-sided valvular dysfunction, or even systemic atrioventricular valve regurgitation, the use of these new technologies has the potential to be very appealing; one study has already proven that percutaneous clipping of a systemic atrioventricular but morphologically tricuspid valve is feasible in patients with ccTGA [67].

14.13 Arrhythmias

A specific chapter in this book will be dedicated to adult patients with CHD. In principle, patients with CHD are at high risk for arrhythmias, especially patients with prior surgeries and Fontan patients. In patients with repaired TOF, risk factors for death and sustained VT include RVH [68]. EKG is an essential diagnostic tool, and the use of Adenosine is also helpful for diagnosing arrhythmias. If the patient is unstable, direct current cardioversion ought to be considered, but it is very important that the staff knows if the patient has levocardia or dextrocardia when placing the pads [45]. Furthermore, patients with CHD are likely to require epicardial wires when implanting permanent devices due to complex anatomy or residual shunts [25].

The Pediatric and Congenital Electrophysiology Society (PACES) and Heart Rhythm Society (HRS) statement on management of arrhythmias in 2014 stated that implantable cardioverter defibrillator (ICD) implantation is indicated for secondary prevention of cardiac arrest due to ventricular fibrillation/ventricular tachycardia (VF/VT) or hemodynamically unstable VT after reversible causes have been excluded [69]. They also recommend ICDs for patients with spontaneous sustained VT who have already undergone a cardiac electrophysiology study and ablation. They also recommend ICDs for patients with a systemic LVEF <35%, biventricular physiology, and NYHA (New York Heart Association) class II–III symptoms. The PACES/HRS guidelines have weaker recommendations for implanting ICDs for primary prevention. For patients with tetralogy of Fallot, appropriate secondary prevention guidelines should be used as the incidence of SCD, VT, or appropriate ICD shock is between 6% and 14% [8]. Use of ICD for primary prevention has yet to be shown to be beneficial.

Cardiac resynchronization therapy (or multisite pacing in patients with a single ventricle) may be useful in patients with ACHD, but this therapy has limited evidence demonstrating its benefit in this population at this time. The details of this therapy will be discussed in another chapter. Small retrospective studies have shown a benefit in a heterogeneous population of patients with CHD [70–72]. The recent PACES/HRS guidelines for arrhythmia management in patients with CHD [69] adapt the existing North American and European heart failure and device therapy guidelines to the CHD population. In terms of implanting CRT, the only class I recommendation they have are for the patients with a systemic LV, EF of ≤35%, sinus rhythm, NYHA II–IV, and LBBB with a QRS ≥150 ms. Other patients, including those with systemic RV and single ventricle, have class IIa and IIb indications depending on their ventricular ejection fraction and the width of their QRS complex [69]. Use of CRT (multisite pacing) may be beneficial in patients with single ventricles, but the evidence is limited [8]. Similarly, there are no good studies

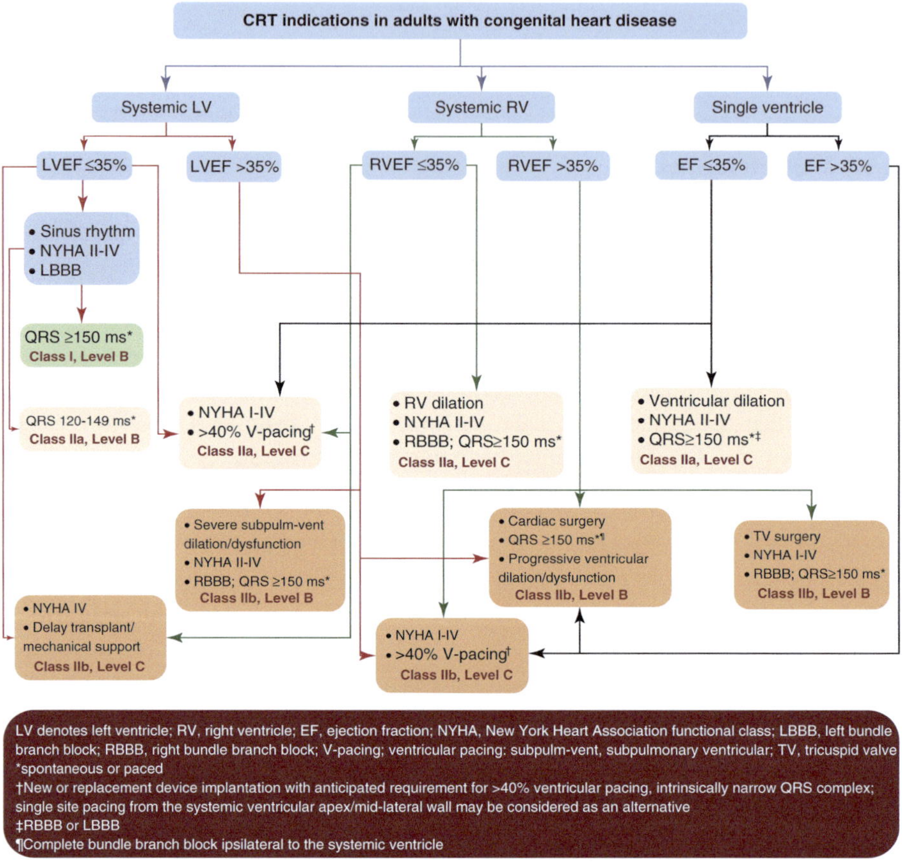

Fig. 14.3 Cited from [69]

for the use of CRT and systemic RV dysfunction and RBBB [8]. Our center has anecdotal success with using CRT in patients with ccTGA; however, patient numbers are small, and further data collection is necessary with this unique population (Fig. 14.3).

Catheter ablation is an accepted procedure in this population, understanding that experience is limited and that repeat procedures for recurrent arrhythmias are common [73]. Maintenance of sinus rhythm is important in most patients with CHD, and class III (amiodarone, dofetilide) are the most accepted agents [73]. If the patient is unstable, then synchronized cardioversion is effective, as long as intra-atrial thrombus is excluded.

If the patient has VT, then cardioversion (synchronized for monomorphic VT, defibrillation for polymorphic or VF) is required. The chronic management of VT/VF involves ICD placement with antiarrhythmic medication and catheter ablation [73].

14.14 Mechanical Support

Mechanical support is a topic discussed in detail in another chapter. The use of mechanical support devices is not common in the current state due to potential barriers, such as pulmonary vascular disease, multiple prior sternotomies, and multiorgan dysfunction. One study showed that while VAD usage is increasing for patients on the heart transplant waitlist for patients with acquired heart disease, the rate of VAD use has not increased for patients with ACHD on the transplant waitlist [74]. Nevertheless, these advanced therapies have been described in ACHD patients [25, 75] and in patients with systemic right ventricles [8].

14.15 Transplantation

A specific chapter in this book is dedicated to transplant. Heart transplantation is not a common outcome for patients with ACHD, but 3% of patients who undergo transplant have CHD. As more and more patients develop end-stage HF with CHD, this will become a more common occurrence. ACHD patients have higher early mortality, but similar long-term survival as those who do not have CHD.ACHD patients have special considerations with regards to transplant. They have sometimes unique and complex anatomy. They are possibly at higher risk due to their previous sternotomies and possible highly sensitized HLA antibodies. They may also have higher incidence of pulmonary hypertension and liver cirrhosis, all of which complicate their pretransplant workup and possibly their organ matching and posttransplant course [76].

References

1. Marelli AJ, Ionescu-Ittu R, Mackie AS, Guo L, Dendukuri N, Kaouache M. Lifetime prevalence of congenital heart disease in the general population from 2000 to 2010. Circulation. 2014;130(9):749–56.
2. Marelli AJ, Mackie AS, Ionescu-Ittu R, Rahme E, Pilote L. Congenital heart disease in the general population: changing prevalence and age distribution. Circulation. 2007;115(2):163–72.
3. Bhatt AB, Foster E, Kuehl K, Alpert J, Brabeck S, Crumb S, et al. Congenital heart disease in the older adult: a scientific statement from the American Heart Association. Circulation. 2015;131:1884–931. https://doi.org/10.1161/CIR.0000000000000204.
4. Opotowsky AR, Siddiqi OK, Webb GD. Trends in hospitalizations for adults with congenital heart disease in the U.S. J Am Coll Cardiol. 2009;54(5):460–7. https://doi.org/10.1016/j.jacc.2009.04.037.
5. Warnes CA, Williams RG, Bashore TM, Child JS, Connolly HM, Dearani JA, et al. ACC/AHA 2008 guidelines for the management of adults with congenital heart disease. J Am Coll Cardiol. 2008;52(23):1890–947. https://doi.org/10.1016/j.jacc.2008.10.001.
6. Baumgartner H, Bonhoeffer P, De Groot NMS, De Haan F, Deanfield JE, Galie N, et al. ESC guidelines for the management of grown-up congenital heart disease (new version 2010). Eur Heart J. 2010;31(23):2915–57.

7. Hunt SA, Abraham WT, Chin MH, Feldman AM, Francis GS, Ganiats TG, et al. 2009 focused update incorporated into the ACC/AHA 2005 guidelines for the diagnosis and management of heart failure in adults. J Am Coll Cardiol. 2009;53(15):e1–90. https://doi.org/10.1161/CIRCULATIONAHA.109.192065.
8. Stout KK, Broberg CS, Book WM, Cecchin F, Chen JM, Dimopoulos K, et al. Chronic heart failure in congenital heart disease: a scientific statement from the American Heart Association. Circulation. 2016;133:770–801.
9. Diller GP, Dimopoulos K, Okonko D, Li W, Babu-Narayan SV, Broberg CS, et al. Exercise intolerance in adult congenital heart disease: comparative severity, correlates, and prognostic implication. Circulation. 2005;112(6):828–35.
10. Wald RM, Marie Valente A, Marelli A. Heart failure in adult congenital heart disease: emerging concepts with a focus on tetralogy of Fallot. Trends Cardiovasc Med. 2015;25(5):422–32. https://doi.org/10.1016/j.tcm.2014.11.011.
11. Moussa NB, Karsenty C, Pontnau F, Malekzadeh-Milani S, Boudjemline Y, Legendre A, et al. Characteristics and outcomes of heart failure-related hospitalization in adults with congenital heart disease. Arch Cardiovasc Dis. 2017;110:1–9. https://doi.org/10.1016/j.acvd.2017.01.008.
12. Alshawabkeh LI, Opotowsky AR. Burden of heart failure in adults with congenital heart disease. Curr Heart Fail Rep. 2016;13(5):247–54. https://doi.org/10.1007/s11897-016-0301-0.
13. Piran S, Veldtman G, Siu S, Webb GD, Liu PP. Heart failure and ventricular dysfunction in patients with single or systemic right ventricles. Circulation. 2002;105(10):1189–94.
14. Khairy P, Ionescu-Ittu R, MacKie AS, Abrahamowicz M, Pilote L, Marelli AJ. Changing mortality in congenital heart disease. J Am Coll Cardiol. 2010;56(14):1149–57. https://doi.org/10.1016/j.jacc.2010.03.085.
15. Raissadati A, Nieminen H, Haukka J, Sairanen H, Jokinen E. Late causes of death after pediatric cardiac surgery: a 60-year population-based study. J Am Coll Cardiol. 2016;68(5):487–98.
16. Dinardo JA. Heart failure associated with adult congenital heart disease. Semin Cardiothorac Vasc Anesth. 2013;17(1):44–54. http://www.ncbi.nlm.nih.gov/pubmed/23264549.
17. Bolger AP, Sharma R, Li W, Leenarts M, Kalra PR, Kemp M, et al. Neurohormonal activation and the chronic heart failure syndrome in adults with congenital heart disease. Circulation. 2002;106(1):92–9.
18. Giannakoulas G, Dimopoulos K, Bolger AP, Tay EL, Inuzuka R, Bedard E, et al. Usefulness of natriuretic peptide levels to predict mortality in adults with congenital heart disease. Am J Cardiol. 2010;105(6):869–73. https://doi.org/10.1016/j.amjcard.2009.11.041.
19. Reardon LC, Williams RJ, Houser LS, Miner PD, Child JS, Aboulhosn JA. Usefulness of serum brain natriuretic peptide to predict adverse events in patients with the eisenmenger syndrome. Am J Cardiol. 2012;110(10):1523–6. https://doi.org/10.1016/j.amjcard.2012.06.061.
20. Lowe BS, Therrien J, Ionescu-Ittu R, Pilote L, Martucci G, Marelli AJ. Diagnosis of pulmonary hypertension in the congenital heart disease adult population: Impact on outcomes. J Am Coll Cardiol. 2011;58(5):538–46. https://doi.org/10.1016/j.jacc.2011.03.033.
21. Fahed AC, Roberts AE, Mital S, Lakdawala NK. Heart failure in congenital heart disease. A confluence of acquired and congenital. Heart Fail Clin. 2014;10(1):219–27.
22. Fahed AC, Gelb BD, Seidman JG, Seidman CE. Genetics of congenital heart disease: the glass half empty. Circ Res. 2013;112(4):707–20.
23. Mcmurray JJV, Adamopoulos S, Anker SD, Auricchio A, Böhm M, Dickstein K, et al. ESC Guidelines for the diagnosis and treatment of acute and chronic heart failure 2012. Eur J Heart Fail. 2012;14(8):803–69.
24. Budts W, Roos-Hesselink J, Rädle-Hurst T, Eicken A, McDonagh TA, Lambrinou E, et al. Treatment of heart failure in adult congenital heart disease: a position paper of the Working Group of Grown-Up Congenital Heart Disease and the Heart Failure Association of the European Society of Cardiology. Eur Heart J. 2016;37(18):1419–27.
25. Ryan TD, Jefferies JL, Wilmot I. Managing heart failure in adults with congenital heart disease. Curr Treat Options Cardiovasc Med. 2015;17(2):376.
26. Babu-Narayan SV, Uebing A, Davlouros PA, Kemp M, Davidson S, Dimopoulos K, et al. Randomised trial of ramipril in repaired tetralogy of Fallot and pulmonary regurgitation: the

APPROPRIATE study (Ace inhibitors for Potential PRevention of the deleterious effects of Pulmonary Regurgitation in Adults with repaired TEtralogy of Fallot). Int J Cardiol. 2012;154(3):299–305. https://doi.org/10.1016/j.ijcard.2010.09.057.

27. Dimopoulos K, Diller GP, Koltsida E, Pijuan-Domenech A, Papadopoulou SA, Babu-Narayan SV, et al. Prevalence, predictors, and prognostic value of renal dysfunction in adults with congenital heart disease. Circulation. 2008;117(18):2320–8. https://doi.org/10.1161/CIRCULATIONAHA.107.734921.
28. Allan CK. Intensive care of the adult patient with congenital heart disease. Prog Cardiovasc Dis. 2011;53(4):274–80. https://doi.org/10.1016/j.pcad.2010.11.002.
29. Giardini A, Balducci A, Specchia S, Gargiulo G, Bonvicini M, Picchio FM. Effect of sildenafil on haemodynamic response to exercise and exercise capacity in Fontan patients. Eur Heart J. 2008;29(13):1681–7.
30. Roy N. Critical care management of the adult patient with congenital heart disease: focus on postoperative management and outcomes. Curr Treat Options Cardiovasc Med. 2015;17(2):1–11.
31. Krieger EV, Valente AM. Heart failure treatment in adults with congenital heart disease: where do we stand in 2014? Heart. 2014;100(17):1329–34.
32. Stefanescu A, Macklin EA, Lin E, Dudzinski DM, Johnson J, Kennedy KF, et al. Usefulness of the Seattle Heart Failure Model to identify adults with congenital heart disease at high risk of poor outcome. Am J Cardiol. 2014;113(5):865–70. http://www.ncbi.nlm.nih.gov/pubmed/24411285.
33. Pignatelli RH, McMahon CJ, Chung T, Vick GW 3rd. Role of echocardiography versus MRI for the diagnosis of congenital heart disease. Curr Opin Cardiol. 2003;18(5):357–65. http://www.ncbi.nlm.nih.gov/pubmed/12960467.
34. Burchill LJ, Huang J, Tretter JT, Khan AM, Crean AM, Veldtman GR, et al. Noninvasive imaging in adult congenital heart disease. Circ Res. 2017;120(6):995–1014. https://doi.org/10.1161/CIRCRESAHA.116.308983.
35. Warnes CA, Bhatt AB, Daniels CJ, Gillam LD, Stout KK. COCATS 4 task force 14: training in the care of adult patients with congenital heart disease. J Am Coll Cardiol. 2015;65(17):1887–98. https://doi.org/10.1016/j.jacc.2015.03.030.
36. Diller GP, Kempny A, Liodakis E, Alonso-Gonzalez R, Inuzuka R, Uebing A, et al. Left ventricular longitudinal function predicts life-threatening ventricular arrhythmia and death in adults with repaired tetralogy of Fallot. Circulation. 2012;125(20):2440–6.
37. Kalogeropoulos AP, Deka A, Border W, Pernetz MA, Georgiopoulou VV, Kiani J, et al. Right ventricular function with standard and speckle-tracking echocardiography and clinical events in adults with D-transposition of the great arteries post atrial switch. J Am Soc Echocardiogr. 2012;25(3):304–12. https://doi.org/10.1016/j.echo.2011.12.003.
38. Cioccari L, Baur H-R, Berger D, Wiegand J, Takala J, Merz TM. Hemodynamic assessment of critically ill patients using a miniaturized transesophageal echocardiography probe. Crit Care. 2013;17(3):R121. http://www.pubmedcentral.nih.gov/articlerender.fcgi?artid=4056104&tool=pmcentrez&rendertype=abstract.
39. Hammoudi N, Hékimian G, Laveau F, Achkar M, Isnard R, Combes A. Three-dimensional transoesophageal echocardiography for cardiac output in critically ill patients: a pilot study of ultrasound versus the thermodilution method. Arch Cardiovasc Dis. 2017;110(1):7–13. http://linkinghub.elsevier.com/retrieve/pii/S1875213616301528.
40. Kilner PJ, Geva T, Kaemmerer H, Trindade PT, Schwitter J, Webb GD. Recommendations for cardiovascular magnetic resonance in adults with congenital heart disease from the respective working groups of the European Society of Cardiology. Eur Heart J. 2010;31(7):794–805.
41. Inuzuka R, Diller GP, Borgia F, Benson L, Tay ELW, Alonso-Gonzalez R, et al. Comprehensive use of cardiopulmonary exercise testing identifies adults with congenital heart disease at increased mortality risk in the medium term. Circulation. 2012;125(2):250–9.
42. Binanay C, et al. Evaluation study of congestive heart failure and pulmonary artery catheterization effectiveness: the ESCAPE trial. JAMA. 2005;294(13):1625–33.

43. Abraham WT, Adamson PB, Bourge RC, Aaron MF, Costanzo MR, Stevenson LW, et al. Wireless pulmonary artery haemodynamic monitoring in chronic heart failure: a randomised controlled trial. Lancet. 2011;377(9766):658–66.
44. Bradley EA, Berman D, Daniels CJ. First implantable hemodynamic monitoring device placement in single ventricle fontan anatomy. Catheter Cardiovasc Interv. 2016;88(2):248–52. https://doi.org/10.1002/ccd.26498.
45. Perry J, Lanzberg M, Franklin W, Webb G, Chang AC. Cardiac intensive care of the adult with congenital heart disease: basic principles in the management of common problems. World J Pediatr Congenit Heart Surg. 2011;2(3):430–44.
46. Dore A, Houde C, Chan KL, Ducharme A, Khairy P, Juneau M, et al. Angiotensin receptor blockade and exercise capacity in adults with systemic right ventricles: a multicenter, randomized, placebo-controlled clinical trial. Circulation. 2005;112(16):2411–6.
47. Doughan ARK, McConnell ME, Book WM. Effect of beta blockers (carvedilol or metoprolol XL) in patients with transposition of great arteries and dysfunction of the systemic right ventricle. Am J Cardiol. 2007;99(5):704–6.
48. Van Der Bom T, Winter MM, Bouma BJ, Groenink M, Vliegen HW, Pieper PG, et al. Effect of valsartan on systemic right ventricular function: a double-blind, randomized, placebo-controlled pilot trial. Circulation. 2013;127(3):322–30.
49. Bouallal R, Godart F, Francart C, Richard A, Foucher-Hossein C, Lions C. Interest of β-blockers in patients with right ventricular systemic dysfunction. Cardiol Young. 2010;20(6):615–9.
50. Dos L, Pujadas S, Estruch M, Mas A, Ferreira-González I, Pijuan A, et al. Eplerenone in systemic right ventricle: double blind randomized clinical trial. the evedes study. Int J Cardiol. 2013;168(6):5167–73. https://doi.org/10.1016/j.ijcard.2013.07.163.
51. Norozi K, Bahlmann J, Raab B, Alpers V, Arnhold JO, Kuehne T, et al. A prospective, randomized, double-blind, placebo controlled trial of beta-blockade in patients who have undergone surgical correction of tetralogy of Fallot. Cardiol Young. 2007;17(4):372–9. http://www.ncbi.nlm.nih.gov/pubmed/17572925.
52. Galiè N, Beghetti M, Gatzoulis MA, Granton J, Berger RMF, Lauer A, et al. Bosentan therapy in patients with Eisenmenger syndrome: a multicenter, double-blind, randomized, placebo-controlled study. Circulation. 2006;114(1):48–54.
53. Shabanian R, Shahbaznejad L, Razaghian A, Kiani A, Rahimzadeh M, Seifirad S, et al. Sildenafil and ventriculo-arterial coupling in fontan-palliated patients: a noninvasive echocardiographic assessment. Pediatr Cardiol. 2013;34(1):129–34.
54. Ringel RE, Peddy SB. Effect of high-dose spironolactone on protein-losing enteropathy in patients with Fontan palliation of complex congenital heart disease. Am J Cardiol. 2003;91(8):1031–2.
55. Mahle WT, Wang A, Quyyumi AA, McConnell ME, Book WM. Impact of spironolactone on endothelial function in patients with single ventricle heart. Congenit Heart Dis. 2009;4(1):12–6.
56. Kouatli AA, Garcia JA, Zellers TM, Weinstein EM, Mahony L. Enalapril does not enhance exercise capacity in patients after Fontan procedure. Circulation. 1997;96(5):1507–12.
57. Ishibashi N, Park I-S, Waragai T, Yoshikawa T, Murakami Y, Mori K, et al. Effect of carvedilol on heart failure in patients with a functionally univentricular heart. Circ J. 2011;75(6):1394–9.
58. Swedberg K, Komajda M, Böhm M, Borer JS, Ford I, Dubost-Brama A, et al. Ivabradine and outcomes in chronic heart failure (SHIFT): a randomised placebo-controlled study. Lancet. 2010;376(9744):875–85.
59. McMurray JJV, Packer M, Desai AS, Gong J, Lefkowitz MP, Rizkala AR, et al. Angiotensin–neprilysin inhibition versus enalapril in heart failure. N Engl J Med. 2014;371(11):993–1004. https://doi.org/10.1056/NEJMoa1409077.
60. Tay ELW, Peset A, Papaphylactou M, Inuzuka R, Alonso-Gonzalez R, Giannakoulas G, et al. Replacement therapy for iron deficiency improves exercise capacity and quality of life in patients with cyanotic congenital heart disease and/or the Eisenmenger syndrome. Int J Cardiol. 2011;151(3):307–12. https://doi.org/10.1016/j.ijcard.2010.05.066.
61. Dimopoulos K, Inuzuka R, Goletto S, Giannakoulas G, Swan L, Wort SJ, et al. Improved survival among patients with Eisenmenger syndrome receiving advanced therapy for pulmonary arterial hypertension. Circulation. 2010;121(1):20–5.

62. Diller GP, Alonso-Gonzalez R, Dimopoulos K, Alvarez-Barredo M, Koo C, Kempny A, et al. Disease targeting therapies in patients with Eisenmenger syndrome: response to treatment and long-term efficiency. Int J Cardiol. 2013;167(3):840–7.
63. Méndez AB, Colchero T, Garcia-Picart J, Vila M, Subirana MT, Sionis A. Unusual case of new-onset heart failure due to cor triatriatum sinister. Eur J Heart Fail. 2013;15(2):237–9.
64. Feldman T, Foster E, Glower DD, Kar S, Rinaldi MJ, Fail PS, et al. Percutaneous repair or surgery for mitral regurgitation. N Engl J Med. 2011;364(15):1395–406. https://doi.org/10.1056/NEJMoa1009355#t=article.
65. Hammerstingl C, Schueler R, Malasa M, Werner N, Nickenig G. Transcatheter treatment of severe tricuspid regurgitation with the MitraClip system. Eur Heart J. 2016;37(10):849–53. https://doi.org/10.1093/eurheartj/ehv710.
66. Taramasso M, Pozzoli A, Guidotti A, Nietlispach F, Inderbitzin DT, Benussi S, et al. Percutaneous tricuspid valve therapies: the new frontier. Eur Heart J. 2017;38:639–47. https://doi.org/10.1093/eurheartj/ehv766.
67. Franzen O, von Samson P, Dodge-Khatami A, Geffert G, Baldus S. Percutaneous edge-to-edge repair of tricuspid regurgitation in congenitally corrected transposition of the great arteries. Congenit Heart Dis. 2011;6(1):57–9. http://www.ncbi.nlm.nih.gov/pubmed/21269414.
68. Valente AM, Gauvreau K, Assenza GE, Babu-Narayan SV, Schreier J, Gatzoulis MA, et al. Contemporary predictors of death and sustained ventricular tachycardia in patients with repaired tetralogy of Fallot enrolled in the INDICATOR cohort. Heart. 2014;100(3):247–53. https://doi.org/10.1136/heartjnl-2013-304958.
69. Khairy P, van Hare GF, Balaji S, Berul CI, Cecchin F, Cohen MI, et al. PACES/HRS expert consensus statement on the recognition and management of arrhythmias in adult congenital heart disease. Can J Cardiol. 2014;30(10):e1–63. https://doi.org/10.1016/j.cjca.2014.09.002.
70. Cecchin F, Frangini PA, Brown DW, Fynn-Thompson F, Alexander ME, Triedman JK, et al. Cardiac resynchronization therapy (and multisite pacing) in pediatrics and congenital heart disease: five years experience in a single institution. J Cardiovasc Electrophysiol. 2009;20(1):58–65.
71. Dubin AM, Janousek J, Rhee E, Strieper MJ, Cecchin F, Law IH, et al. Resynchronization therapy in pediatric and congenital heart disease patients: an international multicenter study. J Am Coll Cardiol. 2005;46(12):2277–83. https://doi.org/10.1016/j.jacc.2005.05.096.
72. Janousek J, Gebauer RA, Abdul-Khaliq H, Turner M, Kornyei L, Grollmuss O, et al. Cardiac resynchronisation therapy in paediatric and congenital heart disease: differential effects in various anatomical and functional substrates. Heart. 2009;95(14):1165–71. http://www.pubmedcentral.nih.gov/articlerender.fcgi?artid=2699215&tool=pmcentrez&rendertype=abstract.
73. Lindsay I, Moore JP. Cardiac arrhythmias in adults with congenital heart disease: scope, specific problems, and management. Curr Treat Options Cardiovasc Med. 2015;17(12):56.
74. Gelow JM, Song HK, Weiss JB, Mudd JO, Broberg CS. Organ allocation in adults with congenital heart disease listed for heart transplant: Impact of ventricular assist devices. J Heart Lung Transplant. 2013;32(11):1059–64. https://doi.org/10.1016/j.healun.2013.06.024.
75. Shah NR, Lam WW, Rodriguez FH, Ermis PR, Simpson L, Frazier OH, et al. Clinical outcomes after ventricular assist device implantation in adults with complex congenital heart disease. J Heart Lung Transplant. 2013;32(6):1–6. http://www.ncbi.nlm.nih.gov/pubmed/23540399.
76. Burchill LJ. Heart transplantation in adult congenital heart disease. Heart. 2016;102(23):1871–7. http://www.ncbi.nlm.nih.gov/pubmed/27836946.

Critical Care Management of the Adult with Eisenmenger Syndrome and Pulmonary Arterial Hypertension Related to Congenital Heart Disease

15

Laura C. Price, Rafael Alonso-Gonzalez, David Alexander, and Konstantinos Dimopoulos

15.1 Introduction

Major advances in the surgical and medical management of congenital heart disease (CHD) in recent decades have meant that an increasing number of children born with CHD survive to adulthood. Lack of early diagnosis and repair in the past resulted in a substantial number of patients, especially those with post-tricuspid shunts (VSD, PDA, ASVD, aorto-pulmonary window), developing pulmonary vascular disease [1]. Even with modern screening and management of CHD, a substantial number of patients present with PAH earlier or later in life. Indeed, pulmonary arterial hypertension (PAH) related to congenital heart disease is still one the most common types of PAH [2].

PAH-CHD shares significant similarities in terms of lung pathology to other types of PAH. Indeed, the Heath and Edwards classification of pulmonary vascular disease (PVD) was described predominantly in PAH-CHD patients, but modified versions of this classification are used to assess and grade all types of PAH [3]. PAH-CHD, however, carries distinct features in terms of pathophysiology and prognosis, and its management requires significant expertise, both in PAH and ACHD [4]. PAH-CHD encompasses a wide spectrum of conditions, broadly classified into four categories (see below), but not all PH associated with CHD is PAH (Table 15.1) [5].

L. C. Price · R. Alonso-Gonzalez · D. Alexander · K. Dimopoulos (✉)
Adult Congenital Heart Centre and National Centre for Pulmonary Hypertension, National Heart and Lung Institute, Imperial College School of Medicine, London, UK

Department of Anaesthetics, Royal Brompton and Harefield NHS Foundation Trust, Royal Brompton Hospital, London, UK
e-mail: Laura.Price@rbht.nhs.uk; D.Alexander@rbht.nhs.uk

E. da Cruz et al. (eds.), *Intensive Care of the Adult with Congenital Heart Disease*, Congenital Heart Disease in Adolescents and Adults,
https://doi.org/10.1007/978-3-319-94171-4_15

Table 15.1 [1, 5]

Types of PAH related to CHD (group 1 of the PH classification)	
1. Eisenmenger syndrome	Large intra- and extra-cardiac defects causing systemic-to-pulmonary shunting, which over time causes severe elevation of pulmonary vascular resistance (PVR) and shunt reversal (pulmonary-to-systemic/bidirectional). Cyanosis, secondary erythrocytosis, and multiple organ involvement are commonly present
2. PAH associated with prevalent systemic-to-pulmonary shunts	Includes moderate to large defects. PVR is mild to moderately increased, with systemic-to-pulmonary shunting and no cyanosis. The defect can be repairable (operable), or not
3. PAH with small/coincidental defects	Marked elevation in PVR in the presence of small cardiac defects, typically a ventricular septal defects <1 cm or atrial septal defect <2 cm in diameter assessed by echo), which are not large enough to account for the development of the elevated PVR. The clinical picture is similar to idiopathic PAH and repair of the defect is contraindicated.
4. PAH after defect correction	Congenital heart disease is repaired, but PAH either persists immediately after correction or develops months or years after repair, in the absence of significant residual lesions
Other types of PH related to CHD	
– Segmental PH	PH affecting parts but not the entire pulmonary vascular tree. Typically encountered in tetralogy of fallot with complex pulmonary atresia. *Included in group 5 of the PH classification*
– Raised PVR in Fontan-type palliation	A low PVR is essential for Fontan-type circulations lacking a subpulmonary ventricle. Any rise in PVR can have a detrimental effect on cardiac output and promote congestion. *Not included in the PH classification*
– Postcapillary PH	Congenital heart disease with left ventricular dysfunction, left-sided valve disease, inflow or outflow tract obstruction, or pulmonary vein stenosis. *Included in group 2 of the PH classification*
– PH in patients with peripheral pulmonary stenoses	Peripheral pulmonary stenoses (PS) can lead to a rise in pressure in the main pulmonary artery, which fulfills the hemodynamic definition of PH. Moreover, peripheral PS may increase flow to non-stenosed segments leading to the development of pulmonary vascular disease, similar to what is observed in chronic thromboembolic PH. *Included in group 4 of the PH classification*

PH significantly affects the prognosis of patients with CHD and is a major risk factor for individuals who require critical care due to deterioration of their underlying disease or around essential surgery or other intervention [6, 7]. A multidisciplinary approach, with significant expertise in CHD, PH, anesthetics, and critical care, is essential in order to optimize the otherwise adverse outcome of PAH-CHD patients who are admitted in intensive care or a high dependency unit.

In this chapter, we provide an overview of the critical care and anesthetic management of adults with PH and in particular PAH-CHD.

15.2 Classification, Pathophysiology, Presentation, and Management of PAH-CHD

15.2.1 Classification

PAH is a common occurrence in patients born with large post-tricuspid shunts (e.g., ventricular septal defects, VSD) who do not undergo reparative surgery in a timely fashion [8]. Large left-to-right shunts cause significant shear stress to the pulmonary vasculature through pressure and volume load and lead to the development of PVD. This, in turn, causes a rise in pulmonary vascular resistance (PVR) and, when PVR reaches near-systemic levels, it causes shunt reversal and cyanosis (Eisenmenger syndrome) [9].

PAH-CHD belongs to group 1 of the international PH classification [5]. It is a heterogeneous group of conditions, with significant variability relating to the severity of the PVD, location and direction of the shunt, and underlying cardiovascular anatomy. The international pulmonary hypertension (PH) guidelines define four major PAH-CHD groups (Table 15.1) [1, 5]. Additional groups of patients with PH associated with CHD include those with postcapillary PH (group 2 of the PH classification), PH associated with pulmonary artery stenosis (group 4), and "segmental PH" affecting some but not all segments of the pulmonary vascular bed, classified within group 5 (multifactorial or unknown mechanisms) [10, 11]. Finally, patients with a Fontan-type circulation often have a raised PVR with "normal" pulmonary arterial pressure due to reduced pulmonary blood flow and the absence of a subpulmonary ventricle; pulmonary vascular disease in Fontan patients is still lacking precise classification in the guidelines [12, 13].

This chapter will focus mainly on PAH-CHD.

15.2.2 Pathology and Pathophysiology

Heath and Edwards studied 67 cases of CHD and 2 cases of idiopathic PH and were the first to provide a detailed histological classification of PVD, based on the type of intimal reaction (none/cellular/fibrous and fibroelastic/plexiform lesion) and the state of the media or arteries and arterioles (hypertrophied/some generalized dilatation/local "dilatation lesions"/pulmonary hemosiderosis/necrotizing arteritis) [3]. Modified versions of the Heath and Edwards classification are still in use to describe and grade PVD, even though lung biopsy is rarely used nowadays to assess the severity of PVD and whether a congenital heart defect can be repaired in patients with borderline hemodynamics; biopsy should be avoided in all patients with significant PH as it carries significant risks [14].

Heath and Edwards described six grades of PVD: grade 4 or above was deemed severe irreversible PVD, even though these and other authors have recognized that PVD is often not homogeneously distributed throughout the lungs, and hence

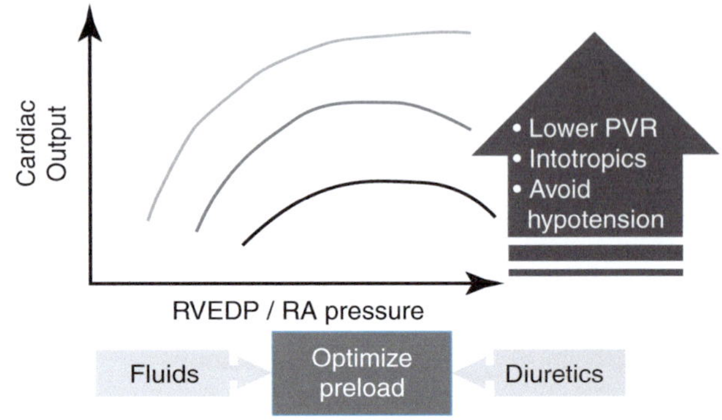

Fig. 15.1 A narrow window for optimizing cardiac output in pulmonary hypertension: the Frank Starling curve [14]. *RVEDP* right ventricular end-diastolic pressure, *RA* right atrium, *PVR* pulmonary vascular resistance

histological findings from limited areas of the lung should be interpreted with caution.

In terms of pathophysiology, the effects of a progressive rise in PVR greatly depend on the ability of the RV to adapt to the increase in afterload. For small increases in afterload, the RV is expected to undergo "homeometric" adaptation, that is, adapt through hypertrophy and an increase in contractility, thus, maintaining cardiac output [14, 15]. However, a greater chronic rise in PVR typically leads to "heterometric" (mal-) adaptation of the RV, with progressive dilatation and loss in contractility, which eventually leads to a drop in cardiac output and right-sided congestive heart failure. Myocardial ischemia, tricuspid regurgitation, and adverse interaction with the left ventricle also contribute to the progressive deterioration, which can be exacerbated by arrhythmias that become more frequent as the right atrium enlarges. This establishes a vicious cycle, which can only be broken by attempts to lower the afterload to the RV, for example, by using PAH therapies. In patients who are in overt heart failure, inotropes for the RV and diuretics to achieve an optimal RV preload are also important, with close monitoring of RA pressure (Fig. 15.1). We discuss the pathophysiology of RV failure further later in this chapter.

In patients with PAH-CHD, especially Eisenmenger syndrome, additional morbidity relates to the congenital heart defect and chronic cyanosis (Fig. 15.2) [6, 16–18]. In fact, Eisenmenger syndrome is a multiorgan disease and special attention should be given to underlying, often occult multiorgan failure, such as renal and hepatic dysfunction, which often become manifest during episodes of acute decompensation and complicate management [19–23].

15.2.3 Clinical Presentation

PAH-CHD is associated with significant morbidity and mortality (Fig. 15.1), which is the combined effect of the CHD, PAH, and chronic cyanosis [1, 24]. Exercise intolerance and reduced cardiovascular reserve are common and not only impact on quality of life but also affect the outcome of any intervention that poses a demand to

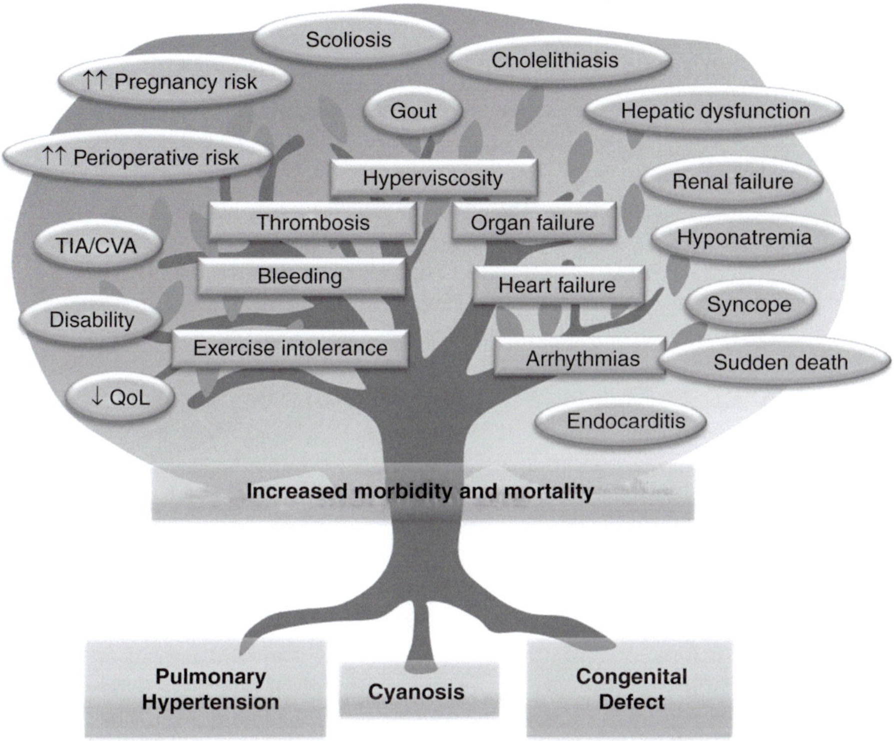

Fig. 15.2 Eisenmenger syndrome: a systemic condition [1]

the cardiovascular system [25, 26]. Studies using cardiopulmonary exercise testing have shown that PAH-CHD patients, and especially patients with Eisenmenger syndrome, have the lowest peak oxygen consumption compared to all other CHD groups; they also demonstrate highly deranged ventilatory response to exercise relating to the reduced pulmonary blood flow and right-to-left shunting [27, 28]. Additional factors impacting on their cardiorespiratory reserve include associated cardiovascular lesions (valve disease, ventricular morphology and function, etc.), restrictive lung defects relating to skeletal abnormalities, previous surgery or significant cardiomegaly, detraining and obesity (e.g., in patients with Down syndrome), arrhythmias, etc. [29–31].

The hematologic effects of cyanotic CHD are well described and are multiple. Erythrocytosis occurs as a response to chronic hypoxia and is considered a compensatory mechanism aimed at increasing the blood's oxygen-carrying capacity and peripheral oxygen delivery [1, 32, 33]. Iron deficiency, which can occur in up to a third of patients, can blunt this compensatory mechanism and adversely affect exercise capacity and tissue oxygenation. Routine venesections have nowadays been abandoned, as severe hyperviscosity symptoms are rare and routine phlebotomy results in chronic and possibly severe iron deficiency, which has been associated with cerebrovascular events and negatively impacts on exercise capacity [34]. Other hematologic effects of cyanotic CHD include a predisposition to thrombosis (e.g., pulmonary artery thrombosis and systemic emboli) but also bleeding, spontaneous or perioperative [17, 35]. This complicates decisions relating to anticoagulation and increases the risk of any invasive procedure.

Heart failure is common in PAH-CHD, which is typically a multiorgan condition, affecting all major organs (e.g., heart, kidneys, liver, gut, brain). Peripheral congestion and ascites is typically the mode of presentation of congestive heart failure in PAH-CHD, which can be exacerbated by arrhythmia or infections (most often lower respiratory tract infections). Endocarditis should always be suspected in patients with signs of sepsis, while a cerebral abscess should be excluded in patients with neurological symptoms. Cholelithiasis is also common in Eisenmenger patients due to the increased red cell count and presents a management dilemma. Indeed, all major surgery should be avoided, whenever possible, in view of the high risk of general anesthesia in this condition and the potential complications related to bleeding and difficult pain management.

15.2.4 General Management Principles and Therapies for Patients with PAH-CHD and Eisenmenger Syndrome

Avoidance of pitfalls and outdated practices, with regular specialist follow-up and use of PAH therapies, is the basis of the management of PAH-CHD. These principles also apply to patients admitted to critical care, who benefit significantly by specialist multidisciplinary care and the use of PAH therapies, oral and parenteral. General management principles include the treatment of congestive heart failure with diuretics and prompt rhythm control (or rate control if prompt cardioversion is too high risk) and reversal of arrhythmias. Yearly flu jabs and the pneumococcal vaccine are strongly recommended, avoiding or promptly treating chest infections that can cause decompensation or precipitate hemoptysis. Good dental and skin hygiene are important, practicing endocarditis prophylaxis for dental procedures in cyanotic patients and those with residual defects in proximity to prosthetic material, prosthetic valves, or prior endocarditis [36]. Pregnancy should be avoided in all PAH patients, as should be any general anesthesia or sedation that is not "essential" [37, 38]. Venesections to "normalize" hematocrit levels are to be avoided unless severe hyperviscosity symptoms are present in the absence of dehydration [1]. Iron deficiency should be diagnosed and treated when appropriate.

PAH therapies currently include medications that work on each of the three pathways responsible for pulmonary vasoconstriction and proliferation: the endothelin pathway, nitric oxide pathway, and prostacyclin pathway. The strongest available evidence in PAH-CHD to date is for Eisenmenger patients using the endothelin receptor antagonist bosentan. The BREATHE-5 study demonstrated bosentan to be safe and resulted in a drop in PVR and an increase in exercise capacity, measured as distance achieved on the 6 min walk test [39–41]. Data are also available for PDE-5 inhibitors in Eisenmenger syndrome (tadalafil and sildenafil) [42–44]. Limited information is available on prostanoids, for example, inhaled iloprost and intravenous epoprostenol, which are, however, the drugs of choice together with inhaled nitric oxide and intravenous sildenafil in intensive care [45–47].

PAH-CHD patients with repaired defects have been included in large trials of PAH therapies together with idiopathic PAH [48, 49]. Extrapolating from the results of these studies, it is generally felt that such patients should be offered PAH therapies, especially as their physiology resembles that of idiopathic PAH. Most experts will also offer PAH therapies to PAH-CHD patients with small (coexistent) cardiac defects (group 3, Table 15.1), as the PAH is felt to be more likely due to intrinsic predisposition of the pulmonary vascular tree towards PVD (similar in pathophysiology to idiopathic PAH) rather than the defect itself.

15.3 Anesthesia and Sedation in PAH-CHD and Eisenmenger Syndrome

15.3.1 Pathophysiology of RV Failure in Patients with PAH

In patients with PAH, including PAH-CHD, an imbalance of endogenous pulmonary vasodilators (nitric oxide (NO), prostaglandin I2, prostacyclin (PG-I2)) and vasoconstrictors such as endothelin-1 and serotonin contributes to pulmonary vasoconstriction, vascular cell proliferation, and thrombus formation [50]. The resulting vessel remodeling increases pulmonary vascular resistance (PVR), leading to RV remodeling and hypertrophy. Patients with PAH can tolerate a raised PVR with a balanced adaptation of RV function for a certain time (homeometric adaptation of the RV) and for many years in some CHD patients, but ultimately RV failure develops (heterometric adaptation), characterized by dilatation of right-sided heart chambers and tricuspid regurgitation (TR). The dilated RV causes deviation of the interventricular septum and compression of the left ventricle (interventricular dependence) reducing systemic ventricular function [51, 52]. Coronary perfusion of the RV, present under normal circumstances during systole and diastole, occurs only in diastole because RV systolic pressure is at systemic levels. In addition, coronary flow during diastole is reduced, because the elevated RV diastolic pressure (due to RV failure) reduces the coronary perfusion gradient and diastole (when myocardial perfusion mainly occurs in hypertrophied pressure-overloaded RVs) is shortened, especially when patients become tachycardic. If untreated, an ongoing downward spiral of failing biventricular function further worsens coronary blood flow and may cause tricuspid regurgitation and arrhythmias of increasing severity, ultimately leading to cardiovascular collapse and death [53].

Pulmonary vascular remodeling reduces the vessel capacitance (i.e., compliance), thereby limiting the unique ability of the pulmonary vascular tree to dilate and "recruit" vasculature when required (e.g., on efforts) in order to maintain a low pulmonary pressure, which is essential to protect the fragile alveolar-capillary barrier and allows cardiac output to increase [54]. Under normal circumstances, vascular recruitment allows increases in cardiac output, which may occur during sympathetic stimulation (e.g., exercise, painful stimuli, laryngoscopy, surgical stress) and increased blood volume (e.g., pregnancy), without increasing RV afterload. In patients with PH, impaired vascular capacitance results in a potentially marked increase in RV afterload.

Clinical presentation of RV failure in PH patients may range from the chronic effects of elevated systemic venous pressure (e.g., peripheral edema, hepatic congestion, ascites) to the more dramatic syndrome of acute RV failure (Fig. 15.1). When not anticipated, this may be a difficult clinical diagnosis to make and challenging to treat. Two concepts are prominent in this context. A "pulmonary hypertensive crisis" describes the syndrome of a hyperacute rise in systolic pulmonary pressure (>50% of systemic pressure) due to any cause [55]. "Acute cor pulmonale" (or, "acute right heart syndrome") describes acute RV failure in the setting of acutely elevated afterload, for example, due to acute pulmonary embolism, acute lung injury, or the effects of positive-pressure ventilation [56].

Acute RV failure may be precipitated by several factors in PH patients in the ICU and perioperative setting (Table 15.2). For example, a critically reduced systemic blood pressure related to systemic vasodilatation secondary to sepsis or intravenous induction of anesthesia may reduce coronary perfusion pressure, inducing RV ischemia, especially if compounded by preload inadequacy

Table 15.2 Potential impact of perioperative and ICU factors on pulmonary vascular/RV function

Anesthetic factors	Surgical factors
Laryngoscopy, extubation	Surgical stress and pain
Sympathetic stimulation	Sympathetic stimulation
Tachycardia	Tachycardia
Hypotension	Surgery mechanics
General versus regional anesthesia	One-lung ventilation
Positive-pressure ventilation	Positioning (Trendelenburg)
High plateau pressure	Pneumoperitoneum
High pCO_2	Hypoxia (HPV), acidosis
Adverse drug effects (see legend)	Cytokine release
Volume overload (fluids)	Endothelial dysfunction (and due to CPB)
	Fluid shifts (pregnancy++)
	Early/late hypotension
Intraoperative hypoxemia	Hemorrhage
Vasopressor requirements	Sepsis

Many factors may precipitate a PH crisis (1) and/or (2) worsen RV function directly. Factors increasing PVR include sympathetic stimuli such as pain and airway instrumentation, endothelial activation (cytokine and endothelin-1 release), effects of hypoxia, hypercapnic acidosis, and positive-pressure ventilation. Anesthetic drugs that may increase PVR include ketamine (causes tachycardia and very minor increases in mPAP) and some of the inhalational agents including desflurane. Inhaled nitrous oxide (N_2O) impairs endothelial function and its prolonged use is associated with adverse cardiovascular outcomes. All intravenous anesthetic induction agents depress myocardial function and reduce SVR to varying degrees. Also protamine and prostaglandin F2alpha increase PVR.

PVR pulmonary vascular resistance, *HPV* hypoxic pulmonary vasoconstriction, CO_2 carbon dioxide, *CPB* cardiopulmonary bypass

(e.g., hypovolemia) or excess (e.g., excessive intravenous fluids). When combined with an increased PVR (e.g., sympathetic stimulation from airway instrumentation or an episode of alveolar hypoxia), a PH crisis may result, with rapidly progressive RV ischemia and failure [57]. This may be compounded by other factors such as dysrhythmias.

Bradycardia can also impair cardiac output and RV coronary perfusion, as the stroke volume in PH is relatively fixed, and the cardiac output (i.e., stroke volume × heart rate) is critically dependent on an adequate heart rate. In addition, the negative inotropic effect of many anesthetic agents (Table 15.2) or increased PVR due to high ventilator pressures can contribute to a drop in cardiac output [58]. Abdominal insufflation with carbon dioxide during laparoscopic surgery may cause acute hypercapnic acidosis, resulting in increased PVR and heart rate, while abdominal distension may lower RV preload [59]. It is also likely that endothelial function may be modulated, directly or indirectly by the release of vasoactive substances induced by inflammation during or after surgery, notably following cardiopulmonary bypass [60].

15.3.2 PH Associated with Cardiothoracic Surgery

Severe RV failure in the setting of cardiothoracic surgery (all subtypes) is associated with an in-hospital mortality of 44–86%, especially with certain procedures, such as repair of congenital heart disease (e.g., Ebstein repair or severe pulmonary regurgitation in patients with severely impaired RV), heart transplantation surgery, valve replacement surgery (mitral more than aortic), and left ventricular assist device insertion (RV failure is a contraindication for LVAD) [61]. In addition, single-lung ventilation, as may be required in thoracic surgery, results in a temporary increase in PVR due to lung compression and increased pulmonary blood flow in the inflated lung. Lung resection is also associated with a loss of lung vessel cross-sectional area. Both of these phenomena may result in PH crises in patients with pre-existing PH [62].

Perioperative PH in the setting of cardiothoracic surgery occurs in two contexts: use of cardiopulmonary bypass (CPB) and as a consequence of lung resection. CPB induces endothelial dysfunction and inflammation, resulting in loss of NO production [63]. Moreover, patients undergoing CPB who receive reversal of heparin with protamine can develop precipitous elevations in PVR due to thromboxane A2 release by circulating protamine-heparin complexes [64].

In adults, the presence of PH is an independent risk factor for mortality around cardiac surgery [65–67]. For example, in mitral valve surgery, preoperative PH is an independent risk factor for perioperative RV failure; therefore, patients are likely to benefit from earlier surgery, before PH occurs [67]. RV failure may also occur in up to 39% of patients requiring left ventricular assist device (LVAD) support [68].

Heart transplantation can be particularly challenging because of a potential mismatch between the PVR in the recipient's lungs and the ability of the donor heart to cope with the recipient's PVR. There are, indeed, strict criteria for deciding which patients will benefit from heart versus heart-lung transplantation. However, even patients deemed suitable for heart transplantation may present with a mild chronic rise in pulmonary pressures, or may develop PH as a result of the CPB on the vascular endothelium. The previously healthy donor RV, which had functioned at low pressures (with a low PVR), now has two challenges. First, the pressures required to perfuse the recipient's lungs are greater than can readily be generated; second, the heart is recovering from ischemic storage (between organ retrieval and implantation); and, thus, the RV is especially compromised. While this situation is not a PH crisis, the RV may fail as it cannot generate high enough pressures (RV afterload mismatch).

Children undergoing surgery for congenital heart disease can be susceptible to PH crises, which may be worsened following surgery and CPB and is treated using inhaled NO [69]. However, with advances in prenatal and neonatal screening, very few children develop pulmonary vascular disease (and PH crises perioperatively) as a result of CHD in developed countries, as congenital lesions are corrected earlier. Indeed, while PH complicated the postoperative care of 16% of patients in a cohort prior to 1994, in a more recent series this occurred in only 2% of children [55, 70]. However, PH following cardiac surgery in children remains an important cause of prolonged intensive care unit (ICU) stay [71].

15.4 Diagnostic Procedures in Patients with PAH-CHD

Diagnostic procedures such as flexible bronchoscopy (FB) and lung biopsy may be indicated in PH patients, albeit very rarely. In general, these should be avoided if at all possible due to the risk of bronchoscopy-associated bleeding, hypoxia and hemodynamic instability, as well as the risks of sedation, including hypoxia and hypercapnic acidosis (due to hypoventilation and partial airway obstruction) on PVR. Suctioning during FB may increase PCWP [72]. PH increases complications following open lung biopsy [73]. Video-assisted thoracoscopic (VATS) lung biopsy, although less invasive, requires one-lung ventilation (OLV), and PH remains an independent risk factor for postoperative complications including death [74].

Right heart catheterization (RHC) in adults with PH (under local anesthesia) is associated with a complication rate of 1%, mostly relating to venous access, arrhythmias, and hypotensive episodes. The overall mortality is 0.055% [75]. In children or adults with learning difficulties requiring general anesthesia, the risk is appreciably higher. For example, in one report of RHC performed under general anesthesia in 70 children with PH (including 23 with PAH), 6% suffered major complications requiring cardiac massage (including 2 dysrhythmias from catheter insertion), resulting in 1 death; although the sample size was small, all patients with major complications had severe PH on pre-catheterization echocardiography [76]. In this context, what might be considered a relatively minor procedure in non-PH patients, may be catastrophic in those with PH, especially when general anesthesia is used.

15.5 Non-cardiac Surgery in Patients with PAH-CHD

Patients with CHD, and especially those with associated PAH, are at increased risk of complications around non-cardiac surgery. The patients at highest risk are infants with a functional single ventricle and patients with suprasystemic PH, left ventricular outflow tract obstruction [77, 78]. Adverse events and perioperative death in CHD patients are frequently related to intraoperative anesthetic care [51]. Studies of non-cardiac surgery in patients with PAH (including PAH-CHD) for procedures including abdominal, gynecological, orthopedic, electrophysiological studies and dental procedures, can be categorized according to their emergency or elective nature and according to operative risk: (1) "low-risk" or "minor" surgery includes endoscopic and superficial procedures; (2) "intermediate-risk" and (3) "high-risk" or "major" surgery includes procedures associated with major aortic/peripheral vascular surgery, laparotomy, and major orthopedic surgery (Table 15.3). Overall 28-day mortality ranges between 7% and 18% and morbidity 14% and 42%, mostly due to RV failure, although other events including renal failure, sepsis, and pneumonia may occur. Certain patient and procedural factors are associated with worse outcomes and are useful when considering the associated mortality risk in PAH-CHD patients undergoing elective surgery (Table 15.3). Emergency surgery carries a prohibitive mortality risk, likely to exceed 50% in some reports, although published numbers are small.

Table 15.3 Risk assessment for invasive procedures in patients with PAH undergoing non-cardiac surgery

Patient factors
NYHA > II
Low 6MWD
High preoperative PVR
Low pulmonary vasoreactivity (cardiothoracic/transplant)
RV dysfunction (echo)
Underlying coronary artery disease
Surgical factors
Emergency surgery
Major surgery
Long operative time >3 h
Laparoscopic surgery (insufflation of carbon dioxide (acidosis), increased intra-abdominal pressure)
Joint replacement surgery (risk of methylmethacrylate embolism)
Head and neck surgery (SVC obstruction)

These patient and surgical factors should be considered, ideally in a formal multidisciplinary meeting setting, to make an assessment of perioperative mortality prior to proceeding with elective surgery. These discussions should involve an experienced PH anesthetist as well as the ACHD/PH clinical teams in attendance

NYHA New York Heart Association, *6MWD* 6-minute walk distance, *PVR* pulmonary vascular resistance, *ACHD* adult congenital heart disease, *PH* pulmonary hypertension

In adults with CHD undergoing non-cardiac surgery, hypotension and desaturation is common following intravenous induction of anesthesia. For example, a report of the 20-year experience of non-cardiac surgery in 33 patients with ES and right-to-left intracardiac shunts in a US center showed that hypotension occurred in 26% of cases and oxygen desaturation in 17% of cases and was most marked in ES patients. Inhalational anesthetic induction resulted in even more marked hypotension than intravenous induction where hypotension was reduced with co-administration of a vasopressor [52]. The planned use of preemptive vasopressor during induction of anesthesia is therefore a key message and remains true in all PAH scenarios with the risk of incipient RV decompensation.

15.5.1 Pregnancy: Cesarean Delivery and PAH-CHD

Pregnancy is extremely high risk for patients with PAH, with several retrospective series in patients with both CHD and non-CHD PAH that are somewhat helpful in understanding the risks. With increasing oxygen demands and a rise in blood volume that occurs from the second trimester onwards, as well as a potential increase in PVR as a result of the pregnancy itself, the already overloaded RV fails to cope. The time immediately following delivery is particularly dangerous in PH, as massive fluid shifts occur after uterine contraction during the third stage of labor, with up to 500ml placental auto-transfusion of maternal blood volume that can precipitate RV failure. Large retrospective series prior to 1998 document obstetric mortality in the region of 30–50%, and more recently as high as 25% [37, 80]. However, more recent studies suggest lower mortality. In a multicenter prospective registry of 26 pregnancies over 3 years, 16 (62%) pregnancies were successful, that is, uncomplicated delivery with healthy babies; 3 (12%) mothers died, and 1 (4%) developed right heart failure requiring urgent heart-lung transplantation [81]. Outcomes were better in women with milder, well-controlled PAH (PVR 6.3 ± 4 Wood units), and in those with responsiveness to calcium channel blockade. In contrast, the women who died or required transplantation had poorly controlled PAH (PVR >21 Wood units) [81]. In an older study of mothers with mainly PAH (NYHA I–III prior to pregnancy), overall mortality was 36%, and cesarean section was associated with a 22% mortality [82]. More recently, Kiely et al. reported on the early use of inhaled iloprost, elective admission in the second trimester, and planned cesarean section (CS) delivery under epidural or combined low-dose spinal and epidural anesthesia (CSE) with good outcomes [83, 84]. Other centers, including the Brompton series, report similar outcomes in 9 women undergoing 12 pregnancies from 1995 to 2010, with 2 maternal deaths (1 related to preeclampsia and 1 to arrhythmia) and no perinatal deaths, with most cases undergoing CS delivery under general anesthesia [85]. In our practice, in this high-risk patient group, we perform elective cesarean delivery at 32–34 weeks using regional or general anesthesia, with the choice of hemodynamic monitoring and anesthetic technique depending on local expertise and experience, with basic hemodynamic monitoring in place (arterial line and invasive central venous pressure monitoring, see below) as a baseline. In other centers, delivery is induced at 32–34 weeks, without cesarean section. Pulmonary artery catheterization is rarely used in practice. Intraoperative transesophageal echocardiography (TEE) to guide beat-to-beat RV function under general anesthesia might be more suited to a cardiac center. Great care is needed with fluid infusions, avoiding excessive blood loss and providing critical monitoring of the third stage of labor, ideally for up to 72 h in a critical care setting. Large bolus dosing of oxytocin (which may cause tachycardia and hypotension and might cause transient increase in PVR) should be avoided, and preemptive use of absorbable B-lynch uterine compression sutures should be considered to minimize the risk of postpartum hemorrhage, which appears to be more common in patients with CHD [86].

15.6 Invasive and Noninvasive Monitoring

The choice of invasive pressure and/or of RV function monitoring is a balance between preference, familiarity, and availability. At a minimum, CVP monitoring and intra-arterial monitoring are recommended, as the onset of RV failure will be detected as a rising right atrial pressure in the setting of systemic hypotension. It could be argued, however, that clinicians should not wait for the onset of RV failure but monitor pulmonary artery pressure and PVR using a pulmonary arterial catheter; monitoring of PCWP will also help differentiate between a pre- or postcapillary cause of acute PH crisis. Measurements of pulmonary arterial pressure alone are unreliable as pressures may be deceiving in the context of a falling cardiac output. In addition, insertion of a PA catheter is not without risk, and development of an intractable arrhythmia during insertion can have devastating effects. Noninvasive monitors, such as PICCO and LIDCO, may be useful to monitor CO postoperatively.

Intraoperative transesophageal echocardiography can be extremely useful for continuously assessing RV function and surrogates of PVR (e.g., pulmonary acceleration time) but requires adequate views and an experienced second operator: it is difficult to monitor the patient, administer anesthesia, and continuously monitor the RV on echocardiography. This approach also requires a full general anesthetic and is not suited for women receiving spinal anesthesia.

On balance, each center with a PH, CHD, and pregnancy and heart disease service should develop and audit its favored approach, depending on local skills and experience. There are currently no direct head-to-head comparison studies on the optimal means of perioperative monitoring.

15.7 Anesthetic Techniques

The choice between general and regional anesthesia is important to consider. General anesthesia (GA) involves administration of gaseous or intravenous drugs to induce central neurological depression and frequently involves endotracheal intubation and positive-pressure ventilation. It might also be associated with an increased

Table 15.4 Key differences between general and regional anesthesia

	Regional anesthesia		General anesthesia
	Spinal (single dose)[a]	Epidural (*continuous*)	General anesthesia
Onset	Rapid	Gradual	Titrated[b]
Impact on SVR	+++	Onset, dose	Onset, dose
Airway manipulation	–	–	++
Ventilation	Spontaneous	Spontaneous	Usually PPV[c]
Anticoagulation	Spinal hemorrhage	Spinal hemorrhage	No risk

[a]Continuous spinal may bridge the effects between single-dose spinal and continuous epidural
[b]A rapid sequence induction is not titrated, but if this is not indicated, GA can be induced gradually
[c]*PPV* positive-pressure ventilation

risk of hemorrhage, notably postpartum [86]. Regional anesthesia consists of neuraxial anesthesia (spinal, epidural, and combined spinal-epidural (CSE)) where drugs are administered in close proximity to the spinal cord and nerve roots and peripheral nerve blocks, for example, brachial plexus block for upper limb surgery. The comparative effects of regional and general anesthesia are outlined in Table 15.4. Both GA and neuraxial blocks have potential adverse pulmonary vascular and RV effects, but it is probably less the case in carefully titrated continuous epidural anesthesia. In addition, airway instrumentation may increase PVR and heart rate via sympathetic stimulation, and positive pressure may reduce RV preload. A marked drop in systemic vascular resistance (SVR) following a single dose of spinal anesthesia may cause systemic hypotension, critically lower RV coronary perfusion, and compromise RV function [57]. In addition, a lowering of the SVR may worsen right-to-left shunting in patients with Eisenmenger syndrome. Acute reductions in SVR are less likely with "low-dose" spinal or CSE techniques.

In a meta-analysis of almost 10,000 general patients without PH, the use of neuraxial blockade reduced postoperative all-cause mortality and morbidity compared to GA, although this may simply relate to avoidance of GA and its inherent risks to PH patients (sympathetic stimulation related to laryngoscopy, airway instrumentation, positive peak airway pressure, potent systemic vasodilators and negative inotropic drugs, etc (Table 15.3)). This is also supported by some PH clinical studies [37, 87]. Consensus among most anesthetists is, therefore, that regional anesthesia is usually preferable to general anesthesia in PH, when surgery permits, but this will also depend on local expertise.

15.7.1 Conduct of Anesthesia

The choice of anesthetic drugs used in patients with PAH is not as important as the manner in which they are used. The overall dose and speed of injection are the most significant factors that impact on their physiological effects. Etomidate is regarded as the drug of choice for the induction of these patients, but usually requires supplementation with an opioid (e.g., fentanyl) to blunt the hypertensive response to intubation. Propofol is an excellent and relatively safe induction agent, but may have significant effects on the SVR as a consequence of vasodilatation, which must be treated aggressively. Ketamine has been reported to worsen the PVR, but has also been used safely in this group of patients.

Any depolarizing/non-depolarizing muscle relaxant can be used; the choice depends on the airways strategy employed. Many of these patients require mechanical ventilation but tolerate it poorly. High airway pressures are deleterious, as are hypoxia and hypercapnia, more so than the general surgical population. Shorter procedures may be better served by allowing spontaneous ventilation, but hypercapnia must be avoided.

During maintenance of anesthesia, total intravenous anesthesia (TIVA) is acceptable (with the proviso that SVR must be maintained), as is inhalational anesthesia. All the current volatile anesthetics are relatively safe in this group of patients. However, nitrous oxide may adversely impact cardiac output through its myocardial depressant effects and may worsen PVR. On emergence from anesthesia, hypoxia, hypercarbia, and pain will all adversely affect pulmonary pressures, and every effort should be made to counteract these effects. If general anesthesia is avoided, and neuraxial anesthesia/analgesia is used, the cardiac consequences of blockade should be treated aggressively [88].

15.8 Pulmonary Hypertensive Crises

These high-risk episodes, with a hyperacute rise of systolic pulmonary pressure (>50% of systemic pressure), may be unpredictable and are extremely high mortality events with rapid cardiovascular collapse; therefore, prompt recognition and aggressive treatment is crucial. Management should aim to: (Step 1) augment SVR to prevent RV ischemia, (Step 2) reduce RV afterload, and (Step 3) improve RV/biventricular function. Hypotension in this setting should be treated aggressively (step 1 above), concurrently with steps 2 and 3, and without stopping pulmonary vasodilators. Fluid challenges should be avoided, and fluid administration should be guided by CVP. The vasopressor noradrenaline (up to 0.5 mcg/kg/min) has been shown to improve coronary blood flow in several models of acute RV failure. Low-dose vasopressin (0.01–0.03 IU/kg/min) may also be useful, although clinical data on this remain limited in PH patients [89]. Within these doses, vasopressin is not only a strong systemic vasoconstrictor but also a pulmonary vasodilator; however, it loses its vasodilator effect when used at higher doses. To acutely reduce RV afterload in a PH crisis, selective inhaled pulmonary vasodilators are, on the whole, preferable to systemic nonselective vasodilators. Inhaled pulmonary vasodilators, including NO, inhaled prostacyclin, and iloprost, reduce PVR following heart transplantation surgery [90–92], pulmonary endarterectomy [93], in LVAD-associated acute RV failure [94], and in mitral valve surgery [95]. Anticipation and careful planning for these episodes is key, especially in the perioperative setting.

15.9 Intensive Care Management of PAH-CHD

Patients with PAH admitted to ICU have an ICU mortality of over 40%, with RV function ultimately being the key determinant of outcome. Additional clinical features predictive of increased ICU mortality in PH include the presence of hyponatremia, renal dysfunction, and tachycardia (reflective of poor RV function) [58]. For any patient with known PAH, including PAH-CHD, close involvement of the CHD and PH teams (a true multidisciplinary approach) is crucial. Pre-existing PAH therapies should not be stopped; alternatives to oral therapies can be used. The principles of ICU management of patients with PAH are previously well reviewed and will depend on the reason for admission, with precipitants of RV failure in critical illness divided into three main categories: [89, 96–98] (a) excessive RV preload, (b) excessive RV afterload, and (c) insufficient myocardial contractility (Fig. 15.1). ICU admission in PAH-CHD patients often relates to the postoperative and posttransplant settings, as well as intercurrent illness and disease (PAH) progression. Ultimately, the decision and extent of monitoring and management will depend on the reversibility of the acute process, and ceilings to care should be discussed in advance, as appropriate (see section below).

ICU management can be considered in steps 1–3 as listed above. In terms of RV preload, venous return is influenced by many factors, including fluids, anesthetic drugs, invasive positive-pressure ventilation (IPPV), and laparoscopic surgery (reducing right-sided venous return). Of the modifiable factors, meticulous fluid management is key, ideally aiming for moderately elevated RV filling pressures with a central venous pressure (CVP) of 8–12 mmHg, thereafter adjusted to optimize RV function and cardiac output. The use of diuretics is a mainstay of ICU management in patients with RV failure, often with intravenous infusion of furosemide, with concurrent potassium-sparing agent (e.g., spironolactone). Serial lactate values, renal function, and superior vena cava saturations (SvO_2) all usefully reflect cardiac output and tissue perfusion, aiming (in patients without a shunt) for normal SvO_2 values. In patients with a shunt, clinicians should modify the target values according to anatomy and prior RHC values, if available.

Secondly, in terms of excessive RV afterload, additional modifiable influences should be sought and managed, for example, pulmonary embolism, pulmonary vasoconstriction due to alveolar hypoxia, hypercapnia, sepsis and acute respiratory distress syndrome (ARDS) (e.g., with endotoxin increasing pulmonary vasoconstriction via interleukin (IL)-6 and serotonin), and elevated airway pressure. Intubation and invasive positive-pressure ventilation (IPPV) may be considered, but are best avoided in PAH patients. If IPPV is unavoidable, strategies to protect the RV should be employed, including the minimal use of positive end-expiratory pressure (PEEP), recruitment maneuvers, with SaO_2 kept above 92%, and ventilator settings adjusted to achieve a lung volume near functional residual capacity and a pCO_2 and pH as close to normal as possible. It is extremely important to avoid hypercapnia and acidosis and to keep a maximum tidal volume of 4–6 mL/Kg and

Table 15.5 Vasoactive drugs for management of acute right ventricular failure and their mechanism of action

	Receptor binding					
Agent	α_1	β_1	β_2	D	V1	Notes
Norepinephrine	++	+				Improves PA/RV coupling in animals [73–75]
Phenylephrine	++					Increases PVR [71, 74, 77]; may induce reflex bradycardia
Epinephrine	++	++	+			[79]
Vasopressin					+	Dose-dependent pulmonary vasodilatation (0.01–0.03 U/min) and vasoconstriction [24, 32, 33]
Dopamine						Risk of arrhythmias
Low (<5 μg/kg/min)		+		++		
Medium (5–10 μg/kg/min)	+	++		++		
High (>10 μg/kg/min)	++	++		++		
Dobutamine		++	+			β_2-Mediated drop in SVR [31]; risk of arrhythmias
Milrinone						Phosphodiesterase-3 inhibitor; inotnopy and pulmonary vasodilatation; drop in LVEDP and SVR [34, 39, 72]; risk of arrhythmias

D Dopaminergic receptor, *LVEDP* Left ventricular end-diastolic pressure, *PA* Pulmonary artery, *PVR* Pulmonary vascular resistance, *RV* Right ventricle, *SVR* Systemic vascular resistance, *V1* Vasopressin receptor 1. + Low to moderate affinity, ++ Moderate to high affinity

a plateau pressure ≤30 mmHg. Alternatives to IPPV include noninvasive ventilation and nasal high flow (Optiflow™), which are well tolerated in PAH, the latter delivering high FiO_2 with low levels of positive pressure (2–3 kPa). When these considerations do not achieve satisfactory improvement in RV function, administration of pulmonary vasodilators may be appropriate, with the agent of choice in the setting of RV failure being intravenous prostacyclin or nitric oxide if the patient is intubated.

Thirdly, reduced RV contractility should be addressed and managed. Loss of RV contractility may relate to overstretching of the RV free wall, metabolic derangements, and insufficient oxygen delivery due to decreased coronary arterial perfusion. It is crucial to understand that, while coronary perfusion occurs throughout the cardiac cycle in normal RVs, in hypertensive RVs coronary perfusion decreases during systole. Hence, an important first aim is to preserve myocardial perfusion by using a vasopressor to restore systemic blood pressure to levels above RV systolic pressure, rather than focusing on fluid balance or the use of inotropes (Table 15.5). Vasopressors are often initiated preemptively, for example, prior to induction of anesthesia or with concurrent use of vasodilating inotropic agents (e.g., milrinone; see below). Inotropes are often needed to augment RV function, with low-dose dopamine and especially dobutamine being common first-line agents. Milrinone (a type 3 PDE inhibitor) is often used in ICU and has attractive inotropic and pulmonary vasodilating properties, with less chronotropic effect than dobutamine (or dopamine) but higher reduction in SVR that, subsequently, will increase the need for higher doses of vasoconstrictors. Calcium sensitizers, such as levosimendan, improve RV function in patients with RV failure. Inhaled milrinone has been used to aide weaning from CPB [99]. Inhaled iloprost may even be more effective than inhaled NO in patients weaning off CPB [100]. Intravenous sildenafil reduces ICU length of stay in children with PH following cardiac surgery and is also used post CPB to wean patients from inhaled NO [101].

Finally, when medical therapy for RV failure in this setting is ineffective, extracorporeal life support (ECLS) should be considered. In practice, this is mainly used as a bridge to definitive therapy (e.g., transplantation or pulmonary endarterectomy). ECLS techniques include veno-venous (VV) and veno-arterial (VA) extracorporeal membrane oxygenation (ECMO) and have been used as a successful bridging therapy in various setting of RV failure, with the VA-ECMO pumping blood from the venous to the arterial circuit to unload the RV, while maintaining systemic oxygenation. VA-ECMO and, more recently, the use of PA-LA paracorporeal assistance, Novalung, have been used in RV failure and in patients awaiting lung transplant for PAH [102–107]. Complications of ECLS include bleeding, infection, thromboembolism, and neurologic sequelae, as well as major psychological effects, which require careful planning and assessment with an experienced team approach.

15.10 Palliative Care and End-of-Life Issues

Patients with PAH requiring intensive care are at high risk of an adverse outcome. This begs the question of which PAH-CHD patients should be offered management in intensive care, that is, who are the patients who are likely to benefit and recover. Reversible causes of deterioration, such as lower respiratory tract infections, arrhythmias, and hemoptysis, may be appropriate reasons to admit, with an aim to reverse the acute pathology, while supporting RV function. Progressive heart failure refractory to medical or other therapy is, however, often not reversible and, unless it is a bridge to transplantation, intensive care may prove futile in patients with severe end-stage PAH.

Risk stratification and prognostication are, thus, important in aiding the decision on whether to offer intensive care and whether a ceiling should be set to minimize discomfort in patients who are unlikely to benefit from invasive cardiovascular and respiratory support. Palliative care input should be sought early in patients with recurrent hospitalizations or in high dependency or critical care, in parallel with life-prolonging interventions. Palliative care teams are valuable in addressing symptoms such as pain, dyspnea, and anxiety. They are also helpful in interacting and supporting the patients' families and introducing end-of life discussions with the patients and their relatives.

15.11 Informed Consent

Clear written consent should be obtained for all procedures under GA or sedation, and the risk-benefit ratio should ideally be agreed in a multidisciplinary team meeting. The above considerations and recommendations should be explained to the patient and caregivers, with sufficient time to reflect and decide on whether to proceed. When possible, a conservative management option should be offered to the patients and the risks and benefits of either approach explained in simple terms.

Conclusion

Significant expertise is required for the management of PAH-CHD patients, especially those who are critically ill. A multidisciplinary approach is essential, especially when the patient is in intensive care, as the pathophysiology of PAH-CHD differs significantly from that of heart failure, or other types of PAH. While all PAH centers should be able to provide critical care to PAH-CHD patients, discussions with regards to palliative care and end-of-life issues should be initiated early. Further work is urgently needed to clarify the optimal approach to anesthesia and intensive care for PAH-CHD patients and the identification of patients who are likely to benefit from an "aggressive" approach, including full resuscitation, mechanical ventilation, and invasive cardiocirculatory support.

Disclosures Dr. Dimopoulos has acted as consultant for Actelion UK, Pfizer UK, and GSK UK and received unrestricted educational grants from Actelion and Pfizer. Dr. Price has acted as a consultant for Actelion UK and GSK UK and has received educational grants from Actelion. Dr Alexander has no disclosures to declare. Dr. Alonso-Gonzalez has acted as consultants for Pfizer Spain and GSK Spain and received unrestricted educational grants from Actelion and GSK.

References

1. Dimopoulos K, Wort SJ, Gatzoulis MA. Pulmonary hypertension related to congenital heart disease: a call for action. Eur Heart J. 2014;35(11):691–700.
2. Health and Social Care Information Centre 1 Trevelyan Square. National Pulmonary Hypertension Audit [Internet]. 2012 [cited 2014 Oct 27]. http://www.hscic.gov.uk/ph.
3. Heath D, Helmholz HF Jr, Burchell HB, Dushane JW, Edwards JE. Graded pulmonary vascular changes and hemodynamic findings in cases of atrial and ventricular septal defect and patent ductus arteriosus. Circulation. 1958;18(6):1155–66.
4. Dimopoulos K, Giannakoulas G, Wort SJ, Gatzoulis MA. Pulmonary arterial hypertension in adults with congenital heart disease: distinct differences from other causes of pulmonary arterial hypertension and management implications. Curr Opin Cardiol. 2008;23(6):545–54.
5. Galiè N, Humbert M, Vachiery J-L, Gibbs S, Lang I, et al. 2015 ESC/ERS Guidelines for the diagnosis and treatment of pulmonary hypertension: the joint task force for the Diagnosis and Treatment of Pulmonary Hypertension of the European Society of Cardiology (ESC) and the European Respiratory Society (ERS) endorsed by: Association for European Paediatric and Congenital Cardiology (AEPC), International Society for Heart and Lung Transplantation (ISHLT). Eur Heart J. 2016;37:67–119.

6. Diller G-P, Dimopoulos K, Broberg CS, Kaya MG, Naghotra US, Uebing A, et al. Presentation, survival prospects, and predictors of death in Eisenmenger syndrome: a combined retrospective and case-control study. Eur Heart J. 2006;27(14):1737–42.
7. Dimopoulos K, Inuzuka R, Goletto S, Giannakoulas G, Swan L, Wort SJ, et al. Improved survival among patients with Eisenmenger syndrome receiving advanced therapy for pulmonary arterial hypertension. Circulation. 2010;121(1):20–5.
8. Wood P. The Eisenmenger syndrome or pulmonary hypertension with reversed central shunt. Br Med J. 1958;2(5098):701–9.
9. Wood P. The Eisenmenger syndrome or pulmonary hypertension with reversed central shunt. Br Med J. 1958;2(5099):755–62.
10. Yamamura K, Nagata H, Ikeda K, Ihara K, Hara T. Efficacy of bosentan therapy for segmental pulmonary artery hypertension due to major aortopulmonary collateral arteries in children. Int J Cardiol. 2012;161(1):e1–3.
11. Schuuring MJ, Bouma BJ, Cordina R, Gatzoulis MA, Budts W, Mullen MP, et al. Treatment of segmental pulmonary artery hypertension in adults with congenital heart disease. Int J Cardiol. 2013;164(1):106–10.
12. Giardini A, Balducci A, Specchia S, Gargiulo G, Bonvicini M, Picchio FM. Effect of sildenafil on haemodynamic response to exercise and exercise capacity in Fontan patients. Eur Heart J. 2008;29(13):1681–7.
13. Hebert A, Mikkelsen UR, Thilen U, Idorn L, Jensen AS, Nagy E, et al. Bosentan improves exercise capacity in adolescents and adults after Fontan operation the TEMPO (treatment with endothelin receptor antagonist in Fontan patients, a randomized, placebo-controlled, double-blind study measuring peak oxygen consumption) study. Circulation. 2014;130(23):2021–30.
14. Dimopoulos K, Diller GP. Pulmonary hypertension in adult congenital heart [Internet]. Springer; 2017 [cited 2017 Sep 2]. http://www.springer.com/us/book/9783319460260.
15. Naeije R, Manes A. The right ventricle in pulmonary arterial hypertension. Eur Respir Rev. 2014;23(134):476–87.
16. Bowater SE, Weaver RA, Beadle RM, Frenneaux MP, Marshall JM, Clift PF. Assessment of the physiological adaptations to chronic hypoxemia in Eisenmenger syndrome. Congenit Heart Dis. 2016;11(4):341–7.
17. Broberg CS, Ujita M, Prasad S, Li W, Rubens M, Bax BE, et al. Pulmonary arterial thrombosis in Eisenmenger syndrome is associated with biventricular dysfunction and decreased pulmonary flow velocity. J Am Coll Cardiol. 2007;50(7):634–42.
18. Daliento L, Somerville J, Presbitero P, Menti L, Brach-Prever S, Rizzoli G, et al. Eisenmenger syndrome. Factors relating to deterioration and death. Eur Heart J. 1998;19(12):1845–55.
19. Dimopoulos K, Diller G-P, Petraco R, Koltsida E, Giannakoulas G, Tay EL, et al. Hyponatraemia: a strong predictor of mortality in adults with congenital heart disease. Eur Heart J. 2010;31(5):595–601.
20. Dimopoulos K, Diller G-P, Koltsida E, Pijuan-Domenech A, Papadopoulou SA, Babu-Narayan SV, et al. Prevalence, predictors, and prognostic value of renal dysfunction in adults with congenital heart disease. Circulation. 2008;117(18):2320–8.
21. Kempny A, Diller G-P, Alonso-Gonzalez R, Uebing A, Rafiq I, Li W, et al. Hypoalbuminaemia predicts outcome in adult patients with congenital heart disease. Heart Br Card Soc. 2015;101(9):699–705.
22. Diller G-P, Alonso-Gonzalez R, Kempny A, Dimopoulos K, Inuzuka R, Giannakoulas G, et al. B-type natriuretic peptide concentrations in contemporary Eisenmenger syndrome patients: predictive value and response to disease targeting therapy. Heart. 2012;98(9):736–42.
23. Hjortshøj CMS, Kempny A, Jensen AS, Sørensen K, Nagy E, Dellborg M, et al. Past and current cause-specific mortality in Eisenmenger syndrome. Eur Heart J. 2017;38(26):2060–7.
24. Kempny A, Hjortshøj CS, Gu H, Li W, Opotowsky AR, Landzberg MJ, et al. Predictors of death in contemporary adult patients with Eisenmenger syndrome: a multicenter study. Circulation. 2017;135(15):1432–40.
25. Kempny A, Dimopoulos K, Uebing A, Moceri P, Swan L, Gatzoulis MA, et al. Reference values for exercise limitations among adults with congenital heart disease. Relation to

activities of daily life—single centre experience and review of published data. Eur Heart J. 2012;33(11):1386–96.

26. Kempny A, Dimopoulos K, Alonso-Gonzalez R, Alvarez-Barredo M, Tutarel O, Uebing A, et al. Six-minute walk test distance and resting oxygen saturations but not functional class predict outcome in adult patients with Eisenmenger syndrome. Int J Cardiol. 2013;168:4784–9.
27. Dimopoulos K, Okonko DO, Diller G-P, Broberg CS, Salukhe TV, Babu-Narayan SV, et al. Abnormal ventilatory response to exercise in adults with congenital heart disease relates to cyanosis and predicts survival. Circulation. 2006;113(24):2796–802.
28. Inuzuka R, Diller G-P, Borgia F, Benson L, Tay ELW, Alonso-Gonzalez R, et al. Comprehensive use of cardiopulmonary exercise testing identifies adults with congenital heart disease at increased mortality risk in the medium termclinical perspective. Circulation. 2012;125(2):250–9.
29. Alonso-Gonzalez R, Borgia F, Diller G-P, Inuzuka R, Kempny A, Martinez-Naharro A, et al. Abnormal lung function in adults with congenital heart disease: prevalence, relation to cardiac anatomy, and association with survival. Circulation. 2013;127(8):882–90.
30. Brida M, Dimopoulos K, Kempny A, Liodakis E, Alonso-Gonzalez R, Swan L, et al. Body mass index in adult congenital heart disease. Heart Br Card Soc. 2017;103(16):1250–7.
31. Dimopoulos K, Kempny A. Patients with Down syndrome and congenital heart disease: survival is improving, but challenges remain. Heart Br Card Soc. 2016;102(19):1515–7.
32. Tay ELW, Peset A, Papaphylactou M, Inuzuka R, Alonso-Gonzalez R, Giannakoulas G, et al. Replacement therapy for iron deficiency improves exercise capacity and quality of life in patients with cyanotic congenital heart disease and/or the Eisenmenger syndrome. Int J Cardiol. 2011;151(3):307–12.
33. Van De Bruaene A, Delcroix M, Pasquet A, De Backer J, De Pauw M, Naeije R, et al. Iron deficiency is associated with adverse outcome in Eisenmenger patients. Eur Heart J. 2011;32(22):2790–9.
34. Ammash N, Warnes CA. Cerebrovascular events in adult patients with cyanotic congenital heart disease. J Am Coll Cardiol. 1996;28(3):768–72.
35. Jensen AS, Idorn L, Thomsen C, von der Recke P, Mortensen J, Sørensen KE, et al. Prevalence of cerebral and pulmonary thrombosis in patients with cyanotic congenital heart disease. Heart Br Card Soc. 2015;101(19):1540–6.
36. Habib G, Lancellotti P, Antunes MJ, Bongiorni MG, Casalta J-P, et al. 2015 ESC Guidelines for the management of infective endocarditis: the task force for the Management of Infective Endocarditis of the European Society of Cardiology (ESC) endorsed by: European Association for Cardio-Thoracic Surgery (EACTS), the European Association of Nuclear Medicine (EANM). Eur Heart J. 2015;36:3075–128.
37. Bédard E, Dimopoulos K, Gatzoulis MA. Has there been any progress made on pregnancy outcomes among women with pulmonary arterial hypertension? Eur Heart J. 2009;30(3):256–65.
38. European Society of Gynecology (ESG), Association for European Paediatric Cardiology (AEPC), German Society for Gender Medicine (DGesGM), Regitz-Zagrosek V, Blomstrom Lundqvist C, Borghi C, et al. ESC Guidelines on the management of cardiovascular diseases during pregnancy: the task force on the Management of Cardiovascular Diseases during Pregnancy of the European Society of Cardiology (ESC). Eur Heart J. 2011;32(24):3147–97.
39. Galiè N, Beghetti M, Gatzoulis MA, Granton J, Berger RMF, Lauer A, et al. Bosentan therapy in patients with Eisenmenger syndrome: a multicenter, double-blind, randomized, placebo-controlled study. Circulation. 2006;114(1):48–54.
40. Gatzoulis MA, Beghetti M, Galiè N, Granton J, Berger RMF, Lauer A, et al. Longer-term bosentan therapy improves functional capacity in Eisenmenger syndrome: results of the BREATHE-5 open-label extension study. Int J Cardiol. 2008;127(1):27–32.
41. Berger RMF, Beghetti M, Galiè N, Gatzoulis MA, Granton J, Lauer A, et al. Atrial septal defects versus ventricular septal defects in BREATHE-5, a placebo-controlled study of pulmonary arterial hypertension related to Eisenmenger's syndrome: a subgroup analysis. Int J Cardiol. 2010;144:373–8.

42. Mukhopadhyay S, Nathani S, Yusuf J, Shrimal D, Tyagi S. Clinical efficacy of phosphodiesterase-5 inhibitor tadalafil in Eisenmenger syndrome—a randomized, placebo-controlled, double-blind crossover study. Congenit Heart Dis. 2011;6(5):424–31.
43. Tay ELW, Papaphylactou M, Diller GP, Alonso-Gonzalez R, Inuzuka R, Giannakoulas G, et al. Quality of life and functional capacity can be improved in patients with Eisenmenger syndrome with oral sildenafil therapy. Int J Cardiol. 2011;149(3):372–6.
44. D'Alto M, Romeo E, Argiento P, Sarubbi B, Santoro G, Grimaldi N, et al. Bosentan-sildenafil association in patients with congenital heart disease-related pulmonary arterial hypertension and Eisenmenger physiology. Int J Cardiol. 2012;155(3):378–82.
45. Fernandes SM, Newburger JW, Lang P, Pearson DD, Feinstein JA, Gauvreau K, et al. Usefulness of epoprostenol therapy in the severely ill adolescent/adult with Eisenmenger physiology. Am J Cardiol. 2003;91(5):632–5.
46. Cha KS, Cho KI, Seo JS, Choi JH, Park YH, Yang DH, et al. Effects of inhaled iloprost on exercise capacity, quality of life, and cardiac function in patients with pulmonary arterial hypertension secondary to congenital heart disease (the Eisenmenger syndrome) (from the EIGER Study). Am J Cardiol. 2013;112(11):1834–9.
47. Yang SI, Chung WJ, Jung SH, Choi DY. Effects of inhaled iloprost on congenital heart disease with Eisenmenger syndrome. Pediatr Cardiol. 2012;33(5):744–8.
48. Pulido T, Adzerikho I, Channick RN, Delcroix M, Galiè N, Ghofrani H-A, et al. Macitentan and morbidity and mortality in pulmonary arterial hypertension. N Engl J Med. 2013;369(9):809–18.
49. Rosenkranz S, Ghofrani H-A, Beghetti M, Ivy D, Frey R, Fritsch A, et al. Riociguat for pulmonary arterial hypertension associated with congenital heart disease. Heart Br Card Soc. 2015;101(22):1792–9.
50. Budhiraja R, Tuder RM, Hassoun PM. Endothelial dysfunction in pulmonary hypertension. Circulation. 2004;109(2):159–65.
51. Stojnic BB, Brecker SJ, Xiao HB, Helmy SM, Mbaissouroum M, Gibson DG. Left ventricular filling characteristics in pulmonary hypertension: a new mode of ventricular interaction. Br Heart J. 1992;68(1):16–20.
52. Vizza CD, Lynch JP, Ochoa LL, Richardson G, Trulock EP. Right and left ventricular dysfunction in patients with severe pulmonary disease. Chest. 1998;113(3):576–83.
53. Via G, Braschi A. Pathophysiology of severe pulmonary hypertension in the critically ill patient. Minerva Anestesiol. 2004;70(4):233–7.
54. West JB. Invited review: pulmonary capillary stress failure. J Appl Physiol Bethesda MD 1985. 2000;89(6):2483–9. discussion 2497.
55. Bando K, Turrentine MW, Sharp TG, Sekine Y, Aufiero TX, Sun K, et al. Pulmonary hypertension after operations for congenital heart disease: analysis of risk factors and management. J Thorac Cardiovasc Surg. 1996;112(6):1600–7. discussion 1607–1609.
56. Jardin F, Dubourg O, Bourdarias JP. Echocardiographic pattern of acute cor pulmonale. Chest. 1997;111(1):209–17.
57. Hickey PR, Retzack SM. Acute right ventricular failure after pulmonary hypertensive responses to airway instrumentation: effect of fentanyl dose. Anesthesiology. 1993;78(2):372–6.
58. Jardin F, Brun-Ney D, Cazaux P, Dubourg O, Hardy A, Bourdarias JP. Relation between transpulmonary pressure and right ventricular isovolumetric pressure change during respiratory support. Cathet Cardiovasc Diagn. 1989;16(4):215–20.
59. Alfonsi P, Vieillard-Baron A, Coggia M, Guignard B, Goeau-Brissonniere O, Jardin F, et al. Cardiac function during intraperitoneal CO2 insufflation for aortic surgery: a transesophageal echocardiographic study. Anesth Analg. 2006;102(5):1304–10.
60. Wort SJ, Evans TW. The role of the endothelium in modulating vascular control in sepsis and related conditions. Br Med Bull. 1999;55(1):30–48.
61. Dávila-Román VG, Waggoner AD, Hopkins WE, Barzilai B. Right ventricular dysfunction in low output syndrome after cardiac operations: assessment by transesophageal echocardiography. Ann Thorac Surg. 1995;60(4):1081–6.

62. Denault A, Deschamps A, Tardif J-C, Lambert J, Perrault L. Pulmonary hypertension in cardiac surgery. Curr Cardiol Rev. 2010;6(1):1–14.
63. Wessel DL, Adatia I, Giglia TM, Thompson JE, Kulik TJ. Use of inhaled nitric oxide and acetylcholine in the evaluation of pulmonary hypertension and endothelial function after cardiopulmonary bypass. Circulation. 1993;88(5 Pt 1):2128–38.
64. Conzen PF, Habazettl H, Gutmann R, Hobbhahn J, Goetz AE, Peter K, et al. Thromboxane mediation of pulmonary hemodynamic responses after neutralization of heparin by protamine in pigs. Anesth Analg. 1989;68(1):25–31.
65. Reich DL, Bodian CA, Krol M, Kuroda M, Osinski T, Thys DM. Intraoperative hemodynamic predictors of mortality, stroke, and myocardial infarction after coronary artery bypass surgery. Anesth Analg. 1999;89(4):814–22.
66. Roques F, Nashef SA, Michel P, Gauducheau E, de Vincentiis C, Baudet E, et al. Risk factors and outcome in European cardiac surgery: analysis of the EuroSCORE multinational database of 19030 patients. Eur J Cardio-Thorac Surg Off J Eur Assoc Cardio-Thorac Surg. 1999;15(6):816–22. discussion 822–823.
67. Ghoreishi M, Evans CF, DeFilippi CR, Hobbs G, Young CA, Griffith BP, et al. Pulmonary hypertension adversely affects short- and long-term survival after mitral valve operation for mitral regurgitation: implications for timing of surgery. J Thorac Cardiovasc Surg. 2011;142(6):1439–52.
68. Romano MA, Cowger J, Aaronson KD, Pagani FD. Diagnosis and management of right-sided heart failure in subjects supported with left ventricular assist devices. Curr Treat Options Cardiovasc Med. 2010;12(5):420–30.
69. Miller OI, Tang SF, Keech A, Pigott NB, Beller E, Celermajer DS. Inhaled nitric oxide and prevention of pulmonary hypertension after congenital heart surgery: a randomised double-blind study. Lancet Lond Engl. 2000;356(9240):1464–9.
70. Lindberg L, Olsson AK, Jögi P, Jonmarker C. How common is severe pulmonary hypertension after pediatric cardiac surgery? J Thorac Cardiovasc Surg. 2002;123(6):1155–63.
71. Pagowska-Klimek I, Pychynska-Pokorska M, Krajewski W, Moll JJ. Predictors of long intensive care unit stay following cardiac surgery in children. Eur J Cardio-Thorac Surg Off J Eur Assoc Cardio-Thorac Surg. 2011;40(1):179–84.
72. Lundgren R, Häggmark S, Reiz S. Hemodynamic effects of flexible fiberoptic bronchoscopy performed under topical anesthesia. Chest. 1982;82(3):295–9.
73. Riley DJ. Risk of surgical lung biopsy in idiopathic interstitial pneumonias. Chest. 2005;127(5):1485–6.
74. Kreider ME, Hansen-Flaschen J, Ahmad NN, Rossman MD, Kaiser LR, Kucharczuk JC, et al. Complications of video-assisted thoracoscopic lung biopsy in patients with interstitial lung disease. Ann Thorac Surg. 2007;83(3):1140–4.
75. Hoeper MM, Lee SH, Voswinckel R, Palazzini M, Jais X, Marinelli A, et al. Complications of right heart catheterization procedures in patients with pulmonary hypertension in experienced centers. J Am Coll Cardiol. 2006;48(12):2546–52.
76. Taylor CJ, Derrick G, McEwan A, Haworth SG, Sury MRJ. Risk of cardiac catheterization under anaesthesia in children with pulmonary hypertension. Br J Anaesth. 2007;98(5):657–61.
77. Gottlieb EA, Andropoulos DB. Anesthesia for the patient with congenital heart disease presenting for noncardiac surgery. Curr Opin Anaesthesiol. 2013;26(3):318–26.
78. Baehner T, Ellerkmann RK. Anesthesia in adults with congenital heart disease. Curr Opin Anaesthesiol. 2017;30(3):418–25.
79. Bennett JM, Ehrenfeld JM, Markham L, Eagle SS. Anesthetic management and outcomes for patients with pulmonary hypertension and intracardiac shunts and Eisenmenger syndrome: a review of institutional experience. J Clin Anesth. 2014;26(4):286–93.
80. Weiss BM, Zemp L, Seifert B, Hess OM. Outcome of pulmonary vascular disease in pregnancy: a systematic overview from 1978 through 1996. J Am Coll Cardiol. 1998;31(7):1650–7.
81. Jaïs X, Olsson KM, Barbera JA, Blanco I, Torbicki A, Peacock A, et al. Pregnancy outcomes in pulmonary arterial hypertension in the modern management era. Eur Respir J. 2012;40(4):881–5.

82. Bonnin M, Mercier FJ, Sitbon O, Roger-Christoph S, Jaïs X, Humbert M, et al. Severe pulmonary hypertension during pregnancy: mode of delivery and anesthetic management of 15 consecutive cases. Anesthesiology. 2005;102(6):1133–7. discussion 5A–6A.
83. Kiely DG, Condliffe R, Webster V, Mills GH, Wrench I, Gandhi SV, et al. Improved survival in pregnancy and pulmonary hypertension using a multiprofessional approach. BJOG. 2010;117(5):565–74.
84. Kiely DG, Condliffe R, Wilson VJ, Gandhi SV, Elliot CA. Pregnancy and pulmonary hypertension: a practical approach to management. Obstet Med. 2013;6(4):144–54.
85. Curry RA, Fletcher C, Gelson E, Gatzoulis MA, Woolnough M, Richards N, et al. Pulmonary hypertension and pregnancy—a review of 12 pregnancies in nine women. BJOG. 2012;119(6):752–61.
86. Cauldwell M, Von Klemperer K, Uebing A, Swan L, Steer PJ, Gatzoulis M, et al. Why is postpartum haemorrhage more common in women with congenital heart disease? Int J Cardiol. 2016;218:285–90.
87. Martin JT, Tautz TJ, Antognini JF. Safety of regional anesthesia in Eisenmenger's syndrome. Reg Anesth Pain Med. 2002;27(5):509–13.
88. Pritts CD, Pearl RG. Anesthesia for patients with pulmonary hypertension. Curr Opin Anaesthesiol. 2010;23(3):411–6.
89. Price LC, Wort SJ, Finney SJ, Marino PS, Brett SJ. Pulmonary vascular and right ventricular dysfunction in adult critical care: current and emerging options for management: a systematic literature review. Crit Care Lond Engl. 2010;14(5):R169.
90. Rajek A, Pernerstorfer T, Kastner J, Mares P, Grabenwöger M, Sessler DI, et al. Inhaled nitric oxide reduces pulmonary vascular resistance more than prostaglandin E(1) during heart transplantation. Anesth Analg. 2000;90(3):523–30.
91. Ardehali A, Hughes K, Sadeghi A, Esmailian F, Marelli D, Moriguchi J, et al. Inhaled nitric oxide for pulmonary hypertension after heart transplantation. Transplantation. 2001;72(4):638–41.
92. Theodoraki K, Tsiapras D, Tsourelis L, Zarkalis D, Sfirakis P, Kapetanakis E, et al. Inhaled iloprost in eight heart transplant recipients presenting with post-bypass acute right ventricular dysfunction. Acta Anaesthesiol Scand. 2006;50(10):1213–7.
93. Kramm T, Eberle B, Krummenauer F, Guth S, Oelert H, Mayer E. Inhaled iloprost in patients with chronic thromboembolic pulmonary hypertension: effects before and after pulmonary thromboendarterectomy. Ann Thorac Surg. 2003;76(3):711–8.
94. Winterhalter M, Fischer S, Tessmann R, Goerler A, Piepenbrock S, Haverich A, et al. Using inhaled iloprost to wean from cardiopulmonary bypass after implanting a left ventricular assist device. Anesth Analg. 2006;103(2):515–6.
95. Rex S, Schaelte G, Metzelder S, Flier S, de Waal EEC, Autschbach R, et al. Inhaled iloprost to control pulmonary artery hypertension in patients undergoing mitral valve surgery: a prospective, randomized-controlled trial. Acta Anaesthesiol Scand. 2008;52(1):65–72.
96. Sztrymf B, Coulet F, Girerd B, Yaici A, Jais X, Sitbon O, et al. Clinical outcomes of pulmonary arterial hypertension in carriers of BMPR2 mutation. Am J Respir Crit Care Med. 2008;177(12):1377–83.
97. Hoeper MM, Granton J. Intensive care unit management of patients with severe pulmonary hypertension and right heart failure. Am J Respir Crit Care Med. 2011;184(10):1114–24.
98. Zamanian RT, Haddad F, Doyle RL, Weinacker AB. Management strategies for patients with pulmonary hypertension in the intensive care unit. Crit Care Med. 2007;35(9):2037–50.
99. Lamarche Y, Perrault LP, Maltais S, Tétreault K, Lambert J, Denault AY. Preliminary experience with inhaled milrinone in cardiac surgery. Eur J Cardio-Thorac Surg Off J Eur Assoc Cardio-Thorac Surg. 2007;31(6):1081–7.
100. Winterhalter M, Simon A, Fischer S, Rahe-Meyer N, Chamtzidou N, Hecker H, et al. Comparison of inhaled iloprost and nitric oxide in patients with pulmonary hypertension during weaning from cardiopulmonary bypass in cardiac surgery: a prospective randomized trial. J Cardiothorac Vasc Anesth. 2008;22(3):406–13.

101. Fraisse A, Butrous G, Taylor MB, Oakes M, Dilleen M, Wessel DL. Intravenous sildenafil for postoperative pulmonary hypertension in children with congenital heart disease. Intensive Care Med. 2011;37(3):502–9.
102. Mydin M, Berman M, Klein A, Tsui S, Dunning J, Valchanov K, et al. Extracorporeal membrane oxygenation as a bridge to pulmonary endarterectomy. Ann Thorac Surg. 2011;92(5):e101–3.
103. Srivastava MC, Ramani GV, Garcia JP, Griffith BP, Uber PA, Park MH. Veno-venous extracorporeal membrane oxygenation bridging to pharmacotherapy in pulmonary arterial hypertensive crisis. J Heart Lung Transplant Off Publ Int Soc Heart Transplant. 2010;29(7):811–3.
104. Rosenzweig EB, Brodie D, Abrams DC, Agerstrand CL, Bacchetta M. Extracorporeal membrane oxygenation as a novel bridging strategy for acute right heart failure in group 1 pulmonary arterial hypertension. ASAIO J Am Soc Artif Intern Organs 1992. 2014;60(1):129–33.
105. Keogh AM, Mayer E, Benza RL, Corris P, Dartevelle PG, Frost AE, et al. Interventional and surgical modalities of treatment in pulmonary hypertension. J Am Coll Cardiol. 2009;54(1 Suppl):S67–77.
106. Strueber M, Hoeper MM, Fischer S, Cypel M, Warnecke G, Gottlieb J, et al. Bridge to thoracic organ transplantation in patients with pulmonary arterial hypertension using a pumpless lung assist device. Am J Transplant Off J Am Soc Transplant Am Soc Transpl Surg. 2009;9(4):853–7.
107. Schmid C, Philipp A, Hilker M, Arlt M, Trabold B, Pfeiffer M, et al. Bridge to lung transplantation through a pulmonary artery to left atrial oxygenator circuit. Ann Thorac Surg. 2008;85(4):1202–5.

Critical Care Management of the ACHD Patient with Arrhythmias and Conduction Disorders

16

Ian Lindsay, Jeremy P. Moore, and Seshadri Balaji

16.1 Acute Tachyarrhythmias

16.1.1 Supraventricular Tachyarrhythmia (SVT)

SVT is the most common tachyarrhythmia in complex ACHD patients, with an estimated 50% lifetime risk entering the third decade of life [1]. There are multiple underlying mechanisms, including intra-atrial reentrant tachycardia (IART), focal atrial tachycardias (related to automatic or non-automatic mechanisms), atrioventricular reciprocating tachycardia (both the conventional form as well as that due to twin AV nodes), atrioventricular (AV) node reentrant tachycardia, and atrial fibrillation. The risk of developing SVT is known to increase with age and the degree of CHD complexity. There are also specific diagnoses and surgical procedures that are associated with a higher risk, such as in patients with d-transposition of the great arteries (DTGA) who have undergone a Mustard or Senning procedure or patients with single-ventricle physiology who have undergone the

I. Lindsay (✉)
Department of Cardiology, Ronald Reagan UCLA Medical Center, Los Angeles, CA, USA
e-mail: ilindsay@mednet.ucla.edu

J. P. Moore
Department of Cardiology, Ronald Reagan UCLA Medical Center, Los Angeles, CA, USA

Department of Pediatric Cardiology, Ronald Reagan UCLA Medical Center, Los Angeles, CA, USA
e-mail: JPMoore@mednet.ucla.edu

S. Balaji
Department of Pediatric Cardiology, OHSU Hospital, Portland, OR, USA
e-mail: balajis@ohsu.edu

E. da Cruz et al. (eds.), *Intensive Care of the Adult with Congenital Heart Disease*, Congenital Heart Disease in Adolescents and Adults,
https://doi.org/10.1007/978-3-319-94171-4_16

Table 16.1 Typical congenital lesions associated with specific arrhythmias and conduction disorders

Dysrhythmia	Typical lesions
Atrial	
IART/AFL	**DTGA, HLHS, single ventricle/heterotaxy**, ASD, TOF, AVSD, PA, TA, DORV, APVR
AF	DTGA, HLHS, single ventricle/heterotaxy, TOF, ASD, AVSD
Pathway	**Ebstein's**, CCTGA, single ventricle/heterotaxy
Ventricular	
VT/VF	**DTGA, TOF**, DORV, CCTGA, AS, coarctation, Ebstein's
Bradycardia	
SND	**DTGA, single ventricle/heterotaxy**, HLHS, PA, APVR
AVB	**CCTGA**, single ventricle/heterotaxy, ASD, AVSD

Most common associations in **Bold**. DTGA association is after Mustard/Senning procedure. *IART* intra-atrial reentrant tachycardia, *AFL* atrial flutter, *AF* strial fibrillation, *VT/VF* ventricular tachycardia/fibrillation, *SND* sinus node dysfunction, *AVB* AV nodal block, *DTGA/CCTGA* D/congenitally corrected transposition of the great arteries, *HLHS* hypoplastic left heart syndrome, *ASD* atrial septal defect, *TOF* tetralogy of Fallot, *AVSD* atrioventricular septal defect, *PA* pulmonary atresia, *DORV* double-outlet right ventricle, *APVR* anomalous pulmonary venous return, *AS* aortic stenosis

atriopulmonary Fontan procedure (Table 16.1) [2]. In the acute setting, SVT can sometimes result in cardiovascular collapse especially if there is an already compromised underlying hemodynamic state. In the subacute and chronic settings, it can also lead to thromboembolism and tachycardia-induced cardiomyopathy.

16.1.2 Intra-atrial Reentrant Tachycardia (IART)

IART is the most common form of SVT in the ACHD population and is particularly prevalent among patients who have undergone atrial level baffling for DTGA (Mustard or Senning procedures) or early iterations of the Fontan procedure [3, 4]. It invariably requires the presence of a centralized obstacle with an adjacent slowly conducting isthmus in order to perpetuate. Central obstacles in the setting of ACHD can include native tissue, such as an AV valve annulus, scar or surgically placed artificial material (such as patches or suture), or fibrosis from chronically altered hemodynamics. On the surface electrocardiogram (ECG), IART may appear as atrial flutter, with a recurring "sawtooth" P-wave at a rate >250 beats per minute and a regular pattern of the ventricular response. Commonly, however, for patients with ACHD, however, IART is characterized by a slower rate with a more discrete appearing P-wave and a long isoelectric interval, which can obscure interpretation (Fig. 16.1). Especially in cases of 2:1 or 3:1 conduction, the diagnosis may be missed entirely as the ventricular rate may be only mildly elevated or even normal (Fig. 16.2).

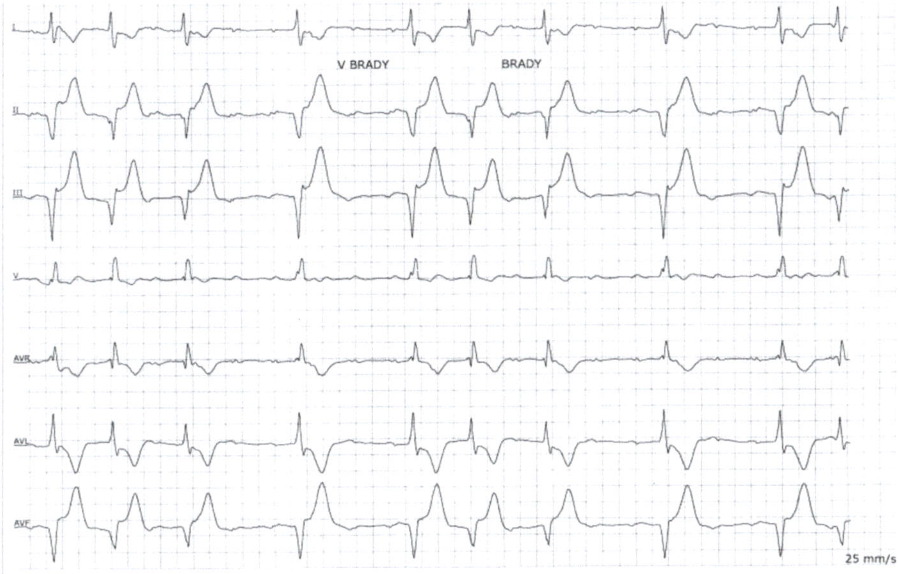

Fig. 16.1 IART with variable ventricular conduction in an adult patient with a single ventricle and lateral tunnel Fontan

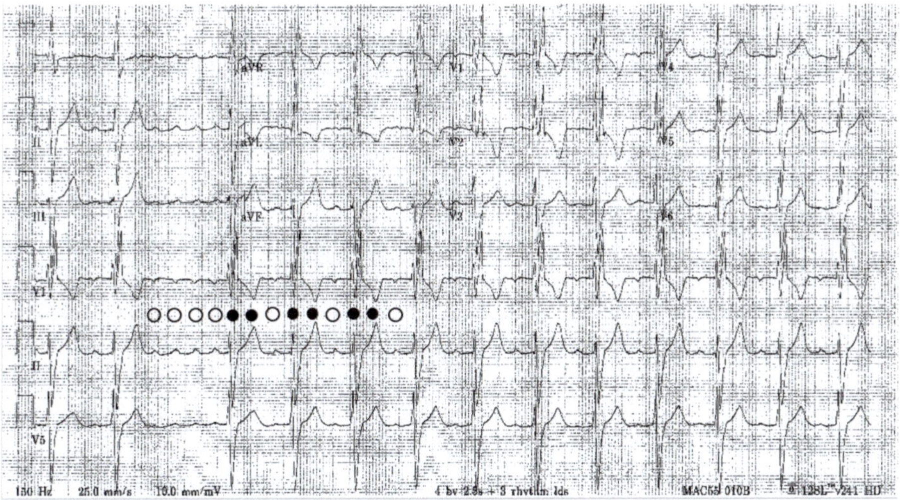

Fig. 16.2 IART with 3:1 ventricular conduction mimicking sinus rhythm in a 20-year-old patient with tetralogy of Fallot with pulmonary atresia. Each dot represents a flutter wave, with only the white dots visible outside the QRS complex or T-wave

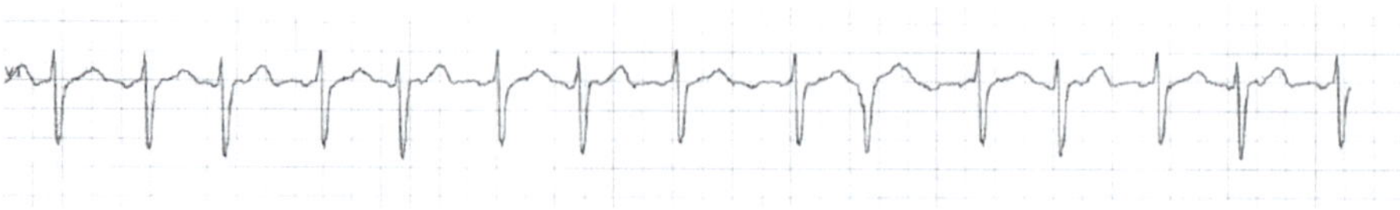

Fig. 16.3 Atrial fibrillation in a 58-year-old patient with double-inlet left ventricle and a lateral tunnel Fontan. Note the absence of a noticeable pattern in the ventricular response ("irregularly irregular ventricular response")

16.1.3 Atrial Fibrillation (AF)

AF is the most common arrhythmia in the adult population without CHD and has well-established risk factors. There is also an increasingly recognized risk in the ACHD population as individuals survive longer into adulthood, and some studies have shown AF to be more prevalent than IART in patients with TOF over the age of 55 years [3]. The risk of AF occurrence aligns with defects that lead to enlargement of the morphologic left atrium, including mitral valve and residual left ventricular lesions, unrepaired ASDs (or those repaired later in life), and palliated complex congenital heart disease [5]. Patients with the most complex congenital anatomy and surgical repair develop AF at a relatively young mean age of 30 years [6]. It has been demonstrated that AF may evolve over time and at a younger age in congenital heart disease patients with more regular atrial tachycardias [6]. AF is characterized by a chaotic and disorganized rhythm within the atria. Triggers of AF classically originate in the pulmonary venous musculature, and the tachyarrhythmia may be perpetuated by chronically remodeled atria. The ECG shows a lack of regular P-waves with irregularly irregular ventricular conduction (Fig. 16.3).

16.1.4 Atrioventricular Reentrant Tachycardia (AVRT)

In the ACHD population, AVRT is most commonly found in patients with Ebstein's anomaly of the tricuspid valve and congenitally corrected transposition of the great arteries (CCTGA) where the prevalence of accessory pathways approaches 20% for the former [7]. It is a typical orthodromic reentrant tachycardia that utilizes an accessory pathway along the tricuspid valve annulus. Patients with heterotaxy syndrome with right atrial isomerism may have twin AV nodes, in which case the sling of tissue connecting them may serve as the supporting pathway. On the ECG, these rhythms are characterized by narrow complex tachycardia with a short RP interval and ventricular rates between 200 and 300 beats per minute.

16.1.5 Automatic Focus Tachycardias

Ectopic atrial tachycardia (EAT) and junctional ectopic tachycardia (JET) are caused by abnormal automaticity in tissue outside the sinus node (atrial tissue in EAT and at the atrioventricular junction in JET). Compared to normal sinus rhythm on ECG, EAT has a distinct P-wave, the same QRS complex, and a faster heart rate. JET typically has warm-up and cooldown periods and has some ECG findings that are similar to VT, such as VA dissociation. Unlike VT, however, there are no fusion beats in JET, and the QRS is the same as sinus rhythm.

16.1.6 Management of SVT

When assessing an ACHD patient in the ICU with acute SVT, the first critical steps are to correctly identify the type of tachycardia and characterize the hemodynamic status. Atrial tachyarrhythmias can almost always be terminated with synchronized direct current cardioversion (DCCV) and less often by overdrive pacing or pharmacological therapy (Table 16.2). For patients in whom SVT has caused significantly decreased cardiac output and hemodynamic compromise, regardless of their risk for thromboembolism, urgent cardioversion of the arrhythmia is recommended. Success rates for termination of SVT have been found to be similar in ACHD patients and non-CHD patients, although they may be somewhat lower for Fontan patients [8]. Care must be taken to adjust the defibrillation pad placement to an anterior-posterior orientation in patients with marked atrial dilation or over the right chest in patients with dextrocardia. All reentrant forms of SVT may also respond to anti-tachycardia pacing [9]. This can be accomplished by temporary rapid pacing through a permanent pacemaker or defibrillator, if present, or with temporary transvenous or esophageal electrodes in patients who can tolerate the arrhythmia during catheter placement. Although semi-invasive, the latter is potentially advantageous in that pacing electrodes are already in place for pacing if there is severe bradycardia due to sinus node dysfunction after effective therapy has been delivered.

Pharmacologic termination is often a preferable option in patients with stable hemodynamic status, as it is less invasive and does not require sedation (Table 16.3). Intravenous adenosine or nondihydropyridine calcium channel blockers (diltiazem and verapamil) may successfully terminate forms of SVT that are dependent on the AV node, as well as for some types of non-automatic focal atrial tachycardia; vagal maneuvers may also be successful in this setting [10]. For IART and atrial fibrillation, current ACHD guidelines would also suggest intravenous ibutilide, 1–2 mg, administered over 10 min as a possible alternative [11]. This has been found to be both highly effective in children and adults with CHD (termination in up to 71% termination of atrial tachyarrhythmias) and superior to oral sotalol, 2 mg/kg in a single dose, which is the only other agent with multiple studies in the CHD population [12]. Importantly, there is a small but significant risk of torsades de pointes with ibutilide administration, and there are studies to suggest that this may be even higher in specific populations, such as African Americans and women [13, 14].

Persistent tachyarrhythmia that is resistant to electrical and pharmacological cardioversion presents a unique challenge. The rapid automatic firing in EAT and JET, for example, persists despite AV nodal blockade (adenosine) or application of direct electrical current, making these arrhythmias particularly difficult to treat. In these cases, especially if there is hemodynamic compromise, invasive emergency

Table 16.2 Characteristics of common antiarrhythmic medications

	Medication	Indication	ECG changes	Comments
Class I—sodium channel blockers				
Ia	Procainamide	Monomorphic VT	Prolongs QRS and QTc	Risk of torsades due to QTc prolongation. Significant side effects with prolonged use, including SLE-like syndrome and blood dyscrasias
Ib	Lidocaine	Monomorphic VT	None	Reduce maintenance infusion in patients with CHF, shock, or hepatic disease. Dose-dependent CNS effects
	Mexiletine	Monomorphic VT	None	Proarrhythmia effect with exacerbation of underlying arrhythmia in 10–15% of patients. GI complaints common
Ic	Flecainide	VT, IART, AF prevention	Prolongs PR and QRS, risk of AVB, and SND	Negative inotrope. Use with caution with decreased ventricular function. Proarrhythmic potential
	Propafenone	VT, IART, AF prevention	Prolongs PR and QRS	Proarrhythmic effect. Prolongs PR and QRS duration. Negative inotrope. Avoid use in patients with SND or overt heart failure
Class II—beta-blockers				
	Metoprolol	IART, AF rate control NSVT prevention	Decreases sinus rate, can prolong PR	Negative inotropic and chronotropic effect. Caution in patients with asthma
	Esmolol	IART, AF rate control	Decreases sinus rate, can prolong PR	Negative inotropic and chronotropic effect. Caution in patients with asthma
Class III—potassium channel blockers				
	Amiodarone	IART, AF cardioversion, prevention	Prolongs QRS and QTc	Significant extra-cardiac end-organ damage with prolonged use. Extreme caution in patients with liver disease or potential for hepatic impairment, such as Fontan patients
	Sotalol	IART, AF cardioversion, prevention VT prevention	Prolongs QTc, risk of sinus bradycardia	Risk of VT and Torsades. Do not initiate if baseline QTc >450 ms. If duration becomes >500 ms, decrease dose or frequency or discontinue. Adjust dose for renal impairment. Requires inpatient cardiac monitoring during initiation
	Ibutilide	IART, AF cardioversion	Prolongs QTc	Risk of VT, torsades
	Dofetilide	IART, AF cardioversion, prevention	Prolongs QTc	Do not initiate if QTc >450 ms (or >500 ms with underlying conduction delay). Risk of Torsades. Adjust dose for renal impairment. Requires inpatient cardiac monitoring during initiation
Class IV—calcium channel blockers				
	Diltiazem	IART, AF cardioversion, prevention	Decreases sinus rate, prolongs PR	Do not use in patients with AF and preexcitation. Negative inotrope

IART intra-atrial reentrant tachycardia, *AF* atrial fibrillation, *VT/VF* ventricular tachycardia/fibrillation, *NSVT* non-sustained ventricular tachycardia, *SND* sinus node dysfunction, *SLE* systemic lupus erythematosus

Table 16.3 Acute management of specific dysrhythmias

Rhythm		DCCV	ATP	Adenosine	Medications
Tachycardia					
	IART	Yes	Yes	No	Ibutilide, amiodarone, sotalol (+ BB, diltiazem for rate control)
	Atrial fibrillation	Yes	No	No	Ibutilide, amiodarone, sotalol (+ BB, diltiazem for rate control)
	AVRT	Yes	Yes	Yes	Flecainide, propafenone, procainamide
	EAT/JET	No	Yes[a]	No	Amiodarone, procainamide, esmolol (+ flecainide, propafenone for EAT)
	Monomorphic VT	Yes	Yes	No	Procainamide, lidocaine, amiodarone, sotalol
	Polymorphic VT/VF	Defibrillation	No	No	
	Torsades de pointes	Defibrillation	No	No	Magnesium sulfate
Bradycardia			**Pacing**	**Mode**	
	AV Block	No	Yes	DDD or VVI	
	Sinus Node Dysfunction	No	Yes	DDD or AAI	Isoproterenol, theophylline, terbutaline

[a]Overdrive pacing to establish AV synchrony

IART intra-atrial reentrant tachycardia, *AVRT* atrioventricular reentrant tachycardia, *EAT* ectopic atrial tachycardia, *JET* junctional ectopic tachycardia, *VT/VF* ventricular tachycardia/fibrillation, *BB* beta-blockers

treatment can be considered, including ECMO support and/or emergency ablation. The congenital electrophysiology team should be intimately involved when these options are being considered.

Patients with CHD have been shown to have a 10–100 times higher rate of thromboembolic complication compared to controls [15, 16]. Sustained IART or AF for 48 h or more, especially in the absence of systemic anticoagulation, is considered a significant risk factor for thromboembolism. In these patients, current guidelines recommend systemic anticoagulation for 3 weeks prior to and 4 weeks after cardioversion [17]. If this is not possible or otherwise undesirable, intracardiac thrombus must be excluded with transesophageal echocardiogram (TEE) prior to electrical or chemical cardioversion. This is especially true in patients who have undergone an atriopulmonary Fontan or other lesions associated with massively dilated atria, and thorough imaging with TEE may be prudent in these patients even in the setting of appropriate anticoagulation.

In instances where patients have converted from SVT to normal sinus rhythm with pharmacological or electrical cardioversion and then return to SVT, there is no role for repeated attempts at cardioversion. Having already proven that conversion is possible, attention must shift to maintaining sinus rhythm with pharmacological therapy.

Initiation of chronic antiarrhythmic therapy often takes place in the ICU after successful cardioversion. In ACHD patients, rhythm control is almost always desirable over rate control, especially in patients with systemic right ventricles or single ventricles [18]. Class III drugs (most commonly sotalol, amiodarone, and dofetilide,) are generally the most effective for maintaining sinus rhythm, although, as a group, they carry proarrhythmic risks. Factors include QTc prolongation with the concurrent risk of torsades de pointes and cardiac arrest, exacerbation of underlying bradyarrhythmia with the first two drugs, non-cardiac end-organ toxicity most notably with amiodarone, and potential contraindications in patients with decreased ventricular function for sotalol. Amiodarone is the most effective medication at maintaining rhythm control in atrial fibrillation and can be used in patients with coronary disease or ventricular dysfunction, but long-term use carries substantial time- and dose-dependent risks [19]. Careful monitoring is vital during initiation of these therapies.

Class I agents (flecainide), while effective, have the potential to slow the flutter rate, which in turn, may make AV nodal conduction easier, and thus can lead to an increase in the ventricular rate. In patients with prior surgical ventricular scar in the setting of congenital heart disease patients, they have been shown to be more proarrhythmic [20]. The same contraindication applies to patients with decreased ventricular function or coronary disease [20].

If rhythm control is not an option due to medication intolerance or refractory arrhythmia, rate control can be achieved with beta-blockers, digoxin, or nondihydropyridine calcium channel blockers. Extreme caution must be taken when using digoxin or calcium channel blockers in the setting of ventricular preexcitation, as their use may promote rapid ventricular conduction and cardiac arrest.

Lastly, similar to acute therapy, anti-tachycardia pacing with a permanent device is an effective means of termination of tachycardia in the outpatient setting. This can be performed either manually in the office or automatically using preprogrammed algorithms that are contained in modern cardiac electronic devices. Pacemaker settings that combine anti-tachycardia pacing with managed ventricular pacing have been shown to decrease progression of permanent or persistent AF in non-CHD patients long-term [21].

16.2 Ventricular Tachycardia (VT) and Ventricular Fibrillation (VF)

VT in ACHD patients is typically reentrant, with a protected isthmus bounded by scar, suture lines, incisions, or valves. This has been most clearly defined for tetralogy of Fallot, where a limited number of isthmuses may exist owing to the underlying anatomy and consistent surgical strategies utilized [22]. Sudden cardiac death (SCD), which is typically due to ventricular arrhythmia, is the second leading cause of death in ACHD patients behind heart failure [23–25]. Specific diagnoses and surgeries are known to increase an individual's risk for SCD. Patients with left ventricular outflow obstruction, DTGA after Mustard or Senning baffle, and TOF are at the highest risk, while those with CCTGA, Ebstein's anomaly, and single-ventricle palliation are at moderately elevated risk [26]. Regardless of their underlying diagnosis, patients with a prior history of SCD and documented sustained VT are at the highest risk for future SCD. The overall incidence of SCD in adults with CHD is approximately 0.1–0.2% per year which is 25–100 times higher than in the general population [26, 27].

VT is characterized by a wide QRS tachycardia that is at least 20% faster than the underlying sinus rate. The pattern of QRS complexes can be described as either monomorphic or polymorphic. When monomorphic, it is helpful to describe the VT morphology as either a right or left bundle branch block pattern, as this is a clue to the ventricular chamber of origin. Pathognomonic findings for monomorphic VT include ventricular-atrial dissociation and the presence of fusion beats, which are variations in the QRS complex that occur when a sinus beat is timed such that it can propagate to the ventricle during VT (Fig. 16.4). These features prove ventricular origin of the tachycardia and should be sought in all cases. This is perhaps of most importance for patients with congenital heart disease where supraventricular tachycardia with aberrancy manifesting as wide complex tachycardia is highly prevalent (Fig. 16.5). For patients with tetralogy of Fallot who present with a wide complex tachycardia and left bundle branch block pattern, VT can be presumed until proven otherwise since these patients invariably have a right bundle branch block pattern in sinus rhythm and with SVT (Fig. 16.4). In general, rapid VT is poorly tolerated and

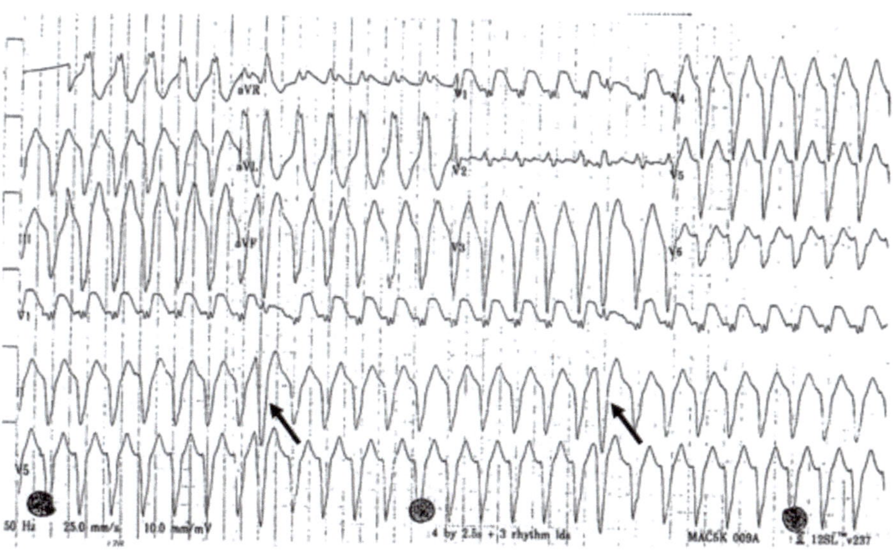

Fig. 16.4 Ventricular tachycardia with left bundle branch block morphology in a patient with repaired TOF. This ECG shows both VA dissociation and fusion beats (arrowhead)

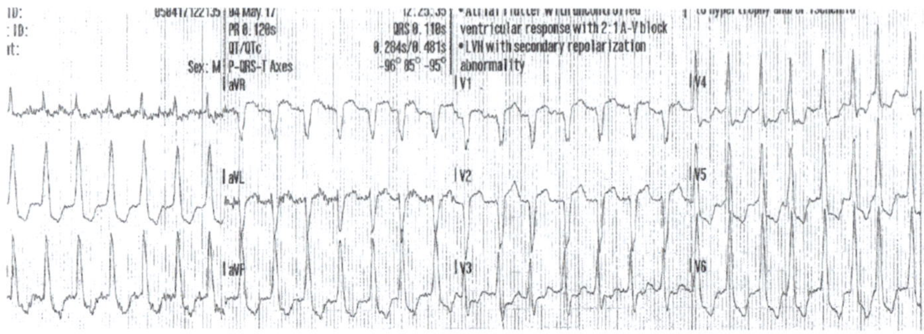

Fig. 16.5 IART with rapid aberrant ventricular conduction in a 33-year-old patient with a surgically repaired ASD

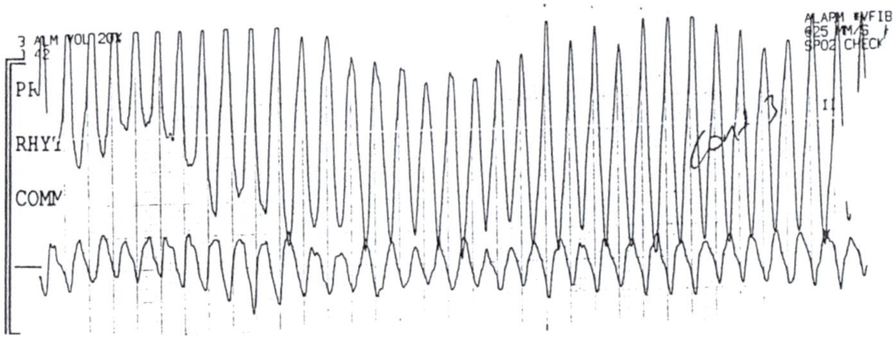

Fig. 16.6 Polymorphic VT in a patient with DORV and a Rastelli repair with decreased RV function due to severe RV-PA conduit stenosis

requires immediate cardioversion. Likewise, immediate defibrillation is required for polymorphic VT/VF (Fig. 16.6).

Torsades de pointes is a specific form of polymorphic VT that occurs in the setting of underlying QT prolongation. It occurs commonly as a result of electrolyte disturbances or QT-prolonging medications that are frequently administered in the intensive care unit. The SADS (sudden arrhythmia death syndromes) Foundation maintains an updated list of medications that prolong the QTc duration on its website (www.sads.org). Torsades is characterized by a continuous change in QRS amplitude and morphology around the isoelectric line. It is poorly tolerated and if allowed to persist will inevitably degenerate to VF, a fatal low-amplitude, and disorganized ventricular rhythm. In addition to standard therapy for polymorphic VT/VF, intravenous magnesium sulfate is uniquely efficacious for the treatment of torsades de pointes.

16.2.1 Non-sustained VT (NSVT)

NSVT is common in critically ill and postoperative patients. It is defined as three or more ventricular beats but less than 30 s in duration and not requiring cardioversion (Fig. 16.7). As with other forms of VT, it can be exacerbated by electrolyte

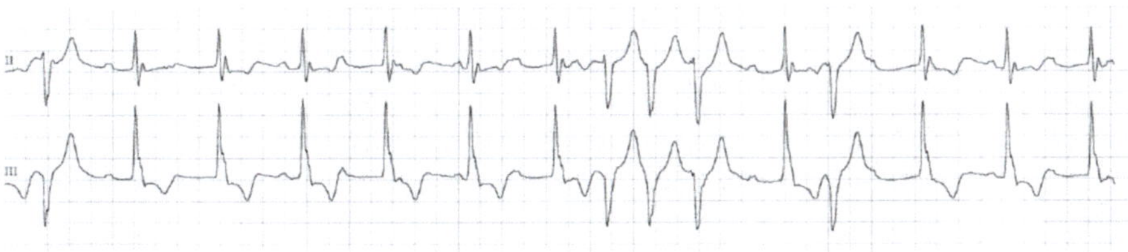

Fig. 16.7 Complete AV block followed by non-sustained ventricular tachycardia in a 45-year-old patient with a bicuspid aortic valve in the postoperative ICU after aortic valve replacement. There is no evidence of intact AV conduction with junctional escape rhythm prior to the NSVT

disturbances, acid-base abnormalities, acute inflammation from surgery, or a mechanical effect of lines or leads in the ventricle. NSVT is generally well tolerated providing that the offending causes are eliminated but is overall weakly associated with sustained VT. This may be especially true for those patients with other risk factors for VT [28]. Beta-blocker therapy is often initiated to decrease the risk of sustained VT, although evidence of efficacy of this approach is lacking in the ACHD population [29].

16.2.2 Management of VT/VF

Unstable monomorphic VT requires immediate electrical cardioversion, and sustained polymorphic VT or VF requires immediate defibrillation, along with standard ACLS-guided care. As in direct current cardioversion for SVT, care must be taken to adjust pad placement according to the heart's position within the chest. Pharmacological treatment may be considered in cases of stable monomorphic VT or recurrent VT/VT storm. Intravenous amiodarone and procainamide are the most effective medications for rapid termination of monomorphic VT. A newer option in the USA is the availability of IV sotalol, but there is, as yet, not much experience with this drug in ACHD patients. Care must be taken to account for the potential decrease in blood pressure caused by these drugs. As with SVT, ECMO can be considered in cases of refractory or recurrent ventricular arrhythmia.

Chronic treatment needs to be quickly initiated to *maintain* sinus rhythm after termination of VT/VF.

ICD placement is the mainstay of therapy for secondary prevention of sudden cardiac death in ACHD patients, unless there is a clearly reversible cause for the event. Most commonly, in-hospital arrests are related to reversible factors and therefore do not warrant ICD placement. On the other hand, for patients admitted to the ICU after a cardiac arrest in the field, device placement generally should occur prior to discharge [30]. It is wise to defer ICD placement until after the patient has demonstrated complete neurologic recovery, as setbacks in neurologic recovery are common after anesthetic exposures.

It is important to remember that in patients with an ICD for prevention or treatment of sudden death due to VT/VF, long-term medical therapy should be considered as an adjunct to ICD therapy in an effort to decrease the number of appropriate

ICD shocks [31–33]. The most commonly used drugs include beta-blockers, amiodarone, and less often sotalol and dofetilide. Another highly effective therapeutic modality is catheter ablation, which is being increasingly utilized especially for patients with tetralogy of Fallot (and in certain situations can be performed in lieu of ICD placement [34]. Finally, unilateral or bilateral stellate ganglionectomy holds promise for the reduction of VT episodes in patients who experience recurrent appropriate shocks despite the above interventions [35]).

16.3 Acute Bradyarrhythmia

16.3.1 Atrioventricular (AV) Block

AV block is characterized by delayed or absent conduction from the atria to the His bundle and ventricles through the AV node. It is most often a result of injury to the conduction system sustained during intracardiac surgical repair; the risk of AV block after specific surgeries is discussed further in the postoperative section of this chapter. Certain forms of CHD that involve congenital abnormalities of the conduction system are predisposed to progressive AV block with time. For example, in CCTGA, the conduction tissue is displaced anteriorly and laterally, with a long and tenuous course of the non-branching His bundle anterior to the pulmonary valve. For this reason, this and other forms of l-looped ventricles are associated with a spontaneous rate of AV block of 1.3% per person-years [36]. Heart block may also develop during pregnancy in the setting of altered volume status and hemodynamics, with obvious implications for both the mother and fetus [37, 38]. On ECG, first-degree AV block is defined as a PR interval greater than 200 ms but with consistent conduction through the AV node. Second-degree type I (Wenckebach) AV block involves progressive prolongation of the PR interval leading to an eventual nonconducted P-wave. Second-degree type II AV block appears as a stable PR interval with intermittently nonconducted P-waves (Fig. 16.8). Third-degree, or complete, AV block is due to a complete absence of conduction through the AV node and shows complete dissociation between ventricular (QRS complex) and atrial (P-wave) conduction (Fig. 16.9).

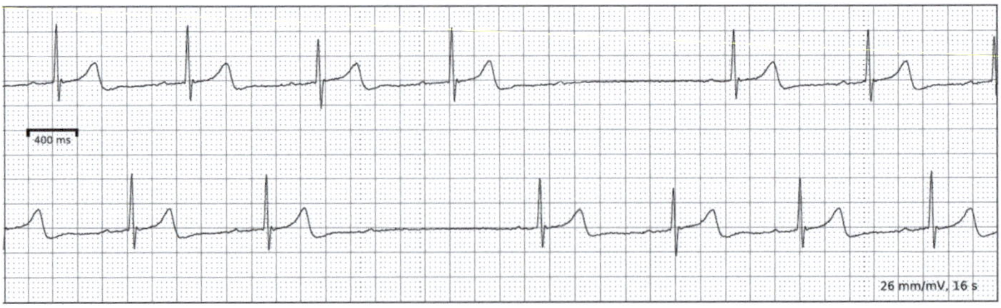

Fig. 16.8 Second-degree AV block type I (Wenckebach) in a 30-year-old patient who has undergone transcatheter device closure of a multi-fenestrated ASD. There is borderline sinus bradycardia as well

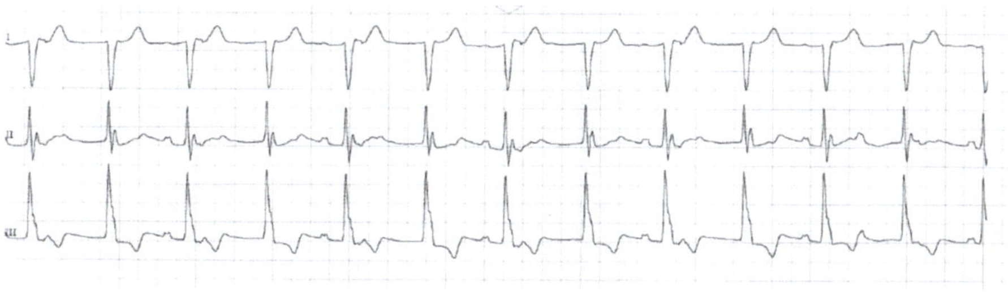

Fig. 16.9 Postoperative complete heart block in a 58-year-old patient with a bicuspid aortic valve who has undergone aortic valve replacement. His native AV conduction recovered before permanent pacemaker placement was required

16.3.2 Sinus Node Dysfunction (SND)

SND can occur congenitally in patients with heterotaxy and left atrial isomerism in whom there is often congenital absence of the sinus node. It is more common, however, as an acute or late postoperative complication, which is discussed in greater detail below. Secondary SND may be due to damage to the vascular supply to the sinus node, surgical incisions in the region of the sinus node complex, and extensive atrial fibrosis due to chronically elevated right atrial pressure. On the surface ECG, SND can appear as marked sinus bradycardia, a junctional escape rhythm with an intrinsic rate that is faster than the dysfunctional sinus node, or as a tachy-brady pattern, with alternating periods of sinus or junctional bradycardia and SVT (Fig. 16.10).

16.3.3 Management of Acute Bradyarrhythmia

Acute bradycardia is often poorly tolerated, especially in palliated single-ventricle patients and those with ventricular dysfunction, and requires rapid intervention in the form of pacing to maintain adequate cardiac output. This can be easily accomplished in patients with a pre-existing permanent pacemaker or in postsurgical patients with temporary epicardial pacing electrodes. For those individuals without pacing electrodes in place, temporary pacing can be accomplished through an externalized ("tempo-perm") transvenous pacing system. For patients with pure sinus node dysfunction, a transesophageal pacing electrode can be positioned to pace the posterior left atrial wall from the lumen of the esophagus. For urgent situations prior to institution of the previously mentioned methods, transcutaneous pacing through defibrillation pads may be required. The last option is reserved for emergencies as it can be painful to the conscious patient, carries the risk of thermal injury to the skin, and is not consistently reliable, especially in larger patients with greater distance between the surface of the skin and the myocardium. Temporary venous lead placement in Fontan patients represents a particularly complicated situation, as the traditional pacing sites have been surgically isolated from the systemic venous system.

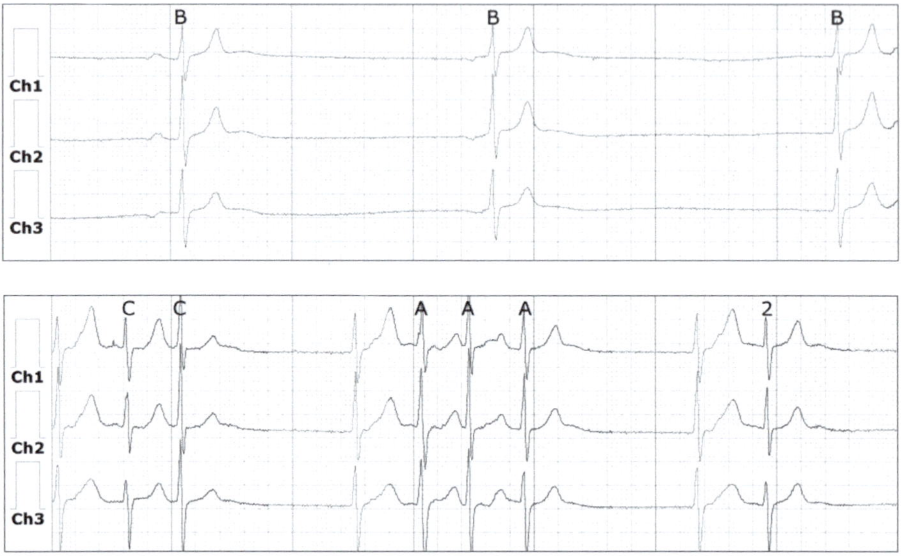

Fig. 16.10 Sinus node dysfunction in a 60-year-old patient after surgical ASD repair. The second ECG shows alternating bradycardia and SVT (tachy-brady syndrome) that can be associated with SND

Nontraditional techniques are often required to access the pulmonary venous atrium in these patients [39], and atrial pacing has even been described from the pulmonary artery [40]. Leadless cardiac pacemakers are a newer technology that may have future implications for ACHD patients, especially those with univentricular anatomy; however experience to date is limited [41, 42]. Currently these devices can only provide VVI pacing.

The pacing mode is dictated by the underlying arrhythmia. For patients with sinus node dysfunction and intact AV conduction, atrial only (AAI) pacing may be adequate. For patients with AV block, with or without sinus node dysfunction, atrial and ventricular or dual-chamber (DDD) pacing is necessary and allows for synchronized conduction between the atria and ventricles. Single site ventricle only (VVI) pacing can be an acceptable temporary alternative but is associated with poorer long-term outcomes, including pacemaker-induced cardiomyopathy.

16.4 Postoperative Arrhythmia

Arrhythmia is one of the most common and consequential complications in the immediate postoperative period after cardiac surgery [43]. Alternatively, arrhythmia management may be the chief reason for the patient being in the ICU setting. Large retrospective reviews of postoperative ICU complications in ACHD patients reveal an overall arrhythmia incidence of 9.4% and as high as 23% in Fontan patients, excluding NSVT [44]. The same study showed 1.9% overall incidence of persistent

AV block requiring permanent pacemaker placement. The risk of arrhythmia is directly related to the underlying CHD diagnosis and procedure performed and can be exacerbated by the complex physiologic response to cardiopulmonary bypass and the frequent need for pharmacological hemodynamic support. The presence of preoperative arrhythmia (14% overall, up to 53% in Fontan patients) increases post-operative risk as well, even if arrhythmia surgery is included in the operation, and preoperative arrhythmia evaluation is therefore essential to minimizing postoperative complications [45, 46]. Likewise, for high-risk surgeries or in patients with preoperative concern for bradyarrhythmia, preoperative surgical planning should include a discussion of placement of permanent epicardial pacing. Arrhythmia is also a well-recognized complication of certain transcatheter interventions, including electrophysiology studies and catheter ablation, as well as certain structural procedures, such as device closure of atrial or ventricular septal defects or transcatheter valve replacement.

16.5 Tachyarrhythmia

SVT is common for all postoperative ACHD patients but especially so in surgeries with incisions or suturing in the atria. For this reason, the highest-risk lesions are ASDs, especially of the sinus venosus type, Ebstein's anomaly of the tricuspid valve, TOF, univentricular hearts after the Fontan procedure, and DTGA after an intra-atrial baffle procedure (Mustard or Senning). Concomitant arrhythmia surgery is often included in these procedures to decrease the acute and long-term arrhythmia burden [47]. As mentioned above, junctional ectopic tachycardia (JET), which commonly develops in younger pediatric patients after surgeries that include VSD closure (or enlargement), is rarely if ever seen in ACHD patients [48]. This is likely due to greater maturity of the cardiac AV nodal myocytes in adults. NSVT is common after all types of intracardiac surgery and is rarely symptomatic or of hemodynamic consequence [49]. Beta-blockers are often initiated, both for their theoretical impact on development of sustained VT and because patients often have other indications for their use, such as hypertension or atrial fibrillation. TOF is most commonly associated with postoperative sustained VT, but there is increased risk whenever there is manipulation or incision of the ventricular body or interventricular septum, including after AV or semilunar valve surgery [50].

In addition to the treatment strategies discussed above, initial evaluation of postoperative tachyarrhythmias should include a review of any offending pharmacological or mechanical agents and any reversible causes of arrhythmia. Postoperative lines, such as pulmonary artery catheters and central venous catheters, can mechanically irritate the atrial or ventricular myocardium and lead to transient supraventricular or ventricular arrhythmia. A clue to this phenomenon is frequent ectopy that is often positional and that is electrocardiographically characterized by morphologies that are overall similar but change slightly from beat to beat. Inotropic agents, such as continuous epinephrine or norepinephrine, can cause sinus tachycardia and also potentiate rapid ventricular conduction during SVT. Milrinone, which is often used in the postoperative period for ventricular support, carries a known risk of arrhythmia [51]. Agents are also frequently used postoperatively that can prolong the QT interval, such as certain antimicrobials as well as psychotropic medications for poor sleep or ICU delirium, and care should be taken to avoid their use in patients who are at higher underlying risk for prolonged QT or torsades de pointes. Lastly, the physiological consequences of cardiopulmonary bypass often include acid-base disturbances, rapid volume shifts, and electrolyte abnormalities, all of which can exacerbate tachycarrhythmias and are potentially correctible.

Almost all antiarrhythmic medications have potentially negative inotropic effects. This can be particularly relevant in the immediate postoperative period when patients often require positive inotropic support to maintain adequate cardiac output. Certain clinical variables, such as longer cardiopulmonary bypass duration or preoperative systemic ventricular dysfunction, may increase this risk. Care must be taken to monitor for these effects or to potentially adjust the treatment strategy to prevent them altogether. The initial bolus of IV amiodarone, for example, can be given at a slower rate. Also, when using calcium channel blockers, ensuring that calcium chloride or calcium gluconate are readily available allows for rapid rescue from any negative inotropic effects.

In addition, especially when using intravenous antiarrhythmic drug therapy in the ICU setting, it is important to be aware of potential side effects of the drug being used. For instance, class 1 drugs such as procainamide (but not lidocaine) and class 3 drugs such as IV ibutilide, or sotalol (and rarely amiodarone), can cause torsades des pointes due to their effect on the QT interval. Intravenous amiodarone should be used carefully (if at all) in patients with compromised liver function or with chronic liver congestion (ass in the Fontan patients) due to its potential for acute liver toxicity. Drug level monitoring is available for a few drugs (such as digoxin, procainamide, and flecainide) and can be useful in the ICU patient.

16.6 Bradyarrhythmia

Any surgery that involves surgical manipulation near the AV node carries an attendant risk for AV block. The congenital lesions most commonly affected by this issue include atrioventricular septal defects, CCTGA, LVOT resection, and those requiring right AV valve replacement. Temporary atrial and ventricular epicardial leads are routinely placed during these procedures to allow for AV pacing. Sinus node dysfunction can occur with any surgery that involves incisions or suturing within the right atrium, and this applies to the vast majority of congenital cardiac surgeries. Specific operations are also associated with an increased prevalence of late postoperative SND (up to 20 years after surgery), including DTGA after Mustard and Senning operation and the early variants of the Fontan procedure (e.g., atriopulmonary Fontan surgery) [52]. Temporary atrial wires can be used to maintain adequate heart rate, assuming that AV node conduction is intact. The use of specific sedatives in the ICU, including dexmedetomidine, has also been shown to increase the rate of postoperative bradyarrhythmia [53].

Temporary SND or AV block due to local edema or irritation presents a challenging problem, as it is often unclear which patients will recover normal sinus rhythm and AV conduction. There is some evidence that certain genetic variants are associated with higher rates of permanent AV block after congenital heart surgery, suggesting a possible future role for genetic testing in prediction of AV node recovery [54]. In non-CHD patients who receive a permanent device, only 30–40% with SND remain pacemaker-dependent for life; this number is much higher, 65–100%, for those with postoperative complete heart block [55]. For these reasons, in patients with postoperative complete heart block, guidelines recommend observing for 5–7 days for resolution of AV block prior to placing a permanent device [56]. There is no data available as to how long to wait before opting for a permanent pacemaker in patients with postoperative sinus node dysfunction. Theophylline and terbutaline are sometimes used to treat SND dysfunction in transplant patients, but there is no evidence regarding efficacy in ACHD patients [57].

16.7 Post-interventional Catheterization Care

Patients who have recently undergone electrophysiology procedures, including catheter ablation or device implantation, rarely require treatment in the ICU. Recurrent SVT after catheter ablation is possible, either from local irritation or due to a second potential arrhythmia that was uncovered after the target arrhythmia was ablated. Unexpected sinus tachycardia in a patient who has just undergone transvenous device placement should prompt an evaluation for lead perforation causing pericardial effusion or tamponade or for a developing hematoma in the device pocket. Transcatheter interventions for structural lesions also carry variable risk for arrhythmia. ASD and VSD device closure, for example, may be complicated by heart block [58]. New ST segment changes or VT in a patient who has just undergone transcatheter semilunar valve replacement should be evaluated for coronary compromise from compression or thromboembolism [59]. Non-sustained VT may also be seen in a significant number of patients after transcatheter pulmonary valve placement [60]. Although the risk for arrhythmia after these procedures is low, and often transient, their development may require device removal and surgical correction of the underlying lesion.

16.8 Device-Related Issues

This final section briefly discusses potential complications with cardiac implantable electronic devices that may require care in the ICU.

16.8.1 Implantable Electronic Device Infections

Bloodstream infections and vegetative endocarditis in the setting of a transvenous pacing or ICD system are a potentially life-threatening complication. This represents a challenging clinic scenario, especially when the patient is dependent on the affected device. There is an increased risk of subacute bacterial endocarditis when transvenous leads are present, and the most recent guidelines include them as an indication for prophylactic antibiotics prior to dental procedures [61]. The Infectious Disease Society of America has published guidelines regarding antimicrobial and surgical management of device infections [62]. In general, if a patient is truly pacemaker-dependent, a "tempo-perm" system can be placed once the infected system has been extracted and kept in place for the duration of antimicrobial therapy. Once the infection has been treated, a new permanent system can be placed. For those patients that require ICD removal, both pharmacological management to decrease the risk of ventricular arrhythmia and an external wearable defibrillator can be utilized until a new permanent system is placed.

16.8.2 Lead Failure

Despite ongoing advancements in device lead technology, pacemaker and ICD leads remain at risk for failure from a number of mechanisms. Lead failure is a rare but serious complication with a reported incidence of 0.28–1.14% [63]. Lead failure may be related to various etiologies, such as progressive fibrosis at the electrode-tissue interface manifesting as exit block, fracture of the conductor coil, disruption of the outer insulation, externalization of the conductor cable, lead dislodgement, and improper pin connections. All of these will manifest similarly as either inappropriate sensing or loss of capture [64] (Fig. 16.11). Both of these scenarios may lead to inappropriate ICD shocks or failure to pace [65]. In the most extreme example, lead fracture can lead to oversensing and ICD storm, in which the patient receives multiple inappropriate shocks in succession (defined as three or more

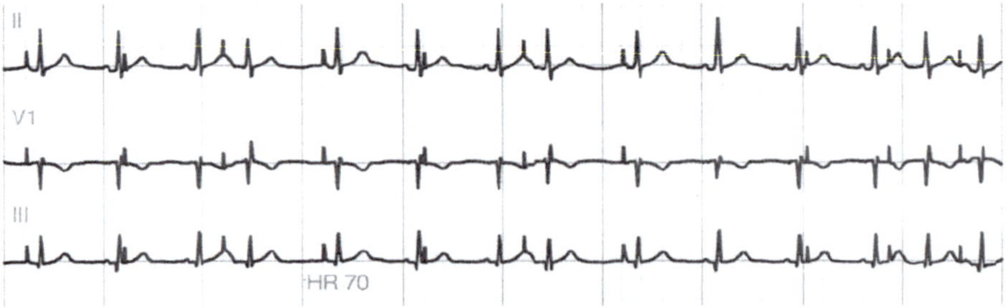

Fig. 16.11 Atrial undersensing in a 34-year-old patient with tricuspid atresia who has undergone an extra-cardiac Fontan. Note the atrial pacing spikes occur regularly at a rate of 60 beats per minute, despite native sinus rhythm. There is evidence of atrial capture, however, with consistent advance of the QRS complex after properly timed atrial pacing

shocks in a 24 h period). Fortunately, newer devices are programmed with algorithms and remote monitoring capability that allows early detection of lead failure and that can alert the patient or provider before the administration of inappropriate shocks. The emergency management for ICD storm is to apply a doughnut magnet over the device, temporarily deactivating all detection capabilities for the device. These magnets are available in all emergency rooms and most, if not all, cardiac intensive care units. Evaluation by the electrophysiology service for the proper device intervention can then ensue.

Conclusion

Dysrhythmias are common in adults with congenital heart disease and have a significant impact on their morbidity and mortality. Rapid identification and treatment of rhythm disturbances is essential to the successful management of ACHD patients in the intensive care unit.

References

1. Bouchardy J, Therrien J, Pilote L, Ionescu-Ittu R, Martucci G, Bottega N, et al. Atrial arrhythmias in adults with congenital heart disease. Circulation. 2009;120(17):1679–86.
2. Khairy P, Fernandes SM, Mayer JE Jr, Triedman JK, Walsh EP, Lock JE, et al. Long-term survival, modes of death, and predictors of mortality in patients with Fontan surgery. Circulation. 2008;117(1):85–92.
3. Khairy P, Aboulhosn J, Gurvitz MZ, Opotowsky AR, Mongeon FP, Kay J, et al. Arrhythmia burden in adults with surgically repaired tetralogy of Fallot: a multi-institutional study. Circulation. 2010;122(9):868–75.
4. Khairy P, Landzberg MJ, Lambert J, O'Donnell CP. Long-term outcomes after the atrial switch for surgical correction of transposition: a meta-analysis comparing the Mustard and Senning procedures. Cardiol Young. 2004;14(3):284–92.
5. Kirsh JA, Walsh EP, Triedman JK. Prevalence of and risk factors for atrial fibrillation and intra-atrial reentrant tachycardia among patients with congenital heart disease. Am J Cardiol. 2002;90(3):338–40.
6. Teuwen CP, Ramdjan TT, Gotte M, Brundel BJ, Evertz R, Vriend JW, et al. Time course of atrial fibrillation in patients with congenital heart defects. Circ Arrhythm Electrophysiol. 2015;8(5):1065–72.
7. Wei W, Zhan X, Xue Y, Fang X, Liao H, Deng H, et al. Features of accessory pathways in adult Ebstein's anomaly. Europace. 2014;16(11):1619–25.
8. Egbe AC, Asirvatham SJ, Connolly HM, Kapa S, Desimone CV, Vaidya VR, et al. Outcomes of direct current cardioversion in adults with congenital heart disease. Am J Cardiol. 2017;119(9):1468–72.
9. Stephenson EA, Casavant D, Tuzi J, Alexander ME, Law I, Serwer G, et al. Efficacy of atrial antitachycardia pacing using the Medtronic AT500 pacemaker in patients with congenital heart disease. Am J Cardiol. 2003;92(7):871–6.
10. Blomstrom-Lundqvist C, Scheinman MM, Aliot EM, Alpert JS, Calkins H, Camm AJ, et al. ACC/AHA/ESC guidelines for the management of patients with supraventricular arrhythmias—executive summary. a report of the American college of cardiology/American heart association task force on practice guidelines and the European society of cardiology committee for practice guidelines (writing committee to develop guidelines for the management of patients with supraventricular arrhythmias) developed in collaboration with NASPE-Heart Rhythm Society. J Am Coll Cardiol. 2003;42(8):1493–531.

11. Khairy P, Van Hare GF, Balaji S, Berul CI, Cecchin F, Cohen MI, et al. PACES/HRS Expert Consensus Statement on the Recognition and Management of Arrhythmias in Adult Congenital Heart Disease: developed in partnership between the Pediatric and Congenital Electrophysiology Society (PACES) and the Heart Rhythm Society (HRS). Endorsed by the governing bodies of PACES, HRS, the American College of Cardiology (ACC), the American Heart Association (AHA), the European Heart Rhythm Association (EHRA), the Canadian Heart Rhythm Society (CHRS), and the International Society for Adult Congenital Heart Disease (ISACHD). Heart Rhythm. 2014;11(10):e102–65.
12. Rao SO, Boramanand NK, Burton DA, Perry JC. Atrial tachycardias in young adults and adolescents with congenital heart disease: conversion using single dose oral sotalol. Int J Cardiol. 2009;136(3):253–7.
13. Gowda RM, Khan IA, Punukollu G, Vasavada BC, Sacchi TJ, Wilbur SL. Female preponderance in ibutilide-induced torsade de pointes. Int J Cardiol. 2004;95(2-3):219–22.
14. Gowda RM, Punukollu G, Khan IA, Wilbur SL, Vasavada BC, Sacchi TJ. Ibutilide for pharmacological cardioversion of atrial fibrillation and flutter: impact of race on efficacy and safety. Am J Ther. 2003;10(4):259–63.
15. Masuda K, Ishizu T, Niwa K, Takechi F, Tateno S, Horigome H, et al. Increased risk of thromboembolic events in adult congenital heart disease patients with atrial tachyarrhythmias. Int J Cardiol. 2017;234:69–75.
16. Hoffmann A, Chockalingam P, Balint OH, Dadashev A, Dimopoulos K, Engel R, et al. Cerebrovascular accidents in adult patients with congenital heart disease. Heart. 2010;96(15):1223–6.
17. Anderson JL, Halperin JL, Albert NM, Bozkurt B, Brindis RG, Curtis LH, et al. Management of patients with atrial fibrillation (compilation of 2006 ACCF/AHA/ESC and 2011 ACCF/AHA/HRS recommendations): a report of the American College of Cardiology/American Heart Association Task Force on Practice Guidelines. J Am Coll Cardiol. 2013;61(18):1935–44.
18. Khairy P, Harris L, Landzberg MJ, Fernandes SM, Barlow A, Mercier LA, et al. Sudden death and defibrillators in transposition of the great arteries with intra-atrial baffles: a multicenter study. Circ Arrhythm Electrophysiol. 2008;1(4):250–7.
19. Roy D, Talajic M, Dorian P, Connolly S, Eisenberg MJ, Green M, et al. Amiodarone to prevent recurrence of atrial fibrillation. Canadian Trial of Atrial Fibrillation Investigators. N Engl J Med. 2000;342(13):913–20.
20. Fish FA, Gillette PC, Benson DW Jr. Proarrhythmia, cardiac arrest and death in young patients receiving encainide and flecainide. The Pediatric Electrophysiology Group. J Am Coll Cardiol. 1991;18(2):356–65.
21. Padeletti L, Purerfellner H, Mont L, Tukkie R, Manolis AS, Ricci R, et al. New-generation atrial antitachycardia pacing (Reactive ATP) is associated with reduced risk of persistent or permanent atrial fibrillation in patients with bradycardia: Results from the MINERVA randomized multicenter international trial. Heart Rhythm. 2015;12(8):1717–25.
22. Zeppenfeld K, Schalij MJ, Bartelings MM, Tedrow UB, Koplan BA, Soejima K, et al. Catheter ablation of ventricular tachycardia after repair of congenital heart disease: electroanatomic identification of the critical right ventricular isthmus. Circulation. 2007;116(20):2241–52.
23. Oechslin EN, Harrison DA, Connelly MS, Webb GD, Siu SC. Mode of death in adults with congenital heart disease. Am J Cardiol. 2000;86(10):1111–6.
24. Avila P, Chaix MA, Mondesert B, Khairy P. Sudden cardiac death in adult congenital heart disease. Card Electrophysiol Clin. 2017;9(2):225–34.
25. Koyak Z, Harris L, de Groot JR, Silversides CK, Oechslin EN, Bouma BJ, et al. Sudden cardiac death in adult congenital heart disease. Circulation. 2012;126(16):1944–54.
26. Silka MJ, Hardy BG, Menashe VD, Morris CD. A population-based prospective evaluation of risk of sudden cardiac death after operation for common congenital heart defects. J Am Coll Cardiol. 1998;32(1):245–51.

27. Gallego P, Gonzalez AE, Sanchez-Recalde A, Peinado R, Polo L, Gomez-Rubin C, et al. Incidence and predictors of sudden cardiac arrest in adults with congenital heart defects repaired before adult life. Am J Cardiol. 2012;110(1):109–17.
28. Wang W, Lian Z, Rowin EJ, Maron BJ, Maron MS, Link MS. Prognostic implications of non-sustained ventricular tachycardia in high-risk patients with hypertrophic cardiomyopathy. Circ Arrhythm Electrophysiol. 2017;10(3):e004604.
29. Giorgberidze I, Saksena S, Krol RB, Munsif AN, Kolettis T, Mathew P, et al. Risk stratification and clinical outcome of minimally symptomatic and asymptomatic patients with nonsustained ventricular tachycardia and coronary disease: a prospective single-center study. Am J Cardiol. 1997;80(5B):3F–9F.
30. Vehmeijer JT, Brouwer TF, Limpens J, Knops RE, Bouma BJ, Mulder BJ, et al. Implantable cardioverter-defibrillators in adults with congenital heart disease: a systematic review and meta-analysis. Eur Heart J. 2016;37(18):1439–48.
31. Khairy P, Landzberg MJ, Gatzoulis MA, Mercier LA, Fernandes SM, Cote JM, et al. Transvenous pacing leads and systemic thromboemboli in patients with intracardiac shunts: a multicenter study. Circulation. 2006;113(20):2391–7.
32. Moore JP, Mondesert B, Lloyd MS, Cook SC, Zaidi AN, Pass RH, et al. Clinical experience with the subcutaneous implantable cardioverter-defibrillator in adults with congenital heart disease. Circ Arrhythm Electrophysiol. 2016;9(9):e004338.
33. Rao M, Goldenberg I, Moss AJ, Klein H, Huang DT, Bianco NR, et al. Wearable defibrillator in congenital structural heart disease and inherited arrhythmias. Am J Cardiol. 2011;108(11):1632–8.
34. Kapel GF, Reichlin T, Wijnmaalen AP, Piers SR, Holman ER, Tedrow UB, et al. Re-entry using anatomically determined isthmuses: a curable ventricular tachycardia in repaired congenital heart disease. Circ Arrhythm Electrophysiol. 2015;8(1):102–9.
35. Buckley U, Yamakawa K, Takamiya T, Andrew Armour J, Shivkumar K, Ardell JL. Targeted stellate decentralization: Implications for sympathetic control of ventricular electrophysiology. Heart Rhythm. 2016;13(1):282–8.
36. Simmons MA, Rollinson N, Fishberger S, Qin L, Fahey J, Elder RW. Modern incidence of complete heart block in patients with l-looped ventricles: does univentricular status matter? Congenit Heart Dis. 2015;10(5):E237–42.
37. Hayward RM, Foster E, Tseng ZH. Maternal and fetal outcomes of admission for delivery in women with congenital heart disease. JAMA Cardiol. 2017;2:664–71.
38. Pillutla P, Nguyen T, Markovic D, Canobbio M, Koos BJ, Aboulhosn JA. Cardiovascular and neonatal outcomes in pregnant women with high-risk congenital heart disease. Am J Cardiol. 2016;117(10):1672–7.
39. Moore JP, Hendrickson B, Brunengraber DZ, Shannon KM. Transcaval puncture for access to the pulmonary venous atrium after the extracardiac total cavopulmonary connection operation. Circ Arrhythm Electrophysiol. 2015;8(4):824–8.
40. Moore JP, Shannon KM. Transpulmonary atrial pacing: an approach to transvenous pacemaker implantation after extracardiac conduit Fontan surgery. J Cardiovasc Electrophysiol. 2014;25(9):1028–31.
41. Reddy VY, Exner DV, Cantillon DJ, Doshi R, Bunch TJ, Tomassoni GF, et al. Percutaneous implantation of an entirely intracardiac leadless pacemaker. N Engl J Med. 2015;373(12):1125–35.
42. Wilson DG, Morgan JM, Roberts PR. "Leadless" pacing of the left ventricle in adult congenital heart disease. Int J Cardiol. 2016;209:96–7.
43. Koyak Z, Achterbergh RC, de Groot JR, Berger F, Koolbergen DR, Bouma BJ, et al. Postoperative arrhythmias in adults with congenital heart disease: incidence and risk factors. Int J Cardiol. 2013;169(2):139–44.
44. Mascio CE, Pasquali SK, Jacobs JP, Jacobs ML, Austin EH 3rd. Outcomes in adult congenital heart surgery: analysis of the Society of Thoracic Surgeons database. J Thorac Cardiovasc Surg. 2011;142(5):1090–7.

45. Brida M, Baumgartner H, Gatzoulis MA, Diller GP. Early mortality and concomitant procedures related to Fontan conversion: quantitative analysis. Int J Cardiol. 2017;236:132–7.
46. Sabate Rotes A, Connolly HM, Warnes CA, Ammash NM, Phillips SD, Dearani JA, et al. Ventricular arrhythmia risk stratification in patients with tetralogy of Fallot at the time of pulmonary valve replacement. Circ Arrhythm Electrophysiol. 2015;8(1):110–6.
47. Giamberti A, Pluchinotta FR, Chessa M, Varrica A, Vitale R, Frigiola A, et al. Surgery for supraventricular tachycardia and congenital heart defects: long-term efficacy of the combined approach in adult patients. Europace. 2016;19:1542–8.
48. Moak JP, Arias P, Kaltman JR, Cheng Y, McCarter R, Hanumanthaiah S, et al. Postoperative junctional ectopic tachycardia: risk factors for occurrence in the modern surgical era. Pacing Clin Electrophysiol. 2013;36(9):1156–68.
49. Marine JE. Nonsustained ventricular tachycardia in the normal heart: risk stratification and management. Card Electrophysiol Clin. 2016;8(3):525–43.
50. Wu MH, Lu CW, Chen HC, Chiu SN, Kao FY, Huang SK. Arrhythmic burdens in patients with tetralogy of Fallot: a national database study. Heart Rhythm. 2015;12(3):604–9.
51. Smith AH, Owen J, Borgman KY, Fish FA, Kannankeril PJ. Relation of milrinone after surgery for congenital heart disease to significant postoperative tachyarrhythmias. Am J Cardiol. 2011;108(11):1620–4.
52. Gelatt M, Hamilton RM, McCrindle BW, Connelly M, Davis A, Harris L, et al. Arrhythmia and mortality after the Mustard procedure: a 30-year single-center experience. J Am Coll Cardiol. 1997;29(1):194–201.
53. Shuplock JM, Smith AH, Owen J, Van Driest SL, Marshall M, Saville B, et al. Association between perioperative dexmedetomidine and arrhythmias after surgery for congenital heart disease. Circ Arrhythm Electrophysiol. 2015;8(3):643–50.
54. Murray LE, Smith AH, Flack EC, Crum K, Owen J, Kannankeril PJ. Genotypic and phenotypic predictors of complete heart block and recovery of conduction after surgical repair of congenital heart disease. Heart Rhythm. 2017;14(3):402–9.
55. Peretto G, Durante A, Limite LR, Cianflone D. Postoperative arrhythmias after cardiac surgery: incidence, risk factors, and therapeutic management. Cardiol Res Pract. 2014;2014:615987.
56. European Society of Cardiology, European Heart Rhythm Association, Brignole M, Auricchio A, Baron-Esquivias G, Bordachar P, et al. 2013 ESC guidelines on cardiac pacing and cardiac resynchronization therapy: the task force on cardiac pacing and resynchronization therapy of the European Society of Cardiology (ESC). Developed in collaboration with the European Heart Rhythm Association (EHRA). Europace. 2013;15(8):1070–118.
57. Kertesz NJ, Towbin JA, Clunie S, Fenrich AL, Friedman RA, Kearney DL, et al. Long-term follow-up of arrhythmias in pediatric orthotopic heart transplant recipients: incidence and correlation with rejection. J Heart Lung Transplant. 2003;22(8):889–93.
58. Rigatelli G, Zuin M, Pedon L, Zecchel R, Dell'Avvocata F, Carrozza A, et al. Clinically apparent long-term electric disturbances in the acute and very long-term of patent foramen ovale device-based closure. Cardiovasc Revasc Med. 2017;18(2):118–22.
59. Loar RW, Qureshi AM, Miyake CY, Valdes SO, Kim JJ, De la Uz CM. Percutaneous pulmonary valve implantation-associated ventricular tachycardia in congenital heart disease. J Interv Cardiol. 2016;29(6):639–45.
60. Prirompríntr B, Silka MJ, Rhodes J, Batra AS. A prospective 5-year study of the frequency of arrhythmias during serial exercise testing and clinical follow-up after Melody valve implant. Heart Rhythm. 2016;13(11):2135–41.
61. Wilson W, Taubert KA, Gewitz M, Lockhart PB, Baddour LM, Levison M, et al. Prevention of infective endocarditis: guidelines from the American Heart Association: a guideline from the American Heart Association Rheumatic Fever, Endocarditis, and Kawasaki Disease Committee, Council on Cardiovascular Disease in the Young, and the Council on Clinical Cardiology, Council on Cardiovascular Surgery and Anesthesia, and the Quality of Care and Outcomes Research Interdisciplinary Working Group. Circulation. 2007;116(15):1736–54.

62. Baddour LM, Epstein AE, Erickson CC, Knight BP, Levison ME, Lockhart PB, et al. Update on cardiovascular implantable electronic device infections and their management: a scientific statement from the American Heart Association. Circulation. 2010;121(3):458–77.
63. Liu J, Brumberg G, Rattan R, Patel D, Adelstein E, Jain S, et al. Longitudinal follow-up of implantable cardioverter defibrillator leads. Am J Cardiol. 2014;113(1):103–6.
64. Swerdlow CD, Kalahasty G, Ellenbogen KA. Implantable cardiac defibrillator lead failure and management. J Am Coll Cardiol. 2016;67(11):1358–68.
65. Garnreiter JM, Pilcher TA, Etheridge SP, Saarel EV. Inappropriate ICD shocks in pediatrics and congenital heart disease patients: risk factors and programming strategies. Heart Rhythm. 2015;12(5):937–42.

Critical Care Management of the ACHD Patient with Endocarditis

17

Laurence Iserin

17.1 Introduction

Admission to the intensive care unit (ICU) is frequently a part of the patient pathway following surgery for infectious endocarditis (IE). In addition, patients with IE may be admitted to the ICU due to IE complications such as heart, renal, or hepatic failure, septic shock, or stroke. In a non-congenital population study, reasons for admission to the ICU in this context were congestive cardiac failure (64%), septic shock (21%), neurological deterioration (15%), and cardiopulmonary resuscitation (9%) [1]. Finally, critically ill patients can acquire IE during an ICU stay due to multiple venous access and CLABSI. CHD population has an increased incidence of IE, and patients often present with numerous risk factors such as comorbidities, prosthesis IE, and *Staphylococcus* sp. infection. Therefore, they can be admitted to the ICU for the same reasons as non-ACHD patients, but every step of their management from diagnosis to medical or surgical treatment can be different from strategies usually utilized with non-ACHD patients with IE [2].

17.2 Cardiac Anatomy Hemodynamics and Vascular Access

Detailed anatomy and surgical repair should be well understood in ACHD patients with IE. A regular follow-up and the knowledge of patient's background and previous interventions can help to determine the probable site of infection. In a previously unknown patient or in a complex patient, echocardiographic assessment by an expert is promptly needed [3].

L. Iserin
ACHD Unit, Cardiology Department and M3C center of reference for complex congenital defects, Hôpital Européen Georges Pompidou, Paris, France
e-mail: laurence.iserin@egp.aphp.fr

E. da Cruz et al. (eds.), *Intensive Care of the Adult with Congenital Heart Disease*, Congenital Heart Disease in Adolescents and Adults,
https://doi.org/10.1007/978-3-319-94171-4_17

Furthermore, in an instable patient admitted to the ICU, several other issues should be discussed within the team:

- Hemodynamic tolerance to the IE within the patient's anatomy and physiology (e.g., operated or not, O_2 saturation objectives, tolerance to volume replacement, and risk of arrhythmias on vasopressors).
- Use of central venous lines (e.g., in a superior cavopulmonary shunt, the line should be withdrawn into the superior vena cava).
- Use of arterial lines (e.g., not reliable on a patient who underwent a Blalock–Taussig shunt).
- Risk of air embolism in case of right-to-left shunt.
- Invasive arterial access may be impossible or else unreliable in upper limbs on the side of a previous Blalock–Taussig shunt.

17.3 Epidemiology

IE is responsible for the highest length of hospital stay when compared to other causes of admission in an ACHD population [4]. In the non-congenital population, admissions for IE represent 3% of admissions in intensive care unit. In ACHD patients though, the risk of endocarditis is much higher than in the general population (11 cases/1000 person-years vs. 3–7 per 100,000 person-years) [5, 6]. Compared to the non-congenital population, its outcome is usually seen as less severe. Nevertheless, in a British tertiary center, the reported IE-related mortality is 6.9 % [7] (vs. 4% in a "historical cohort") [8] but rated as high as 16% in the Dutch CONCOR registry (vs. 20% in-hospital mortality in the non-congenital population, rising up to 50% in critically ill patients) [9]. This increasing frequency and severity can be explained by the growing population with complex and multiple diseases and by the increase of devices such as percutaneous valve implantations, implantable cardiac defibrillators, and pacemakers [10, 11].

Risk of men with ACHD to develop IE is higher than in women, one of the possible speculated causes being the difference in dental hygiene between men and women.

The commonest affected sites vary according to different studies: within non-operated lesions, ventricular septal defects (VSD) are the most frequently affected anomalies, followed by aortic stenosis and bicuspid aortic valve; among operated lesions, tetralogy of Fallot and atrioventricular septal defects are the commonest [8, 12, 13]. In the recent CONCOR study, the main affected defect for IE is pulmonary atresia with VSD. In this same cohort including more than 15,000 patients, independent predictors of IE in this specific population were baseline valve-containing prosthetics, multiple defects, previous IE, and gender [5, 9].

Finally, patients with 22q11 deletions (10% of conotruncal defects) have variable depressed immunological status; they are therefore at higher risk of cardiac postoperative infection, but the weight of this comorbidity in IE is not fully elucidated [14].

17.4 Prophylaxis

As this chapter focuses on critically ill patients, prophylaxis is rarely an issue. Nevertheless, it is important to emphasize that the European and American societies [3, 15] have recommended antibiotic prophylaxis restricted to high-risk dental procedures in patients at highest risk for IE. High-risk dental procedures are the ones that require manipulation of the gingival or periapical region of the teeth or perforation of the oral mucosa [16].

Patients at the highest risk for IE are those (1) with any prosthetic valve, including a transcatheter valve, or those in whom any prosthetic material was used for cardiac valve repair, (2) patients with a previous episode of IE, and (3) patients with CHD. The latter includes any type of cyanotic CHD and any type of CHD repaired with a prosthetic material, whether placed surgically or by percutaneous techniques, up to 6 months after the index procedure or lifelong if any residual shunt or valvular regurgitation remains. Recommendations in the USA extend this strategy to transplanted patients with valvular disease. In the UK, the NICE group does not recommend any antibiotic prophylaxis considering that the risk–benefit balance of this strategy has not been reliably established [17].

Also, in the European and American recommendations, systematic antibiotic prophylaxis is not advised for non-dental procedures. Pre-procedure (surgical or interventional) antibiotic therapy is only needed when invasive procedures are performed in the context of infection. Notwithstanding this, preoperative antibiotic therapy to prevent on-site infection is routinely given in different surgical procedures including cardiac surgery, implantation of electronic devices, and gynecologic and visceral surgery; such recommendations arise from scientific societies rather than established guidelines [18, 19].

17.5 Antecedent Events

Cardiac surgery itself is a risk factor for endocarditis. In the CONCOR cohort, about half of the patients (1389/2427) who underwent congenital heart surgery after age 18 years had valvular surgery performed [20].

Early postoperative IE is classified as endocarditis occurring during the first postoperative year (mainly due to *Staphylococcus aureus* or coagulase negative). Late postoperative IE occurs after 1 year (mainly due to streptococcus and other bacteria found in native valve endocarditis).

The percutaneous pulmonary valve implantation (PPVI) with the bovine jugular valve (BJV) has been described in several studies [21–23] as a favorable substrate for IE. This prosthetic material also used as a surgical material (Venpro tube) carries a high risk of early and late IE, suggesting that the substrate for future infections may be related to the tissue rather than the method of implantation. Compared to non-bovine valves, the PPVI with BJV carries a higher risk of IE. A recent meta-analysis evaluating right-sided endocarditis and comparing the incidence and outcomes in patients with a surgical and percutaneous pulmonary valve confirmed a higher incidence of IE for BJV compared with other valves (5.4% vs. 1.2%) [24].

Interventional closure of atrial septal defects or ventricular septal defects, stent implantation, or closure of patent ductus arteriosus may also be complicated by infective endocarditis, but except if a residual leak is present, IE occurs exclusively during the 6 months post-procedure [9]. Bacteremia with risk of IE can also occur during uncomplicated vaginal delivery (1–5%) and in patients having had insertion of a contraceptive device.

In young patients, piercing, tattooing, acne, or intravenous drug abuse can be a source of infection as well [25].

Education of each patient is crucial. As a prevention strategy, in our team we give cards to high-risk patients with the antibiotic prophylaxis guidelines and also with the mention that "blood cultures should be done in case of unexplained fever" [26].

17.6 Diagnostic in Critically Ill Patients

The modified Duke criteria are most commonly used nowadays for the diagnosis of endocarditis (Table 17.1) [27]. The diagnosis of IE is based on clinical signs and echocardiogram, although auscultation is of poor contribution in ACHD patients. IE should be suspected in all patients with CHD presenting with fever or newly manifesting heart failure. Transthoracic echocardiography (TTE) is used as the first imaging step, but transesophageal echocardiography (TEE) may be necessary depending on patient habitus and echogenicity and also allows the detection of smaller lesions in left heart endocarditis.

The recent ESC recommendation had recently emphasized the contribution of CT scanner or even 18F-fluorodeoxyglucose positron emission tomography/computed tomography in congenital patients [28], but the latter technique cannot be applied in an unstable patient. Conversely, the CT scanner can easily assess patients for suspected cardiac abscess and the presence of systemic or pulmonary emboli (Figs. 17.1 and 17.2), especially in complex anatomy. The CT scanner in ACHD provides important data on the detailed anatomy, the presence of abscess or even dehiscent patches, and should be, in our view, routinely performed as preoperative assessment in ACHD patients.

Not infrequently, in ACHD patients, diagnosis of IE can be difficult. Firstly, the distinction between right and left endocarditis is not always possible. In the case of cyanotic disease, emboli can be in the systemic or pulmonary circulation. In patients with unclosed VSD, pulmonary emboli are the rule, but the aortic valve can be infected by proximity to the defect. In case of right heart IE with pulmonary emboli, the diagnosis is often made late as patients are often treated for recurrent pulmonary infection.

Table 17.1 Definition of terms used in the proposed modified Duke criteria for the diagnosis of infective endocarditis (IE) (From Li)

Major criteria
Blood culture positive for IE
• Typical microorganisms consistent with IE from two separate blood cultures:
Viridans streptococci, *Streptococcus bovis*, HACEK group, *Staphylococcus aureus*, or community-acquired enterococci, in the absence of a primary focus
• Microorganisms consistent with IE from persistently positive blood cultures, defined as follows:
At least two positive cultures of blood samples drawn >12 h apart
All of the three or a majority of more than four separate cultures of blood (with the first and last sample drawn at least 1 h apart)
• Single positive blood culture for *Coxiella burnetii* or antiphase I IgG antibody titer >1:800
Evidence of endocardial involvement
• Echocardiogram positive for IE
(TEE recommended in patients with prosthetic valves, rated at least "possible IE"
by clinical criteria, or complicated IE [paravalvular abscess]; TTE as the first test in other patients), defined as follows:
Oscillating intracardiac mass on valve or supporting structures, in the path of regurgitant jets, or on implanted material in the absence of an alternative anatomic explanation
Abscess
New partial dehiscence of prosthetic valve and new valvular regurgitation (worsening or changing of preexisting murmur not sufficient)
Minor criteria
• *Predisposition*
Predisposing heart condition or injection drug use
• *Fever* (temperature >38 °C)
• *Vascular phenomena*: major arterial emboli, septic pulmonary infarcts, mycotic aneurysm, intracranial hemorrhage, conjunctival hemorrhages, and Janeway's lesions
• *Immunologic phenomena*: glomerulonephritis, Osler's nodes, Roth's spots, and rheumatoid factor
• *Microbiological evidence*: positive blood culture but does not meet a major criterion as noted above or serological evidence of active infection with organism consistent with IE

Diagnosis of IE is made by the association of two major criteria, one major criterion and three minor criteria, or five minor criteria. IE is declared possible if one major criterion and one minor criterion are met or if three minor criteria are present

TEE may not be as contributive as in non-congenital patients. For example, pulmonary IE in prosthesis in particular is not well assessed by TEE; in case of cyanotic patients with systemic to pulmonary anastomosis, IE visualization of vegetations by TTE or TEE is unlikely. In these circumstances, the use of CT scanner can facilitate the identification of vegetations in a conduit as well as the presence of emboli [29–31].

As far as bacteriologic diagnosis is concerned, the rules are the same as in non-congenital patients. A specific situation can be found in a pulmonary prosthetic IE (surgical or percutaneous valve) with severe obstruction and non-identified bacteria. As a lifesaving procedure, we have in three occasions performed interventional catheterization to open the valve, in order to restore hemodynamic balance. During the procedure, blood cultures into the pulmonary artery can then be performed, bypassing the "lung filter."

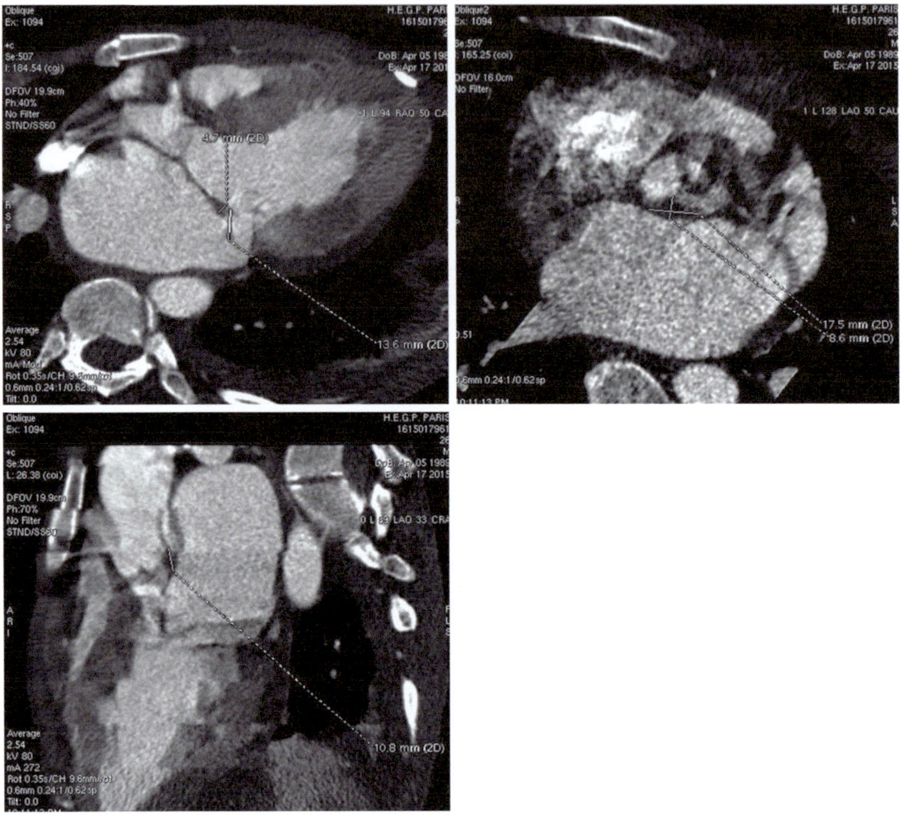

Fig. 17.1 CT scanner on a patient with bicuspid aortic valve. Aortic and mitral vegetations, with aortic posterior abscess (Courtesy of Dr. G. Soulat and Pr. E. Mousseaux, Vascular Radiology, HEGP)

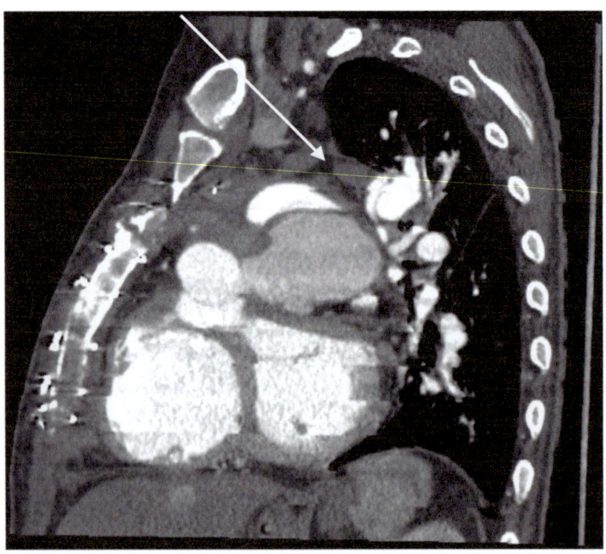

Fig. 17.2 CT scanner of a patient with operated tetralogy of Fallot with pulmonary bioprosthesis and septic false aortic aneurysm (*arrow*) (Courtesy of Dr. G Soulat and Pr. E Mousseaux, Vascular Radiology, HEGP)

17.7 Screening Patients at High Risks upon Admission

Patients with left heart IE, HF, peri-annular complications, and/or *S. aureus* infection are at the highest risk of death and need surgery in the active phase of the disease. When three of these factors are present, the odds of demise reach 79% [1, 32]. In pulmonary valve IE, symptoms of an obstructed valve can be misleading (e.g., chest pain, low blood pressure, renal failure).

17.8 Neurological Evaluation

Clinical evaluation of patients with suspected IE is crucial as altered mental status at IE onset, which is associated with brain injury, is a major determinant of short-term outcome.

Systematic MRI is recommended in left-sided IE as neurological complications of IE are numerous and can contraindicate cardiac surgery. In this scenario brain MRI may reveal cerebral abnormalities in up to 80% of patients, including cerebral embolism in 50%, most of the patients being asymptomatic [33].

Management of neurological complications of endocarditis is identical to non-ACHD patients, keeping in mind, though, that ACHD patients although young have a high incidence of preexisting cerebral lesions, either due to post-operative insults or to silent embolic events (e.g., in cyanotic patients). In non-ACHD patients, a recent cohort study reported that a period of heightened stroke risk becomes apparent several months before the diagnosis of IE and lasts for several months afterward, but there is no data to support the same process in ACHD patients [34–36].

17.9 Causative Pathogens

As in the general population, *Staphylococcus* sp. and *Streptococcus* sp. are responsible for 80–90% of IE cases. The difference is rather between *Staphylococcus aureus*, more related to healthy or operated patients, and *Streptococcus* being predominant in native lesions [3, 12]. *Staphylococcus aureus* is a highly destructive microorganism and identified in several studies as a risk factor for larger vegetations and for mortality. Nevertheless, it is not by itself an indication for surgery as previously thought. As in non-congenital patients, blood culture-negative IE occurs in up to 30% of case, supposedly because of the previous antibiotic use. Culture negativity can also be related to slow-growing microorganisms such as *Brucella*, *Coxiella burnetii*, *Bartonella*, *Tropheryma whipplei*, *Mycoplasma*, or *Legionella* or, rarely, fungi. Complementary and specific serologies and histopathological specimen analysis can be done if no bacteria are found on repeated blood cultures [37].

17.10 Empirical Therapy

In critically ill patients (septic shock), once blood cultures are taken, treatment of IE should be immediately started, before microorganism identification. As it might be an emergency decision, we support the recommendations for empirical therapy, within the mindset that targeted therapy once the microorganism is identified remains the goal.

In the ESC recommendations [3], the initial choice of empirical treatment depends on several considerations:

1. Whether the patient has received previous antibiotic therapy
2. Whether the infection affects a native valve or a prosthesis and if so, when surgery was performed (early vs. late PVE)
3. The place of the infection (community, nosocomial, or non-nosocomial healthcare-associated IE) and knowledge of the local epidemiology, especially for antibiotic resistance and specific genuine culture-negative pathogens

In community-acquired native valve or late prosthetic valve (≥12 months postsurgery) endocarditis, in order to cover staphylococci, streptococci, and enterococci, the use of ampicillin with (flu) cloxacillin or oxacillin with gentamicin (or in case of allergy, vancomycin with gentamicin) is recommended.

For patients with early PVE (<12 months postsurgery) or nosocomial and non-nosocomial healthcare-associated endocarditis, in order to cover methicillin-resistant staphylococci, enterococci, and, ideally, non-HACEK Gram-negative pathogens, vancomycin with gentamicin added with rifampin (only in case of PVE and delayed for 4–5 days after the beginning of vancomycin) is recommended.

In the US recommendations, objectives are the same but cephalosporins (cefepime in NVE or ceftriaxone in late PVE) are recommended rather than penicillin [15]. If subsequent blood culture results or other laboratory methodologies define a pathogen, then empirical therapy should be revised to focused therapy that is recommended for the specific identified pathogen.

17.11 Complications and Surgical Indications During the Acute Phase

As in non-ACHD patients, left-sided IE acute main complications are heart failure, uncontrolled sepsis or thromboembolic events, and neurologic complications. In this group, by analogy cyanotic disease should be seen as potential right and left heart IE. These life-threatening complications are themselves considered as indications for surgery, but caregivers should keep in mind that surgery is not always feasible in complex disease (especially in univentricular physiology or in cyanotic patients with or without pulmonary hypertension such as Eisenmenger syndrome).

Classical risk factors for surgical mortality in non-ACHD patients (such as diabetes) are not always present in ACHD patients, but these may have a high frequency of preexisting renal or hepatic impairment [30]. Furthermore, in this population severely underweight BMI is associated with increased unplanned cardiac operation and reoperation for bleeding, whereas obesity is associated with increased risk of wound infection.

There are, even in non-ACHD patients, no firm recommendations on the timing of surgery during the acute phase as it represents a dilemma between the high risk of the operation during an uncontrolled sepsis and the benefit of preventing heart failure or thromboembolic events. Further, more recent studies have shown that the embolic risk of the vegetations is maximal during the first days of diagnosis and treatment.

Recently, published data suggest that after an ischemic stroke surgery indicated for heart failure, uncontrolled infection, abscess, or persisting high emboli risk should not be delayed, provided that the patient is not comatose or has no severe deficit. Surgery should be postponed for 2–3 weeks for patients with intracranial hemorrhage [38, 39]. Endovascular treatment is recommended for cerebral mycotic aneurysms, if there is no severe mass effect [40].

In non-congenital patients, multidisciplinary strategies for management of IE cases by intensivists , cardiologists, infectious disease specialists, and cardiac surgeons have been found to improve survival [41–43]. This kind of approach is mandatory with ACHD patients, and the team should also include ACHD specialists, physicians, and surgeons. Adapted recommendations for ACHD patients for the timing of surgery are summarized in Table 17.2.

17.12 Choice of Surgical Substitute

In young adults with ACHD, cryopreserved or sterilized homografts are often used both in order to reduce the risk of persistent or recurrent infection, especially in the presence of annular abscesses, and to avoid mechanical prosthesis in young adults. However, mechanical prostheses and xenografts have led to similar results in terms of persistent or recurrent infection. Ross procedure may be used in children or adolescents to facilitate growth and in young adults for extended durability. The surgery should be reserved to experienced congenital surgeons, integrity of pulmonary valve should be checked, and this long surgery is often not suitable in unstable patients [39].

Cardiac transplantation may be considered in extreme cases where repeated operative procedures have failed to eradicate persistent or recurrent IE. We have this experience in two patients with very good long-term results.

The specific case of obstructed pulmonary valve is a very high-risk situation, and cardiac catheterization might be an option to relieve the obstruction and allow a delayed surgical procedure upon clinical stability.

Table 17.2 Indications for surgery in acute phase of IE for ACHD patients (adapted from Eur Heart J, 2015)

(A) In left-sided valve infective endocarditis (or cyanotic patients)	
Heart failure	
Aortic or mitral NVE or PVE with severe acute regurgitation, obstruction, or fistula causing refractory	Emergency
Aortic or mitral NVE or PVE with severe regurgitation or obstruction causing symptoms of HF or echocardiographic signs of poor hemodynamic tolerance	Urgent
Uncontrolled infection	
Locally uncontrolled infection (abscess, false aneurysm, fistula, enlarging vegetation)	Urgent
Infection caused by fungi or multiresistant organisms	Urgent/ elective
Persisting positive blood cultures despite appropriate antibiotic therapy and adequate control of septic metastatic foci	Urgent
PVE caused by staphylococci or non-HACEK Gram-negative bacteria	Urgent/ elective
Prevention of embolism	
Aortic or mitral NVE or PVE with persistent vegetations .10 mm after one or more embolic episode despite appropriate antibiotic therapy	Urgent
Aortic or mitral NVE with vegetations .10 mm, associated with severe valve stenosis or regurgitation, and low operative risk	Urgent
Aortic or mitral NVE or PVE with isolated very large vegetations (.30 mm)	Urgent
Aortic or mitral NVE or PVE with isolated large vegetations (.15 mm) and no other indication for surgery	Urgent
(B) In right-sided valve infective endocarditis	
Uncontrolled infection Microorganisms difficult to eradicate (e.g., persistent fungi) or bacteremia for 7 days (e.g., *S. aureus*, *P. aeruginosa*) despite adequate antimicrobial therapy	Elective
Persistent tricuspid valve vegetations .20 mm after recurrent pulmonary emboli with or without concomitant right heart failure	Urgent/ elective
Hemodynamic compromise	
Right HF secondary to severe tricuspid regurgitation with poor response to diuretic therapy	Urgent/ elective
Obstructive pulmonary valve (especially in a previously small or stenosed conduit. This can also be an indication of interventional catheter as lifesaving procedure)	Emergency

Emergency surgery: surgery performed within 24 h
Urgent surgery: within a few days
Elective surgery: after at least 1–2 weeks of antibiotic therapy

17.13 Anticoagulants

In left-sided IE, cessation of oral anticoagulants is recommended with a surrogate administration of subcutaneous heparin. This is recommended specifically in unstable patients with a high risk of hemorrhagic stroke. In pulmonary or tricuspid IE without shunts, there are no firm recommendations, bearing in mind that in some patients obstruction of the pulmonary valve may occur after cessation of antiplatelet therapy [23].

Conclusion

A number of issues are still unsolved in the management of severe IE, both in non-ACHD population and in the ACHD population, with various defects and surgical repairs. Comorbidities are different (younger population but renal pulmonary and hepatic fragility). Recent data support the creation of multidisciplinary endocarditis teams that ought to be inclusive of the ACHD team experts.

References

1. Mirabel M, Sonneville R, Hajage D, Novy E, Tubach F, Vignon P, Perez P, Lavoué S, Kouatchet A, Pajot O, Mekontso-Dessap A, Tonnelier JM, Bollaert PE, Frat JP, Navellou JC, Hyvernat H, Hssain AA, Timsit JF, Megarbane B, Wolff M, Trouillet JL, ENDOREA Study Group. Long-term outcomes and cardiac surgery in critically ill patients with infective endocarditis. Eur Heart J. 2014;35(18):1195–204.
2. Price S, Jaggar SI, Jordan S, et al. Adult congenital heart disease: intensive care management and outcome prediction. Intensive Care Med. 2007;33:652–9.
3. Habib G, Lancellotti P, Antunes MJ, Bongiorni MG, Casalta JP, Del Zotti F, Dulgheru R, El Khoury G, Erba PA, Iung B, Miro JM, Mulder BJ, Plonska-Gosciniak E, Price S, Roos-Hesselink J, Snygg-Martin U, Thuny F, Tornos Mas P, Vilacosta I, Zamorano JL. 2015 ESC guidelines for the management of infective endocarditis: The Task Force for the Management of Infective Endocarditis of the European Society of Cardiology (ESC). Eur Heart J. 2015;36(44):3075–128.
4. Cedars A, Benjamin L, Burns SV, Novak E, Amin A. Clinical predictors of length of stay in adults with congenital heart disease. Heart. 2017;103(16):1258–63.
5. Verheugt CL, Uiterwaal CS, van der Velde ET, Meijboom FJ, Pieper PG, Veen G, Stappers JL, Grobbee DE, Mulder BJ. Turning 18 with congenital heart disease: prediction of infective endocarditis based on a large population. Eur Heart J. 2011;32:1926–34.
6. Mourvillier B, Trouillet JL, Timsit JF, et al. Infective endocarditis in the intensive care unit. Clinical spectrum and prognostic factors in 228 consecutive patients. Intensive Care Med. 2004;30:2046–52.
7. Tutarel O, Alonso-Gonzalez R, Montanaro C, Schiff R, Uribarri A, Kempny A, Grübler MR, Uebing A, Swan L, Diller GP, Dimopoulos K, Gatzoulis MA. Infective endocarditis in adults with congenital heart disease remains a lethal disease. Heart. 2018;104:161–5.
8. Li W, Somerville J. Infective endocarditis in the grown-up congenital heart (GUCH) population. Eur Heart J. 1998;19:166–73.
9. Kuijpers JM, Koolbergen DR, Groenink M, Peels KCH, Reichert CLA, Post MC, Bosker HA, Wajon EMCJ, Zwinderman AH, Mulder BJM, Bouma BJ. Incidence, risk factors, and predictors of infective endocarditis in adult congenital heart disease: focus on the use of prosthetic material. Eur Heart J. 2017;38(26):2048–56.
10. Marelli AS, Mackie R, Ionescu-Ittu E, Rahme L. Pilote: congenital heart disease in the general population: changing prevalence and age distribution. Circulation. 2007;115(2):163–72.
11. Morris CD, Reller MD, Menashe VD. Thirty-year incidence of infective endocarditis after surgery for congenital heart defect. JAMA. 1998;279:599–603.
12. Ishiwada N, Niwa K, Tateno S, et al. Causative organism influences clinical profile and outcome of infective endocarditis in pediatric patients and adults with congenital heart disease. Circ J. 2005;69:1266–7.
13. Baek JE, Park SJ, Woo SB, Choi JY, Jung JW, Kim NK. Changes in patient characteristics of infective endocarditis with congenital heart disease: 25 years experience in a single institution. Korean Circ J. 2014;44:37–41.

14. Morsheimer M, Brown Whitehorn TF, Heimall J, Sullivan KE. The immune deficiency of chromosome 22q11.2 deletion syndrome. Am J Med Genet A. 2017;173(9):2366–72.
15. Baddour LM, Wilson WR, Bayer AS, et al. Infective endocarditis in adults: diagnosis, antimicrobial therapy, and management of complications: a scientific statement for healthcare professionals from the American Heart Association. Circulation. 2015;132:1435–86.
16. Tubiana S, Blotière PO, Hoen B, Lesclous P, Millot S, Rudant J, Weill A, Coste J, Alla F, Duval X. Dental procedures, antibiotic prophylaxis, and endocarditis among people with prosthetic heart valves: nationwide population based cohort and a case crossover study. BMJ. 2017;358:j3776.
17. Thornhill MH, Dayer M, Lockhart PB, McGurk M, Shanson D, Prendergast B, Chambers JB. A change in the NICE guidelines on antibiotic prophylaxis. Br Dent J. 2016;221(3):112–4.
18. Ban KA, Minei JP, Laronga C, et al. American College of Surgeons and Surgical Infection Society: surgical site infection guidelines, 2016 update. J Am Coll Surg. 2017;224:59–74.
19. Sandoe JA, Barlow GV, Chambers JB, et al. Guidelines for the diagnosis, prevention and management of implantable cardiac electronic device infection. Report of a joint working party project on behalf of the British Society of Antimicrobial Chemotherapy, British Heart Rhythm Society, British Cardiovascular Society, British Heart Valve Society, and British Society of Echocardiography. J Antimicrob Chemother. 2015;70(2):325–59.
20. Verheugt CL, Uiterwaal CS, Vaartjes I, van der Velde ET, Zomer AC, Meijboom FJ, Pieper PG, Post MC, Vliegen HW, Hazekamp MG, Grobbee DE, Mulder BJ. Chance of surgery in adult congenital heart disease. Eur J Prev Cardiol. 2017;24(12):1319–27.
21. Jalal Z, Galmiche L, Lebeaux D, Villemain O, Brugada G, et al. Selective propensity of bovine jugular vein material to bacterial adhesions: an in-vitro study. Int J Cardiol. 2015;198:201–5.
22. Malekzadeh-Milani S, Ladouceur M, Iserin L, Bonnet D, Boudjemline Y. Incidence and outcomes of right-sided endocarditis in patients with congenital heart disease after surgical or transcatheter pulmonary valve implantation. J Thorac Cardiovasc Surg. 2014;148(5):2253–9.
23. Malekzadeh-Milani S, Ladouceur M, Patel M, Boughenou FM, Iserin L, Bonnet D, Boudjemline Y. Incidence and predictors of Melody® valve endocarditis: a prospective study. Arch Cardiovasc Dis. 2015;108(2):97–106.
24. Sharma A, Cote AT, Hosking MCK, Harris KC. A systematic review of infective endocarditis in patients with bovine jugular vein valves compared with other valve types. JACC Cardiovasc Interv. 2017;10(14):1449–58.
25. Yu CH, Minnema BJ, Gold WL. Bacterial infections complicating tongue piercing. Can J Infect Dis Med Microbiol. 2010;21:e70–4.
26. Gatzoulis. Adult congenital heart disease: education, education, education. Nat Clin Pract Cardiovasc Med. 2006;3(1):2–3.
27. Li JS, Sexton DJ, Mick N, Nettles R, Fowler VG Jr, Ryan T, Bashore T, Core GR. Proposed modifications to the Duke criteria for the diagnosis of infective endocarditis. Clin Infect Dis. 2000;30(4):633–8.
28. Pizzi MN, Dos-Subirà L, Roque A, Fernández-Hidalgo N, Cuéllar-Calabria H, Pijuan Domènech A, Gonzàlez-Alujas MT, Subirana-Domènech MT, Miranda-Barrio B, Ferreira-González I, González-López JJ, Igual A, Maisterra-Santos O, García-Dorado D, Castell-Conesa J, Almirante B, Escobar Amores M, Tornos P, Aguadé-Bruix S. (18)F-FDG-PET/CT angiography in the diagnosis of infective endocarditis and cardiac device infection in adult patients with congenital heart disease and prosthetic material. Int J Cardiol. 2017;248:396–402.
29. Gomes A, Glaudemans AWJM, Touw DJ, van Melle JP, Willems TP, Maass AH, Natour E, NHJ P, RJH B, van Geel PP, RHJA S, van Assen S, Sinha B. Diagnostic value of imaging in infective endocarditis: a systematic review. Lancet Infect Dis. 2017;17(1):e1–e14.
30. Baumgartner P, Bonhoeffer NM, Groot D, et al. ESC Guidelines for the management of grown-up congenital heart disease (new version 2010). Eur Heart J. 2010;31(23):2915–57.
31. Feuchtner GM, Stolzmann P, Dichtl W, et al. Multislice computed tomography in infective endocarditis: comparison with transesophageal echocardiography and intraoperative findings. J Am Coll Cardiol. 2009;53:436–44.
32. Olmos C, Vilacosta I, Habib G, Maroto L, Fernández C, et al. Risk score for cardiac surgery in active left-sided infective endocarditis. Heart. 2017;103(18):1435–42.

33. Duval X, Iung B, Klein I, IMAGE (Resonance Magnetic Imaging at the Acute Phase of Endocarditis) Study Group, et al. Effect of early cerebral magnetic resonance imaging on clinical decisions in infective endocarditis: a prospective study. Ann Intern Med. 2010;152:497–504.
34. Cantier M, Mazighi M, Klein I, Desilles JP, Wolff M, et al. Neurologic complications of infective endocarditis: recent findings. Curr Infect Dis Rep. 2017;19(11):41.
35. Merkler AE, Chu SY, Lerario MP, Navi BB, Kamel H. Temporal relationship between infective endocarditis and stroke. Neurology. 2015;85(6):512–6.
36. Yanagawa B, Pettersson GB, Habib G, Ruel M, Saposnik G, Latter DA, Verma S. Surgical management of infective endocarditis complicated by embolic stroke: practical recommendations for clinicians. Circulation. 2016;134(17):1280–92.
37. Fournier PE, Thuny F, Richet H, et al. Comprehensive diagnostic strategy for blood-negative endocarditis: a prospective study of 819 cases. Clin Infect Dis. 2010;51:131–40.
38. Barsic B, Dickerman S, Krajinovic V, et al. International Collaboration on Endocarditis – Prospective Cohort Study (ICE-PCS) investigators. Influence of the timing of cardiac surgery on the outcome of patients with infective endocarditis and stroke. Clin Infect Dis. 2013;56:209–17.
39. AATS Surgical Treatment of Infective Endocarditis Consensus Guidelines Writing Committee Chairs, Pettersson GB, Coselli JS, Writing Committee, Hussain ST, Griffin B, Blackstone EH, Gordon SM, SA LM, Woc-Colburn LE. The American Association for Thoracic Surgery (AATS) consensus guidelines: Surgical treatment of infective endocarditis: Executive summary. J Thorac Cardiovasc Surg. 2017;153(6):1241–58.
40. Steiner T, Juvela S, Unterberg A, European Stroke Organization, et al. European Stroke Organization guidelines for the management of intracranial aneurysms and subarachnoid haemorrhage. Cerebovasc Dis. 2013;35:93–112.
41. Legrand M, Pirracchio R, Rosa A, et al. Incidence, risk factors and prediction of post-operative acute kidney injury following cardiac surgery for active endocarditis: an observational study. Crit Care. 2013;17:R220.
42. Botelho-Nevers E, Thuny F, Casalta JP, Richet H, Gouriet F, Collart F, Riberi A, Habib G, Raoult D. Dramatic reduction in infective endocarditis-related mortality with a management-based approach. Arch Intern Med. 2009;169:1290–8.
43. Chirillo F, Scotton P, Roco F, et al. Impact of a multidisciplinary management strategy on the outcome of patients with native valve infective endocarditis. Am J Cardiol. 2013;112:1171–6.

The Critically Ill Pregnant ACHD Patient 18

Lucia Baris and Jolien W. Roos-Hesselink

18.1 Introduction

Heart disease is globally a major cause of maternal mortality. Maternal mortality due to cardiac disease in the UK was reported to be 23 per 100,000 births in the period 1985–2014, with an incidence of 51 per 100,000 births in the period 2009–2014 alone [1]. These numbers are only expected to increase further due to increasing maternal age, an increasing incidence of metabolic syndrome, and the increased life expectancy of women with congenital heart disease (CHD).

Adult women with CHD form an emerging entity, mainly due to improvements in surgical techniques, anesthesia, pediatric diagnostic possibilities, and intensive care medicine, resulting in today's high quality of care. The majority of these women want to start a family and have the ability to become pregnant. However, maternal cardiac complications occur in approximately 12% of these pregnancies and are therefore not to be taken lightly [2].

Most of the knowledge regarding the management of cardiac disease and cardiac emergencies during pregnancy is not based on evidence from randomized clinical trials, but is derived from small consecutive series, expert opinion, case reports, and registries.

As the incidence of cardiac disease during pregnancy increases, it is important that physicians and clinical staff identify patients at low risk and reassure them, but they also have to be aware of the potentially devastating complications associated with pregnancy in high-risk patients.

In this chapter, we will elaborate on the care for and the management of the critically ill pregnant patient with CHD. In addition, the specific management during pregnancy will be discussed.

L. Baris · J. W. Roos-Hesselink (✉)
Department of Cardiology, Erasmus University, Rotterdam, The Netherlands
e-mail: l.baris@erasmusmc.nl; j.roos@erasmusmc.nl

E. da Cruz et al. (eds.), *Intensive Care of the Adult with Congenital Heart Disease*, Congenital Heart Disease in Adolescents and Adults,
https://doi.org/10.1007/978-3-319-94171-4_18

18.2 Cardiovascular Adaptations in Normal Pregnancy and Labor

Pregnancy induces major hemodynamic changes in order to provide the developing fetus with an adequate blood supply. Women with cardiac disease may not be capable of adapting to these changes adequately. In order to understand the hemodynamic burden placed upon the already diseased heart of women with CHD, the most extensive changes are summarized below.

18.2.1 Blood Volume

During the first trimester, plasma volume and red blood cell mass will increase. This increase continues until it reaches a steady state during the third trimester. Primarily due to physiological sodium retention, about 6–8 L of water will be retained and distributed among the intra- and extracellular spaces as well as the fetal circulation and the amniotic fluid. This will eventually result in a 30–50% increase in plasma volume in pregnant women compared to nonpregnant women. Because the plasma volume expansion is relatively greater than the increase in the red blood cell volume, most women in their third trimester have a so-called physiologic anemia of pregnancy [3–5].

18.2.2 Cardiac Output

The cardiac output rises 30–50% during normal pregnancy. This elevation results from changes in three factors that determine cardiac output: preload increases due to the above-described rise in plasma volume, afterload reduces due to the decline in systemic vascular resistance, and the maternal heart rate rises up to 20 beats per minute [4, 5].

18.2.3 Peripheral Vascular Resistance and Blood Pressure

Early in gestation, maternal peripheral vascular resistance falls as a result of the low-resistance uteroplacental circulation, decreased mean aortic pressure, and endogenous hormones. In the first and second trimester, the fall in systemic vascular resistance, which exceeds the increase in cardiac output, leads to a drop in both systolic and, especially, diastolic blood pressure [4]. After the second trimester, blood pressure rises again.

18.2.4 Labor and Delivery

The most extensive fluctuations in hemodynamic parameters occur during labor, delivery, and the immediate postpartum period. Uterine contractions increase the venous return, and cardiac output may rise by a further 25% due to this increase in preload but also due to increased sympathetic stimulation (pain, anxiety).

18.2.5 Postpartum Period

During the early postpartum period, cardiac output increases as a result of a blood shift from the contracting uterus to the systemic circulation and increased preload due to caval decompression [4]. The hemodynamic changes that occurred during pregnancy resolve slowly after delivery, with the most recovery during the first 2 weeks postpartum. In general, more gradual hemodynamic shifts occur in the months thereafter, and full recovery of the prepregnancy hemodynamic status is said to be at about 5–6 months postpartum [6].

18.3 Pregnancy in Women with Congenital Heart Disease

Prepregnancy counseling of all women with CHD is very important and should start early. The modified World Health Organization (mWHO) classification (Table 18.1) is a validated instrument to make an accurate individual risk assessment possible for patients with CHD and is used to predict the risk of maternal cardiac complications during pregnancy [7, 8]. It divides patients into five groups, based on their underlying cardiac condition. It ranges from mWHO class I, which consists of patients with no increased risk of mortality and a very low risk of morbidity, to mWHO class IV in which a pregnancy is considered life-threatening and therefore contraindicated.

Prepregnancy counseling should address issues like maternal, obstetric and fetal risks, drug use, maternal life expectancy, risk of recurrence of the congenital defect in the offspring, and the impact of pregnancy on the maternal condition. In all patients, an echocardiogram and an exercise test should be performed preferably prepregnancy.

18.4 Cardiac Medications During Pregnancy

Many women with CHD require cardiac medications, especially in the case of arrhythmias and heart failure but also in those with a mechanical valve prosthesis. However, not all drugs can be safely administered to pregnant women, due to teratogenicity or other unwanted effects for especially the fetus. Also, the hemodynamic changes that occur during pregnancy influence the pharmacokinetics, requiring dose adjustments in some cases. Table 18.2 summarizes recommendations for use during pregnancy of the most important cardiovascular drugs [9].

18.5 Heart Failure

Heart failure is the most prevalent cardiac complication in pregnant women with CHD and accounts for elevated incidences of fetal and maternal morbidity and maternal mortality [10]. The incidence varies within the literature but can be estimated to be approximately 13% but is highly dependent on the underlying cardiac condition [11]. Patients that are particularly at risk are those with pulmonary hypertension with or without Eisenmenger syndrome, patients with impaired systemic

Table 18.1 Modified WHO classification of maternal cardiovascular risk

	Risk	Diagnosis	Pregnancy	Delivery
mWHO I	No detectable increased risk of maternal mortality and no/mild increase in morbidity	Uncomplicated, small or mild: • Pulmonary stenosis • PDA • Mitral valve • Mitral valve prolaps Repaired simple lesions (A5D/VSD, PDA, PAPVR) Atrial or ventricular ectopic beats	Follow-up by cardiologist twice during pregnancy	After uncomplicated pregnancy: as usual Otherwise, as class II
mWHO II	Small increased risk of maternal mortality or moderate increase in morbidity	Unrepaired ASD or VSD Repaired tetralogy of Fallot Most arrhythmias	**Follow-up by cardiologist and obstetrician:** At 12 weeks, 20 weeks (+ echocardiography) and 30 weeks Aortic diameter >40 mm: Echocardiography every 4–8 weeks (or advanced imaging) Frequent monitoring up to monthly	**Multidisciplinary team decides on:** • Timing of delivery • Mode of induction • Mode of delivery • Anesthesia **Postpartum monitoring:** 24, 48 or 72 h in case of moderate increased risk of heart failure or arrhythmia
mWHO II–III		Mild systemic ventricular impairment Hypertrophic cardiomyopathy Native or tissue valvular heart disease Marfan <40 mm BAV <45 mm Repaired coarctation		
mWHO III	Significantly increased risk of maternal mortality or severe morbidity.	Mechanical valve Systemic right ventricle Fontan circulation Cyanotic heart disease (unrepaired) Other complex con genital heart disease Marfan 40–45 mm or BAV 40–50 mm		
mWHO IV	Extremely high risk of maternal mortality or severe morbidity	Pulmonary arterial hypertension of any cause Severe systemic ventricular dysfunction Previous peripartum cardiomyopathy with any residual impairment of left ventricular function Severe mitral stenosis, severe aortic stenosis Marfan >45 mm or BAV >50 mm Native severe coarctation	Pregnancy contra-indicated. If pregnancy occurs, care for as class III	

Table 18.2 Cardiac medication during pregnancy

Drug	Teratogenicity	Recommendations
ASA	No known teratogenicity in humans	Maximum dosage of 100 mg a day
Clopidogrel	Unknown in humans	Not recommended
Ticagrelor	Unknown in humans, in high dosages teratogenic in animals	Not recommended
Heparin	No known teratogenicity in humans	Recommended in pregnancy
Low-moleculair-weight heparin	Unknown in humans, no known teratogenicity in animals	Recommended in pregnancy if benefits outweigh the risks
Coumarines	Teratogenic in first trimester	Contra-indicated during first trimester, usage during second and third trimester only if benefits outweigh the risks
B-blockers	No known teratogenicity in humans and animals. Possible fetal bradycardia and hypotensia.	Recommended in pregnancy if benefits outweigh the risks. Exception: Atenlol, contra-indicated
Nitrates	Unknown in humans, no known teratogenicity in animals	Recommended in pregnancy if benefits outweigh the risks
Statines	Unknown in humans, possibly teratogenic	Contra-indicated in pregnancy
ACE-inhibitors	Teratogenic in humans, especially during second and third trimester (IUGR, neonatal longhypoplasia, skull hypoplasia)	Usage during first trimester not recommended, usage during second and third trimester contra-indicated
Aldosterone antagonists	Unknown in humans, possible teratogenicity in animals	Not recommended
Calcium channel blockers	Unknown in humans, especially during first trimester. No known teratogenicity in animals	Usage during first trimester not recommended, usage during second and third trimester only if benefits outweigh the risks
Furosemide	No known teratogenicity in humans, possible teratogenicity in animals	Recommended in pregnancy if benefits outweigh the risks
Thiazide diuretics	Unknown in humans, no known teratogenicity in animals	Recommended in pregnancy if benefits outweigh the risks
AT2-antagonists	Teratogenic in humans, especially during second and third trimester (IUGR, neonatal longhypoplasia, skull hypoplasia)	Usage during first trimester not recommended, usage during second and third trimester contra-indicated
NOACs	Unknown in humans, teratogenic in animals	Contra-indicated
Dopamine	Unknown in humans, possible teratogenicity in animals	Recommended in pregnancy if benefits outweigh the risks
Dobutamine	Unknown in humans, possible teratogenicity in animals	Recommended in pregnancy if benefits outweigh the risks
Phosphodiesterase inhibitors	Unknown in humans, no known teratogenicity in animals	Recommended in pregnancy if benefits outweigh the risks
Noradrenaline	Unknown in humans, decreased placental perfusion	Not recommended in pregnancy

(continued)

Table 18.2 (continued)

Drug	Teratogenicity	Recommendations
Adenosine	Unknown in humans and animals	Recommended in pregnancy if benefits outweight the risks
Amiodarone	Unknown in humans, possible teratogenicity in animals	Recommended in pregnancy if benefits outweigh the risks
Digoxine	No known teratogenicity in humans, unreliable serum levels. Higher dosage needed in pregnancy.	Recommended in pregnancy
Flecainide	Unknown in humans, possible teratogenicity in animals	Recommended in pregnancy if benefits outweigh the risks

ventricular function, and patients with severe left heart obstruction. Most cases of heart failure occur during the end of the second trimester, during labor and delivery, and especially during the early postpartum period. Delivery and the postpartum period are considered high-risk periods due to an extra increase in cardiac stress from pain, anxiety, uterine contractions, and autotransfusion from the uterus directly postpartum [12].

18.5.1 Management During Pregnancy

In the case of heart failure occurring during pregnancy, a multidisciplinary team (consisting of a cardiologist, obstetrician, perinatologist, and if necessary, an intensivist, anesthesiologist, and cardiac surgeon) in a tertiary center should decide on the management plan.

When a woman suffers from acute heart failure during pregnancy, the pharmacological management should follow the guidelines for nonpregnant patients with a few exceptions. Management should always be individualized and determined by the abovementioned multidisciplinary team, taking into account the fetal viability and the severity of the maternal condition. Choices are to be made between immediate delivery if the fetus is already viable or continuation of the pregnancy with support therapy in the case of fetal non-viability [13, 14]. In general, pregnancy termination has advantages for the maternal condition and should therefore always be considered. Of course, this cannot be done independently from fetal viability, and the wish of the patient and her partner should always be the priority. The ethical dilemmas associated with termination of pregnancy for maternal health indications are not to be underestimated, and patients and their families should always be involved in the decision-making process.

Table 18.2 summarizes the recommendations for use during pregnancy of the most important heart failure medication. Figure 18.1 depicts a flow diagram for the treatment and management of acute heart failure in pregnant patients with congenital heart disease. A few specific conditions will be discussed below.

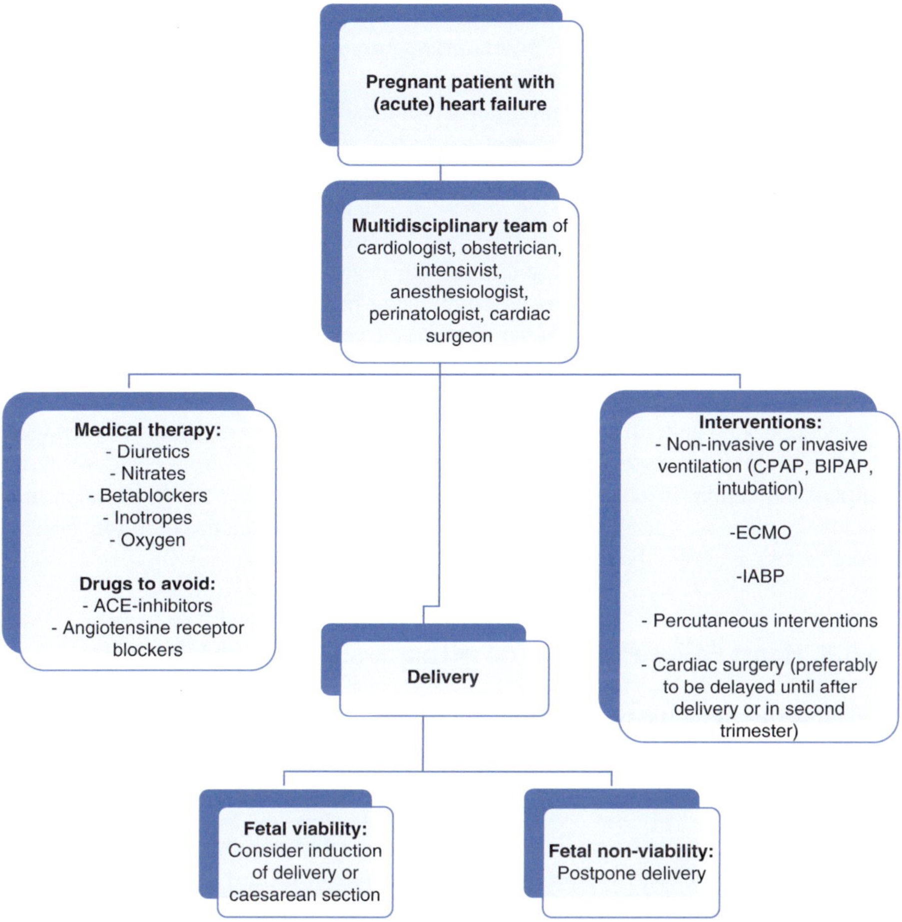

Fig. 18.1 Management of heart failure in pregnancy

18.5.2 Heart Failure in Patients with a Fontan Circulation

Women with a Fontan palliation have a univentricular circulation, and the hemodynamic overload during pregnancy places them at increased risk of heart failure and arrhythmias. As with women with a systemic right ventricle, incidences of complications vary within the literature. The cardiac complication rate in women with a Fontan circulation varies between 9% and 65%, and most common complications are atrial tachyarrhythmias and heart failure.

Atrial tachyarrhythmias can be devastating complications for patients with a Fontan circulation and should be tackled immediately by means of pharmacological therapy or electric cardioversion (ECV). These will be discussed later in Sect. 18.10.

Fetal complication rates are also high and vary between 14% and 100% within the literature, with miscarriage, prematurity, intrauterine growth retardation, and neonatal death being the most common [15–18].

These numbers point out the importance of intensive monitoring of Fontan patients during pregnancy and during the early postpartum period, as the cardiac, obstetric, and neonatal adverse event rates are high. Heart failure in these patients should be treated as mentioned above, with the important sidenote that their pulmonary circulation is solely dependent on an adequate venous return. Treatment with diuretics should therefore be done extra carefully and under close supervision, to avoid intravascular volume depletion. The pulmonary low-flow state in Fontan patients gives them an increased risk for thrombotic events. Regarding anticoagulation therapy for these patients during pregnancy, there is no consensus as to whether this is mandatory and which regimen should be given [15–18]. However, it is advised to be very cautious in these patients, and general anticoagulation therapy is advised in pregnant women with a Fontan circulation, especially in the case of arrhythmias or diminished systemic ventricular function. In general, it is advised that monitoring up until 48 h postpartum should take place or, if indicated by the maternal condition, longer as required. If heart failure occurs, it should be treated as mentioned above [14, 19].

18.5.3 Heart Failure in Patients with a Systemic Right Ventricle

Women with a systemic right ventricle (after Mustard/Senning surgery or congenitally corrected TGA) are at increased risk of an assortment of adverse cardiac and fetal events.

The incidence of cardiac complications during pregnancy and the postpartum period varies within the literature from 14% to 36%. Most common cardiac complications are atrial tachyarrhythmias (14–22%) and heart failure (7–14%).

Atrial tachyarrhythmias are, as in women with a Fontan circulation, a serious complication in pregnant women with a systemic right ventricle and should be immediately treated with pharmacological therapy or electric cardioversion. These will be discussed later in Sect. 18.10.

Many patients (between approximately 25% and 50%) with a systemic right ventricle experience a NYHA class deterioration during pregnancy, as do many healthy pregnant women. However, between 8% and 75% of the women with a systemic right ventricle, the NYHA class deterioration persists postpartum.

In addition to adverse cardiac events, women with a systemic right ventricle are also at increased risk of fetal adverse events during pregnancy. Especially premature birth (<37 weeks) is a very common complication and happens in about 31–71% of pregnancies. Approximately 18% of these babies are born before the 34th week of pregnancy.

No recurrences of heart disease in the offspring are reported in the literature, although high rates of late fetal mortality (approximately 7.8%) and perinatal mortality (between 3.9% and 14%) are reported which are mostly secondary to the high rate of prematurity [19–22].

These numbers show that pregnant patients with a systemic right ventricle have high risks of cardiac and fetal/neonatal adverse events and should therefore be monitored extensively during their pregnancy and in the postpartum period. Current guidelines and recommendations concerning management of heart failure during pregnancy in patients with a systemic right ventricle are derived from small consecutive studies and expert opinion. As for the patients with a Fontan circulation, it is advised that these patients remain monitored until 48 h postpartum or, if indicated by the maternal condition, longer as required.

18.5.4 Heart Failure in Patients with Severe Left Ventricular Obstruction

In patients with congenital aortic valve stenosis, the increase in cardiac output that occurs during pregnancy will result in an increase in left ventricular outflow tract obstruction gradient. Due to the increase in cardiac output and afterload, there is a high risk of heart failure, even in the case of good ventricular function beforehand. Therefore, intensive monitoring and management in these patients is advised. When symptoms of heart failure occur, the first step is bed rest with conventional heart failure treatment. In the case of unsatisfactory response, an intervention should be considered. Emergency delivery should be considered if the fetus is viable, so that the prepregnancy hemodynamic state is restored. In the case of fetal non-viability, percutaneous balloon valvotomy or valve replacement surgery can be performed during pregnancy [23]. It should be noted that the majority of patients require elective valve replacement after pregnancy either way; therefore, balloon valvuloplasty should be regarded as a palliative procedure to enable the pregnancy to be carried to term without the need for cardiac surgery during pregnancy [23, 24]. More on surgical or percutaneous valvular interventions can be found in Sect. 18.14.

18.5.5 Management in the Postpartum Period

In the postpartum period, there are no limitations concerning drug use, and patients with heart failure can then be treated according to the guidelines for nonpregnant patients. However, during the early postpartum stages, large volume shifts occur which makes the intravascular and extravascular volumes in these patients difficult to control and which makes them prone to heart failure or to worsening of existing heart failure. Women with a history of heart failure or women who have experienced heart failure during their pregnancy should be monitored intensively postpartum during at least 48 h at a cardiac care facility, to ensure that the most major fluid shifts and accompanying complications can be managed safely [11, 25].

18.6 Acute Myocardial Infarction

Acute myocardial infarction (AMI) is rare in pregnant women, although pregnancy is a period of increased risk compared to the nonpregnant situation. Due to increasing maternal age at the onset of pregnancy and increasing prevalence of risk factors such as obesity and smoking, myocardial ischemic event rates are increasing. The incidence of AMI in pregnancy ranges in literature from 3 to 100 per 100,000 births. It is associated with high rates of maternal and fetal mortality and morbidity, with maternal mortality rates up to 50% [16]. Specific risk factors include pregnancy-induced hypertensive disorder (PIHD) and (pre-)eclampsia but also the commonly known risk factors for atherosclerosis such as diabetes and hypertension, older age of the mother (>35 years), and a smoking history.

In pregnancy, AMI is less often caused by atherosclerotic lesions than it is in the general population. In a significant proportion of patients, spontaneous coronary artery dissection is the cause for the AMI in pregnancy, with incidences in the literature varying between 27% and 43% [26–28]. This is hypothesized to be caused by a different underlying pathophysiological mechanism related to pregnancy-induced hemodynamic or hormonal changes that affect the different linings of the arterial wall [27]. Also, pre-existing or pregnancy-induced hypertension could play an important role in the etiology. Also thrombotic lesions are more often the cause of myocardial infarction, compared with the nonpregnant state. Due to hormonal changes, pregnancy induces a hypercoagulable state which makes women more prone to thromboembolic complications.

The management of AMI in pregnant women is challenging [25]. In general, the treatment is the same as outside pregnancy; however, a treatment plan should be individualized, as maternal and fetal needs may conflict. Choices can be made between conservative pharmacological treatment, percutaneous coronary interventions (PCI), and coronary artery bypass graft surgery (CABG), the latter two of which will be discussed under Sect. 18.14. Overall, it is advised that women with acute ST-elevation myocardial infarction during pregnancy should undergo immediate coronary angiography and, when applicable and possible, percutaneous (or surgical) treatment of the lesion(s).

Spontaneous coronary artery dissection that does not involve the left main, and without ongoing chest pain or ongoing ischemia on electrocardiogram, can be treated conservatively [29, 30].

It might be beneficial to postpone delivery to reduce the immediate requirement of high cardiac output after AMI. Also, epidural anesthesia, left lateral position, instrumental delivery, or cesarean section should be considered when AMI occurs around the time of delivery [30].

In the case of hemodynamic instability with cardiogenic shock, support therapy with intra-aortic balloon pumps or extracorporeal membrane oxygenation is possible and will be discussed later under Sects. 18.13 and 18.14.

In women who receive an intracoronary stent, dual antiplatelet therapy (DAPT) is indicated. When choosing the right type of stent, pregnancy duration should be taken into account. This will be further elaborated later in this chapter. Dual antiplatelet therapy can be given during pregnancy; however, it should be discontinued around the time of delivery to reduce the risk of major hemorrhagic events. Aspirin is safe in low dose, but there is not good evidence on the use of clopidogrel [30].

18.7 Mechanical Valve Thrombosis

During the hypercoagulable state of pregnancy, women with a mechanical heart valve (MHV) are at increased risk of mechanical valve thrombosis (MVT). All pregnant patients with a MHV presenting during pregnancy with complaints should be suspected of having MVT. MVT is a potentially life-threatening complication in patients with prosthetic valves and can be either obstructive or nonobstructive. Symptoms can vary depending on the size of the thrombus or the obstructive character, but patients usually present with dyspnea, fatigue, signs of acute heart failure, systemic embolization, palpitations, and diminished prosthetic valve sounds [11]. Transesophageal echocardiography and advanced imaging can be used as diagnostic tools. Patients with a MHV in mitral position have a higher risk of MVT than those with MHV in aortic position, due to the low-flow conditions surrounding the mitral valve. The reported incidence of symptomatic, obstructive MVT ranges from 0.3% to 1.3% per year in the general population, but higher rates are observed in the case of sub-therapeutic anticoagulation therapy [31]. In pregnancy, warfarin or other vitamin K antagonists can be harmful for the fetus during week 6–9 and especially when high dosages are necessary (see Table 18.2). Unfortunately there is still no consensus with respect to the best strategy [32].

18.7.1 Management

The ESC guidelines (2012) and the AHA/ACC guidelines (2014) both provide recommendations for the treatment of mechanical valve thrombosis in pregnant women, albeit conflicting at several points [33, 34]. The recommendations are summarized in Fig. 18.2. The treatment of choice for left-sided mechanical valve thrombosis in a hemodynamically stable patient is intravenous heparin. When this treatment fails or when the patient is or becomes hemodynamically unstable, emergency valve replacement surgery should take place, if possible (in the case of fetal viability) right after emergency cesarean section. In the case of a critical situation in which emergency surgery is not an option (e.g., in a regional center with an unstable patient that is unfit for transport), fibrinolytic therapy can be considered. However, due to the high risk of embolization (10%) and the risk of subplacental bleeding, fibrinolysis is not a treatment of first choice. In the case of right-sided mechanical valve thrombosis, however, fibrinolysis is the treatment of first choice, either before or after treatment with intravenous heparin.

18.8 Pulmonary Arterial Hypertension

Pregnancy in women with pulmonary hypertension and Eisenmenger syndrome is associated with high rates of maternal mortality, with incidences varying between 5% and 56% in the literature. It is classified as a mWHO IV class condition, and

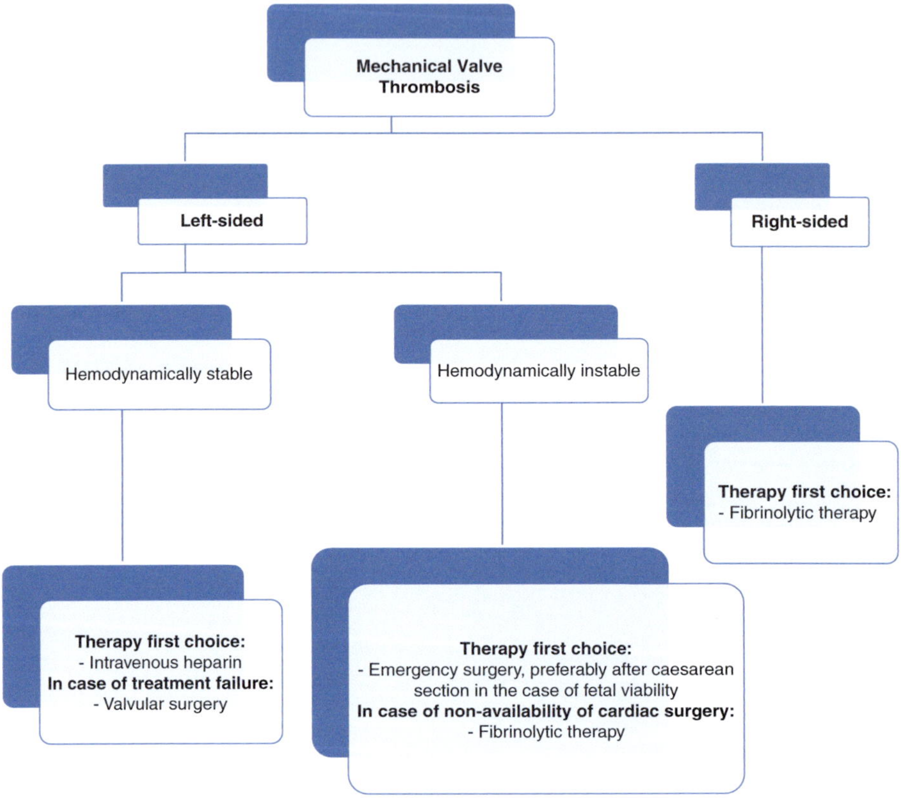

Fig. 18.2 Management of MVT in pregnancy

pregnancy is therefore considered contraindicated. However, despite extensive pre-pregnancy counseling and the advice to not become pregnant, pregnancy remains a choice of the woman in question, and some women with pulmonary hypertension still do become pregnant. If pregnancy does occur and the patient will not terminate, intensive monitoring and management should be carried out by specialists in pulmonary hypertension and pregnancy. A recent study suggests that higher pulmonary pressures are associated with more serious complications [35].

18.8.1 Management

Most of the maternal deaths occur in the third trimester or postpartum, mainly because of pulmonary hypertensive crises when vascular resistance increases. Invasive monitoring during the last trimester, labor, and delivery is therefore recommended with hospitalization up until at least 1 week postpartum, as the postpartum period is a very high-risk period for the occurrence of pulmonary hypertensive crisis. Ideally therefore, patients should be monitored for at least 6 months after delivery. In case of WHO functional class IV or severe ventricular impairment, parenteral prostaglandins are recommended. Intravenous infusion of prostacyclin (epoprostenol) has been mostly used during delivery and postpartum to decrease pulmonary pressure in order to manage pulmonary hypertensive crises [36]. Intensive monitoring during labor and delivery is recommended; in the case of extremely high pulmonary pressures, invasive monitoring (e.g., Swan-Ganz catheter) should be considered. Further evaluation is needed concerning new drugs such as the oral phosphodiesterase inhibitor sildenafil and the endothelin receptor antagonist bosentan during pregnancy [37], as the adverse effects for the fetus are not quite clear. However, in the case of extreme maternal pulmonary arterial hypertension, it can be decided to continue or even start this medication as it lowers the high risk of maternal mortality and is thereby beneficial for the fetus as well.

18.9 Ascending Aortic Dissection

Several congenital and genetic disorders affect the thoracic aorta, making it vulnerable for events such as acute or chronic aortic dissection. All patients with known aortic pathology or conditions associated with aortic pathology should therefore undergo careful prepregnancy counseling and preferably imaging of the entire aorta. For these patients, a crisis plan should be composed to ensure adequate measures will be taken in the case of type A aortic dissection during pregnancy, like an emergency surgery, anesthesia (CPB), and postoperative care plan. Also, prepregnancy surgery should be considered depending on the diameter of the aorta and the underlying condition [38]. Aortic diameter should be corrected for body surface area (BSA) in patients of short stature (such as patients with Turner syndrome). Patients at risk for aortic dissection should get regular echocardiographic checkups during pregnancy, preferably every 4–12 weeks (up to 6 months postpartum), and strict blood pressure control should be implemented. In the case of progressive aortic dilatation during pregnancy, corrective surgery with the fetus in utero should be considered if nonviable. Nevertheless, cesarean section of a viable fetus prior to cardiac or aortic surgery is always preferable. As seen in Table 18.1, the modified World Health Organization classification classifies patients with Marfan syndrome and ascending aortic dilatation of 45 mm or higher at such a high risk that pregnancy is contraindicated. In these cases, prepregnancy surgery should be considered. In Table 18.3, the recommendations are summarized for prepregnancy surgery and aortic diameter in patients with forms of aortic pathology. In the case of the high rates of aortic dissections in the direct family of the patient, it should be considered to perform prepregnancy surgery when aortic diameter is ≥40 mm in patients with Loeys-Dietz, SMAD3, and Ehlers-Danlos syndrome and Marfan syndrome. Recommendations on mode of delivery can be found in Sect. 18.18.

In patients with Turner syndrome, an aortic size index (ASI) of ≥25 mm/m^2 (corrected for body surface area (BSA)) is regarded as cutoff value above which aortic surgery should be considered. Aortic size indices of 25 mm or greater with associated malformations such as bicuspid aortic valve or coarctation of the aorta

Table 18.3 Indications for prepregnancy aortic surgery

Condition	Negative family history of aortic dissections (mm)	Positive family history of aortic dissections (mm)
Marfan syndrome	≥45	≥40
Loeys-Dietz syndrome	≥45	≥40
Ehlers-Danlos syndrome (type IV)	≥45	≥40
SMAD-3	≥42	≥40
Isolated bicuspid aortic valve	≥50	≥45

are considered very high risk, and in these women, pregnancy is contraindicated. However, there is no evidence that prepregnancy aortic surgery lowers the risks of aortic rupture associated with pregnancy in patients with Turner syndrome. Therefore, current guidelines recommend that pregnancy should be contraindicated in patients with Turner syndrome and with ASI ≥25 mm/m^2 and associated cardiac malformations, independent of whether surgical correction has taken place or not.

Patients presenting with symptoms of type A aortic dissection, with or without known aortic pathology, should receive immediate echocardiography and if necessary advanced imaging such as computed tomography or magnetic resonance. Dissection of the ascending aorta during pregnancy is an indication for emergency surgery independent of fetal viability. When the fetus is viable, cesarean delivery should take place followed by immediate aortic surgery [38]. In the case of fetal non-viability, surgery should be performed as soon as possible with the fetus in utero.

18.10 Arrhythmias

18.10.1 Supraventricular Tachycardia

During pregnancy, supraventricular tachyarrhythmias (SVT) are relatively common and are mostly benign; however, in patients with cardiac disease, for instance, in Fontan patients, the impact of a SVT can be devastating. In this case or in the case of sustained SVT, with or without hemodynamic instability, immediate treatment is required as this poses a threat to both the maternal and fetal condition. In case of AV-nodal reentry tachyarrhythmias, vagal maneuvers are the first choice of treatment, followed by adenosine intravenously in case of treatment failure. Sotalol can be used for rhythm control in atrial fibrillation, as well as digoxin or calcium channel antagonists. In case of hemodynamic instability, or if pharmacological treatment has failed, electric cardioversion (ECV) should be performed.

In the case of atrial fibrillation, the indications for oral anticoagulation are generally the same as in the nonpregnant population [11, 25] with the sidenote that the hypercoagulable state of pregnancy can be considered as an extra risk factor for thrombotic events. The CHA_2DS_2-VASc score is a widely used tool for estimating the stroke risks in atrial fibrillation, and it is our advice that an extra point be added for pregnancy to this score. Especially during the first trimester, there is a preference for low-molecular-weight heparin instead of warfarin due to teratogenic effects. The recommendations concerning the most common anti-arrhythmic drugs are summarized in Table 18.2. Figure 18.3 depicts a summary of the management and treatment of sustained supraventricular tachycardia in pregnancy.

18.10.2 Ventricular Tachycardia

Fortunately, ventricular tachycardia (VT) during pregnancy is rare. However, when it occurs, it can be life-threatening and requires immediate therapeutic actions. In hemodynamically stable patients with sustained ventricular tachycardia, the treatment of first choice is pharmacological in the form of beta-blockers or amiodarone in case of monomorphic VT. In the case of hemodynamic instability or (witnessed) cardiac arrest due to ventricular tachycardia or ventricular fibrillation, immediate

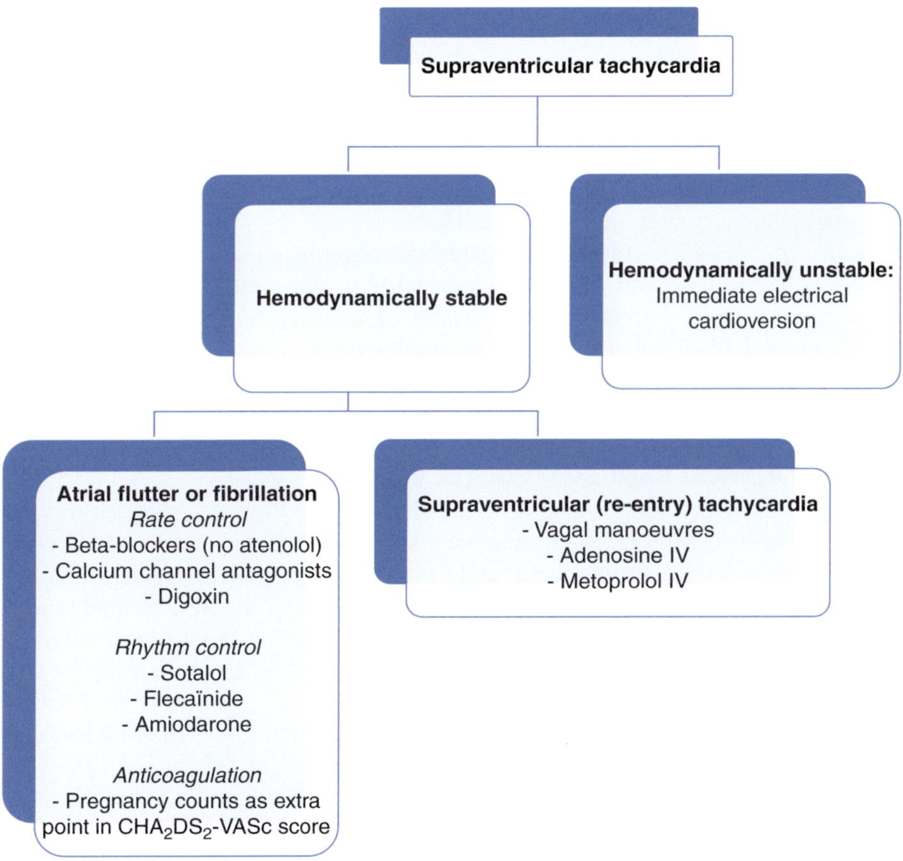

Fig. 18.3 Management of SVT in pregnancy

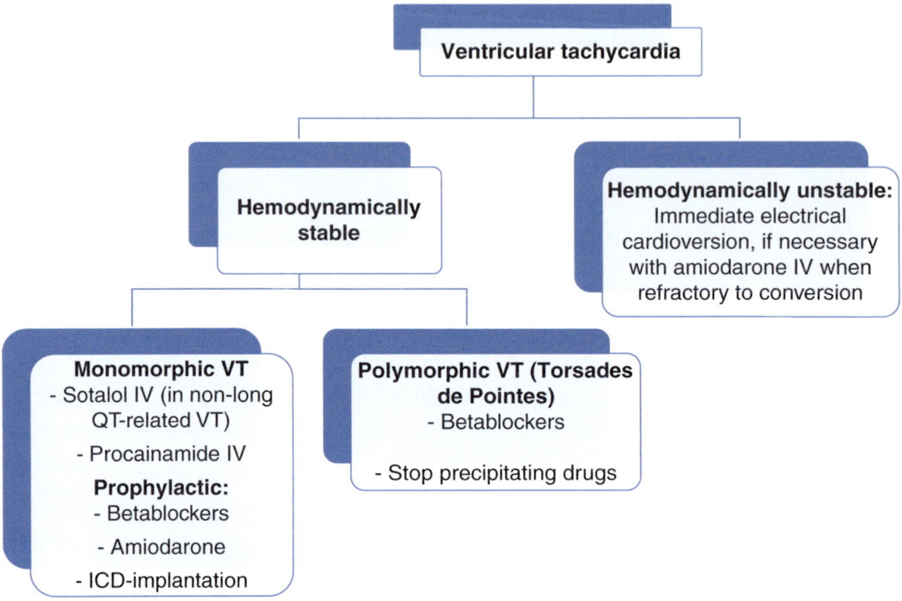

Fig. 18.4 Management of VT in pregnancy

defibrillation is indicated [11, 25]. The management and treatment of ventricular tachyarrhythmias is summarized in Fig. 18.4.

When the tachyarrhythmia is drug-resistant, radiofrequency ablation should be considered. However, radiation exposure to the fetus should be taken into account when considering the timing of intervention. Implantation of a cardioverter-defibrillator (ICD) during pregnancy is considered safe, although data is limited [11].

18.11 Electrical Cardioversion (ECV)

Electrical cardioversion (ECV) during pregnancy is considered a safe and effective treatment for maternal arrhythmias. Fetal monitoring is advised during and after the ECV as the ECV can sometimes cause a hypertonic uterus resulting in fetal bradycardia. However, this complication is quite rare, and the uterus is usually not affected by the electrical current. As many arrhythmias during pregnancy in women with CHD, especially those with complex malformations, have potential devastating consequences, the possible complications of ECV do not outweigh the benefit of rapid termination of the maternal tachyarrhythmia [39].

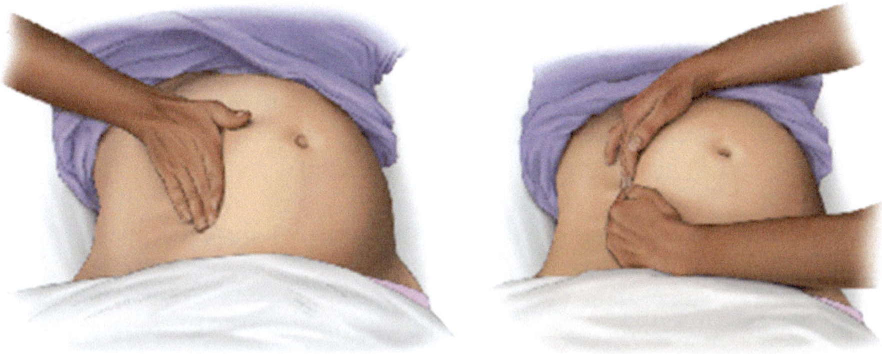

Fig. 18.5 Manual left uterine displacement (Figure courtesy of the American Heart Association)

18.12 Cardiopulmonary Resuscitation and Defibrillation

Cardiac arrest during pregnancy is rare and can result from cardiac and noncardiac causes, such as myocardial infarction, acute heart failure, aortic dissection, myocarditis, ventricular tachyarrhythmias, amniotic fluid embolism, sepsis, (pre-)eclampsia, and pulmonary embolism, as well as hypermagnesemia from magnesium sulfate supplementation by obstetricians for (pre-)eclampsia.

Cardiopulmonary resuscitation (CPR) during pregnancy consists of basic life support (BLS) and advanced cardiac life support (ACLS), as it does in the nonpregnant population. After 20 weeks of pregnancy duration or in the case of a visible gravid uterus, manual left uterine displacement should be performed in order to relieve aortocaval compression, as depicted in Fig. 18.5. As the fetal condition in the situation of maternal cardiopulmonary arrest and resuscitation is inferior to the condition of the mother, fetal monitors are not useful [40].

When CPR is not successful after 4 min, emergency cesarean section should be performed immediately with the aim of maternal resuscitation (due to diminished aortocaval compression and sudden autotransfusion from the uterus) and is therefore independent of fetal viability [40].

18.13 Extracorporeal Circulation

Extracorporeal membrane oxygenation (ECMO) for cardiopulmonary failure during pregnancy is an emerging form of support therapy. Despite very limited data, it is considered an effective and relatively safe treatment for both the mother and the fetus. In a recently published review, the overall maternal survival rate was 77.8%, and the fetal survival rate was 65.1%, based on 45 pregnant patients treated with extracorporeal life support for various underlying conditions. While ECMO is associated with high risks of bleeding or thrombotic complications, the potential benefits for the pregnant patient and her unborn child can outweigh these risks [41].

18.14 Surgical and Percutaneous Interventions

18.14.1 Cardiac Surgery with Cardiopulmonary Bypass

Cardiac surgery with cardiopulmonary bypass is relatively safe for pregnant women in terms of maternal morbidity and mortality, with mortality rates being comparable to those in the nonpregnant population. However, high rates of fetal mortality (around 20%) and morbidity (especially late neurological impairment) are reported. Cardiac surgery is therefore only indicated in pregnant patients when there are no other therapeutic options. In the case of fetal viability, it is recommended to deliver before surgery, possibly after a course of corticosteroids for fetal lung development. During surgery, the fetal heart rate and uterine tone and contractions (CTG) should be monitored in addition to standard monitoring by the anesthesiologist. Also, hemodilution during cardiopulmonary bypass should be avoided to maximize oxygen delivery to the fetus [25]. Other specific techniques may be of benefit for the fetus such as pulsatile flow during cardiopulmonary bypass, normothermic perfusion, and the avoidance of hypocapnia, as this induces placental vasoconstriction and thus fetal hypoxia [25].

18.14.2 Percutaneous Interventions

Percutaneous interventions during pregnancy are considered safe and effective but are nevertheless invasive and should therefore be performed only when there are no other treatment options with comparable results. In the case of timing semi-elective intervention, the fourth month of pregnancy is regarded as the best time to intervene, as the fetal organogenesis is then completed. Also, it is advised to minimize the exposure of radiation during the procedures, independent of pregnancy duration. When possible, echocardiography should replace radiation-based imaging as much as possible during the procedures. In the case of an obvious gravid uterus or pregnancy duration of 20 weeks or more, the patient should be positioned in the left lateral position during PCI. Also, it is advisable to create intra-arterial or intravenous access above diaphragm level due to possible aortocaval compression [25].

18.15 Percutaneous Coronary Interventions

Drug-eluting stents (DES) are the first choice of intracoronary stents in pregnancy, as they are associated with low risks of stent thrombosis. However, the pregnancy term should be taken into account for this. When the AMI occurs during third trimester, the upcoming delivery should be taken into account in the decision of if and which intracoronary stent will be used. There is no evidence for bridging with unfractionated or low-molecular-weight heparin, and there is also no preference for thrombolytic therapy in the management of AMI, especially due to the high risks of bleeding [30]. In all scenarios, aspirin in low dose is safe and should be continued.

18.16 Percutaneous Balloon Valvuloplasty

Balloon valvuloplasty for severe aortic or mitral stenosis during pregnancy can be performed in case of symptomatic patients in whom pharmacological therapy and bed rest give no relief of symptoms or in whom there is actual heart failure with or without left ventricular dilatation. However, with balloon valvuloplasty, there is always a risk of the occurrence of severe acute valvular regurgitation and therefore the need for emergency cardiac surgery. As mentioned above, cardiac surgery with cardiopulmonary bypass is associated with high rates of fetal adverse outcomes and should be avoided when possible. In the case of fetal viability, it is always recommended to perform a cesarean section prior to balloon valvuloplasty or valvular surgery. In the case of fetal non-viability and a valvular intervention being clinically inevitable, the patient and her family should be made aware of the risk of acute severe valvular regurgitation and the possible need for emergency surgery [23].

18.17 Intra-aortic Balloon Pumps (IABP)

The use of an IABP in the case of cardiac failure during pregnancy is considered safe. It is advised that the patient should be positioned in the left lateral position to reduce caval compression during the whole duration of treatment [30].

18.18 Delivery

In all patients with CHD, the preferred mode of delivery is vaginal. Cesarean section is primarily reserved for obstetric indications, with the exception of patients with a severely dilated (≥45 mm) or dissected aorta, severe heart failure, or anticoagulant use in preterm labor [42]. Epidural anesthesia is generally recommended in order to reduce sympathetic stimulation (pain, anxiety) and thereby cardiac workload. To minimize caval compression, the patient should be preferably positioned in the left lateral position during labor and delivery. In high-risk patients, delivery should take place in a tertiary center with specialist multidisciplinary care. Current guidelines no longer advise routine use of antibiotic prophylaxis [25].

References

1. Knight M, Nair M, Tuffnell D, Kenyon S, Shakespeare J, Brocklehurst P, Kurinczuk JJ, editors. On behalf of MBRRACE-UK. Saving lives, improving mothers' care—surveillance of maternal deaths in the UK 2012–14 and lessons learned to inform maternity care from the UK and Ireland Confidential Enquiries into Maternal Deaths and Morbidity 2009–14. Oxford: National Perinatal Epidemiology Unit, University of Oxford; 2016.
2. Balint OH, Siu SC, Mason J, Grewal J, Wald R, Oechslin EN, et al. Cardiac outcomes after pregnancy in women with congenital heart disease. Heart. 2010;96:1656–61.
3. Lund CJ, Donovan JC. Blood volume during pregnancy. Significance of plasma and red cell volumes. Am J Obstet Gynecol. 1967;98:394.
4. Katz R, Karliner JS, Resnik R. Effects of a natural volume overload state (pregnancy) on left ventricular performance in normal human subjects. Circulation. 1978;58:434.
5. Capeless EL, Clapp JF. Cardiovascular changes in early phase of pregnancy. Am J Obstet Gynecol. 1989;161:1449.
6. Steer PJ, editor. Heart disease and pregnancy. London: The Royal College of Obstetricians and Gynaecologists; 2006. ISBN: 1-04752-30-6
7. Van Hagen IM, Boersma E, Johnson MR, Thorne SA, Parsonage WA, Subías PE, et al. Global cardiac risk assessment in the Registry of Pregnancy and Cardiac disease: results of a registry from the European Society of Cardiology. Eur J Heart Fail. 2016;18:523–33.
8. Thorne S, MacGregor A, Nelson-Piercy C. Risks of contraception and pregnancy in heart disease. Heart. 2006;92:1520–5.
9. www.farmacotherapeutischkompas.nl
10. Van Hagen IM, Cornette J, Johnson MR, Roos-Hesselink JW. Managing cardiac emergencies in pregnancy. Heart. 2016;0:1–15.
11. Ruys TPE, Roos-Hesselink JW, Hall R, Subirana-Domènech MT, Grando-Ting J, Estensen M, et al. Heart failure in pregnant women with cardiac disease: date from the ROPAC. Heart. 2014;100:231–8.
12. Drenthen W, Pieper PG, Roos-Hesselink JW, et al. Outcome of pregnancy in women with congenital heart disease: a literature review. J Am Coll Cardiol. 2007;49:2303–11.
13. Hilfiker-Kleiner D, Westhoff-Bleck M, Gunter HH, et al. A management algorithm for acute heart failure in pregnancy. The Hannover experience. Eur Heart J. 2015;36:769–70.
14. McMurray JJ, Adamopoulos S, Anker SD, et al. ESC Guidelines for the diagnosis and treatment of acute and chronic heart failure 2012: The Task Force for the Diagnosis and Treatment of Acute and Chronic Heart Failure 2012 of the European Society of Cardiology. Developed in collaboration with the Heart Failure Association (HFA) of the ESC. Eur Heart J. 2012;33:1787–847.
15. Drenthen W, Pieper PG, Roos-Hesselink JW, van Lottum WA, Voors AA, Mulder BJ, et al. Pregnancy and delivery in women after Fontan pallitation. Heart. 2006;92:1290–4.
16. Zentner D, Kotevski A, King I, Grigg L, d'Udekem Y. Fertility and pregnancy in the Fontan population. Int J Cardiol. 2016;208:97–101.
17. Khan A, Kim YY. Pregnancy in complex CHD: focus on patients with Fontan circulation and patients with a systemic right ventricle. Cardiol Young. 2015;25:1608–14.
18. Gouton M, Nizard J, Patel M, Sassolas F, Jimenez M, Radojevic J, et al. Maternal and fetal outcomes of pregnancy with fontan circulation: a multicentric observation study. Int J Cardiol. 2015;187:84–9.
19. Canobbio MM, Morris CD, Graham TP, Landzberg MJ. Pregnancy outcomes after atrial repair for transposition of the great arteries. Am J Cardiol. 2006;98:668–72.
20. Metz T, Jackson GM, Yetman AT. Pregnancy outcomes in women who have undergone an atrial switch repair for congenital d-transposition of the great arteries. Am J Obstet Gynecol. 2011;205:273.e1–5.

21. Drenthen W, Pieper PG, Ploeg M, Voors AA, Roos-Hesselink JW, Mulder BJM, et al. Risk of complications during pregnancy after Senning or Mustard (atrial) repair of complete transposition of the great arteries. Eur Heart J. 2005;26:2588–95.
22. Guedes A, Mercier LA, Leduc L, Berube L, Marcotte F, Dore A. Impact of pregnancy on the systemic right ventricle after a Mustard operation for transposition of the great arteries. JACC. 2004;44(2):433–7.
23. Myerson SG, Mitchell AR, Ormerod OJ, Banning AP. What is the role of balloon dilatation for severe aortic stenosis during pregnancy? J Heart Valve Dis. 2005;14:147–50.
24. Presbitero P, Boccuzzi GG, Oakley C. Percutaneous therapy. In: Oakley C, Warnes CA, editors. Heart disease in pregnancy (second edition). Oxford: Blackwell Publishing Group; 2007. p. 304–15.
25. Regitz-Zagrosek V, Blomstrom Lundqvist CB, Borghi C, Cifkova R, Ferreira R, et al. ESC Guidelines on the management of cardiovascular diseases during pregnancy. The Task Force on the Management of Cardiovascular Diseases during Pregnancy of the European Society of Cardiology (ESC). Eur Heart J. 2011;32:3147–97.
26. Roth A, Elkayam U. Acute myocardial infarction associated with pregnancy. J Am Coll Cardiol. 2008;52:171–80.
27. Petitti DB, Sidney S, Quesenberry CP Jr, Bernstein A. Incidence of stroke and myocardial infarction in women of reproductive age. Stroke. 1997;28:280.
28. Elkayam U, Jalnapurkar S, Barakkat MN, et al. Pregnancy-associated acute myocardial infarction: a review of contemporary experience in 150 cases between 2006 and 2011. Circulation. 2014;129:1695.
29. Yip A, Saw J. Spontaneous coronary artery dissection: a review. Cardiovasc Diagn Ther. 2015;5:37–48.
30. Ismail S, Wong C, Rajan P, Vidovic MI. ST-elevation acute myocardial infarction in pregnancy: 2016 update. Clin Cardiol. 2017;40:399–406.
31. Dürrleman N, Pellerin M, Bouchard D, et al. Prosthetic valve thrombosis: twenty-year experience at the Montreal Heart Institute. J Thorac Cardiovasc Surg. 2004;127:1388.
32. Van Hagen IM, Roos-Hesselink JW, Ruys TPE, Merz WM, Goland S, Gabriel H, et al. Pregnancy in women with a mechanical heart valve: data of the European Society of Cardiology Registry of Pregnancy and Cardiac Disease (ROPAC). Circulation. 2015;132:132–42.
33. Vahanian A, Alfieri O, Andreotti F, Antunes MJ, Barón-Esquivias G, Baumgartner H, et al. Guidelines on the management of valvular heart disease (version 2012) . The Joint Task Force on the Management of Valvular Heart Disease of the European Society of Cardiology (ESC) and the European Association for Cardio-Thoracic Surgery (EACTS). Eur Heart J. 2012;33:2451–96.
34. Nishimura RA, Otto CM, Bonow RO, Ruiz CE, Carabello BA, Skubas NJ, et al. 2014 AHA/ACC guideline for the management of patients with valvular heart disease: executive summary. A report of the American College of Cardiology/American Heart Association Task Force on Practice Guidelines. Circulation. 2014;129:2440–92.
35. Sliwa K, Van Hagen IM, Budts W, Swan L, Sinagra G, Caruana M, et al. Pulmonary hypertension and pregnancy outcomes: data from the Registry of Pregnancy and Cardiac Disease (ROPAC) of the European Society of Cardiology. Eur J Heart Fail. 2016;18:1119–28.
36. Tabarsi N, Levy R, Rychel V, Kiess M, Swinston J, Oakes J, Grewal J. Pregnancy among women with pulmonary arterial hypertension: a changing landschape? Int J Cardiol. 2014;177:490–1.
37. Galie N, Humbert M, Vachiery JL, Gibbs S, Lang I, Torbicki A, et al. 2015 ESC/ERS Guidelines for the diagnosis and treatment of pulmonary hypertension: The Joint Task Force for the Diagnosis and Treatment of Pulmonary Hypertension of the European Society of Cardiology (ESC) and the European Respiratory Society (ERS): Endorsed by: Association of European Pediatric and Congenital Cardiology (AEPC), International Society for Heart and Lung Transplantation (ISHLT). Eur Heart J. 2016;37:67–119.
38. Stewart FM. Marfan's syndrome and other aortopathies in pregnancy. Obstet Med. 2013;6:112–9.

39. Tromp CHN, Nanne ACM, Pernet PJM, Tukkie R, Bolte AC. Elektrical cardioversion during pregnancy: safe or not? Neth Hear J. 2011;19(3):134–6.
40. Jeejeebhoy FM, Zelop CM, Lipman S, Carvalho B, Joglar J, Mhyre JM, et al. Cardiac arrest in pregnancy. a scientific statement from the American Heart Association. Circulation. 2015;132:1747–73.
41. Agerstrand C, Abrams D, Biscotti M, Moroz L, Rosenzweig EB, D'Alton M, et al. Extracorporeal membrane oxygenation for cardiopulmonary failure during pregnancy and postpartum. Ann Thorac Surg. 2016;102:774–9.
42. Ruys TPE, Roos-Hesselink JW, Pijuan-Domènech A, Vasario E, Gaisin IR, Lung B. Is a planned caesarean section in women with cardiac disease beneficial? Heart. 2015;101:530–6.

Part III

Specific Management Topics

Advanced Cardiac Support in Adults with Congenital Heart Disease

19

Scott R. Auerbach and Andreas Brieke

19.1 Introduction

Survival of children born with congenital heart disease (CHD) has been improving for decades, thanks to improvements in surgical techniques and postoperative care [1, 2]. Adults with congenital heart disease (ACHD) now outnumber children with CHD [3–5]. As survival into adulthood has increased, so has the complexity and severity of CHD in addition to the association of heart failure (HF) in ACHD [3]. ACHD HF is unique compared to non-ACHD HF in adults, and its evaluation and management were outlined in a statement by the American Heart Association [6]. ACHD HF is less likely to be primarily ischemic. There are heterogeneous anatomic lesions. Many have failing systemic right ventricles (RV) that are not designed to pump against systemic resistance. Additionally, anemia, cyanosis, HF multiplied across decades, chronotropic incompetence, and a higher risk of arrhythmias complicate the disease course. There is lack of evidence-based data to guide medical treatments, interventions, and surgical therapies. Management requires individualization based on a patient's anatomy, physiology, and comorbidities. When acute or end-stage HF manifests in ACHD, mechanical circulatory support (MCS) may be required to support the systemic and/or pulmonary circulations and recover end-organ function.

S. R. Auerbach (✉)
Department of Pediatrics, Heart Institute, Aurora, CO, USA
e-mail: scott.auerbach@childrenscolorado.org

A. Brieke
Heart Failure Program, University of Colorado Hospital, Aurora, CO, USA

E. da Cruz et al. (eds.), *Intensive Care of the Adult with Congenital Heart Disease*,
Congenital Heart Disease in Adolescents and Adults,
https://doi.org/10.1007/978-3-319-94171-4_19

19.2 Characteristics of ACHD Patients Requiring Ventricular Assist Device (VAD) Support

ACHD HF is most commonly associated with pressure and volume overload lesions, abnormal ventriculo-ventricular interactions, systemic RV in a biventricular circulation, and functionally univentricular hearts (FUH) with either a morphologic RV or left ventricle (LV). Chronic arrhythmias and high risk of sudden cardiac death complicate the clinical course [7]. Chronotropic incompetence due to sinus node dysfunction can result in a chronic volume load that contributes to ventricular dysfunction [8]. Atrial arrhythmias, such as atrial flutter, can go unrecognized for long periods of time and directly, or indirectly, contribute to progression to end-stage heart failure [9]. When surgical correction or palliation is not available for an individual patient and medical options have been exhausted, MCS should be considered.

The variety of lesions and their risk of hospital admission for a first HF event are shown in Table 19.1 [10]. Of the various ACHD lesions, tetralogy of Fallot (TOF), D-transposition of the great arteries (D-TGA), congenitally corrected transposition of the great arteries (CC-TGA), and functionally univentricular heart (FUH) are the most likely to result in HF. Additional risk factors for ACHD HF include prior surgery, reoperation, and pacemaker implantation [10, 11]. Such CHD and their various palliative surgeries result in a myriad of challenges for MCS compared to non-ACHD HF. The arterial switch is associated with a dilated aortic root and/or

Table 19.1 Independent risk factors for first HF admission in adulthood

	HR	95% CI
Patient characteristics		
Multiple defects	2.2	1.7–2.9
Main defect		
Ventricular septal defect	–	–
Atrial septal defect	1.1	0.7–1.7
Aortic coarctation	0.4	0.2–0.9
Tetralogy of Fallot	2.1	1.3–3.6
Aortic stenosis	1.9	1.0–3.4
Pulmonary stenosis	0.6	0.3–1.4
Bicuspid aortic valve	0.7	0.4–1.5
AVSD	2.7	1.5–5.1
Marfan syndrome	0.8	0.3–2.2
TGA	5.0	2.5–9.9
Patent arterial duct	0.6	0.2–1.7
Ebstein malformation	0.7	0.2–2.2
ccTGA	5.2	1.8–15.4
PA + VSD	3.0	1.2–7.4
FUH/DILV	11.4	5.9–22.0
Other	3.1	2.2–6.1
Interventions in childhood		
Surgery	2.5	1.8–3.5
Reoperation	1.8	1.2–2.6
Pacemaker implantation	3.1	1.5–6.3

HR hazard ratio, 95% CI *95%* confidence interval

aortic insufficiency requiring intervention at the time of LVAD placement [12–18]. Failure to address aortic insufficiency at the time of VAD implant can result in circular VAD flow and inefficient support [19]. Additionally, arrhythmias, pulmonary hypertension, valve or conduit stenosis or insufficiency, complicated systemic and pulmonary venous drainage, ventricular trabeculations, and adhesions at the time of surgery may be present. These complications will need to be addressed prior to, or at the time, of VAD placement.

19.3 Systemic RV in a Biventricular Circulation

D-TGA following atrial switch and unrepaired CC-TGA both have the unique anatomy of a RV in the systemic position and a sub-pulmonary morphologic LV. The systemic RV is predisposed to systemic AV valve dysfunction and pump failure. The large number of trabeculations in the RV can cause VAD inflow cannula obstruction. Screening for residual lesions prior to VAD placement is crucial. D-TGA patients following atrial switch are at risk for atrial baffle obstruction and residual shunts, which must be identified prior to the placement of the VAD. If multiple residual lesions are found and VAD support is required, consideration should be given to the use of a total artificial heart (TAH) rather than a systemic ventricular assist device (SVAD) alone. Extensive atrial suture lines following atrial switch predispose to complicating atrial arrhythmias.

19.4 Functionally Univentricular Hearts

Patients with heart failure due to a FUH can present with systemic ventricular systolic dysfunction, with failure of the Fontan circulation despite preserved ventricular function, or with both ventricular dysfunction and Fontan circuit failure. Failure of the Fontan vascular circuit is typically caused by elevation in pulmonary vascular resistance in the setting of passive blood flow through the pulmonary vascular bed, regardless of systemic pump function. This impairment in pulmonary venous return results in systemic venous hypertension, preload deprivation, and low cardiac output. Systemic venous hypertension results in chronic pleural effusions, renal insufficiency, liver fibrosis or cirrhosis, protein losing enteropathy, ascites, peripheral edema, peripheral chronic venous insufficiency, and/or plastic bronchitis [20–22]. Chronotropic incompetence and/or AV dyssynchrony can also contribute to reductions in cardiac output [8]. Formation of systemic venous-to-pulmonary venous collateral vessels can result in cyanosis [21]. Aortopulmonary collateral vessels may be present, adding a volume load to the FUH, and are a source of bleeding in the operating room [23, 24].

MCS for the failing Fontan circuit alone is challenging. Patients with Fontan failure but preserved ventricular systolic function are unlikely to benefit from a SVAD alone, as the SVAD will likely still be derived of preload due to inadequate passive flow through the Fontan circuit. The Berlin Heart EXCOR has been used as a sub-pulmonary ventricle after creation of a "new chamber" between the superior and inferior vena cava in a patient with Fontan failure but preserved ventricular function (Fig. 19.1), resulting in resolution of ascites and improvement in renal function to the point that the patient could be listed for heart transplantation [25]. Creation of such a chamber may not be possible in all patients, and the use of a TAH

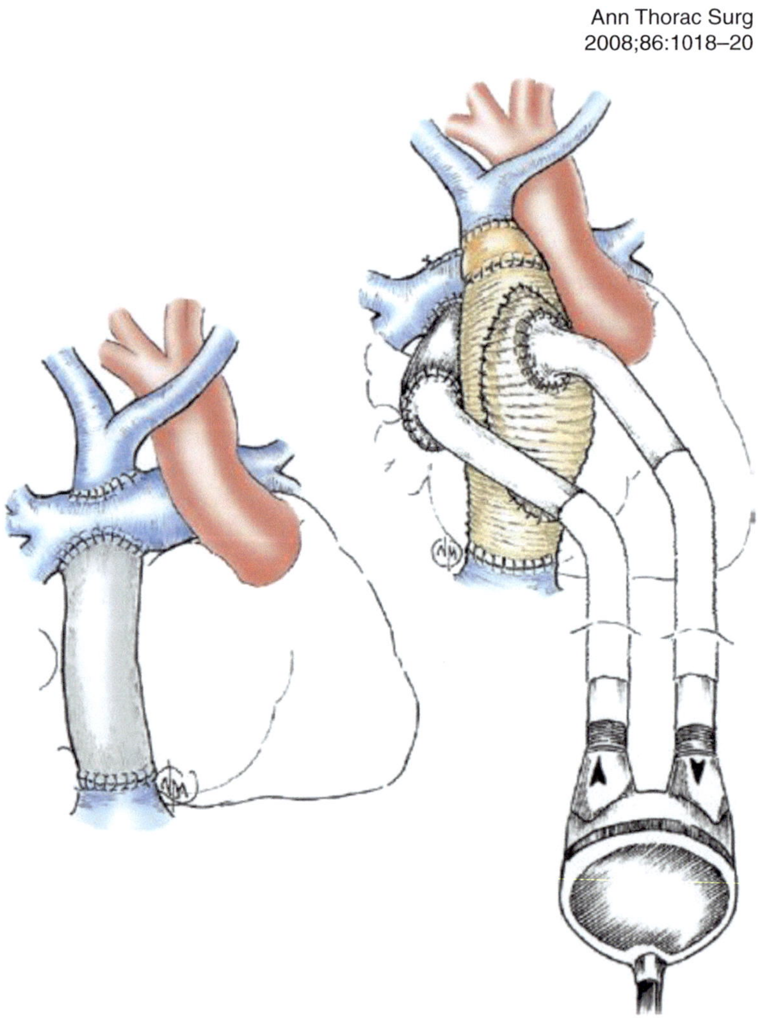

Fig. 19.1 Schematic view of the implantation of the Berlin heart on the right circulation. Left sketch shows the cavopulmonary anastomosis and the extracardial conduit with a Gore-Tex graft (W. L. Gore & Associates, Flagstaff, AZ). Right sketch shows the implantation of the arterial cannula in the proximal stump of the extracardiac conduit, the capacity chamber created with an enlarging patch of Dacron in a Dacron graft (Vascutek Terumo, Wadenswil, Switzerland) and the connection of the superior vena cava in the capacity chamber with enlargement patch of xenopericardium. The venous cannula is inserted in the capacity chamber. Both cannula are brought percutaneously and connected to a paracorporeal ventricle

is another possible consideration for VAD support in Fontan failure. Fontan patients with ventricular systolic dysfunction may be candidates for SVAD support alone, and there are reports of successful bridge to transplantation with multiple devices [26–28]. A thorough evaluation of both anatomy and physiology of each individual patient is critical prior to deciding on the best device option and should include advanced imaging with some combination of MRI, CT, and cardiac catheterization.

19.5 Comorbidities Specific to the Adult with Congenital Heart Disease Population

Optimizing outcomes of MCS requires careful attention to the details of patient selection. Adults with congenital heart disease not only have anatomic problems specific to their heart disease, but they also can present with non-cardiac disease specific to the adult age group. New cardiac issues can develop with time, especially valvular abnormalities which might impose an obstacle to the use of systemic ventricular assist devices (Table 19.2). Progression of heart disease can cause secondary organ problems that can complicate medical and device management. Furthermore, these patients can develop medical problems unrelated to their heart disease which can impose challenges utilizing durable MCS devices, as happens in non-ACHD adults requiring assist devices (Table 19.2).

19.6 Strategy for MCS

The strategy for the use of durable mechanical circulatory support is individualized to the patients and is divided in three groups:

Bridge to transplant (BTT): patients listed for transplantation with severe hemodynamic compromise that are unlikely to survive to transplant without mechanical-assisted circulation to transplantation

Destination therapy (DT): patients with heart failure refractory to medical management but who are ineligible for transplant and require long-term mechanical support

Bridge to recovery/decision to transplant (BTD): a patient with potentially reversible cardiomyopathy requiring imminent mechanical support or in whom candidacy for transplant cannot be determined at that time

19.7 Indications for Mechanical Circulatory Support

The need for MCS in patients with advanced HF arrives when the cardiac impairment reaches the point of insufficient end-organ perfusion, or severe physical impairment. Patients are either refractory to optimal medical therapy, dependent on inotropic support, or dependent on temporary MCS (i.e., IABP, Impella, TandemHeart, ECMO). The classification by the NYHA grading leaves a wide spectrum for interpretation of the patient's clinical status and is not always helpful in

Table 19.2 Risk management of cardiac and noncardiac comorbidities in patients considered for durable mechanical circulatory support devices (J Heart Lung Transplant. 2013 Feb;32(2):157–87)

Disease/issue	Recommendation (all expert opinion only)
Cardiac	
Coronary artery disease	CT scan to localize bypass grafts, delay implantation in the setting of acute MI
Bioprosthetic AVR	If functioning no intervention needed
Mechanical AVR	Replacement with bioprosthetic AVR or surgical closure
Aortic regurgitation	More than mild requires surgical intervention
Aortic stenosis	Consider bioprosthetic AVR for any degree of aortic stenosis if more than mild aortic insufficiency is also present
Aortic root disease	Patients with known vascular and or coronary disease should have a preoperative assessment of the ascending aorta
Mitral valve stenosis	Valve replacement with tissue valve if moderate or worse stenosis present
Mitral valve insufficiency	Routine mitral valve repair or replacement for severe MR is not recommended unless ventricular recovery is expected
Mechanical mitral valve replacement	Presence of mechanical mitral valve requires higher maintenance INR
Moderate or greater tricuspid valve regurgitation	Surgical repair to be considered at the time of implant
Infective endocarditis	Valvular endocarditis or infection of an implanted ICD or pacemaker with active bacteremia is a contraindication to MCS
Intracardiac shunts	Atrial defects should be closed at the time of implant, LVAD unknown in this setting off ventricular septal defect or free wall rupture is not recommended
Intracardiac thrombus	Presence needs to be excluded by echo or CT
Atrial arrhythmia	Atrial arrhythmias are not a contraindication to MCS, consider AV node ablation in the presence of refractory atrial tachyarrhythmias within need of appropriate pacemaker placement
Ventricular arrhythmia	Patients with refractory ventricular arrhythmia should not be considered for LV support alone
Noncardiac	
Peripheral vascular disease	Relative contraindication based on the extent of the disease
Pulmonary hypertension	All patients require hemodynamic invasive assessment of the pulmonary vascular resistance
Neurologic function	In the presence of significant neurologic disease with dementia, neurologic consultation should be obtained. All patients considered for MCS should have a Doppler examination of extracranial arteries. Patients with a history of a stroke should have a baseline CT scan or MRI of the brain performed. Patients with neuromuscular disease which compromises the ability to care for the external system components or to ambulate should not be considered for MCS
Coordination and hematologic disorders	Patients with abnormalities and baseline assessment off the coagulation parameters should have a hematologic consultation especially with a history of thrombophilia. Patients with a clinical syndrome of HIT should have confirmatory testing
Malignancies	Patients with a history of cancer in long-term remission should be considered candidates for MCS. Patients with a recent history of treated cancer and life expectancy of over 2 years may be candidates for destination therapy. MCS is not recommended for patients with active malignancy and life expectancy of less than 2 years

Table 19.2 (continued)

Disease/issue	Recommendation (all expert opinion only)
Diabetes mellitus	All patients should be screened for diabetes mellitus and the potential presence of end-organ damage. The presence of diabetes-related proliferative retinopathy, poor glycemic control, severe neuropathy, vasculopathy, or peripheral neuropathy can be a relative contraindication to MCS
Pregnancy	MCS in the setting of active pregnancy is not recommended, and the use of contraception in women of childbearing age after MCS is recommended
Advanced age	Patients over the age of 60 should undergo a thorough evaluation of the presence of other clinical risk factors that may decrease survival or quality of life after MCS
Psychosocial	
Psychological and psychiatric	Patient should undergo a comprehensive evaluation which needs to include:
	Assessment of her general demographic information
	Physical functioning
	Psychological and psychiatric status
	Behavior and coping
	Family and support network
	Financial situation
	Screening for cognitive dysfunction
	MCS is contraindicated in patients who:
	Are physically unable to operate the pump
	Are unable to report signs and symptoms of device malfunction
	Live in an unsafe environment
	Have active psychiatric illness that requires long-term institutionalization or makes him/her unable to care for maintenance of the device
Tobacco use	Previous tobacco use should not preclude placement of an emergent pump for BTT, but patients cannot be active on the transplant list until 6 months of abstinence has been proven
Alcohol and substance abuse	Active substance abuse, including alcohol, is a contraindication for MCS therapy. The patient should be abstinent for a period of time as defined by the implanting program

hospitalized patients. Therefore, the approach to MCS in ACHD must be individualized, and the Interagency Registry for Mechanically Assisted Circulatory Support (INTERMACS) classification system is a more useful tool to determining timing and eligibility for VAD therapy. The INTERMACS classification (Table 19.3) was developed to capture the clinical scenarios from cardiogenic shock (INTERMACS 1) to ambulatory end-stage heart failure patient (INTERMACS4-7) [29].

Temporary MCS is most likely to be utilized in the setting of cardiogenic shock (INTERMACS 1) or in heart failure that is thought to be reversible [30]. The ISHLT MCS guidelines state that "use of temporary mechanical support should be strongly considered in patients with multi-organ failure, sepsis, or on mechanical ventilation to allow successful optimization of clinical status and neurologic assessment prior to placement of a long-term MCS device (Level of evidence C)" [31]. Temporary support can either be percutaneously or surgically placed (Tables 19.4 and 19.5) [32, 33]. Once the patient has been stabilized and end-organ function either normalized or preserved, patients can move on to be candidates for a durable mechanical circulatory

Table 19.3 INTERMACS level of limitation at the time of implant (J Heart Lung Transplant. 2009 Jun;28(6):535–41)

INTERMACS profile descriptions	Time frame for intervention
Profile 1: Critical cardiogenic shock	
Patients with life-threatening hypotension despite rapidly escalating inotropic support critical organ hypoperfusion, often confirmed by worsening acidosis and/or lactate levels. "*Crash* and bum"	Definitive intervention needed within hours
Profile 2: Progressive decline	
Patient with declining function despite intravenous inotropic support may be manifest by worsening renal function, nutritional depletion, and inability to restore volume balance. "Siding on inotropes." Also describes declining status in patients unable to tolerate inotropic therapy	Definitive intervention needed within few days
Profile 3: Stable but inotrope dependent	
Patient with stable blood pressure, organ function, nutrition, and symptoms on continuous intravenous inotropic support (or a temporary circulatory support device or both), but demonstrating repeated failure to wean from support due to recurrent symptomatic hypotension or renal dysfunction. "Dependent stability"	Definitive intervention elective over a period of weeks to few months
Profile 4: Resting symptoms	
Patient can be stabilized close to normal volume status but experiences daily symptoms of congestion at rest or during ADL. Doses of diuretics generally fluctuate at very high levels. More intensive management and surveillance strategies should be considered, which may in some cases reveal poor compliance that would compromise outcomes with any therapy. Some patients may shuttle between 4 and 5	Definitive intervention elective over a period of weeks to few months
Profile 5: Exertion intolerant	
Comfortable at rest and with ADL but unable to engage in any other activity, living predominantly within the house. Patients are comfortable at rest without congestive symptoms, but may have underlying refractory elevated volume status, often with renal dysfunction. If underlying nutritional status and organ function are marginal, patients may be more at risk than INTERMACS 4, and require definitive intervention	Variable urgency, depends upon maintenance of nutrition, organ function, and activity
Profile 6: Exertion limited	
Patient without evidence of fluid overload is comfortable at rest, and with activities of daily living and minor activities outside the home, but fatigues after the first few minutes of any meaningful activity. Attribution to cardiac limitation requires careful measurement of peak oxygen consumption, in some cases with hemodynamic monitoring to confirm severity of cardiac impairment. "Walking wounded"	Variable, depends upon maintenance of nutrition, organ function, and activity level
Profile 7: Advanced NYHA III	
A placeholder for more precise specification in future; this level includes patients who are without current or recent episodes of unstable fluid balance, living comfortably with meaningful activity limited to mild physical exertion	Transplantation or circulatory support may not currently be indicated
Modifiers for profiles	
TCS—Temporary circulatory support can modify only patients in hospital (other devices would be INTERMACS devices) Includes WBP, ECMO, TandemHeart Levitronix, BVS 50DQ or AB50C0, Impella	Possible profiles to modify 1, 2, 3 in hospital

Table 19.3 (continued)

INTERMACS profile descriptions	Time frame for intervention
A—Arrhythmia can modify any profile. Recurrent ventricular tachyarrhythmias that have recently contributed substantially to clinical compromise. This includes frequent ICD shock or requirement for external defibrillator, usually more than twice weekly	Any profile
FF—Frequent flyer can modify only outpatients, designating a patient requiring frequent emergency visits or hospitalizations for diuretics, ultrafiltration, or temporary intravenous vasoactive therapy	3 if at home, 4,5,6. A frequent flyer would rarely be profile 7

Table 19.4 Suggested indication for percutaneous mechanical circulatory support (25861963; J Am Coll Cardiol. 2015 May 19;65(19):e7–e26)

Indication	Comments
Complications of AMI	Ischemic mitral regurgitation is particularly well suited to these devices as the hemodynamic disturbance is usually acute and substantial. Acutely depressed LV function from large AMI during and after primary PCI is an increasing indication for temporary MCS use. Cardiogenic shock from RV infarction can be treated with percutaneous right ventricular support.
Severe heart failure in the setting of nonischemic cardiomyopathy	Examples include severe exacerbation of chronic systolic heart failure as well as acutely reversible cardiomyopathies such as fulminant myocarditis, stress cardiomyopathy, or peripartum cardiomyopathy. In patients presenting in INTERMACS profiles 1 or 2, MCS can be used as a bridge to destination VAD placement or as a bridge to recovery if the ejection fraction rapidly improves.
Acute cardiac allograft failure	Primary allograft failure (adult or pediatric) may be due to acute cellular or antibody-mediated rejection, prolonged ischemic time, or inadequate organ preservation.
Posttransplant RV failure	Acute RV failure has several potential causes, including recipient pulmonary hypertension, intraoperative injury/ ischemia, and excess volume/blood product resuscitation. MCS support provides time for the donor right ventricle to recover function, often with the assistance of inotropic and pulmonary vasodilator therapy.
Patients slow to wean from cardiopulmonary bypass following heart surgery	Although selected patients may be transitioned to a percutaneous system for additional weaning, this is rarely done.
Refractory arrhythmias	Patients can be treated with a percutaneous system that is somewhat independent of the cardiac rhythm. For recurrent refractory, ventricular arrhythmias, ECMO may be required for biventricular failure.
Prophylactic use for high-risk PCI	Particularly in patients with severe LV dysfunction (EF <20% to 30% and complex coronary artery disease involving a large territory) (sole-remaining vessel, left main, or three-vessel disease).
High-risk or complex ablation of ventricular tachycardia	Similar to HR-PCI, complex VT ablution can be made feasible with percutaneous support. MCS use allows the patient to remain in VT longer during arrhythmia mapping without as much concern about systemic hypoperfusion.
High-risk percutaneous valve interventions	These evolving procedures may be aided with the use of MCSs.

Table 19.5 Various long-term and short-term mechanical circulatory support devices in oommercBl use or ongoing clinical strides (Lee et al. Hanyang Med Reviews 2014)

Device type	Cover name and manufacturer	Device characteristics	US FDA approval status
Durable devices			
First-generation pulsatile flow extracorporeal device	Thoratec PVAD	Pneumatic pump, BiVAD capable, short- to intermediate-term support	US FDA approved for BTT (1995) postcardiotomy recovery (1998)
	Berlin Heart Excor VAD	Pneumatic pump, BiVAD capable, intermediate term support	US FDA approved child version under Humanitarian Device Exemption (HDE) (2008)
First-generation pulsatile flow intracorporeal device	Thoratec Heart Mate IP, Heart Mate VE, XVE	Pneumatic pump, electric vented pump intermediate to long term support	Heart Mate XVE approved for BTT (2001) DT (2003), rarely used nowadays
	Thoratec IVAD	Implantable version of Thoratec PVAD, short- to intermediate-term support only FDA-approved implantable BiVAD	US FDA approved BTT/ postcardiotomy recovery (2004)
Second-generation continuous axial flow device	Thoratec Heart Mate II	Axial flow pump	US FDA approved for BTT (2008) DT (2010)
	MicroMed DeBakey VAD	Axial flow pump	US FDA approved child version under HDE (2005)
	Jarvik 200	Axial flow pump size with intracardiac location, postauricular cable capable	US FDA permitted usage under investigational device exemption (IDE)
Third-generation continuous centrifugal pump	Berlin Heart Incor VAD	Magnetically suspended axial flow pump	Not approved in the USA
	Heartware HVAD	Hydromagnetically suspended centrifugal pump, intrapericardial location	US FDA approved BTT (2012) On clinical trial for DT
	Terumo Duraheart	Magnetically suspended centrifugal pump	US FDA permitted usage under IDE
	Thoratec Heart Mate III	Magnetically suspended centrifugal pump, smaller size, intrathoracic location	On clinical trial
Total artificial heart	Syncardia TAH	Pneumatic pump, replaces both of the ventricle and four heart valves	US FDA approved for BTT (2004)
	AbioCor TAH	Motor-driven hydraulic pumping system	US FDA approved under HDE who are ineligible to heart transplantation or LVAD for DT

Table 19.5 (continued)

Device type	Cover name and manufacturer	Device characteristics	US FDA approval status
Temporary device			
Surgically implanted	Abiomed AB5000	Pneumatic pump, BiVAD capable, ambulatory version of BVS 5000	US FDA approved for BTR (2003)
	Abiomed BVS 5000	Pneumatic pump, BiVAD capable	US FDA approved for BTR (2003)
	Levtronix CentriMag	Magnetically suspended centrifugal pump, BiVAD capable	US FDA approved for BTD/BTR for 6 h for LV support, 30 days for RV support under HDE
	Biomedicus	Motor-driven centrifugal pump, BiVAD capable	US FDA approved for BTD or BTR for 6 h for LV support, 30 days for RV support
Percutaneously implanted	Tandem Heart	Motor-driven centrifugal pump, interatrial septal puncture needed	US FDA approved for BTD/BTR for 6 h for LV support or support for high-risk intervention
	Impella	Motor microaxial pump located within a catheter implanted retrograde into the left ventricle	Impella 2.5 is US FDA approved for BTD/BTR for 6 h for LV support or support for high-risk intervention

PVAD paracorporeal ventricular assist device, *BiVAD* biventricular assist device, *BTT* bridge to transplant, *DT* destination therapy, *BTR* bridge to recovery

support device [34]. The utilization of temporary and permanent support is a dynamic process and was summarized by the ISHLT guidelines in 2013 (Fig. 19.2) [31].

Patients in INTERMACS profile 1 do far worse compared to profiles 2 and 3. Many programs have abandoned implantation of these sick patients without stabilization with temporary MCS, such as extracorporeal membranous oxygenation (ECMO), prior to durable VAD implantation [31, 35]. VAD implantation in INTERMACS profiles 4–7 is outside the scope of this text.

19.8 ACHD VAD Outcomes

The ACHD population accounted for only 0.7% of patients (n = 126) reported as receiving VAD support in the INTERMACS registry [36]. Most had a morphologic left systemic ventricle (n = 63), followed by a morphologic right systemic ventricle (n = 45) and single ventricle (n = 17). Compared to non-ACHD, ACHD were more likely to be younger, undergo device implantation as bridge to transplant, and require BIVAD or TAH support. Overall, there was no difference in INTERMACS profile for ACHD and non-ACHD. However, more ACHD on BiVAD/TAH support were

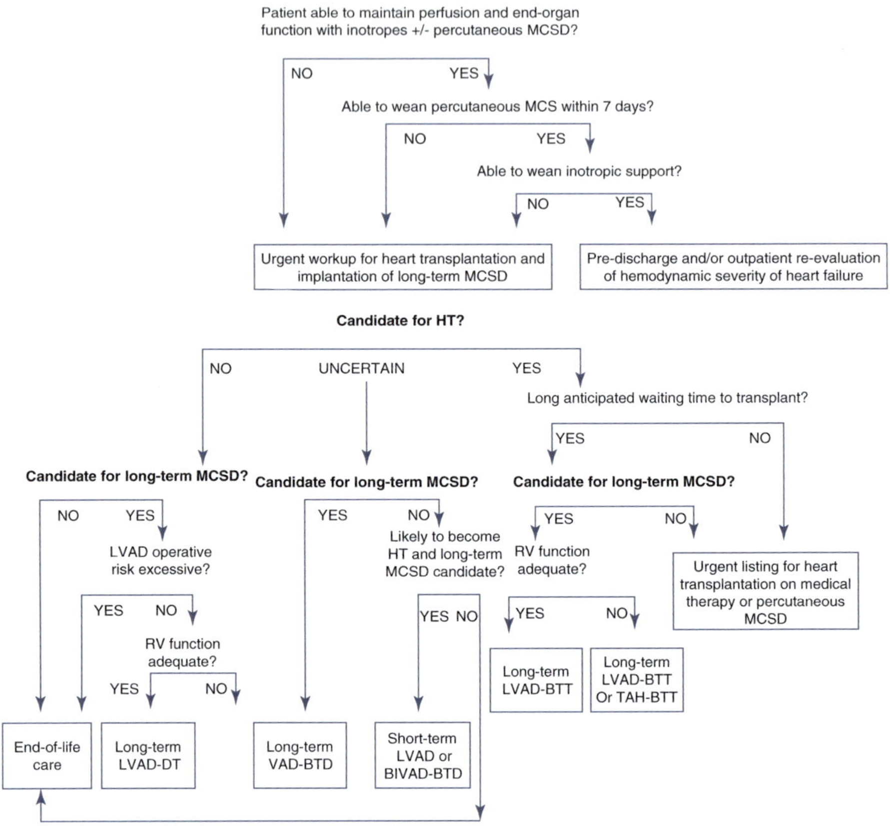

Fig. 19.2 Approach to mechanical circulatory support devices: BTT and DT. **MCSD* mechanical circulatory support device, *HT* heart transplant, *RV* right ventricle, *LVAD* left ventricular assist device, *BIVAD* biventricular assist device, *TAH* total artificial heart, *DT* destination therapy, *BTD* bridge to decision, and *BTT* bridge to transplantation

INTERMACS profile 1 compared with ACHD on a systemic ventricular assist device (SVAD) alone. While overall survival was worse in the ACHD group, there was no difference in survival for ACHD on LVAD. The difference in survival was caused by worse survival in ACHD on BiVAD/TAH (Fig. 19.3), highlighting the need to initiate VAD support prior to the onset of cardiogenic shock [36]. Adverse events (AE) during VAD support were more common in ACHD and are discussed below.

19.9 Contraindications to VAD Placement

Temporary MCS is contraindicated for patients with non-cardiac forms of shock, clinical futility, or multi-organ failure. The majority of temporary devices support systemic ventricular function only and have device-specific limitation in terms of size and mode of placement which need to be considered in each individual patient and might create patient-specific contraindications [37]. ECMO should be utilized

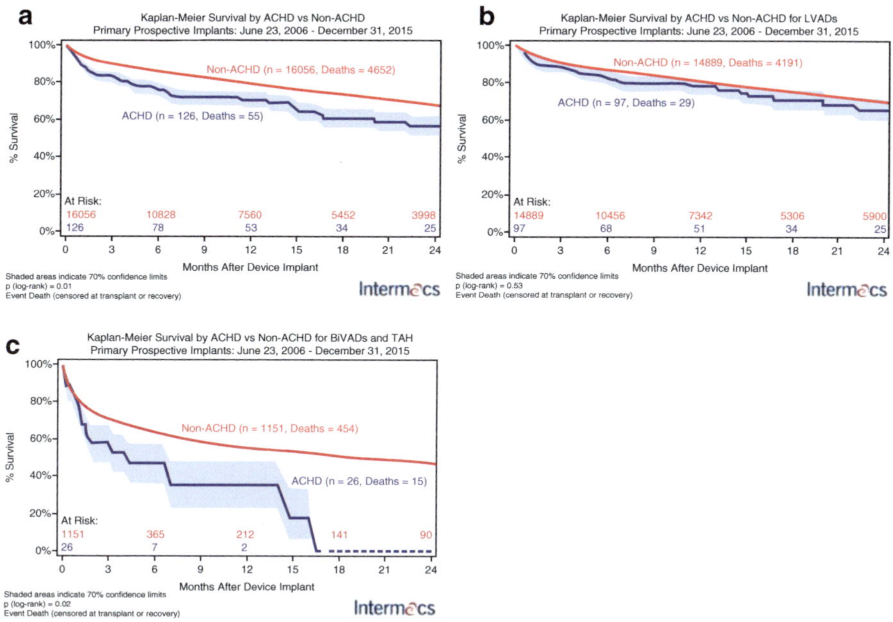

Fig. 19.3 (**a**) Kaplan-Meier survival after MCS implantation for all ACHD compared with all non-ACHD patients. (**b**) Kaplan-Meier survival after VAD implantation for all ACHD compared with all non-ACHD patients. (**c**) Kaplan-Meier survival after BiVAD and TAH implantation for all ACHD compared with all non-ACHD patients. All patients were censored at the time of transplant or recovery (MCS explanation)

in patients with respiratory failure. The implantation of a permanent MCS device carries a significant risk in terms of complications. Some of these complications are more predictable and common when certain clinical or psychosocial features are present prior to implantation. Every implant center develops its own internal list of relative and absolute contraindications (Table 19.6).

19.10 Pre-implant Evaluation and Patient Selection

The workup prior to implant of a durable MCS device is similar to the evaluation of candidacy for heart transplantation. There is no universally accepted protocol specifically for a durable VAD available, so an example of data required for the evaluation is shown in Table 19.7. Medical evaluation specific to ACHD includes a thorough evaluation of arrhythmia-induced ventricular dysfunction, residual lesions, and AV valve function. Treatment of arrhythmias may alleviate the need for MCS. Interventional and surgical options prior to MCS may include removal pressure and volume loads by occlusion of collateral vessel or shunts, balloon valvuloplasty or angioplasty, percutaneous valve placement, conduit or valve replacement, or AV valve repair. Fontan conversion with a maze procedure may be a better option than MCS in patients with an atriopulmonary connection [38].

Table 19.6 Contraindications for implantation of durable mechanical circulatory support devices

Contraindications for implantation of durable MCS	
Relative	Absolute

Age above 80
Chronic kidney disease (e.g., persistent creatinine level above 3.0 mg/dL)
Chronic malnutrition
Obesity (BMI >40)
Mechanical ventilation
Abdominal aneurysm (>5 cm) or severe peripheral vascular disease
Heparin-induced thrombocytopenia
Inability to tolerate aspirin
Frailty out of proportion to cardiac disease
	Potentially reversible cause of heart failure (e.g., fulminant myocarditis, where temporary MCS may be more appropriate)
	Active systemic infection or major chronic risk for infection
	Multisystem organ failure (may be appropriate for temporary MCS, e.g., ECMO or Impella, so assess reversibility and stabilization)
	Prohibitively high surgical risk for successful implantation
	Recent or evolving stroke
	Coexisting terminal conditions—life expectancy less than 2 years
	  Cancer with poor prognosis
	  Cirrhosis, portal hypertension
	  Severe pulmonary dysfunction, O2 dependence not heart failure related
	Neurological deficits or cognitive issues impairing the ability to manage the device following the implant
	Significant underlying psychiatric illness impairing the ability to manage the device following the implant
	Ongoing substance abuse (alcohol, IV drugs, methamphetamine, cocaine)
	Lack of social support that may impair the ability to maintain or operate VAD
	Inability to tolerate anticoagulation with warfarin

Table 19.7 Workup sheet for placement of durable mechanical circulatory support (internal)

Laboratory	CBC with differential, CMP, uric acid, LDH, PT, PTT, INR, prealbumin, HCV, HBV, HIV, PSA (males), pregnancy test (females), iron studies, TSH, HGA1C, ABO, BNP, troponin, CK, hemoccults, spot urine for albumin/creatinine ratio, urine analysis
Consultations	Cardiothoracic surgery, social work, family meeting with VAD coordinator, financial counselor, palliative care, dental consult
Technical studies	Right-heart catheterization with vasodilatory challenge, hepatic wedge pressure if indicated, assessment of collateral burden (aortopulmonary; venovenous)
	Fontan specific: liver CT or MRI
	Liver biopsy if cirrhosis is suspected
	Ischemia evaluation if indicated
	Pulmonary function tests
	ECG
	Device interrogation (ICD, BiV pacer)
	Coronary angiogram if indicated
	2D echocardiography with assessment for interatrial shunt, TEE if suboptimal windows
	First-pass right-heart nuclear ventriculography or cardiac CT to evaluate RV function if no other imaging study leads to a sufficient result
	Abdominal ultrasound
	Duplex ultrasound of the carotid arteries
	Duplex ultrasound of the lower extremity arteries (plus ABI)
	Chest X-ray PA and lateral
	Pulmonary function tests with bronchodilator challenge if indicated
	Colon cancer screening (<50, hemoccult, >50 colonoscopy or colonography
	Breast cancer screening >40 years (female)
	CT chest if indicated to assess ascending aorta or RV to sternum relationship
	Exercise tolerance test to assess maximal oxygen consumption (VO2max)

Once the medical evaluation is complete, a thorough evaluation of the social situation, substance abuse history, and financial situation has to be performed. In the United States, regulatory agencies require that patients be evaluated by a palliative care team prior to VAD implantation, especially for destination therapy. Once this evaluation process has been completed, patients need to be discussed in a multispecialty selection meeting to determine the appropriate strategy and candidacy for the patient. The unique features of ACHD patients described above need to be taken into account during this process.

19.11 Timing for Placement of a Durable Mechanical Circulatory Support Device

Timing of implant is a critical component of optimizing outcomes. Over the years, certain risk scores were developed in order to judge the operative mortality of non-ACHD LVAD placement. However, these scoring systems have not been validated in the ACHD population [39–41]. The most critical ACHD assessment tool is the INTERMACS classification system (Table 19.3), which identifies clinical features of patients with end-stage heart failure at various stages of disease to optimize timing of VAD implantation [29]. Durable VAD outcomes in patient labeled INTERMACS 1 (crash and burn) have significantly worse survival compared to INTERMACS 2 (sliding on inotropes) or INTERMACS 3 (stable on inotropes). Due to this finding, LVAD implantation has decreased in INTERMACS 1 patients [42]. These patients are usually best managed by stabilization with temporary devices (intra-aortic balloon pump, TandemHeart, Impella, CentriMag) or ECMO to recover end-organ function prior to durable VAD placement [37, 43].

19.12 Device Types

The type of device chosen must be tailored to an individual patient and depends on the chosen strategy for the individual (BTD vs. BTT vs. DT). Commonly used devices are shown in Table 19.5. In general, temporary devices and ECMO are utilized in situations for which recovery is anticipated, as a bridge to interventional therapy or as a bridge to a durable VAD. Durable devices are typically used as BTT, BTD, or DT. Situations with potential for recovery may include postoperative ventricular dysfunction, sepsis, myocarditis, medically refractory arrhythmias, or transient ischemia. If temporary support does not result in ventricular recovery, conversion to a durable VAD can be performed if the anatomy is amenable (Fig. 19.2). ECMO can be utilized if there is concern that lung function may be inadequate for gas exchange or if it will allow for more rapid initiation of MCS. ECMO is not commonly utilized after ACHD surgery, and survival is just under 50% if ECMO is required postoperatively [44]. While ECMO can effectively stabilize patients with cardiogenic shock and recover end-organ function prior to placement of a durable VAD, temporary VAD may be more appealing than ECMO when coming out of the operating room if lung function is intact. A temporary VAD (percutaneous or surgically placed) avoids exposure to the large artificial surface of the oxygenator. Oxygenator exposure results in more heat loss, inflammatory response, platelet activation, and consumption of coagulation factors. If lung function becomes inadequate, some temporary VAD systems allow for insertion of an oxygenator into the circuit. Fortunately, over the last several years, oxygenators have become more compact, decreasing the surface area for blood exposure [45]. Outside of the postoperative period, progressive HF in ACHD may be suitable for treatment with percutaneous VAD support. Devices such as the Impella, the TandemHeart, or the CentriMag can be considered for percutaneous systemic ventricular or sub-pulmonary ventricular support if patient anatomy is appropriate.

19.13 Preparing for the Operating Room (Table for Studies)

Optimization of the clinical status is essential to ensure a good outcome and avoid adverse events. End-organ dysfunction related to sub-pulmonary ventricular failure such as volume overload, renal dysfunction, and coagulopathy should be treated if possible. If resolution does not occur, BiVAD support is likely necessary. In patients with severe sub-pulmonary atrioventricular (AV) valve regurgitation or ventricular failure, intractable arrhythmias, transplant graft failure, or failed Fontan physiology, the decision should be made to proceed with a biventricular support strategy. The decision to use systemic or biventricular support can at times be unclear. Assessment of clinical factors that can affect sub-pulmonary ventricular function is critical. Echocardiographic (TAPSE, 1.5 cm, RV size/LV size), hemodynamic (RVSWI <300 mmHg*mL/m^2, PAPI<1.85, CVP/PW > 0.62), and biological (total bilirubin ≥ 2 mg/dL, AST $\geq$ 80 IU/l, creatinine ≥ 2.3 mg/dL) parameters of sub-pulmonary ventricular function need to be assessed and optimized before proceeding with placement of a systemic VAD [46–50]. Temporary VAD support for the sub-pulmonary ventricle in patients with an elevated PVRI and/or any of the above risk factors should be readily available. Malnutrition in the setting of end-stage heart failure is often encountered and is most often not amenable to a rapid correction. Malnutrition is clearly related to operative recovery and impaired wound healing. Therefore, even temporary nutritional supplementation with a feeding tube should be considered. Any infection must be treated aggressively, and the presence of an active infection, especially bloodstream infections, is a contraindication for placement of a durable VAD. The type of hemodynamic monitoring to be placed in the operating room should be determined for each individual patient in the preoperative planning phase. Additionally, postoperative bleeding should be anticipated and the blood bank alerted to the potential need for large volumes of blood products.

19.14 Intraoperative Decision-Making

Determination of the optimal location to place a device in a patient with a systemic right ventricle is challenging. TEE guidance along with the use of a needle to confirm the location of the systemic right ventricle and to aid in resection of right ventricular trabeculations may be necessary [6, 51–53]. If VAD output is suboptimal when coming off cardiopulmonary bypass, there should be a high index of suspicion for cannula obstruction. Adjustment of cannula positioning and/or additional resection of trabeculae may be necessary and can result in normalization of VAD flow and function [53]. If there is no evidence of cannula obstruction, assessment of the adequacy of the sub-pulmonary ventricular function is critical and requires inclusion of data from invasive monitoring, transesophageal echocardiography, and the device. Chronotropic incompetence should be treated with drugs or temporary pacing. A high central venous pressure (defined by INTERMACS as >16 mmHg) with low cardiac output is consistent with sub-pulmonary ventricular failure, especially if associated with moderate or greater tricuspid regurgitation and RV dilation. In this setting, continuous flow device monitors are likely to show low pulsatility and flow, while pulsatile devices will demonstrate incomplete filling. If there is a shift of the interventricular septum toward the systemic ventricle, the cause of the sub-pulmonary ventricular dysfunction could be the excessive septal shift. In this case, the settings of the continuous flow device should be adjusted (decrease the RPM) to allow for better filling of the systemic ventricle. If unresponsive to changes in device settings, the treatment should include escalation of inotropic support, inhaled nitric oxide, and possibly a temporary sub-pulmonary VAD. Persistent elevation of CVP with low output, unresponsive changes in inotropic support, pacing, initiation of inhaled nitric oxide, or adjustment of RPM, should result in temporary sub-pulmonary VAD placement. Prior to leaving the operating room, ICD or pacemaker settings should return to their appropriate settings. Consultation with an electrophysiology team should be performed if deviation from the preoperative ICD/pacemaker plans needs to be made.

19.15 VAD-Specific Postoperative Care

The initial stabilization of the ACHD VAD patient will be dependent on events that occur in the operating room. Involvement of the intensivist and VAD physician with the surgical team in the operating room when coming off cardiopulmonary bypass helps to ensure a smooth transition to the ICU setting. The general transition from the operating room to the intensive care setting is discussed elsewhere in this text.

Invasive hemodynamic monitoring, including systemic arterial blood pressure, pulmonary artery pressure, and central venous pressure, is critical for patient management and troubleshooting. The device itself provides invasive monitoring, and each device can give indications of inadequate preload or excessive afterload. It is even possible to diagnose cardiac tamponade based on continuous flow pump waveforms evaluation. Noninvasive monitoring is similar to what has been described elsewhere in this text with few exceptions. Patients with systemic continuous flow devices are typically pulseless. Therefore, pulse oximetry is unreliable, and noninvasive blood pressure measurements must be taken using the Doppler method to obtain a mean arterial pressure. Once arterial blood pressure monitoring is no longer necessary, noninvasive blood pressure measurements should be performed prior to removing arterial lines to ensure correlation.

Upon return to the intensive care unit, control of bleeding is of the highest priority. Extensive postoperative bleeding should be anticipated in ACHD patients, and a large volume of blood products, including packed red blood cells, fresh frozen plasma, cryoprecipitate, and activated factor 7, should be available from the blood bank. Anticoagulation, required to prevent pump thrombosis and stroke, should not be initiated until control of bleeding is confirmed. Each individual center should develop an anticoagulation protocol and initiate anticoagulation between 24–48 h after surgery [54]. Anticoagulation is typically initiated with heparin, but alternative anticoagulants such as bivalirudin can be used when heparin is contraindicated. In adults, bivalirudin has been shown to be efficacious in the setting of heparin-induced thrombocytopenia [55, 56].

Managing continuous flow devices requires a thorough understanding of the type of device implanted, the device's sensitivity to preload and afterload, and the potential for adverse events [36, 57–59]. Determining the etiology of device output abnormalities requires the incorporation of multiple different forms of data from physical examination, hemodynamic monitoring, laboratory evaluation, and device data (continuous flow device waveforms, power consumption, and flow or pulsatile flow device pump filling and emptying). Figure 19.3 shows an algorithm for evaluation of low output/hypotension for patients with continuous flow devices [60]. This algorithm helps in differentiating sub-pulmonary ventricular failure from hypovolemia, bleeding, tamponade, cannula obstruction, low pump speed, vasodilating medications, and sepsis. Specific complications can be recognized by incorporation of multiple different forms of patient data. Patterns of patient data in various complications of pulsatile and continuous flow devices are shown in Tables 19.8 and 19.9, respectively [59]. If resuscitation is necessary, resuscitation algorithms for continuous flow devices and the TAH should be followed (Figs. 19.4 and 19.5) [60].

Table 19.8 Recognizing pulsatile flow left ventricular assist device complications

	Heart rate	Central venous pressure	Echocardiogram	Pump changes	Treatment
RV failure	↑	↑↑	RV dysfunction	Poor filling	Inotropes, pulmonary vasodilators, consider RVAD
Thrombus	No change	No change	No change	No change	Pump change
Tamponade	↑↑	↑↑	Underfilled LV	Poor filling	Exploration
Hypervolemia	No change	↑↑	LV distension	Full fill, decreased ejection	Increase rate, diuresis
Hypovolemia	↑↑	↓	Potential suction events	Poor filling	Fluid, evaluate right heart

RV right ventricular, *LV* left ventricular, *VAD* ventricular assist device

Table 19.9 Recognizing continuous-flow left ventricular assist device complications

	Heart rate	Central venous pressure	Echocardiogram	Pump changes for HM II	Pump changes for Heartware ventricular assist device	Treatment
Right-heart failure	↑	↑↑	RV dysfunction, poor LV filling	Decreased PI and watts	Decreased amplitude and watts	Inotropes, pulmonary vasodilators, consider decreasing RPM, or right ventricular assist device
Thrombus	NC	NC	LV dilation, failed ramp study (HM II)	Increased watts and flow	Increased watts and flow	Heparin or pump exchange
Tamponade	↑	↑↑	Poor LV filling	Suction, decreased PI and flow	Suction, decreased amplitude and flow	Exploration
Hypervolemia	NC	↑	LV distension	Increased watts and flow	Increased watts and flow	Consider increasing RPM, diuresis
Hypovolemia	↑↑	↓	Poor filling, suction	Suction, decreased PI	Suction, decreased amplitude	Fluid, evaluate right heart, ±decrease RPM

HM II HeartMate II, *LV* left ventricular, *NC* no change, *PI* pulsatility index, *RPM* revolutions per minute, *VAD* ventricular assist device

Defibrillation and chest compressions can be performed in all device types except the TAH. Table 19.10 shows device-specific differences in performing resuscitation in patients on MCS [60].

Sub-pulmonary ventricular failure can happen at any point post-VAD placement, and its management is similar to what was described above (intraoperative decision-making). Inotropic support should be escalated. A combination of milrinone and epinephrine is commonly used. Milrinone's pulmonary vasodilating properties are beneficial in this setting. However, its systemic vasodilating properties can result in hypotension, and milrinone has been associated with arrhythmias in adults [61]. The degree of renal impairment must be taken into account when dosing milrinone, as supra-therapeutic milrinone levels in the adult population correlate with renal dysfunction with milrinone dosing at 0.2 mcg/kg/min [62]. Epinephrine in low doses (0.02–0.05 mcg/kg/min) may be the best catecholamine option for increasing contractility of right ventricles [63, 64]. Sub-pulmonary ventricular afterload can be reduced

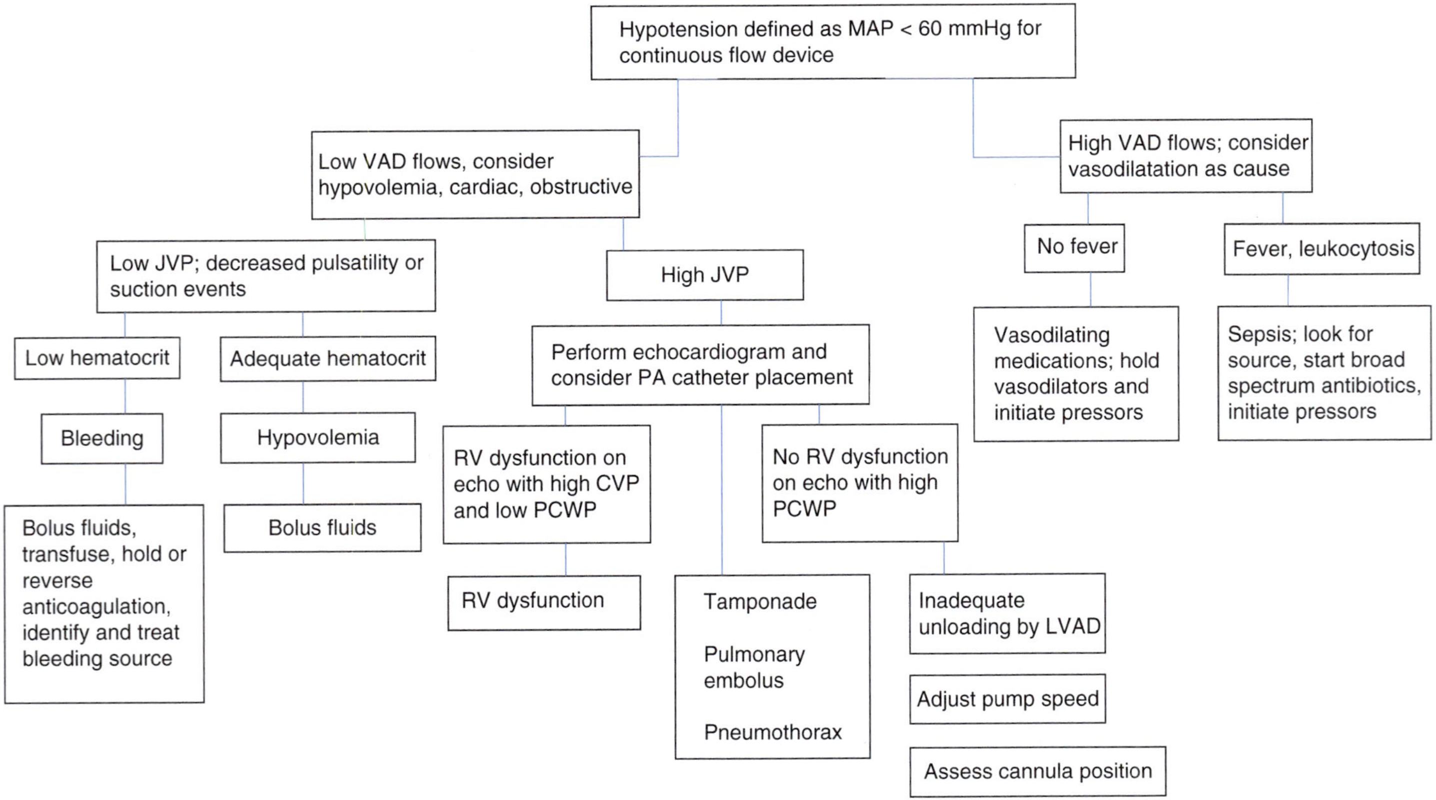

Fig. 19.4 Algorithm for assessment of hypotension after implant. *CVP* central venous pressure, *JVP* jugular venous pressure, *LVAD* left ventricular assist device, *MAP* mean arterial pressure, *PA* pulmonary artery, *PCWP* pulmonary capillary wedge pressure, *RV* right ventricular, *VAD* left ventricular assist device

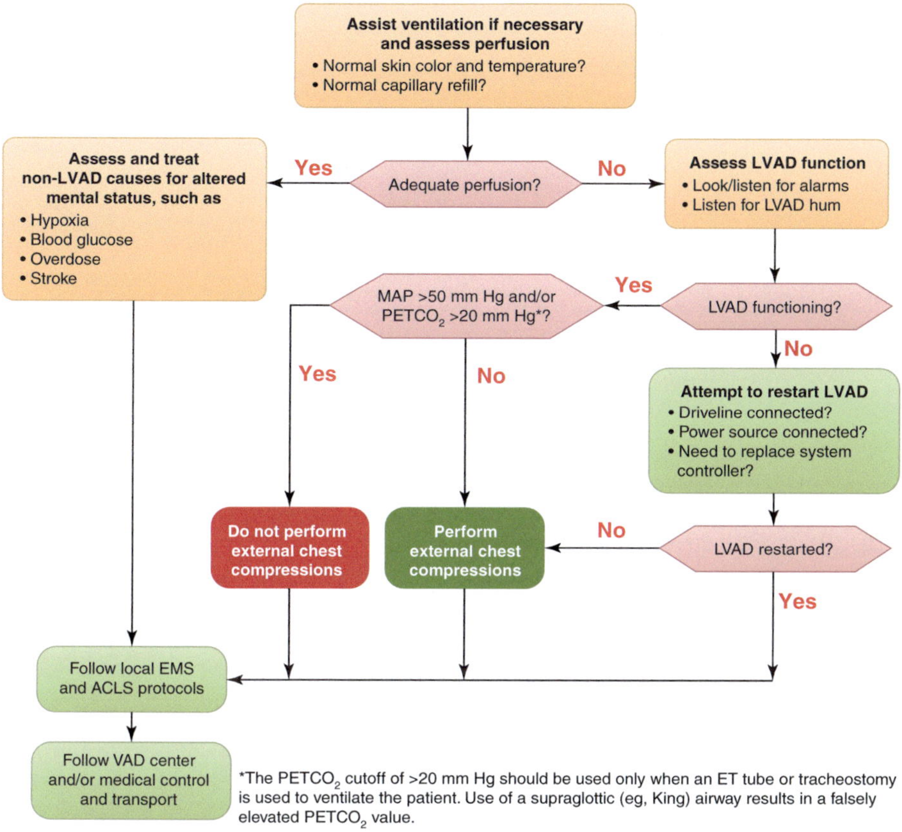

Fig. 19.5 Algorithm showing response to a patient with a left ventricular assist device (LVAD) with unresponsiveness or other altered mental status. *ACLS* indicates advanced cardiovascular life support, *EMS* emergency medical services, *ET* endotracheal tube, *MAP* mean arterial pressure, *Petco2* partial pressure of end-tidal carbon dioxide, and *VAD* ventricular assist device

Table 19.10 Basic differences in performing resuscitation in patients with mechanical circulatory support

Mechanical support type	Perfusion (pulse check)	ECG	Defibrillation/ cardioversion	Chest compressions	ACLS drugs
p-RVAD	Pulsatile	Present	Acceptable	Acceptable	Acceptable
p-LVAD	Pulsatile	Present	Acceptable	Acceptable	Acceptable
p-BiVAD	Pulsatile	Present	Acceptable	Acceptable	Acceptable
cf-RVAD	Pulsatile	Present	Acceptable	Acceptable	Acceptable
cf-LVAD	Absent pulsatile	Present	Acceptable	Acceptable	Acceptable
cf-BiVAD	Absent pulsatile	Present	Acceptable	Acceptable	Acceptable
TAH	Pulsatile	Absent	Unacceptable	Unacceptable	Unacceptable

ACLS indicates advanced cardiovascular life support, *BiVAD* biventricular assist device, *cf* continuous flow, *LVAD* left ventricular assist device, *p* pulsatile, *RVAD* right ventricular assist device, and *TAH* total artificial heart

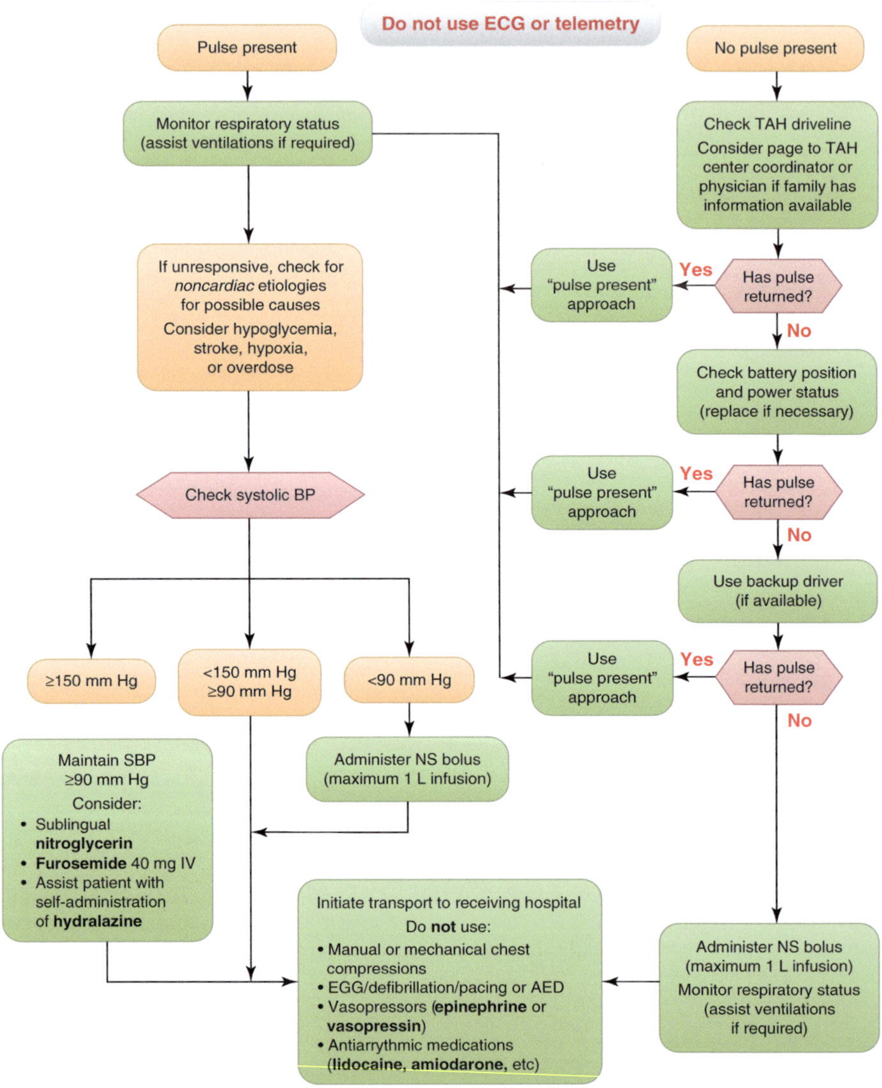

Fig. 19.6 Algorithm showing response to a patient with a total artificial heart (TAH) with altered mental status, unresponsiveness, or respiratory distress. *AED* indicates automated external defibrillator, *BP* blood pressure, *IV* Intravenous, *NS* normal saline, and *SBP* systolic blood pressure

with inhaled nitric oxide [65–67] and phosphodiesterase 5 inhibitors [68, 69]. Echocardiography should evaluate the position of the IVS. If the septum is shifted toward the systemic ventricle, the RPMs on the devices should be lowered to improve sub-pulmonary ventricular geometry, which may improve contractility. Volume overload often contributes to acute RV failure. A continuous infusion of a loop diuretic may help avoid large swings in intravascular volume, while providing a reduction in filling pressures and subsequent improvement in ventricular performance (Fig. 19.6).

Any continuous flow device patient with evidence of hemolysis, high power consumption, and/or new heart failure symptoms should be evaluated for pump thrombosis. The recognition and management of pump thrombosis are shown in Fig. 19.7 and Table 19.9 [59]. Diagnosing pump thrombosis requires a combination of clinical findings, which may include changes in device log file reports, heart failure, high device power consumption, and hemolysis. Echocardiography with escalating device RPM performed in a patient with pump thrombosis may show a lack of reduction in systemic ventricular size. CT of the chest with angiography can allow visualization of the thrombus. Once confirmed, pump thrombosis is initially treated with discontinuation of long-acting anticoagulants and initiation of heparin. The definitive treatment is typically surgical pump exchange or transplantation. However, the risk-benefit ratio may not be in favor of going to the operating room in all cases, and medical management may be considered in select patients [70, 71].

Blood pressure control is a critical component of avoiding pump thrombosis and strokes, as mean arterial pressures >90 mmHg have been associated with a higher risk of stroke in continuous flow device patients. Centers should have a protocolized approach to BP reduction, as hemorrhagic stroke risk has been shown to be lower in centers with such a protocol [70, 72].

While MCS outcomes have improved over time with advancement of technology and increased clinical experience (Fig. 19.8), adverse events (AE) occur in nearly 80% of adult VAD patients by 30 months post-implant (Fig. 19.9) [35]. Therefore,

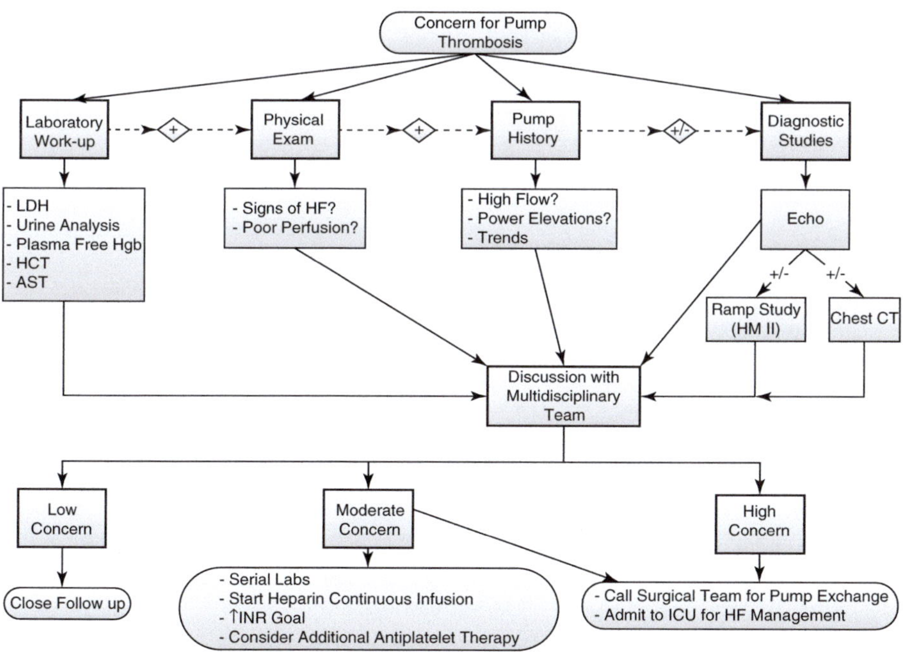

Fig. 19.7 Proposed guidelines for evaluating pump thrombosis in durable, continuous-flow devices. *ACT* activated clotting time, *HCT* hematocrit, *HF* heart failure, *Hgb* hemoglobin, *HR* heart rate, *LDH* lactate dehydrogenase

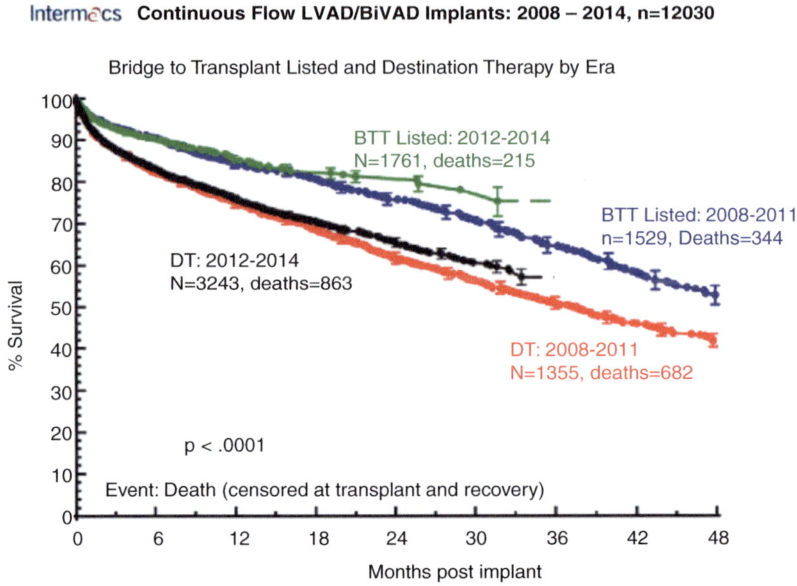

Fig. 19.8 Actuarial survival curves stratified by implant strategy and era. *BTT* bridge to transplant, *DT* destination therapy. The depiction is as shown in Fig. 19.6

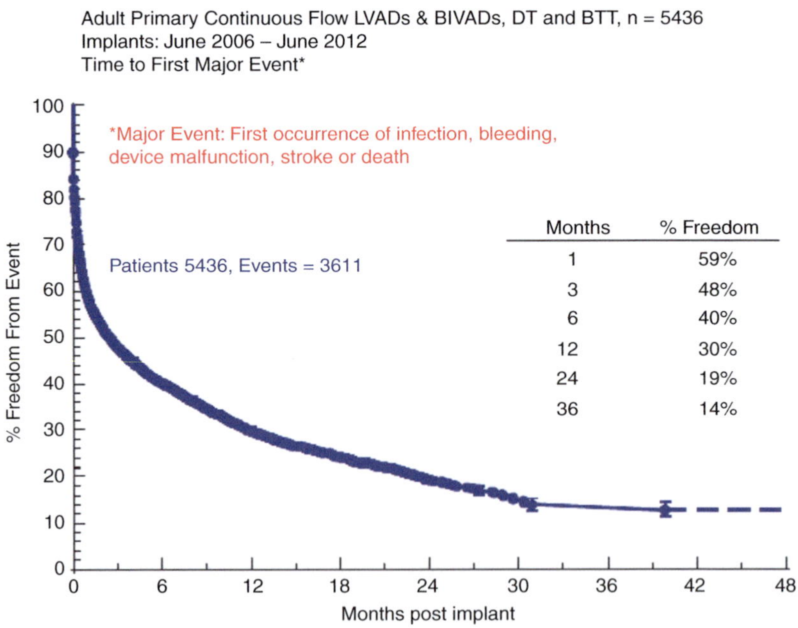

Fig. 19.9 Actuarial freedom from any of the following adverse events: infection, bleeding, device malfunction, stroke, or death. Error bars indicate ±1 standard error. *BIVAD* biventricular assist device, *BTT* bridge to transplant, *DT* destination therapy, *LVAD* left ventricular assist device

there has been an increased focus on preventing AE. INTERMACS has developed standardized definitions of AE which have reached wide acceptance in the field. The incidence of AE in the INTERMACS registry differs significantly between ACHD and non-ACHD patients (Table 19.11) [73]. ACHD are more likely to develop infection, arrhythmias, hepatic dysfunction, renal dysfunction, respiratory failure, and hospital readmission post-VAD than non-ACHD. ACHD with BiVAD support are more likely to develop bleeding, hepatic dysfunction, infection, neurologic dysfunction, renal dysfunction, respiratory failure, device malfunction, and rehospitalization than ACHD LVAD patients.

Table 19.11 Adverse event rates compared between ACHD and non-ACHD patients after the implantation of mechanical circulatory support devices

		ACHD		Non-AEHD		
Event	Period[a]	Events	AE rate[b]	Events	AE rate[b]	*p*-Value
Arterial non-CNS	Early	1	0.3	134	0.4	0.75
thromboembolism	Late	2	0.1	36	0.04	0.04
Bleeding	Early	52	16.1	8461	19.6	0.16
	Late	26	1.9	7305	3.3	0.006
Cardiac arrhythmia	Early	33	10.2	4814	11.2	0.62
	Late	29	2.1	2332	1.0	<0.001
Hepatic dysfunction	Early	18	5.6	687	1.6	<0.001
	Late	12	0.9	440	0.2	<0.001
Infection	Early	64	19.8	7300	16.9	0.21
	Late	85	6.2	9035	4.0	<0.001
Myocardial infarction	Early			55	0.1	
	Late			56	0.03	
Neurologic dysfunction	Early	18	5.6	1997	4.6	0.43
	Late	20	1.5	2710	1.2	0.39
CVA	Early	11	3.4	1079	2.5	0.31
	Late	12	0.9	1623	0.7	0.50
Other SAE	Early	62	19.2	5676	13.2	0.003
	Late	27	2.0	4200	1.9	0.77
Pericardial drainage	Early	5	1.6	941	2.2	0.44
	Late			29	0.01	
Psychiatric episode	Early	12	3.7	1087	2.5	0.18
	Late	6	0.4	679	0.3	0.36
Rehospitalization	Early	66	20.5	8869	20.6	0.97
	Late	244	17.9	34,995	15.6	0.03
Renal dysfunction	Early	34	10.5	1845	4.3	<0.001
	Late	15	1.1	1008	0.4	<0.001
Respiratory failure	Early	49	15.2	3430	8.0	<0.001
	Late	27	2.0	1133	0.5	<0.001
Venous thromboembolism	Early	7	2.2	715	1.7	0.48
	Late			148	0.07	
Wound dehiscence	Early	2	0.6	225	0.5	0.81
	Late			74	0.03	

ACHD adult congenital heart disease, *AE* adverse event, *CNS* central nervous system, *CVA* cerebrovascular accident, *SAE* serious adverse event

[a]Early = within 3 months of device implantation. Late = ≥3 months after device implantation.

[b]Rates per 100 patient-months. ACHD early follow-up, 322.47 months; ACHD late follow-up, 1364.13 months; non-ACHD early follow-up, 43,119.34 months; non-ACHD late follow-up, 224,374.69 months

A multidisciplinary team approach is required to ensure proper intensive care and transition out of the ICU setting. Transplant/VAD surgeons, intensivists, ACHD cardiologists, ICU nurses, transplant/VAD coordinators, step-down unit nurses, pharmacists, psychologist/psychiatrists, social workers, and dieticians should all be involved in the management of these complex patients early in the postoperative period. Early extubation should be a goal in patients with stable sub-pulmonary ventricular function without pulmonary hypertension. Early mobilization, early initiation of enteral nutrition, and excellent wound/driveline care are all critical components of avoiding adverse events and beginning of the rehabilitative process.

References

1. Boneva RS, Botto LD, Moore CA, Yang Q, Correa A, Erickson JD. Mortality associated with congenital heart defects in the United States: trends and racial disparities, 1979–1997. Circulation. 2001;103:2376–81.
2. Khairy P, Ionescu-Ittu R, Mackie AS, Abrahamowicz M, Pilote L, Marelli AJ. Changing mortality in congenital heart disease. J Am Coll Cardiol. 2010;56:1149–57.
3. Marelli AJ, Mackie AS, Ionescu-Ittu R, Rahme E, Pilote L. Congenital heart disease in the general population: changing prevalence and age distribution. Circulation. 2007;115:163–72.
4. Marelli AJ, Ionescu-Ittu R, Mackie AS, Guo L, Dendukuri N, Kaouache M. Lifetime prevalence of congenital heart disease in the general population from 2000 to 2010. Circulation. 2014;130:749–56.
5. van der Bom T, Mulder BJ, Meijboom FJ, van Dijk AP, Pieper PG, Vliegen HW, Konings TC, Zwinderman AH, Bouma BJ. Contemporary survival of adults with congenital heart disease. Heart. 2015;101:1989–95.
6. Ross HJ, Law Y, Book WM, Broberg CS, Burchill L, Cecchin F, Chen JM, Delgado D, Dimopoulos K, Everitt MD, Gatzoulis M, Harris L, Hsu DT, Kuvin JT, Martin CM, Murphy AM, Singh G, Spray TL, Stout KK, American Heart Association Adults with Congenital Heart Disease Committee of the Council on Cardiovascular Disease in the Young, Council on Cardiovascular and Stroke Nursing, Council on Functional Genomics and Translational Biology, and American College of Cardiology. Transplantation and mechanical circulatory support in congenital heart disease: a scientific statement from the American Heart Association. Circulation. 2016a;133:802–20.
7. Verheugt CL, Uiterwaal CS, van der Velde ET, Meijboom FJ, Pieper PG, van Dijk AP, Vliegen HW, Grobbee DE, Mulder BJ. Mortality in adult congenital heart disease. Eur Heart J. 2010;31:1220–9.
8. Norozi K, Wessel A, Alpers V, Arnhold JO, Binder L, Geyer S, Zoege M, Buchhorn R. Chronotropic incompetence in adolescents and adults with congenital heart disease after cardiac surgery. J Card Fail. 2007;13:263–8.
9. Khairy P, Van Hare GF, Balaji S, Berul CI, Cecchin F, Cohen MI, Daniels CJ, Deal BJ, Dearani JA, Groot N, Dubin AM, Harris L, Janousek J, Kanter RJ, Karpawich PP, Perry JC, Seslar SP, Shah MJ, Silka MJ, Triedman JK, Walsh EP, Warnes CA, PACES/HRS Expert Consensus Statement on the Recognition and Management of Arrhythmias in Adult Congenital Heart Disease: developed in partnership between the Pediatric and Congenital Electrophysiology Society (PACES) and the Heart Rhythm Society (HRS). Endorsed by the governing bodies of PACES, HRS, the American College of Cardiology (ACC), the American Heart Association (AHA), the European Heart Rhythm Association (EHRA), the Canadian Heart Rhythm Society (CHRS), and the International Society for Adult Congenital Heart Disease (ISACHD). Heart Rhythm. 2014;11:e102–65.

10. Zomer AC, Vaartjes I, van der Velde ET, de Jong HM, Konings TC, Wagenaar LJ, Heesen WF, Eerens F, Baur LH, Grobbee DE, Mulder BJ. Heart failure admissions in adults with congenital heart disease; risk factors and prognosis. Int J Cardiol. 2013;168:2487–93.
11. Norozi K, Wessel A, Alpers V, Arnhold JO, Geyer S, Zoege M, Buchhorn R. Incidence and risk distribution of heart failure in adolescents and adults with congenital heart disease after cardiac surgery. Am J Cardiol. 2006;97:1238–43.
12. Ma K, Li S, Hu S, Hua Z, Yang K, Yan J, Zhang H, Chen Q, Zhang S, Qi L. Neoaortic valve regurgitation after arterial switch: ten years outcomes from a single center. Ann Thorac Surg. 2016;102:636–42.
13. Hanke JS, ElSherbini A, Avsar M, Horke A, Schmitto JD. Left ventricular assist device implantation in a patient with congenitally corrected transposition of the great arteries. Artif Organs. 2015;39:1069–71.
14. Gregoric ID, Kosir R, Smart FW, Messner GN, Patel VS, La Francesca S, Cervera RD, Frazier OH. Left ventricular assist device implantation in a patient with congenitally corrected transposition of the great arteries. Tex Heart Inst J. 2005;32:567–9.
15. Shim MS, Jun TG, Yang JH, Park PW, Kang IS, Huh J, Song JY. Current expectations of the arterial switch operation in a small volume center: a 20-year, single-center experience. J Cardiothorac Surg. 2016;11:34.
16. Lo Rito M, Fittipaldi M, Haththotuwa R, Jones TJ, Khan N, Clift P, Brawn WJ, Barron DJ. Long-term fate of the aortic valve after an arterial switch operation. J Thorac Cardiovasc Surg. 2015;149:1089–94.
17. Villafane J, Lantin-Hermoso MR, Bhatt AB, Tweddell JS, Geva T, Nathan M, Elliott MJ, Vetter VL, Paridon SM, Kochilas L, Jenkins KJ, Beekman RH 3rd, Wernovsky G, Towbin JA. D-transposition of the great arteries: the current era of the arterial switch operation. J Am Coll Cardiol. 2014;64:498–511.
18. Michalak KW, Moll JA, Moll M, Dryzek P, Moszura T, Kopala M, Mludzik K, Moll JJ. The neoaortic root in children with transposition of the great arteries after an arterial switch operation. Eur J Cardiothorac Surg. 2013;43:1101–8.
19. Bhagra S, Bhagra C, Ozalp F, Butt T, Ramesh BC, Parry G, Roysam C, Woods A, Robinson-Smith N, Wrightson N, MacGowan GA, Schueler S. Development of de novo aortic valve incompetence in patients with the continuous-flow HeartWare ventricular assist device. J Heart Lung Transplant. 2016;35:312–9.
20. Khairy P, Fernandes SM, Mayer JE Jr, Triedman JK, Walsh EP, Lock JE, Landzberg MJ. Long-term survival, modes of death, and predictors of mortality in patients with Fontan surgery. Circulation. 2008;117:85–92.
21. Rychik J, Goldberg DJ. Late consequences of the Fontan operation. Circulation. 2014;130:1525–8.
22. Khambadkone S, Li J, de Leval MR, Cullen S, Deanfield JE, Redington AN. Basal pulmonary vascular resistance and nitric oxide responsiveness late after Fontan-type operation. Circulation. 2003;107:3204–8.
23. Whitehead KK, Harris MA, Glatz AC, Gillespie MJ, DiMaria MV, Harrison NE, Dori Y, Keller MS, Rome JJ, Fogel MA. Status of systemic to pulmonary arterial collateral flow after the fontan procedure. Am J Cardiol. 2015;115:1739–45.
24. Bhatt AB, Foster E, Kuehl K, Alpert J, Brabeck S, Crumb S, Davidson WR Jr, Earing MG, Ghoshhajra BB, Karamlou T, Mital S, Ting J, Tseng ZH, American Heart Association Council on Clinical Cardiology. Congenital heart disease in the older adult: a scientific statement from the American Heart Association. Circulation. 2015;131:1884–931.
25. Pretre R, Haussler A, Bettex D, Genoni M. Right-sided univentricular cardiac assistance in a failing Fontan circulation. Ann Thorac Surg. 2008;86:1018–20.
26. Niebler RA, Ghanayem NS, Shah TK, De La Rosa BA, Zangwill S, Brosig C, Frommelt MA, Mitchell ME, Tweddell JS, Woods RK. Use of a HeartWare ventricular assist device in a patient with failed Fontan circulation. Ann Thorac Surg. 2014;97:e115–6.

27. Morales DL, Adachi I, Heinle JS, Fraser CD Jr. A new era: use of an intracorporeal systemic ventricular assist device to support a patient with a failing Fontan circulation. J Thorac Cardiovasc Surg. 2011;142:e138–40.
28. Frazier OH, Gregoric ID, Messner GN. Total circulatory support with an LVAD in an adolescent with a previous Fontan procedure. Tex Heart Inst J. 2005;32:402–4.
29. Stevenson LW, Pagani FD, Young JB, Jessup M, Miller L, Kormos RL, Naftel DC, Ulisney K, Desvigne-Nickens P, Kirklin JK. INTERMACS profiles of advanced heart failure: the current picture. J Heart Lung Transplant. 2009;28:535–41.
30. Rihal CS, Naidu SS, Givertz MM, Szeto WY, Burke JA, Kapur NK, Kern M, Garratt KN, Goldstein JA, Dimas V, Tu T, Society for Cardiovascular Angiography and Interventions (SCAI); Heart Failure Society of America (HFSA); Society of Thoracic Surgeons (STS); American Heart Association (AHA), and American College of Cardiology (ACC). 2015 SCAI/ACC/HFSA/STS clinical expert consensus statement on the use of percutaneous mechanical circulatory support devices in cardiovascular care (Endorsed by the American Heart Association, the Cardiological Society of India, and Sociedad Latino Americana de Cardiologia Intervencion; Affirmation of Value by the Canadian Association of Interventional Cardiology-Association Canadienne de Cardiologie d'intervention). Catheter Cardiovasc Interv. 2015a;85:E175–96.
31. Feldman D, Pamboukian SV, Teuteberg JJ, Birks E, Lietz K, Moore SA, Morgan JA, Arabia F, Bauman ME, Buchholz HW, Deng M, Dickstein ML, El-Banayosy A, Elliot T, Goldstein DJ, Grady KL, Jones K, Hryniewicz K, John R, Kaan A, Kusne S, Loebe M, Massicotte MP, Moazami N, Mohacsi P, Mooney M, Nelson T, Pagani F, Perry W, Potapov EV, Eduardo Rame J, Russell SD, Sorensen EN, Sun B, Strueber M, Mangi AA, Petty MG, Rogers J, International Society for Heart and Lung Transplantation. The 2013 International Society for Heart and Lung Transplantation Guidelines for mechanical circulatory support: executive summary. J Heart Lung Transplant. 2013;32:157–87.
32. Rihal CS, Naidu SS, Givertz MM, Szeto WY, Burke JA, Kapur NK, Kern M, Garratt KN, Goldstein JA, Dimas V, Tu T, Society for Cardiovascular Angiography and Interventions (SCAI); Heart Failure Society of America (HFSA); Society for Thoracic Surgeons (STS); American Heart Association (AHA); American College of Cardiology (ACC). 2015 SCAI/ACC/HFSA/STS clinical expert consensus statement on the use of percutaneous mechanical circulatory support devices in Cardiovascular Care (Endorsed by the American Heart Association, The Cardiological Society of India, and Sociedad Latino Americana de Cardiologia Intervencionista; Affirmation of Value by the Canadian Association of Interventional Cardiology-Association Canadienne de Cardiologie d'intervention). Catheter Cardiovasc Interv. 2015b;85:1112–4.
33. Lee SJ, Hong SG. Current status of heart transplantation and left ventricular assist device: major changes in the last decade. Hanyang Med Rev. 2014;34:185.
34. Nagpal AD, Singal RK, Arora RC, Lamarche Y. Temporary mechanical circulatory support in cardiac critical care: a state of the art review and algorithm for device selection. Can J Cardiol. 2017;33:110–8.
35. Kirklin JK, Naftel DC, Pagani FD, Kormos RL, Stevenson LW, Blume ED, Myers SL, Miller MA, Baldwin JT, Young JB. Seventh INTERMACS annual report: 15,000 patients and counting. J Heart Lung Transplant. 2015;34:1495.
36. VanderPluym CJ, Cedars A, Eghtesady P, Maxwell BG, Gelow JM, Burchill LJ, Maltais S, Koehl DA, Cantor RS, Blume ED. Outcomes following implantation of mechanical circulatory support in adults with congenital heart disease: an analysis of the Interagency Registry for Mechanically Assisted Circulatory Support (INTERMACS). J Heart Lung Transplant. 2018;37(1):89–99.
37. Rihal CS, Naidu SS, Givertz MM, Szeto WY, Burke JA, Kapur NK, Kern M, Garratt KN, Goldstein JA, Dimas V, Tu T, Society for Cardiovascular Angiography and Interventions (SCAI); Heart Failure Society of America (HFSA); Society for Thoracic Surgeons (STS); American Heart Association (AHA); American College of Cardiology (ACC). 2015 SCAI/ACC/HFSA/STS clinical expert consensus statement on the use of percutaneous mechanical circulatory support devices in cardiovascular care: endorsed by the American Heart

Association, the Cardiological Society of India, and Sociedad Latino Americana de Cardiologia Intervencion; Affirmation of Value by the Canadian Association of Interventional Cardiology-Association Canadienne de Cardiologie d'intervention. J Am Coll Cardiol. 2015c;65: e7–e26.
38. Morales DL, Dibardino DJ, Braud BE, Fenrich AL, Heinle JS, Vaughn WK, McKenzie ED, Fraser CD Jr. Salvaging the failing Fontan: lateral tunnel versus extracardiac conduit. Ann Thorac Surg. 2005;80:1445–51; discussion 1451–2
39. Lietz K, Long JW, Kfoury AG, Slaughter MS, Silver MA, Milano CA, Rogers JG, Naka Y, Mancini D, Miller LW. Outcomes of left ventricular assist device implantation as destination therapy in the post-REMATCH era: implications for patient selection. Circulation. 2007;116:497–505.
40. Cowger J, Sundareswaran K, Rogers JG, Park SJ, Pagani FD, Bhat G, Jaski B, Farrar DJ, Slaughter MS. Predicting survival in patients receiving continuous flow left ventricular assist devices: the HeartMate II risk score. J Am Coll Cardiol. 2013;61:313–21.
41. Levy WC, Mozaffarian D, Linker DT, Sutradhar SC, Anker SD, Cropp AB, Anand I, Maggioni A, Burton P, Sullivan MD, Pitt B, Poole-Wilson PA, Mann DL, Packer M. The Seattle Heart Failure Model: prediction of survival in heart failure. Circulation. 2006;113:1424–33.
42. Kirklin JK, Naftel DC, Kormos RL, Stevenson LW, Pagani FD, Miller MA, Baldwin JT, Young JB. Fifth INTERMACS annual report: risk factor analysis from more than 6,000 mechanical circulatory support patients. J Heart Lung Transplant. 2013;32:141–56.
43. Abu Saleh WK, Jabbari OA, Guha A, Loebe M, Bruckner BA. Treatment strategies for patients with an INTERMACS I profile. Methodist Debakey Cardiovasc J. 2015;11:4–8.
44. Acheampong B, Johnson JN, Stulak JM, Dearani JA, Kushwaha SS, Daly RC, Haile DT, Schears GJ. Postcardiotomy ECMO support after high-risk operations in adult congenital heart disease. Congenit Heart Dis. 2016;11:571–755.
45. Lequier L, Horton SB, McMullan DM, Bartlett RH. Extracorporeal membrane oxygenation circuitry. Pediatr Crit Care Med. 2013;14:S7–12.
46. Kukucka M, Stepanenko A, Potapov E, Krabatsch T, Redlin M, Mladenow A, Kuppe H, Hetzer R, Habazettl H. Right-to-left ventricular end-diastolic diameter ratio and prediction of right ventricular failure with continuous-flow left ventricular assist devices. J Heart Lung Transplant. 2011;30:64–9.
47. Kormos RL, Teuteberg JJ, Pagani FD, Russell SD, John R, Miller LW, Massey T, Milano CA, Moazami N, Sundareswaran KS, Farrar DJ, HeartMate IICI. Right ventricular failure in patients with the HeartMate II continuous-flow left ventricular assist device: incidence, risk factors, and effect on outcomes. J Thorac Cardiovasc Surg. 2010;139:1316–24.
48. Morine KJ, Kiernan MS, Pham DT, Paruchuri V, Denofrio D, Kapur NK. Pulmonary artery pulsatility index is associated with right ventricular failure after left ventricular assist device surgery. J Card Fail. 2016;22:110–6.
49. Matthews JC, Koelling TM, Pagani FD, Aaronson KD. The right ventricular failure risk score a pre-operative tool for assessing the risk of right ventricular failure in left ventricular assist device candidates. J Am Coll Cardiol. 2008;51:2163–72.
50. Argiriou M, Kolokotron SM, Sakellaridis T, Argiriou O, Charitos C, Zarogoulidis P, Katsikogiannis N, Kougioumtzi I, Machairiotis N, Tsiouda T, Tsakiridis K, Zarogoulidis K. Right heart failure post left ventricular assist device implantation. J Thorac Dis. 2014;6(Suppl 1):S52–9.
51. Jouan J, Grinda JM, Bricourt MO, Iserin L, Fabiani JN. Non-pulsatile axial flow ventricular assist device for right systemic ventricle failure late after Senning procedure. Int J Artif Organs. 2009;32:243–5.
52. Neely RC, Davis RP, Stephens EH, Takayama H, Khalpey Z, Ginns J, Lee SH, Chen J. Ventricular assist device for failing systemic ventricle in an adult with prior mustard procedure. Ann Thorac Surg. 2013;96:691–3.
53. Joyce DL, Crow SS, John R, St Louis JD, Braunlin EA, Pyles LA, Kofflin P, Joyce LD. Mechanical circulatory support in patients with heart failure secondary to transposition of the great arteries. J Heart Lung Transplant. 2010;29:1302–5.

54. Maltais S, Kilic A, Nathan S, Keebler M, Emani S, Ransom J, Katz JN, Sheridan B, Brieke A, Egnaczyk G, Entwistle JW 3rd, Adamson R, Stulak J, Uriel N, O'Connell JB, Farrar DJ, Sundareswaran KS, Gregoric I, Investigators PS. PREVENtion of HeartMate II pump thrombosis through clinical management: the PREVENT multi-center study. J Heart Lung Transplant. 2017;36:1–12.
55. Morshuis M, Boergermann J, Gummert J, Koster A. A modified technique for implantation of the HeartWare left ventricular assist device when using bivalirudin anticoagulation in patients with acute heparin-induced thrombocytopenia. Interact Cardiovasc Thorac Surg. 2013;17:225–6.
56. Garland C, Somogyi D. Successful implantation of a left ventricular assist device in a patient with heparin-induced thrombocytopenia and thrombosis. J Extra Corpor Technol. 2014;46:162–5.
57. Slaughter MS, Pagani FD, Rogers JG, Miller LW, Sun B, Russell SD, Starling RC, Chen L, Boyle AJ, Chillcott S, Adamson RM, Blood MS, Camacho MT, Idrissi KA, Petty M, Sobieski M, Wright S, Myers TJ, Farrar DJ, HeartMate IICI. Clinical management of continuous-flow left ventricular assist devices in advanced heart failure. J Heart Lung Transplant. 2010;29:S1–39.
58. Moazami N, Fukamachi K, Kobayashi M, Smedira NG, Hoercher KJ, Massiello A, Lee S, Horvath DJ, Starling RC. Axial and centrifugal continuous-flow rotary pumps: a translation from pump mechanics to clinical practice. J Heart Lung Transplant. 2013;32:1–11.
59. Byrnes J, Villa C, Lorts A. Ventricular assist devices in pediatric cardiac intensive care. Pediatr Critical Care Med. 2016;17:S160–70.
60. Peberdy MA, Gluck JA, Ornato JP, Bermudez CA, Griffin RE, Kasirajan V, Kerber RE, Lewis EF, Link MS, Miller C, Teuteberg JJ, Thiagarajan R, Weiss RM, O'Neil B, American Heart Association Emergency Cardiovascular Care Committee, Council on Cardiopulmonary Critical Care, Perioperative, Resuscitation, Council on Cardiovascular Diseases in the Young, Council on Cardiovascular Surgery and Anesthesia, Council on Cardiovascular and Stroke Nursing and Council on Clinical Cardiology. Cardiopulmonary resuscitation in adults and children with mechanical circulatory support: a scientific statement from the American Heart Association. Circulation. 2017;135:e1115–34.
61. Cuffe MS, Califf RM, Adams KF Jr, Benza R, Bourge R, Colucci WS, Massie BM, O'Connor CM, Pina I, Quigg R, Silver MA, Gheorghiade M. Outcomes of a prospective trial of intravenous Milrinone for exacerbations of chronic heart failure I. Short-term intravenous milrinone for acute exacerbation of chronic heart failure: a randomized controlled trial. JAMA. 2002;287:1541–7.
62. Hasei M, Uchiyama A, Nishimura M, Mashimo T, Fujino Y. Correlation between plasma milrinone concentration and renal function in patients with cardiac disease. Acta Anaesthesiol Scand. 2008;52:991–6.
63. Maslow AD, Regan MM, Schwartz C, Bert A, Singh A. Inotropes improve right heart function in patients undergoing aortic valve replacement for aortic stenosis. Anesth Analg. 2004;98:891–902, table of contents
64. Apitz C, Honjo O, Friedberg MK, Assad RS, Van Arsdell G, Humpl T, Redington AN. Beneficial effects of vasopressors on right ventricular function in experimental acute right ventricular failure in a rabbit model. Thorac Cardiovasc Surg. 2012;60:17–23.
65. Chang JC, Sawa Y, Ohtake S, Fukushima N, Nishimura M, Kagizaki K, Ohata T, Yamaguchi T, Matsuda H. Hemodynamic effect of inhaled nitric oxide in dilated cardiomyopathy patients on LVAD support. ASAIO J. 1997;43:M418–21.
66. Argenziano M, Choudhri AF, Moazami N, Rose EA, Smith CR, Levin HR, Smerling AJ, Oz MC. Randomized, double-blind trial of inhaled nitric oxide in LVAD recipients with pulmonary hypertension. Ann Thorac Surg. 1998;65:340–5.
67. Lovich MA, Pezone MJ, Wakim MG, Denton RJ, Maslov MY, Murray MR, Tsukada H, Agnihotri AK, Roscigno RF, Gamero LG, Gilbert RJ. Inhaled nitric oxide augments left ventricular assist device capacity by ameliorating secondary right ventricular failure. ASAIO J. 2015;61:379–85.

68. Klodell CT Jr, Morey TE, Lobato EB, Aranda JM Jr, Staples ED, Schofield RS, Hess PJ, Martin TD, Beaver TM. Effect of sildenafil on pulmonary artery pressure, systemic pressure, and nitric oxide utilization in patients with left ventricular assist devices. Ann Thorac Surg. 2007;83:68–71. discussion 71
69. Hamdan R, Mansour H, Nassar P, Saab M. Prevention of right heart failure after left ventricular assist device implantation by phosphodiesterase 5 inhibitor. Artif Organs. 2014;38:963–7.
70. Najjar SS, Slaughter MS, Pagani FD, Starling RC, McGee EC, Eckman P, Tatooles AJ, Moazami N, Kormos RL, Hathaway DR, Najarian KB, Bhat G, Aaronson KD, Boyce SW, Investigators HBTAT. An analysis of pump thrombus events in patients in the HeartWare ADVANCE bridge to transplant and continued access protocol trial. J Heart Lung Transplant. 2014;33:23–34.
71. Stulak JM, Sharma S, Maltais S. Management of pump thrombosis in patients with left ventricular assist devices. Am J Cardiovasc Drugs. 2015;15:89–94.
72. Teuteberg JJ, Slaughter MS, Rogers JG, McGee EC, Pagani FD, Gordon R, Rame E, Acker M, Kormos RL, Salerno C, Schleeter TP, Goldstein DJ, Shin J, Starling RC, Wozniak T, Malik AS, Silvestry S, Ewald GA, Jorde UP, Naka Y, Birks E, Najarian KB, Hathaway DR, Aaronson KD, ADVANCE Trial Investigators. The HVAD left ventricular assist device: risk factors for neurological events and risk mitigation strategies. JACC Heart Fail. 2015;3:818–28.
73. VanderPluym JH, Robertson CM, Joffe AR, Conway J, Rebeyka IM, Ross DB, Garcia Guerra G, Al Aklabi MM, Buchholz H. Neurologic, neurocognitive, and functional outcomes in children under 6 years treated with the Berlin Heart Excor Ventricular Assist Device. ASAIO J. 2017b;63:207–15.

Transplant Evaluation and Acute Posttransplant Care of the Adult with Congenital Heart Disease

20

Vanessa Wong and Juan Alejos

20.1 Introduction

As of 2010 there were approximately 2.4 million people in the United States living with congenital heart disease of which 1.4 million are adults [1]. With the advancement in prenatal detection, early surgical intervention, and improved medical management, more children with congenital heart disease are living into adulthood. While there has been significant advancement in palliative and corrective surgical repairs of congenital heart disease, congestive heart failure still remains a significant cause for morbidity and mortality in adults with congenital heart disease. As a result, 10–20% of adults with congenital heart disease may require heart transplantation, and they account for approximately 3% of all adult heart transplants [2]. Although congenital heart disease is a small percentage of causes for heart transplant, the percentage of heart transplants for adults with congenital heart disease has nearly doubled in the last 18 years and will likely continue to increase as more children with congenital heart disease survive into adulthood. Much of the transplant evaluation is similar in adults with congenital heart disease and those without; however, there are unique pathologic and physiologic characteristics of those with congenital heart disease that require special consideration in the evaluation process prior to listing for heart transplantation and the postoperative care after transplantation. In this chapter we will discuss the evaluation process for transplant and the immediate postoperative management of the adult congenital heart disease population who receive a heart transplantation.

V. Wong · J. Alejos (✉)
UCLA Mattel Children's Hospital, Los Angeles, CA, USA
e-mail: jalejos@mednet.ucla.edu

E. da Cruz et al. (eds.), *Intensive Care of the Adult with Congenital Heart Disease*, Congenital Heart Disease in Adolescents and Adults,
https://doi.org/10.1007/978-3-319-94171-4_20

20.2 Transplant Evaluation

In 2006, the first guidelines of listing criteria for heart transplantation were published by the International Society for Heart and Lung Transplantation (ISHLT). While these guidelines provided clear recommendations for the different steps to take in the evaluation process, they did not take into account the adult congenital heart disease population. Thus, in 2016 the ISHLT updated these guidelines to specifically address some key aspects missing from the original 2006 guidelines including providing recommendations for patients with congenital heart disease. In the evaluation process, there are multiple factors that help determine ideal candidacy for transplantation especially in patients with congenital heart disease as their physiology leads to unique consequences on other organ systems. Therefore, the evaluation process requires a multidisciplinary approach to thoroughly evaluate and exclude any potential comorbidities that can affect the perioperative risk or long-term survival. The following are guidelines for the transplant evaluation process for this unique group of patients.

20.3 Selection Criteria

As with adults without congenital heart disease, the first step in the evaluation process is determining the severity of heart failure. Those patients with class IIIb/VI heart failure symptoms who are receiving optimal medical therapy and have no other identifiable reversible causes for heart failure should be considered for transplant evaluation [3]. Heart failure survival scores [HFSS] can also be used to help guide clinicians in making decisions for consideration of transplant listing, but should not be used alone [4]. A 1-year survival of <80% (calculated using the Seattle Heart Failure Model) or a HFSS in the medium- to high-risk range can be used at cutoffs to guide transplant listing [4]. In addition to selection criteria, there are also contraindications to transplantation for those without congenital heart disease that can be extrapolated to those with congenital heart disease as well. Some of the absolute contraindications include those with systemic illness with a life expectancy less than 2 years despite heart transplant and significant pulmonary hypertension with PVR >6 woods units [3]. Figure 20.1 provides an overview of absolute and relative contraindications to heart transplant as outlined by Macini and Lietz in their article on Selection of Cardiac Transplant Candidates in 2010. Once a patient has been identified as a potential heart transplant candidate, the following evaluations based on the 2016 updated ISHLT guidelines should take place.

20.4 Infectious Disease Evaluation

Screening for specific active or latent infections and management of those infections is important prior to heart transplantation. All candidates are screened for human immunodeficiency viral infection (HIV), *Trypanosoma cruzi* infection (Chagas disease), hepatitis B and C viral infections (HBV and HCV), Epstein-Barr

Fig. 20.1 Contraindications to Heart Transplant

Absolute contraindications

- Systemic illness with a life expectancy < 2 y despite HT, including
  - Active or recent solid organ or blood malignancy within 5 y (eg. leukemia, low-grade neoplasms of prostate with persistently elevated prostate-specific antigen)
  - AIDS with frequent opportunistic infections
  - Systemic lupus erythematosus, sarcoid, or amyloidosis that has multisystem involvement and is still active
  - Irreversible renal or hepatic dysfunction in patients considered for only HT
  - Significant obstructive pulmonary disease (F_{EV_1} <1 L/min)
- Fixed pulmonary hypertension
  - Pulmonary artery systolic pressure >60 mm Hg
  - Mean transpulmonary gradient >15 mm Hg
  - Pulmonary vascular resistance >6 Wood units

Relative contraindications

- Age > 72 y
- Any active infection (with exception of device-related infection in VAD recipients)
- Active peptic ulcer disease
- Severe diabetes mellitus with end-organ damage (neuropathy, nephropathy, or retinopathy)
- Severe peripheral vascular or cerebrovascular disease
  - Peripheral vascular disease not amenable to surgical or percutaneous therapy
  - Symptomatic carotid stenosis
  - Ankle brachial index <0. 7
  - Uncorrected abdominal aortic aneurysm >6 cm
- Morbid obesity (body mass index >35 kg/m^2) or cachexia (body mass index <18 kg/m^2)
- Creatinine >2.5 mg/dL or creatinine clearance <25 mL/min*
- Bilirubin >2.5 mg/dL, serum transaminases >3×, INA >1.5 off warfarin
- Severe pulmonary dysfunction with F_{EV_1} <40% normal
- Recent pulmonary infarction within 6 to 8 wk
- Difficult-to-control hypertension
- Irreversible neurological or neuromuscular disorder
- Active mental illness or psychosocial instability
- Drug, tobacco, or alcohol abuse within 6 mo
- Heparin-induced thrombocytopenia within 100 d

INR indicates international normalized ratio.
*May be suitable for HT if inotropic support and hemodynamic management produce a creatinine <2 mg/dL and creatinine clearance >50 mL/min.
Transplantation may also be advisable as combined heart-kidney transplantation.

viral infection (EBV), cytomegalovirus infection (CMV), toxoplasmosis, and tuberculosis [4, 5]. In addition, vaccination history and the presence of serologic protection for the live vaccines are assessed as live vaccines are contraindicated after transplant [4]. Specifically, patients are screened for varicella, mumps, measles, rubella, and herpes zoster titers [4]. If the patient serology is negative, immunization is recommended ideally 3–4 weeks prior to transplantation [4].

20.5 Immunocompatibility and Allosensitization Testing

ABO blood group typing is required by the United Network for Organ Sharing or UNOS on two separate occasions prior to transplantation [5]. Allosensitization is also extremely important and even more important in patients with congenital heart disease as they have often had prior blood exposures secondary to previous cardiac bypass and the use of human homograft material for certain congenital heart defect palliations or repairs [6]. Screening for the presence of anti-donor HLA antibodies is accomplished by using panel reactivity antibody (PRA) testing which can give insight to the clinician regarding the likelihood of humoral rejection after transplantation [5]. A PRA >10% is considered positive and requires repeat testing every 1–2 months [5]. PRA testing should also be repeated 2 weeks after the patient receives any blood transfusion [5].

20.6 Special Procedures

20.6.1 Cardiopulmonary Stress Testing

As part of the transplant evaluation, every adult congenital heart patient should have cardiopulmonary stress testing, a right heart catheterization, and advanced imaging to better evaluate complex cardiac anatomy. Cardiopulmonary stress testing is routinely used in non-congenital heart disease patients as a guide for transplantation listing. Cutoffs for predicting 1-year mortality with peak oxygen consumption (VO2) of ≤14 mL/kg/min (or ≤12 mL/kg/min for those taking a beta-blocker) have been used to guide listing in patients without congenital heart disease [4]. Unfortunately, prospective studies to evaluate peak oxygen consumption in adult congenital heart disease patients with heart failure have not been done [7]. Thus, the results of cardiopulmonary stress testing should be used in addition to other factors when determining listing.

20.6.2 Heart Catheterization

In addition to the use of data from standard echocardiograms, it is important for all transplant candidates to undergo a right heart catheterization to evaluate hemodynamics. It is even more important for congenital heart patients to have a cardiac catheterization as part of their transplant evaluation not only to obtain hemodynamic data but also to assess for pulmonary hypertension as well as evaluate for aortopulmonary collaterals which can complicate the transplant and lead to significant surgical bleeding.

Elevated pulmonary artery pressures can lead to early right heart graft failure and has been associated with increased morbidity and mortality after heart transplantation. Patients without congenital heart disease have been shown to have an increased 3-month mortality of 17.9% with a pulmonary vascular resistance >2.5 wood units compared to a mortality of 6.9% in patients with pulmonary vascular resistance ≤2.5 wood units [8]. In children with congenital heart disease who have elevated pulmonary pressures, heart transplantation has been feasible when the administration of vasodilators or inotropes can decrease the pulmonary vascular disease [9]. Therefore, it is important to perform vasoreactivity testing at the time of cardiac catheterization in those patients with elevated pulmonary artery pressures to determine the reversibility of their pulmonary vascular disease.

It has been shown that the volume overload from aortopulmonary collaterals has been associated with primary graft failure after transplantation in this population [10]. Thus, in addition to obtaining hemodynamic data, it may be beneficial to not only assess for aortopulmonary collaterals but also attempt coil embolization of these collaterals in order to reduce the burden of volume overload and reduce surgical bleeding at the time of transplantation.

20.6.3 Advanced Imaging

Congenital heart patients are unique in that at the time of transplantation evaluation they have likely undergone at least one if not several previous sternotomies for palliative procedures. Previous sternotomies and surgeries lead to adhesions that can cause increased bleeding and prolonged ischemic time of the graft at the time of transplantation and can therefore have an adverse effect on outcomes [11]. Therefore, it is important to evaluate intrathoracic anatomy using either cardiac magnetic resonance imaging or chest computed tomography. In addition, many adults with congenital heart disease have thrombosis of veins and/or arteries due to repeated bypass cannulation as well as multiple cardiac catheterizations. Evaluation of the major upper and lower extremity vessels is helpful in surgical planning as well as trying to maintain patency of these vessels for future cardiac catheterization and biopsies.

20.7 Comorbidities

There are several comorbidities that should be screened for as part of the transplant evaluation. These comorbidities are either absolute or relative contraindications to transplant and are outlined previously in Fig. 20.1. In those patients who have undergone single ventricle palliation with a Fontan procedure, it is especially important to evaluate liver function prior to consideration of transplant as these patients may benefit not only from a heart transplantation but a combined heart-liver transplant. There is increasing evidence that cirrhosis of the liver is a long-term and frequent complication in those patients who have undergone a Fontan procedure [12]. The passive Fontan circulation physiology leads to venous congestion, and this combined with low cardiac output induces hypoxic stress that can trigger inflammation, fibrosis, and subsequent cirrhosis [13]. Therefore, evaluation of liver function and anatomy should be done and include liver function tests (e.g., AST, ALT, bilirubin, international normalized ratio (INR), and albumin), imaging (e.g., liver ultrasound, liver elastography), and possible liver biopsy at the time of cardiac catheterization. In addition, utilizing an Model for End-Stage Liver Disease excluding international normalized ratio (MELD-XI) score may help provide information for those Fontan patients with more significant liver disease as a higher MELD-XI score in Fontan patients has demonstrated earlier sudden death, death from heart failure, and earlier heart transplantation [14].

20.8 Other Considerations

20.8.1 Tobacco and Substance Use

It is well known that tobacco exposure is associated with significant cardiovascular disease including coronary artery disease. In those patients being listed for transplant, it is imperative that they have ceased smoking for at least 6 months prior to transplantation as a cardiac allograft is especially vulnerable to tobacco exposure and has been shown to have increased incidence of coronary vasculopathy and decreased survival [5]. For those who are actively using illicit substances (including alcohol), consideration for transplantation is contraindicated.

20.8.2 Psychosocial Evaluation

Compliance with medications after transplantation is imperative for the long-term preservation of the cardiac allograft. There are four important areas that the psychosocial evaluation should address—compliance, comprehension, quality of life, and social evaluation [5]. Therefore, a psychosocial evaluation before transplant listing is important to evaluate the candidate's ability to comply with instructions including medication compliance and to assess the patient's ability to give informed consent [5].

20.9 Immediate Posttransplant Care

The acute postoperative heart transplant period is a critical time with significant hemodynamic changes and immunological changes. During this time, management of these critically ill patients includes both general medical management of a postoperative patient and management of transplant-specific issues including immunosuppression.

20.10 Monitoring

The 2010 ISHLT Guidelines for Heart Transplant Care outline specific immediate postoperative monitoring parameters. As donor dysfunction is common immediately postoperatively, it is important to monitor hemodynamics to ensure the graft is able to generate enough cardiac output. As recommended by the ISHLT guidelines [15], the following table outlines the monitoring recommendations for all postoperative heart transplant recipients. Direct measuring of right atrial pressure and left atrial pressure allows the physician to determine whether there is right ventricular, left ventricular, or biventricular dysfunction immediately following the transplantation. Measurement of pulmonary artery pressure is also especially useful in patients with pulmonary hypertension prior to transplantation.

Continuous ECG monitoring	Intermittent measurement of cardiac output
Arterial pressure monitoring	Intraoperative transesophageal echocardiogram
Direct measurement of right atrial pressure or central venous pressure	Continuous assessment of urinary output
Measurement of left atrial or pulmonary artery wedge pressure	Continuous measurement of arterial oxygen saturation

Adapted from the 2010 ISHLT Guidelines for Heart Transplant Care [5]

20.11 Graft Failure

According the ISHLT early graft failure incidence is 3.8% with 3.6% of patients dying and 0.1% of patients requiring re-transplantation [16]. In addition, the data suggests that patients who are transplanted for congenital and valvular etiologies have the highest incidence of early graft failure in the first 5 days posttransplant [16]. Primary graft dysfunction (PGD) presents in the first 24 h postoperatively and may present as right, left, or biventricular dysfunction and is a life-threatening complication of transplantation; definitions are provided in the table below [17]. It manifests as severe hemodynamic instability with hypotension and low cardiac output in the presence of adequate filling pressures [18]. PGD can range from mild to severe, and management requires hemodynamic support with inotropic support to mechanical support (extracorporeal membrane oxygenation, ventricular assist device, intra-aortic balloon pump) (Table 20.1).

20.12 Right Ventricular Failure

After cardiac transplantation the right ventricle is more likely to have dysfunction than the left ventricle as the recipient often has elevated pulmonary vascular resistance that the new graft has to cope with. In transplant patients without congenital heart disease, their elevated pulmonary vascular resistance is secondary to volume overload from heart failure. In adult congenital heart patients, however, they often develop pulmonary hypertension due to the vascular remodeling that is caused by increased pulmonary blood flow, increased pressures from left to right shunting, and sheer stress [19]. It is estimated that about 5-10% of congenital heart disease patients will develop pulmonary hypertension [19]. Therefore, it is important to recognize that after heart transplant, this group of patient is at an increased risk of having right ventricular failure. Many of these patients may already be on pharmacologic agents to treat pulmonary hypertension prior to transplantation, which may need to be continued postoperatively. Treatment of immediate right ventricular dysfunction,

Table 20.1 Definition and grading of primary graft dysfunction

Grade	Left or biventricular	Right ventricular	Support
Mild	RA >15 mmHg, PAW >20 mmHg, CI <2.0 L/min/m^2 (lasting >1 h)	RA >15 mmHg, PAWP <15 mmHg, CI <2.0 L/min/m^2	Low-dose inotropic infusion
	Or	*Plus*	
	LVEF 40–50%	TPG <15 mmHg and/or PA Sys <50 mmHg	
Moderate	RA >15 mmHg, PAW >20 mmHg, CK 2.0 L/min/m^2, MAP <70 mmHg (lasting >1 h)	RA >15 mmHg, PAWP <15 mmHg, CK 2.0 L/min/m^2, MAP <70 mmHg (lasting >1 h)	High-dose inotropic support (inotrope score >10)
	Or	*Plus*	*Or*
	LVEF <40%	TPG <15 mmHg and/or PA Sys <50 mmHg	IABP
Severe	As above	As above	Mechanical circulatory support beyond IABP
	Plus	*Plus*	
	LVAD or BiVAD (e.g., ECMO)	RVAD	

Inotrope score: dopamine (×1)+dobutamine (×1)+amrinone (×1)+milrinone (×15)+epinephrine (×100)+norepinephrine (×100) with each drug dosed in mcg/kg/min

however, is managed by optimizing preload, achieving hemodynamic stability with the use of inotropes/vasopressors and possibly RV assist devices or ECMO, maintaining atrial-ventricular synchrony, and utilization of ventilatory support [15]. If the patient is hemodynamically stable, pulmonary vasodilators (e.g., nitroglycerine, nitroprusside, and nitric oxide) can be used to help decrease pulmonary pressures [15]. The figure below outlines the ISHLT guidelines for treatment of acute right ventricular failure.

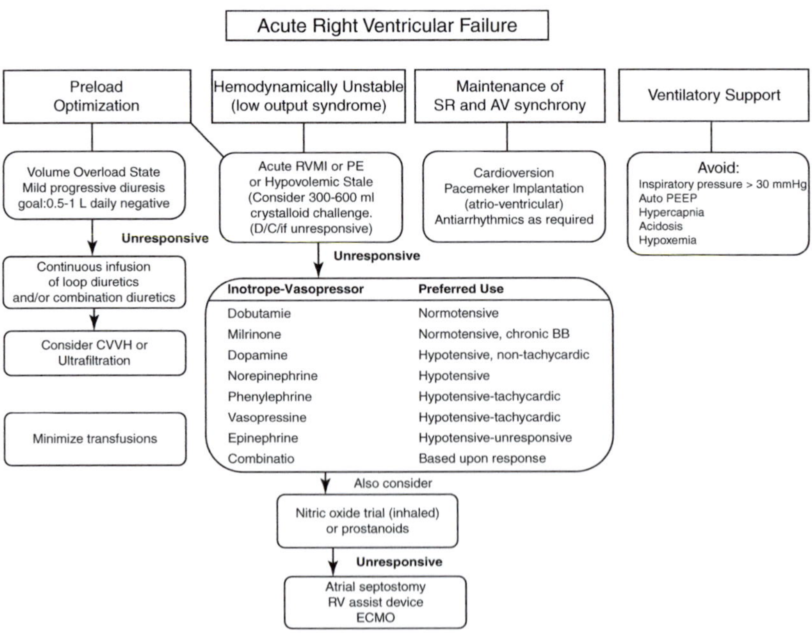

Table 20.2 Properties of intravenous vasoactive drugs used after heart transplantation

	Peripheral vasoconstriction	Cardiac contractility	Peripheral vasodilation	Chronotropic effect	Arrhythmia risk
Isoproterenol	0	++++	+++	++++	++++
Dobutamine	0	+++	++	+	+
Dopamine	++	+++	+	+	+
Epinephrine	+++	++++	+	++	+++
Milrinone/enoximone	0	+++	+	++	++
Norepinephrine	++++	+++	0	+	+
Phenylephrine	++++	0	0	0	0
Vasopressin	++++	0	0	0	0

Adapted and reprinted with permission from Costanzo MR et al. [15]

20.13 Vasoactive Drug Use

Inotropic and vasoactive drugs are routinely used postoperatively to help support cardiac output in the setting of ventricular dysfunction. It is common that the transplanted heart will have some degree of ventricular dysfunction in the immediate postoperative period for several reasons which can be anything from post-bypass inflammation, reperfusion injury, fluid shifts, or primary graft failure as described above. The ISHLT recommends a combination of pharmacologic therapies to help support ventricular function with continuous infusions of isoproterenol alone, isoproterenol +/− dopamine, dobutamine +/− dopamine, and/or milrinone [15]. Alpha-adrenergic agonists phenylephrine, norepinephrine, or epinephrine can be used to maintain mean arterial blood pressure, and vasopressin can be added in cases of vasodilatory shock [15]. Table 20.2 outlines the different vasoactive drugs and their effects.

20.14 Postoperative Management of Rhythm Disturbances

Arrhythmias frequently occur after orthotropic heart transplantation and include bradyarrhythmias (50%), atrial fibrillation (5–24%), atrial flutter (12–30%), other SVT (12–17%), and sustained ventricular tachycardia and ventricular fibrillation (<2%) [20]. The type of operative technique used for anastomosis of the graft can affect the type of arrhythmia seen postoperatively. The bicaval anastomosis better preserves right atrial anatomy and function and may minimize trauma to the SA node [20]. In addition, the transplanted heart is denervated which leads to loss of the autonomic nervous system's ability to change the heart's electrophysiologic properties. Sinus bradycardia and junctional bradycardia are commonly seen, and therefore the use of chronotropic agents (isoproternol and theophylline) as well as atrial and ventricular pacing can be useful to maintain the heart rate between 90 and 100 bpm [15]. If the bradycardia does not resolve within 2 weeks after transplantation, there should be concern for graft ischemia or rejection [20]. A permanent pacemaker becomes an indication if the bradycardia does not resolve 3 weeks after transplantation [15]. Early rejection can also lead to arrhythmias, in particular ventricular tachycardia; thus, providers should consider early rejection if a patient develops a ventricular tachycardia posttransplant. These patients should undergo a cardiac catheterization with endomyocardial biopsy [15]. For the tachyarrhythmias, treatment should be aimed at rate control using beta-blockers, calcium channel blockers, sotalol, and amiodarone [15]. Patients with evidence of reentry circuits or ectopic foci may benefit from catheter ablation [20]. It is important to remember that due to the denervation of the cardiac allograft, certain antiarrhythmics may not have the same effect on the transplanted heart. In particular, digoxin and atropine will not have a chronotropic effect on the transplanted heart.

20.15 Perioperative Infection Prophylaxis

Minimizing infection postoperatively is extremely important for decreasing morbid and mortality after transplantation. Patients are susceptible to a myriad of infections given that they will be receiving significant immunosuppression postoperatively. In addition, certain congenital heart defects are associated with functional asplenia, and special consideration regarding antibiotic choice should be given to these patients as they are often at risk for infection with encapsulated organisms. Fontan patients also have impaired immune systems, especially those with protein losing enteropathy. Bacterial infections are the most commonly encountered infections postoperatively, and antibiotics, especially against skin flora, should be given preoperatively. If the donor was infected with a bacterial infection at the time of transplant, a course of appropriate antibiotics should be given to the recipient following transplantation [15]. Prophylaxis against CMV should also be started within 24 to 48 hours after transplantation [15]. An intermediate- and high-risk patient should receive IV ganciclovir, whereas low-risk patients can receive acyclovir [15]. Antifungal as well as antiprotozoal prophylaxis is also recommended and includes initiation of nystatin oral solution or clotrimazole lozenges and trimethoprim/sulfamethoxazole [15].

20.16 Immunosuppression

Allograft rejection is a common cause of early mortality, and thus initiation of immunosuppression early is important. A fine balance between under-immunosuppression and over-immunosuppression is key to avoid rejection and consequences of over-immunosuppression including kidney disease and malignancy. Immunosuppression regimens are generally thought of in three different categories: induction, maintenance, and immunosuppression for rejection. For the purposes of this chapter, immunosuppression for rejection will not be discussed.

20.16.1 Induction Immunosuppression

According to the ISHLT data registry, about 50% of transplant patients receive induction immunosuppression [15]. Induction immunosuppression that has been used in heart transplant recipients includes rabbit antithymocyte globulin (rATG), horse antithymocyte globulin (hATG), IL-2 receptor antagonists (basiliximab or daclizumab), anti-CD3 antibodies (muromonab), and anti-CD52 antibodies (alemtuzumab), with ATG and IL-2 receptor antagonists being the most commonly used agents [21]. ATGs are polyclonal antibodies that bind to T and B cells and cause T and B cell depletion, whereas IL-2 receptor antagonists are monoclonal antibodies that bind to the IL-2 receptor on T cells and inhibit their proliferation and differentiation [21]. There is not a clear answer on which induction agent is better, and the choice may vary depending on the transplant center. A study done in 2006 by Augero et al. found greater survival in patients who received induction therapy with an IL-2 receptor antagonist and maintenance immunosuppression with mycophenolate mofetil and tacrolimus [22]. However, other studies have shown that induction with ATG may prevent acute cellular rejection better than induction with an IL-2 receptor antagonist [21]. There still remains controversy as to whether induction immunosuppression should be used in all heart transplant recipients; however, some benefits may include earlier reduction of corticosteroid use and delayed initiation of calcineurin inhibitors [21]. Induction therapy thus should be considered in patients at high risk of renal dysfunction in order to delay starting a calcineurin inhibitor. It should also be considered in patients with preformed anti-HLA antibodies and donor-specific antibodies.

20.16.2 Maintenance Immunosuppression

Maintenance immunosuppression usually consists of corticosteroids, a calcineurin inhibitor (cyclosporin or tacrolimus), and an antimetabolite (azathioprine or mycophenolate mofetil).

Corticosteroids affect both the innate and adaptive immunity; calcineurin inhibitors inhibit calcineurin in T cells, which prevents proliferation and differentiation of T cells; and the antimetabolites inhibit the cell cycle of T and B lymphocytes [21]. The m-Tor inhibitors (everolimus and sirolimus) which inhibit the enzyme m-TOR found in T and B lymphocytes are also used as well and especially in those patients with chronic kidney disease [21]. The utilization of a calcineurin inhibitor remains the standard for maintenance immunosuppression with the addition of mycophenolate mofetil, everolimus, or sirolimus to assist in reducing the onset and progression of cardiac allograft vasculopathy [15].

References

1. Gilboa SM, Devine OJ, Kucik JE, Oster ME, Riehle-Colarusso T, Nembhard WN, Xu P, Correa A, Jenkins K, Marelli AJ. Congenital heart defects in the United States: estimating the magnitude of the affected population in 2010. Circulation. 2016;134(2):101–9.
2. Goldberg SW, Fisher SA, Wehman B, Mehra MR. Adults with congenital heart disease and heart transplantation: optimizing outcomes. J Heart Lung Transplant. 2014;33(9):873–7.
3. Mancini D, Lietz K. Selection of cardiac transplantation candidates in 2010. Circulation. 2010;122(2):173–83.
4. Mehra MR, Canter CE, Hannan MM, Semigran MJ, Uber PA, Baran DA, Danziger-Isakov L, Kirklin JK, Kirk R, Kushwaha SS, Lund LH. The 2016 International Society for Heart Lung Transplantation listing criteria for heart transplantation: a 10-year update. J Heart Lung Transplant. 2016;35(1):1):1–23.
5. Mehra MR, Kobashigawa J, Starling R, Russell S, Uber PA, Parameshwar J, Mohacsi P, Augustine S, Aaronson K, Barr M. Listing criteria for heart transplantation: International Society for Heart and Lung Transplantation guidelines for the care of cardiac transplant candidates—2006. J Heart Lung Transplant. 2006;25(9):1024–42.
6. Hoyel L, et al. Heart transplantation in adults with congenital heart disease. Arch Cardiovasc Dis. 2017;110:346. https://doi.org/10.1016/j.acvd/2017.01.002
7. Burchill LJ. Heart transplantation in adult congenital heart disease. Heart. 2016;102(23):1871–7.
8. Costard-Jäckle A, Fowler MB. Influence of preoperative pulmonary artery pressure on mortality after heart transplantation: testing of potential reversibility of pulmonary hypertension with nitroprusside is useful in defining a high risk group. J Am Coll Cardiol. 1992;19(1):48–54.
9. Giglia TM, Humpl T. Preoperative pulmonary hemodynamics and assessment of operability: is there a pulmonary vascular resistance that precludes cardiac operation? Pediatr Crit Care Med. 2010;11:S57–69.
10. Krishnan US, Lamour JM, Hsu DT, Kichuk MR, Donnelly CM, Addonizio LJ. Management of aortopulmonary collaterals in children following cardiac transplantation for complex congenital heart disease. J Heart Lung Transplant. 2004;23(5):564–9.
11. Morrow WR, Frazier E, Naftel DC. Survival after listing for cardiac transplantation in children. Prog Pediatr Cardiol. 2000;11(2):99–105.
12. Lindsay I, Johnson J, Everitt MD, Hoffman J, Yetman AT. Impact of liver disease after the Fontan operation. Am J Cardiol. 2015;115(2):249–52.
13. Rychik J, Veldtman G, Rand E, Russo P, Rome JJ, Krok K, Goldberg DJ, Cahill AM, Wells RG. The precarious state of the liver after a Fontan operation: summary of a multidisciplinary symposium. Pediatr Cardiol. 2012;33(7):1001–12.
14. Assenza GE, Graham DA, Landzberg MJ, Valente AM, Singh MN, Bashir A, Fernandes S, Mortele KJ, Ukomadu C, Volpe M, Wu F. MELD-XI score and cardiac mortality or transplantation in patients after Fontan surgery. Heart. 2013;99(7):491–6.
15. Costanzo MR, Dipchand A, Starling R, Anderson A, Chan M, Desai S, Fedson S, Fisher P, Gonzales-Stawinski G, Martinelli L, McGiffin D, Smith J, Taylor D, Meiser B, Webber S, Baran D, Carboni M, Dengler T, Feldman D, Frigerio M, Kfoury A, Kim D, Kobashigawa J, Shullo M, Stehlik J, Teuteberg J, Uber P, Zuckermann A, Hunt S, Burch M, Bhat G, Canter C, Chinnock R, Crespo-Leiro M, Delgado R, Dobbels F, Grady K, Kao W, Lamour J, Parry G, Patel J, Pini D, Towbin J, Wolfel G, Delgado D, Eisen H, Goldberg L, Hosenpud J, Johnson M, Keogh A, Lewis C, O'Connell J, Rogers J, Ross H, Russell S, Vanhaecke J, International Society of Heart and Lung Transplantation Guidelines. The International Society of Heart and Lung Transplantation Guidelines for the care of heart transplant recipients. J Heart Lung Transplant. 2010;29(8):914–56.
16. Lund LH, Edwards LB, Kucheryavaya AY, Benden C, Dipchand AI, Goldfarb S, Levvey BJ, Meiser B, Rossano JW, Yusen RD, Stehlik J. The Registry of the International Society for Heart and Lung Transplantation: thirty-second official adult heart transplantation report—2015; focus theme: early graft failure. J Heart Lung Transplant. 2015;34(10):1244.

17. Chew HC, Kumarasinghe G, Iyer A, Hicks M, Gao L, Doyle A, Jabbour A, Dhital K, Granger E, Jansz P, Hayward C. Primary graft dysfunction after heart transplantation. Curr Transplant Rep. 2014;1:257–65.
18. Iyer A, Kumarasinghe G, Hicks M, Watson A, Gao L, Doyle A, Keogh A, Kotlyar E, Hayward C, Dhital K, Granger E. Primary graft failure after heart transplantation. J Transplant. 2011;2011:1, Article ID 175768, 9 p
19. Rodriguez-Lopez J. Pulmonary hypertension in adult congenital heart disease. Curr Treat Options Cardiovasc Med. 2014;16(8):1–2.
20. Stecker EC, Strelich KR, Chugh SS, Crispell K, McAnulty JH. Arrhythmias after orthotopic heart transplantation. J Card Fail. 2005;11(6):464–72.
21. Söderlund C, Rådegran G. Immunosuppressive therapies after heart transplantation—the balance between under-and over-immunosuppression. Transplant Rev. 2015;29(3):181–9.
22. Agüero J, Almenar L, Martínez-Dolz L, Chamorro C, Moro J, Rueda J, Arnau MA, Zorio E, Izquierdo M, Salvador A. Influence of immunosuppression regimen on heart transplantation survival. Transplant Proc. 2006;38(8):2550–2.

Cardiovascular Disease and Acute Coronary Syndrome in the Adult Patient with Congenital Heart Disease

21

Jordan D. Awerbach, Wayne J. Franklin, Ronald A. Bronicki, and Peter R. Ermis

21.1 Introduction

Outcomes for congenital heart disease (CHD) have improved significantly over time. Owing to this success, adults with CHD now outnumber children. As the size and age of this population continues to increase, greater numbers of patients will develop significant coronary artery disease (CAD) leading to a myocardial infarction (MI). The presentation of MI can be varied, from a subtle worsening of routine anginal chest pain to complete cardiovascular collapse. The clinician must be able to assess cardiovascular risk in the adult patient, rapidly identify an acute MI, and initiate guideline-based therapies to resolve ischemia and reperfuse myocardium while still salvageable.

21.2 Cardiovascular Disease

Cardiovascular disease (CVD) is the leading cause of death worldwide and has been so in developed countries like the USA (United States of America) for nearly a century. One in three US citizens is diagnosed with CVD. Of this group, 16.5 million (6.3%) have CAD, yet this accounts for half of all CVD-related deaths [1].

J. D. Awerbach (✉) · W. J. Franklin · P. R. Ermis
Section of Pediatric Cardiology, Department of Pediatrics, Baylor College of Medicine, Texas Children's Hospital, Houston, TX, USA
e-mail: wjf@bcm.edu; prermis@texaschildrens.org

R. A. Bronicki
Section of Critical Care Medicine and Cardiology, Department of Pediatrics, Baylor College of Medicine, Texas Children's Hospital, Houston, TX, USA
e-mail: rxbronic@texaschildrens.org

E. da Cruz et al. (eds.), *Intensive Care of the Adult with Congenital Heart Disease*, Congenital Heart Disease in Adolescents and Adults,
https://doi.org/10.1007/978-3-319-94171-4_21

The significance of CAD in the adult congenital heart disease (ACHD) population is becoming increasingly recognized. In a retrospective analysis of ACHD deaths over time, Pillutla et al. reported that MI overtook arrhythmia as the leading cause of death in noncyanotic ACHD patients after 1990 [2]. The prevalence of CAD in the ACHD population is estimated to be between 4.5 and 14% [3, 4] with overall mortality increasing fivefold in the presence of CAD [5]. An angiographic study by Giannakoulas et al. of 250 ACHD patients referred for reasons other than suspected CAD found that 9.2% had stenosis of greater than 50% in a major coronary vessel (mean age 51.4 years) [3, 6]. These data indicate that CAD is as prevalent, and possibly more so, in the ACHD population compared to the general population.

21.2.1 Risk Factors for Cardiovascular Disease

The term "risk factor" was first penned by the investigators of the Framingham Heart Study in 1961 [7]. Since then, numerous population-based studies have underscored the modifiable and nonmodifiable risk factors that contribute to the development of CAD. A large population-based study of a young ACHD cohort (median age 26 years) from Belgium reported at least one modifiable cardiovascular risk factor present in 80% of patients, with hypertension and hyperlipidemia being the most common [8]. With the growing ACHD population, discussions about cardiovascular risk between the patient and their congenital cardiologist are of paramount importance. In the general US population, only about half of patients hospitalized for MI report have been told they were at risk for a heart attack [1].

In patients with noncyanotic CHD, cardiovascular risk is also related to the type of cardiac lesion. For example, coarctation of the aorta is associated with a significant CAD risk, possibly owing to the increased incidence of chronic hypertension in this group. Severe atherosclerotic plaques have been demonstrated in patients with a history of coarctation on autopsy [4]. Many noncyanotic CHD lesions are also associated with inherent anatomic coronary abnormalities or require manipulation of the coronaries during surgical repair or palliation, placing these patients at additional risks for nonatherosclerotic coronary complications. Coronary translocation also results in sympathetic denervation of the artery and creates an increased long-term CAD risk. Abnormal vasoreactivity and increased intimal thickness of the coronary arteries have been demonstrated in patients after arterial switch operation [9].

Cyanotic CHD patients have historically been thought to be protected against the development of CAD. This is related to a number of anti-atherosclerotic factors, including hypocholesterolemia, hyperbilirubinemia, reduced platelet counts, and an increased bioavailability of nitric oxide [3, 6]. Indeed, there was no angiographic evidence of CAD found in any of the cyanotic patients evaluated in the Giannakoulas study [3]. However, emerging evidence has raised questions about chronic hypoxia causing endothelial dysfunction and a prothrombotic state, and CAD has been reported in a small series of patients with Eisenmenger syndrome [6].

In the following section, we present a brief overview of pertinent cardiac risk factors as they relate to the ACHD population. Multiple scoring systems exist to assist the clinician in predicting risk of an initial cardiovascular event. We support using the Pooled Cohort Equation to estimate 10-year and lifetime risks of first atherosclerotic CVD (ASCVD) event, as recommended by the 2013 American College of Cardiology (ACC)/American Heart Association (AHA) guidelines (http://tools.acc.org/ascvd-risk-estimator) [10]. It is important to note that this estimation is validated only in Caucasian and African American men and women aged 40–79. Although its use in other populations may under- or overestimate risk to some degree, it nevertheless provides a good starting point for addressing CVD risk in these populations as well.

21.2.1.1 Modifiable Risk Factors

Blood Pressure

Globally, hypertension is the most significant risk factor for CVD. Nearly one billion people worldwide carry this diagnosis, and up to half of CVD-related deaths are attributable to hypertension [11]. The degree of blood pressure (BP) elevation is directly related to CVD risk. For patients aged 40–70, CVD risk doubles for each 20 mmHg increase in systolic BP or 10 mmHg increase in BP between 115/75 and 185/115 mmHg [12]. The 2017 ACC/AHA hypertension guidelines lowered the definition of high BP from previous recommendations and target a goal BP <130/80 mmHg in all adult populations [13]. Lifestyle modifications should be recommended to all patients, and antihypertensive medications initiated at a BP ≥140/90 mmHg in low-risk populations and ≥130/80 mmHg in high-risk populations (inclidling patients with clinical ASCVD, an estimated 10-year CVD risk ≥10%, diabetes, and chronic kidney disease).

30–50% of ACHD patients have hypertension [6]. Patients with a history of coarctation of the aorta are at the highest risk for developing hypertension and CAD. 30-year survival in patients with coarctation is 72%, with CAD being the leading cause of death [14]. The overall prevalence of hypertension in this group is estimated to be at least 35%. Typically, these patients develop isolated systolic hypertension, though diastolic hypertension can rarely be seen [14, 15]. Age at the time of repair plays a significant role in the risk of long-term hypertension. While hypertension may develop in only a minority of patients repaired in infancy, it is almost universally seen in those who are repaired after the first decade of life [16]. Patients who have undergone repair with a subclavian flap technique or use of a prosthetic graft, and those with continued arch hypoplasia after repair, may also be at an increased risk of hypertension [15, 17].

Cholesterol

Elevated low-density lipoprotein (LDL) cholesterol is a significant risk factor for atherogenesis and one of the strongest causes of cardiac morbidity and mortality [12]. This is perhaps best exemplified in patients with familial hypercholesterolemia who can have angiographic evidence of diffuse atherosclerotic plaque formation by early childhood. High-density lipoprotein (HDL) cholesterol, on the other hand, is cardioprotective. Each increase in HDL levels by 1 mg/dL may reduce CVD risk by 2–3% [12].

Reducing LDL cholesterol levels has become a basis of both primary and secondary CVD prevention. Goal LDL levels are outlined by the ATP III guidelines and vary depending on the presence of known CAD or CAD equivalents (e.g., diabetes), or by the number of CAD risk factors present [18] Along with lifestyle modifications, statins have become the mainstay of therapy. The effectiveness of statin-mediated reductions in LDL in preventing both primary and secondary cardiovascular events has been well established in multiple large-scale randomized controlled trials [12, 19]. Patients at the lowest risk for cardiovascular events appear to derive the greatest risk reduction, arguing for early and intensive intervention [20].

Very limited data exist on the prevalence of dyslipidemia in the ACHD population. In ACHD patients with established CAD, the prevalence of hyperlipidemia was between 10 and 75%. As previously described, cyanotic patients typically have lower cholesterol levels owing to their chronic hypoxemia [6]. LDL and HDL targets for ACHD patients should follow the same guidelines as the general population [18].

Smoking

In the USA, all-cause mortality is three times higher for smokers compared to never smokers, with an average of 13–15 years of life lost and a two- to fourfold increase in CAD risk [1, 12]. Smoking is one of the leading causes of premature death throughout the world. CVD risk begins to increase with exposure to even a few cigarettes per day, and those routinely exposed to secondhand smoke also see a 25–30% increase in heart disease risk [12]. While US smoking rates have declined, tobacco use continues to rise globally and is directly responsible for five million deaths annually [1]. Smoking cessation decreases excess CAD risk by 50% within 2 years and approaches that of never smokers by 5 years [12]. Smoking rates in the ACHD population appear to be lower than that of the general population, with estimates from 13 to 20% [21]. Geography likely plays a role in this, with increased prevalence in regions with overall higher smoking rates for the general population.

Obesity

Few health problems have as far-reaching effects as obesity. Obesity increases risks for hypertension, CVD, diabetes, renal disease, depression, musculoskeletal disease, sleep apnea, cancer, and all-cause mortality. Roughly 20% of children and over one-third of adults in the USA are obese [1]. Higher rates are seen in black and Hispanic populations and in women [22]. Excess weight or frank obesity has been seen in half of young adults with moderate or complex CHD undergoing cardiac surgery [23]. In the Belgian study, one-third of ACHD patients were overweight or obese. ACHD patients in the study were overall more physically active than the general population, although a significant percentage (37.8%) reported not participating in any sport activity [8]. Physical inactivity is a major risk factor for ischemic heart disease and all-cause mortality. Some CHD patients face competitive sports restrictions during childhood. Many become restricted from even low to moderate intensity athletics due to fears on the part of the patient or parent, and this can translate into a more sedentary lifestyle as an adult. Emphasizing the need for regular physical activity and addressing any concerns is important in the care of CHD patients of any age.

Diabetes

From 1980 to 2014, the number of people worldwide with diabetes rose from 108 to 422 million. Diabetes has become a global epidemic. It is responsible for at least 1.5 million deaths annually, over 40% of which occur in patients <70 years old [24]. The risk of CVD is 2–3 times greater in patients with diabetes. In part this is due to the prevalence of associated risk factors seen in diabetes: 75–85% of patients have hypertension, 70–80% have elevated LDL cholesterol, and 60–70% are obese [1]. Costs associated with diabetes care in the USA include $176 billion in medical costs and an additional $69 billion lost productivity. Limited ACHD data suggests the prevalence of diabetes in the ACHD population is equal to the general population [6, 8].

Glucose control, with a goal hemoglobin A1c <7%, is recommended for most patients with diabetes and is associated with a decreased risk of microvascular complications (nephropathy, neuropathy, and retinopathy). However, evidence for reductions in macrovascular complications (CAD and stroke) is lacking. Tight glycemic control may decrease the risk of nonfatal myocardial infarction (MI) but has not yet been shown to decrease cardiovascular or all-cause mortality [25–27]. This underscores the need to optimize other cardiovascular risk factors when present in this vulnerable population.

21.2.1.2 Nonmodifiable Risk Factors

Age, gender, and family history play significant roles in cardiovascular risk. The overall prevalence of vascular disease prior to age 60 is low, about 3.5%. After this time, risk rises exponentially with each additional decade of life [28]. Women, owing to the cardioprotective effects of estrogen, are at inherently less risk than men. The risk of a heart attack in women is about 20% lower until menopause, after which time gender differences become equal. MI risk also increases with a family history of a first-degree relative with premature CAD (defined as <55 years in males and <65 years in females). A premature cardiovascular event in one or both parents doubles the risk of heart attack in men and increases the risk in women by 70% [1, 29].

21.2.1.3 Novel Risk Factors

Up to 20% of people experiencing their first cardiovascular event do so in the absence of a major cardiovascular risk factor [12]. Thus, there is a continued need for novel tools in the assessment of cardiovascular risk. Linking inflammatory biomarkers (such as high sensitivity C-reactive protein (hsCRP), interleukin-1, interleukin-6 and ST2) to increased atherogenesis has been the focus of much of this research. The best studied of these biomarkers is hsCRP. Multiple large prospective cohorts have established that elevated hsCRP adds to cardiovascular risk as much as, if not more than, hypertension and dyslipidemia. Ridker et al. demonstrated that patients with elevated hsCRP but low LDL cholesterol had an increased risk of cardiovascular events above that of patients with high LDL but low hsCRP [12]. Cardiovascular risk assessment with CRP is divided into low, moderate, and high risk based on levels of <1, 1–3, and >3 mg/L, respectively. It remains unclear if CRP itself is directly atherogenic or if it only denotes the inflammation associated with atherosclerosis. Limited evidence in ACHD patients suggests elevated hsCRP is correlated with increased heart failure symptoms and cardiovascular mortality [30]. However, hsCRP has also been shown to be elevated in the setting of chronic hypoxia [31], and its prognostic value in cyanotic CHD is less clear.

Coronary artery calcium (CAC), as detected by computed tomography (CT) scan, is strongly associated with CAD and with predicting the risk of future cardiac events, particularly in those patients who are deemed "intermediate" risk by more traditional assessments [32]. As the degree of calcification increases, the sensitivity of CAC detection decreases while specificity increases. A CAC score of <100 is considered low risk, whereas a score of >400 is considered high risk for coronary events. CAC screening in patients with intermediate ASCVD risk can help guide risk reduction therapy and the need for further interventions. Cardiac calcification in the ACHD population has only been evaluated postmortem in a series of seven patients. Three of the patients were above age 50 and had the presence of atherosclerotic calcifications. Interestingly, two of the patients examined had Eisenmenger syndrome and were without evidence of coronary or cardiac calcifications [33].

21.3 Acute Coronary Syndrome

Each year approximately 800,000 US adults will have a heart attack, equating to one person every 40 s. Of this group, 14% will die from their MI [1]. Although the incidence and mortality rates for MI have dropped over the last 50 years [34], this decline has plateaued over the past decade [35].

Acute coronary syndrome (ACS) encompasses the diagnoses of MI, which can be further subdivided into ST-elevation MI (STEMI) and non-ST-elevation ACS (NSTE-ACS), the latter of which includes non-ST-elevation MI (NSTEMI) and unstable angina (UA). Like MI, UA represents progression or rupture of a coronary plaque, although it does not ultimately lead to myocardial necrosis. The clinical presentation of MI requires patients to meet two out of three basic criteria upon presentation: a clinical story consistent with anginal chest pain or its equivalent, elevated cardiac biomarkers, and ECG changes reflective of acute ischemia.

The initial care of patients with ACS starts with prompt recognition of the signs and symptoms by both patients and medical professions. People experiencing an MI routinely do not seek care for up to 2 h after symptom onset [36, 37]. Delayed presentation is more often seen in women, the elderly, blacks, and patients of lower socioeconomic status [38]. Many patients do not seek care because they feel they are not at risk for a heart attack or fear being wrong, or because their symptoms do not fit a preconceived notion of MI symptoms. Up to one-third of patients will present with symptoms other than typical anginal chest pain [37].

Only about 60% of patients experiencing an MI are transported to the hospital via Emergency Medical Services (EMS) [37, 39]. Since 2004, intense efforts have been put forth by the ACC and AHA to improve community awareness of available EMS services and to protocolize the EMS triage and treatment of patients experiencing ACS. For example, identification of a STEMI by EMS should initiate a sequence of events that triggers prehospital activation of the cardiac catheterization lab in patients suitable to undergo percutaneous coronary intervention (PCI). These efforts have improved the delivery of care and reduced total ischemic time and mortality in patients experiencing ACS [37, 38].

The ACHD population faces a unique challenge in receiving appropriate ACS care. Many ACHD patients are cared for at pediatric institutions, and many adult institutions that routinely take care of ACS patients may be uncomfortable caring for ACHD patients. There may be temptation to deviate from routine STEMI treatment and uncertainty in taking these patients to the catheterization laboratory for PCI. All pediatric institutions caring for ACHD patients should have an algorithm in place that is in line with ACC/AHA management guidelines (Fig. 21.1). This

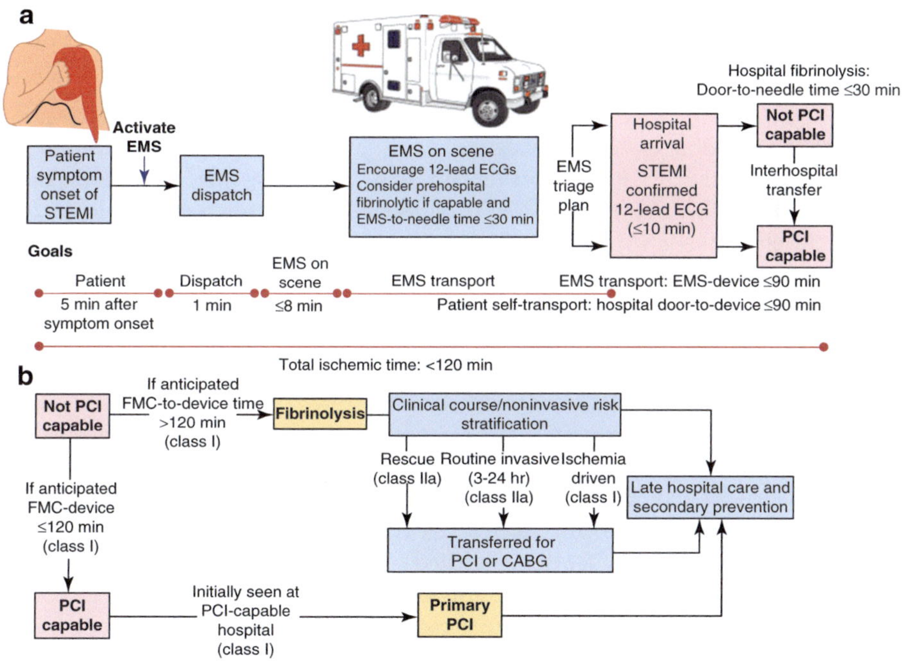

Fig. 21.1 (**a**) ACC/AHA goals in patients with STEMI and (**b**) STEMI reperfusion strategies (From Mega JL, Morrow DA. ST-Elevation Myocardial Infarction: Management. In: *Braunwald's Heart Disease a Textbook of Cardiovascular Medicine*. Tenth Edition. Elsevier Inc.; 2015:1095–1154. Special credits to: Armstrong PW, Collen D, Antman E: Fibrinolysis for acute myocardial infarction: The future is here and now. *Circulation* 107:2533, 2003; and O'Gara PT, Kushner FG, Ascheim DD, et al.: 2013 ACCF/AHA guideline for the management of ST-elevation myocardial infarction: A report of the American College of Cardiology Foundation/American Heart Association Task Force on Practice Guidelines. *JACC* 61:e78, 2013)

should include the activation of appropriate pediatric and/or adult interventional cardiology teams for patients with STEMI with a goal of ≤90–120 min to initial stent deployment.

21.3.1 Pathophysiology

The events leading to ACS typically begin with either acute rupture or superficial erosion of the fibrous cap overlying an atherosclerotic plaque. This exposes the lipid-rich, thrombogenic core to circulating platelets, which adhere and form so-called white clots overlying the site of plaque rupture [40]. At the same time, numerous vasoconstrictive mediators are released leading to further reductions in blood flow. White thrombi are nonocclusive but unstable and may embolize. They are the typical clots seen in patients with NSTE-ACS. With rapid activation of the coagulation cascade, a rich layer of fibrin can be deposited on top of the platelet-rich thrombus leading to completely occlusive "red clots" characteristic of STEMI [41]. These pathophysiologic differences form the basis of the different therapeutic strategies employed in NSTE-ACS versus STEMI patients.

21.3.2 Presentation of Chest Pain in Patients with ACS

Anginal chest pain is typically characterized as an intense, substernal tightness or pressure. Many patients will report feeling as if something was standing on their chest and may report an impending sense of doom. The pain often radiates to the left side of the chest, the left shoulder, and down the left arm. Atypical presentations are more common in certain populations, including women, the elderly, and patients with diabetes. These patients may present with isolated neck or epigastric pain, or significant dyspnea without chest pain. Symptoms associated with ACS include respiratory distress, diaphoresis, lightheadedness, nausea, and vomiting. Patients with a history of angina may be considered to have progressed to UA if their symptoms (either chest pain or their anginal equivalent) are significantly worsened as compared to previous episodes, or begin occurring at rest or with a significantly lessened degree of activity.

Patients can appear markedly distressed from numerous causes of noncardiac chest pain that must be rapidly distinguished from ACS-related pain. Reproducible chest pain is often reassuring for a musculoskeletal cause but rarely can be seen in ACS. Ripping or tearing chest pain that radiates to the back may be indicative of aortic dissection, especially if there is a recent history of trauma involving a sudden deceleration, such as a high-speed car accident. A history of prolonged immobilization, either due to recent surgery or travel, combined with sharp and pleuritic chest pain points toward a pulmonary embolism. Chest pain that is worse when supine is suggestive of pericarditis, especially in a patient with recent infectious symptoms or who has recently undergone cardiac surgery.

21.3.3 Electrocardiogram

The 12-lead electrocardiogram (ECG) can be the most vital piece of information obtained by the clinician during the initial assessment of ACS. Patients with concern for ACS should have an ECG performed within 10 min of arrival to an emergency department. Transmural ischemia from complete occlusion of a coronary artery will result in ST-elevations in the underlying ECG territory (in the absence of significant collateral circulation). Over the ensuing hours to days, the ST segments may normalize followed by the development of T-wave inversions. In patients with a previous MI, new ST-elevations or normalization of previously established T-wave inversions can be indicative of a new ACS event. The pattern of myocardial depolarization is different when myocardial injury is limited to the subendocardium and instead results in the ST depression characteristic of NSTE-ACS [42]. With resultant myocardial cell death, pathologic Q-waves become visible on the ECG over the ensuing weeks post-injury. Q-wave formation can be seen with both STEMI and NSTEMI.

The combination of ischemic chest pain symptoms with ST changes indicative of acute ischemia should immediately trigger activation of an ACS reperfusion algorithm. In the absence of a left bundle branch block (LBBB), ECG changes consistent with MI are [43]:

- ST-elevation:
  - New elevation at the J point in at least two contiguous leads of ≥2 mm in men or ≥1.5 mm in women in leads V2–V3
  - ≥1 mm in other contiguous chest leads or limb leads
- ST depression:
  - New horizontal or down-sloping ST depression ≥0.5 mm in two contiguous leads
  - T-wave inversion ≥0.1 mm in two contiguous leads with prominent R wave or R/S ratio >1

Complete occlusion of the circumflex artery can result in a misleading picture. This typically causes ischemia in the infero-basal ("posterior") myocardium with resultant ST depression seen on the anterior chest leads (leads V1–V3) on ECG. ST-elevation can be seen with placement of posterior leads V7–V9 [43].

The presence of a new LBBB has been considered a surrogate of ST-elevation. However, this should be taken within the context of the entire patient presentation. It is often the case that the LBBB is assumed to be new due to lack of a previous ECG for comparison. Diagnostic criteria for STEMI in the presence of a LBBB were initially proposed by Sgarbossa et al. [44] and subsequently modified by Smith et al. [45]. These can also be applied to patients with bundle branch blocks secondary to ventricular pacing. The modified Sgarbossa criteria are satisfied if any one of the following are true and have a sensitivity of 80% and specificity of 99% for ACS [45, 46]:

- Concordant ST-elevation of ≥1 mm in at least 1 lead
- Concordant ST depression of ≥1 mm in leads V1–V3

- Proportionally excessive discordant ST changes, defined as ST-elevation or depression of ≥1 mm in at least 1 lead that is ≥25% of the height of the preceding S or R-wave, respectively

Numerous ECG changes associated with CHD can confound the diagnosis of acute ischemia. ECG changes that can mimic the findings of MI can be seen in patients with early repolarization, ventricular hypertrophy, cardiomyopathy, pre-excitation, and Brugada syndrome. ST-elevation is often seen postoperatively after PCI or cardiac surgery, or in patients with pericarditis (postoperative or infectious). Pericarditis should be suspected with diffuse ST-elevation that does not follow a single coronary distribution; PR segment depression is often seen as well.

21.3.4 Cardiac Biomarkers

Cardiac troponin (measured as either troponin T or troponin I) is the gold standard for diagnosing myocardial injury and necrosis. Patients presenting to the emergency room with suspected ACS should have a troponin measured either by rapid point-of-care testing or via a central lab with a goal of less than 60 min from patient arrival to obtaining the result [39]. Troponin can become elevated within 2–4 h of symptoms but may not be detectable in the blood for as long as 8–12 h post-onset (Fig. 21.2). Thus, a single negative troponin upon presentation does not rule out ACS and should be repeated within 4–8 h of symptom onset in high-risk patients. Values typically peak within 24–48 h. Normalization of troponin values is slow, and elevated levels may continue to be seen for as long as 2 weeks post-MI. Additionally, the degree of peak troponin elevation has prognostic implications, with higher levels indicating a larger territory of necrosis and a higher mortality in patients with ACS [39].

It is important to note that while an elevated troponin signifies myocardial damage, it is nonspecific with respect to etiology. Troponin elevations can be seen in numerous conditions outside of ACS, including heart failure, sepsis, pulmonary embolism, myocarditis, and cardiac trauma. In these situations, serial troponin measurements are helpful, with elevations >20% above baseline likely representing new myocardial injury or necrosis [47]. Patients with renal disease often have elevated circulating levels of troponin T. Measurement of troponin I may be more sensitive for detecting acute ischemia in this population [36]. Multiple assays of variable sensitivity exist for the measurement of troponin I. Thus, providers should be familiar with the cut-off for abnormal troponin I elevations (above the 99th percentile) at their institution. The troponin T assay is currently made by a single manufacturer.

Creatine kinase-MB (CK-MB) is also contained within cardiac muscle but is less specific than troponin for cardiac injury or necrosis. It may still be sent if troponin testing is unavailable but is otherwise unnecessary in the initial evaluation of suspected ACS. An initially positive CK-MB is of limited prognostic value, and discordant results should always favor the troponin testing [48]. CK-MB has a significantly shorter half-life than troponin, which does give it indications in specific

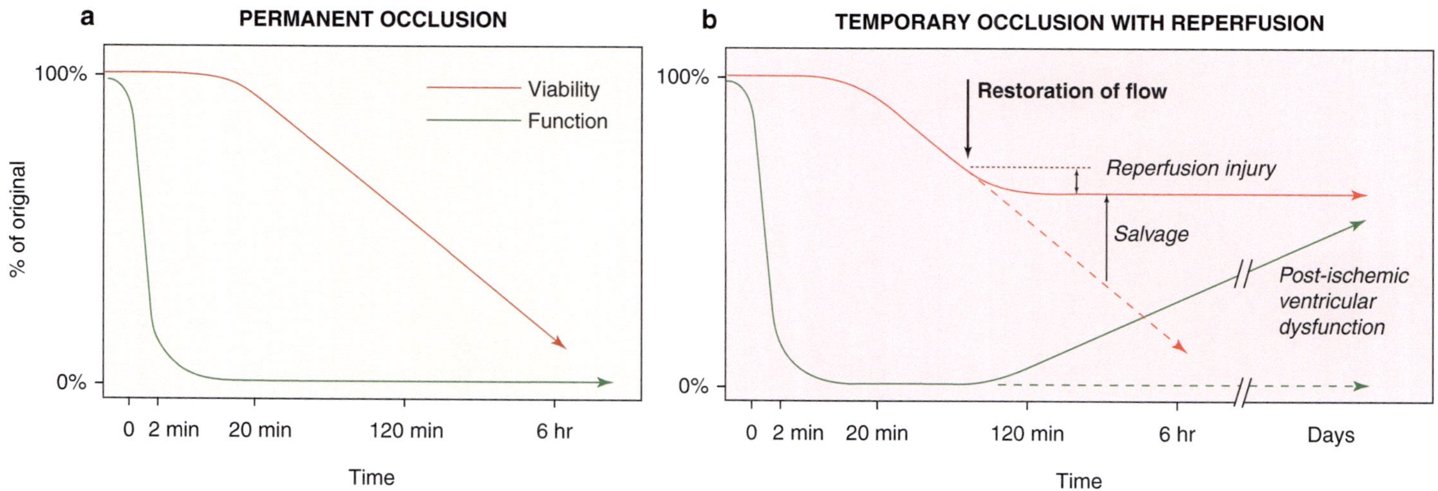

Fig. 21.2 (**a**) Myocardial viability and function are completely lost without reperfusion, and (**b**) with reperfusion some myocardium can be salvaged (Reproduced from Schoen FJ, Mitchell RN. The Heart. In: Kumar V, Abbas AK, Aster JC, eds. *Robbins and Cotran Pathologic Basis of Disease*. Ninth. Saunders; 2015:523–578)

circumstances. CK-MB elevations after the initial presentation can be diagnostic of reinfarction or infarct extension, as well as for periprocedural MI [36]. Since CK-MB is present in noncardiac tissues and in skeletal muscle, in particular, it should always be measured with total creatine kinase to aid in the interpretation of elevated values.

21.3.5 Additional Imaging

Other imaging modalities are rarely necessary to diagnose ACS but can have important prognostic information and may be helpful in evaluating other diagnoses. Noninvasive imaging can permit the clinician to document the presence of CAD and the risk of plaque rupture, better localize the affected myocardium and extent of infarcted territory, and evaluate the degree of residual ischemia after therapies have been initiated [49]. Demonstration of newly depressed function and loss of myocardial viability are consistent with ischemia; the absence of these essentially rules out an MI [43].

A chest radiograph is almost always obtained in the emergency room. The presence of pulmonary edema may be an indication of an elevated left ventricular filling pressure and depressed cardiac function. A widened mediastinum should raise concern for aortic dissection. Echocardiography can be used to assess systolic and diastolic dysfunction and to evaluate for areas of regional wall motion abnormalities. CT angiography is diagnostic for pulmonary embolism and aortic dissection. In patients with suspected ACS, CT coronary angiography can document high-risk plaques that are likely to rupture [49]. Magnetic resonance imaging (MRI) can assess myocardial perfusion, function, and viability. MRI is of high utility in patients with ECG changes and biomarker elevations suspected of having myocarditis. Radionucleotide imaging can directly assess myocardial viability [43].

21.3.6 Initial Medical Therapies

21.3.6.1 Analgesia

Morphine is the drug of choice for ischemic pain relief. In addition to analgesia, it can reduce sympathetic tone and anxiety and thereby myocardial oxygen demand. Its venodilating properties can also improve pulmonary edema and air hunger. Intravenous doses of 4–8 mg should be used initially, followed by additional 2–8 mg every 5–15 min until symptoms resolve or side effects preclude further administration [37].

21.3.6.2 Nitroglycerin

Nitroglycerin is a potent venodilator that decreases preload and may increase coronary blood flow. Sublingual nitroglycerin can be used to relieve chest pain due to ACS, though it generally does not improve the extent of myocardial injury [37]. It is contraindicated in patients with hypotension, especially with concomitant bradycardia, in patients with suspected right ventricular infarction (who are preload dependent), and in patients with recent phosphodiesterase inhibitor use [37, 38].

Use of nonsteroidal anti-inflammatory drugs (NSAIDs) should be avoided during ACS treatment. They have been associated with increases in cardiovascular mortality and morbidities, including reinfarction, ventricular rupture, renal injury, and heart failure [37, 38].

21.3.6.3 Oxygen

It was previously common practice for all patients presenting with suspected ACS to be placed on oxygen. However, supplemental oxygen likely has a limited effect in patients without significant hypoxemia. Concerns have emerged about the risks of inappropriate use of oxygen in patients with ACS, which may increase coronary vascular resistance and have potential mortality implications [37, 47]. Knowledge of the underlying structural anatomy in ACHD patients presenting with potential ACS and of their baseline oxygen saturations (for cyanotic patients) is important. In patients with shunting lesions, supplemental oxygen administration may increase pulmonary perfusion, leading to significant respiratory distress and compromised systemic perfusion for those patients presenting with MI-induced heart failure.

21.3.6.4 Aspirin

The mortality benefit of aspirin when received within the first 24 h of MI symptoms was established by the Second International Study of Infarct Survival (ISIS-2) [39]. A loading dose of 162–325 mg should be administered, preferably as a non-enteric form that can be chewed to allow for rapid absorption through the buccal mucosa. Patients should then continue a daily maintenance dose of 75–100 mg indefinitely [37, 47]. Higher doses are rarely indicated and significantly increase gastrointestinal bleeding risk.

21.3.6.5 Beta-Blockers

Initiation of oral beta-blocker therapy within the first 24 h of presentation is recommended for all patients without evidence of decompensated heart failure (often defined by the presence of pulmonary edema) or a low cardiac output state. Beta-blockers reduce myocardial demand and the size of the infarct territory, as well as the frequency of ventricular arrhythmias [38, 47]. Chronic therapy helps to prevent postischemic ventricular remodeling and reduces mortality. Those patients with left ventricular dysfunction and stable heart failure symptoms appear to derive the greatest benefit. Recommended drugs for which proven mortality data exist include metoprolol, carvedilol, and bisoprolol. A cardioselective beta-blocker can be chosen in patients with asthma or COPD to limit the risk of adverse pulmonary events. Patients with initial contraindications should be continuously reevaluated for initiation and continuation at hospital discharge. Intravenous beta-blocker use should be limited to patients presenting with demand ischemia in the setting of a hypertensive emergency [37, 38]. Beta-blockers are contraindicated in cocaine-induced ACS.

21.3.6.6 Angiotensin-Converting Enzyme (ACE) Inhibitors

In conjunction with beta-blocker therapy, ACE inhibitors reduce cardiac morbidity and mortality. The best outcomes are seen in higher-risk patients, including those with anterior MI or with an ejection fraction (EF) <40% post-MI [37]. ACE inhibitor therapy should be initiated within the first 24 h of presentation and continued indefinitely following discharge. Angiotensin receptor blockers (ARBs) can be given to patients intolerant of ACE inhibitors. ACE inhibitor or ARB use should be emphasized in patients with diabetes and/or chronic kidney disease [47].

21.3.6.7 Statins

Initiation of statin therapy lowers morbidity and mortality in patients with ACS, including the risk of recurrent cardiovascular events and the need for coronary revascularization. Intensive therapy, such as with atorvastatin 80 mg daily, is preferred with a goal of reducing LDL cholesterol levels by ≥50% [37, 47]. Administration of a statin on presentation may play an acute role in plaque stabilization. Statins given prior to PCI have demonstrated reductions in periprocedural MI and in 30-day mortality [50]. Rare complications of statin therapy include hepatic dysfunction and myopathies.

21.3.7 Treatment of STEMI

Rapid relief of coronary obstruction and resultant myocardial reperfusion is at the center of STEMI care. Complete vessel occlusion is seen in 90% of patients presenting with STEMI. While it is the case that higher-grade stenoses are more likely to precipitate a STEMI, most patients will have insignificant vessel occlusion (<50%) in the months leading up to the event. The amount of salvageable myocardium begins to decrease as early as 15 min after ischemia begins [51]. In addition to the duration of ischemia, the viability of the myocardium depends upon an interplay of multiple other factors, such as myocardial demand and the overall burden of CAD. In those patients with significant chronic coronary obstruction, collateral vessels have often developed that can mitigate the extent of ischemia.

21.3.7.1 Percutaneous Coronary Intervention

Primary PCI is the preferred treatment for patients who can undergo intervention at a high-quality PCI center within 90–120 min of presentation and are within 12 h of symptom onset. However, the greatest in-hospital and long-term mortality benefits are seen when reperfusion takes place within the first few critical hours (Fig. 21.3). The risk of 1-year mortality increases by 8% per every 30 min delay to PCI [38]. ACC/AHA goals for time from first medical contact to deployment of first device are <90 min for patients transported directly to a PCI-capable facility and <120 min when patients present at non-PCI-capable hospitals (Fig. 21.2) [37]. PCI is superior to fibrinolytic therapy in terms of restoration of normal (thrombolysis in myocardial infarction (TIMI) grade 3) flow, bleeding risks, incidence of reinfarction, and death [37, 52]. However, these benefits wane, and mortality rises as the duration of ischemia increases [53, 54]. The highest-risk patients derive the greatest mortality benefit from primary PCI. Patients who present in or develop cardiogenic shock or severe heart failure at any point during their hospitalization should undergo PCI. It should also be considered in patients with significant contraindications to thrombolytics and in those with ongoing evidence of ischemia at 12–24 h post-symptom onset [37].

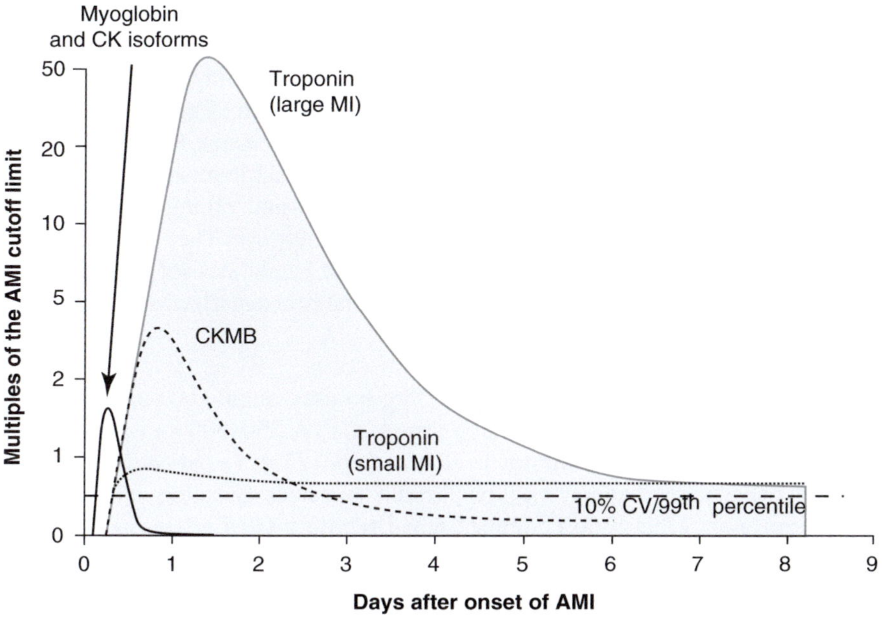

Fig. 21.3 Time course of biomarker elevations in acute myocardial infarction (Reproduced from Jaffe AS, Babuin L, Apple FS. Biomarkers in Acute Cardiac Disease. *JACC*. 2006;48(1):1–11)

Coronary stent implantation is superior to angioplasty alone and should be performed at the time of PCI. Options include bare metal stents (BMS) and drug-eluting stents (DES). DESs are preferred as they are associated with a decreased rate of restenosis, which is as high as 30% after BMS placement [55]. However, placement of a DES necessitates at least 1 year of dual antiplatelet therapy (DAPT) to minimize the risk of stent thrombosis. The risk of thrombosis for BMSs is greatest in the initial few weeks after placement, and thus short-term DAPT (typically 1 month) is safer in this group. Determining who is a good candidate for prolonged DAPT during acute STEMI management remains a challenge for providers [37]. Newer generations of DESs have been found to have a lower thrombosis risk. Further investigations are needed to determine the safety of shorter courses of DAPT in patients receiving these devices [56].

21.3.7.2 Antiplatelet Therapy

All patients undergoing PCI should be treated with DAPT with a combination of aspirin and a $P2Y_{12}$ inhibitor (either oral clopidogrel, prasugrel, or ticagrelor). $P2Y_{12}$ inhibitor use is associated with improvements in cardiovascular outcomes and reduced adverse events during hospitalization. In the CURE trial, clopidogrel use was shown to reduce the risk of MI, stroke, and cardiovascular death by 20% [57]. Clopidogrel use is mainly limited by the fact that as many as 30% of patients have gene polymorphisms that are associated with reduced drug efficacy. Prasugrel and ticagrelor are often preferred given their greater potency and more reliable efficacy. Prasugrel is associated with an increased risk of noncardiac bleeding and is contraindicated in patients with increased bleeding risk, including the elderly, those weighing <60 kg, and in patients with a history of prior stroke or transient ischemic attack [37]. Ticagrelor is a reversible $P2Y_{12}$ blocker that has a rapid onset and delivers near-complete blockade of the $P2Y_{12}$ receptor [55]. More recently the first intravenous $P2Y_{12}$ inhibitor, cangrelor, was also approved for use in PCI [58]. Prior to the introduction of $P2Y_{12}$ inhibitors, GP IIb/IIIa receptor inhibitors (abciximab, tirofiban, or eptifibatide) were routinely used in patients undergoing PCI. However, their use has largely been supplanted by $P2Y_{12}$ inhibitor use. They are rarely indicated but can be considered in patients who are not candidates for $P2Y_{12}$ use and have a large thrombus burden or unsuccessful initial revascularization [37].

21.3.7.3 Anticoagulation

Unfractionated heparin, given as 50–70 IU/kg boluses, should be administered at the time of PCI. Goal-activated clotting time (ACT) is 250–300 s (200–250 s if a glycoprotein (GP) IIb/IIIa inhibitor is administered) [55]. In patients with higher bleeding risks, monotherapy with bivalirudin (a direct thrombin inhibitor) has shown equivalent efficacy to combined heparin with a GP IIb/IIIa inhibitor (and thus concomitant GP IIb/IIIa use should be avoided). Bivalirudin can also be used safely in patients with renal dysfunction. Fondaparinux, an indirect factor Xa inhibitor, is also associated with a lower bleeding risk than heparin but has been shown to increase the risk of catheter thrombosis and should not be used as monotherapy in patients undergoing PCI [37].

21.3.7.4 Fibrinolysis

Fibrinolytic therapy should be administered to patients presenting within 12 h of symptom onset and in whom PCI is either not available or will be delayed longer than 90–120 min [37]. Contraindications predominantly involve an assessment of bleeding risk (Table 21.1). Although the mortality benefit seen with fibrinolytic therapy extends throughout the first 12 h of symptoms, it is most pronounced when administered within the first several hours of ischemia [59, 60]. Prehospital fibrinolytic therapy can be safely administered by EMS and is associated with reductions of up to an hour in time to reperfusion and a 17% risk reduction in all-cause mortality [37]. The overall efficacy of fibrinolytics is less than PCI. Restoration of TIMI grade 2 or 3 flow is seen in as many as 85% of patients [37].

Streptokinase was the original thrombolytic agent; however it is no longer available in the USA. Although inexpensive and effective, it is highly antigenic and can elicit a significant allergic response with repetitive exposure [38]. Fibrin-specific agents are now preferred and include tenecteplase, reteplase, and alteplase. All have shown equivalent mortality reductions [61]. Tenecteplase is the easiest to administer and may be given as a single, weight-based bolus over 5–10 min. Alteplase has a much shorter half-life and must be administered as a combined bolus and infusion over 90 min.

Relief of chest pain and significant improvement in ST-elevation on ECG provide reliable noninvasive markers of restoration of coronary blood flow. Reperfusion arrhythmias can also be seen and provide additional evidence of restored blood flow

Table 21.1 Contraindications and cautions for fibrinolytic therapy in STEMI

Absolute contraindications
• Any prior ICH
• Known structural cerebral vascular lesion (e.g., arteriovenous malformation)
• Known malignant intracranial neoplasm (primary or metastatic)
• Ischemic stroke within 3 months – EXCEPT acute ischemic stroke within 4.5 h
• Suspected aortic dissection
• Active bleeding or bleeding diathesis (excluding menses)
• Significant closed-head or facial trauma within 3 months
• Intracranial or intraspinal surgery within 2 months
• Severe uncontrolled hypertension (unresponsive to emergency therapy)
• For streptokinase, prior treatment within the previous 6 months
Relative contraindications
• History of chronic, severe, poorly controlled hypertension
• Significant hypertension on presentation (SBP >180 mmHg or DBP >110 mmHg)
• History of prior ischemic stroke >3 months
• Dementia
• Known intracranial pathology not covered in absolute contraindications
• Traumatic or prolonged (>10 min) CPR
• Major surgery (<3 weeks)
• Recent (within 2–4 weeks) internal bleeding
• Noncompressible vascular punctures
• Pregnancy
• Active peptic ulcer
• Oral anticoagulant therapy

ICH intracranial hemorrhage, *SBP* systolic blood pressure, *DBP* diastolic blood pressure, *CPR* cardiopulmonary resuscitation
From O'Gara PT, Kushner FG, Ascheim DD, et al. 2013 ACCF/AHA Guideline for the Management of ST-Elevation Myocardial Infarction. JACC. 2013;61(4):e78–e140

[38]. Resolution of >70% of ST-elevation in the lead with the greatest initial change combined with a complete absence of chest pain is strongly indicative of TIMI grade 3 flow. Failure of ST segment elevation to resolve by more than 50% within 2 h of fibrinolytic therapy suggests continued abnormal flow and should prompt consideration for rescue PCI therapy [37]. Patients who develop cardiogenic shock or severe heart failure should also be referred for rescue PCI. Even after successful post-fibrinolytic reperfusion, it is reasonable to refer stable patients for angiography and potential PCI. This approach has demonstrated significant reductions in 30-day and 1-year risks of recurrent MI or death when performed within 24 h. In stable patients PCI should be delayed for 2–3 h post-fibrinolytic administration to reduce the risk of bleeding [38].

Patients receiving fibrinolytic therapy should also receive aspirin and clopidogrel loads. Maintenance clopidogrel should be continued for at least 14 days and up to 1 year and aspirin continued indefinitely. Patients should also be started on anticoagulation. A heparin infusion can be given for the first 48 h, after which time it is preferable to convert to a subcutaneous regimen, either enoxaparin or fondaparinux. Enoxaparin dosing must be adjusted in patients with renal dysfunction, and fondaparinux is contraindicated with a creatinine clearance of less than 30 mL/min. Patients who develop heparin-induced thrombocytopenia may be converted to bivalirudin [37].

21.3.7.5 Coronary Artery Bypass Graft (CABG) Surgery

Excluding stable patients who are not candidates for either PCI or fibrinolysis, CABG is rarely indicated as the primary reperfusion strategy during ACS. More commonly, CABG is utilized when the coronary anatomy is unfavorable for PCI. This has often included left main coronary artery disease and multivessel disease (involving either the proximal left anterior descending and one additional coronary or three-vessel disease). Although a CABG has been thought of as the preferred treatment of left main coronary disease, outcomes for treatment by either PCI or a CABG are equivalent [62]. Patients with extensive, multivessel disease clearly benefit from a CABG [63]. A CABG is also recommended for patients that require repair of MI-induced structural defects, such as papillary muscle or ventricular free-wall rupture.

21.3.7.6 Complications After STEMI

Cardiogenic shock is seen in 5–8% of patients with STEMI [38] and portends a poor prognosis. It may occur either due to severe left ventricular failure or from mechanical complications such as ventricular free-wall rupture. Unstable patients presenting in cardiogenic shock or severe heart failure should undergo emergent revascularization when possible; use of an intra-aortic balloon pump or left ventricular assist device may be required for hemodynamic support in the post-procedure period [37]. Mortality rises exponentially in patients with an EF <40% after reperfusion [38]. In the absence of sustained ventricular arrhythmias, implantable cardioverter defibrillator (ICD) placement during the hospitalization is not recommended, as it has not been shown to reduce cardiovascular mortality. Function and heart failure symptoms should be reevaluated at least 40 days after STEMI and ICD placement considered for patients with continued risk of sudden death (EF ≤30% or ≤35% with significant heart failure-related exercise limitations) [37].

Involvement of the right ventricle and right ventricular failure is seen in up to one-third of patients with STEMI. Patients with isolated right ventricular infarction often present with hypotension, clear lungs, and jugular venous distension. The ECG may show ST-elevations in precordial leads V1 and V4R. Patients with right ventricular infarction and dysfunction are preload dependent; nitrates and diuretics are contraindicated [37].

Mechanical complications are rarely seen today, occurring in <1% of patients presenting with STEMI [64]. They are most often seen within the first 24 h, but may occur at any time during the first week following MI. Complications may include mitral valve papillary rupture, ventricular septal rupture, rupture of the left ventricular free wall, and left ventricular aneurysms. Except for left ventricular aneurysm, these complications are poorly tolerated and quickly lead to hemodynamic instability. Medical management is associated with a grim prognosis. Emergent surgical intervention is generally warranted but is also high risk with operative mortality rates of at least 20–40% [37, 64].

Ventricular arrhythmias are frequently seen early in the course of STEMI. Ventricular ectopy and nonsustained, hemodynamically stable rhythm disturbances do not require treatment or the initiation prophylact therapy (such as lidocaine) [38]. The incidence appears to be lower in patients treated with PCI over fibrinolytic therapy and when beta-blockers are initiated early in the course of hospitalization [37]. The associated mortality risk increases with late-onset ventricular tachycardia or fibrillation, and placement of an ICD is recommended in patients with these arrhythmias occurring more than 48 hours post-STEMI (except in cases where a transient etiology is identified and can be treated) [37]. Bradycardia and atrioventricular conduction blocks may also be seen and are more common with inferior MI. Complete heart block occurs in 3.7% of patients with an inferior MI and a small percentage of those with anterior MI [37]. In inferior MI, there is often a gradual progression to high-grade heart block that is hemodynamically well tolerated. Conversely, patients with large anterior infarctions may have a sudden progression to complete heard block and become unstable [38].

Noncardiac complications of STEMI most often include bleeding or thromboses. Both minor and major bleeds are associated with worse outcomes, including longer hospitalizations, recurrent cardiovascular events, and increased risk of death [37]. The most commonly seen bleeding is from the site of vascular access for PCI and can typically be managed conservatively. Major bleeds such as intracranial hemorrhage are associated with an in-hospital mortality as high as 20% [37]. Risk factors for bleeding include advanced age (>75 years), female gender, use of fibrinolytic therapy, and the presence of diabetes or severe renal dysfunction [37]. Heparin-induced thrombocytopenia (HIT) is a rare but serious complication associated with very high rates of thrombosis. If HIT is suspected, all heparin products should be discontinued, and patients should be switched to an alternative agent, such as bivalirudin, fondaparinux, or argatroban, while testing is being performed.

21.3.7.7 Out-of-Hospital Cardiac Arrest

Nearly 70% of STEMI deaths occur out of the hospital, most often in the setting of a ventricular fibrillation (VF) sudden cardiac arrest. The risk is greatest in the first hour after symptom onset [37, 38]. Only a minority of patients have a shockable rhythm upon EMS arrival, but it is these patients who have the greatest likelihood of neurologically intact survival [37]. Median hospital survival is only about 8% for all out-of-hospital arrests, but is as high as 22% for those patients found to be in VF [37]. Therapeutic hypothermia is associated with improved neurologic outcomes and should be initiated as soon as possible [37]. Patients found to have STEMI should undergo PCI after initial stabilization.

21.3.8 NSTE-ACS

The majority of ACS patients today (70%) present with NSTE-ACS [47]. While risk reduction strategies have helped reduce the overall rate of MI in the USA, a disproportionately greater decrease in the incidence of STEMI versus NSTE-ACS has resulted from these preventative therapies [65]. At the same time, the incidence of NSTE-ACS has increased as the American population has aged and developed increased comorbidities. Troponin assays have also become increasingly more sensitive, leading to greater numbers of patients diagnosed with NSTEMI who would have previously been classified as UA [49]. In-hospital mortality for all comers with ACS is as low as 2–2.5% and is overall higher in STEMI versus NSTE-ACS [66]. However, the combination of advanced age, increased comorbidities, and the presence of more extensive coronary disease seen in patients with NSTE-ACS is associated with higher long-term mortality over patients post-STEMI [49, 67].

21.3.8.1 Initial Management

Once NSTE-ACS has been identified, rapid risk assessment forms the cornerstone of treatment and determines if patients should undergo an initially invasive strategy (angiography with planned revascularization within 48 h of presentation) versus medical management (an "ischemia-guided" strategy). Fibrinolytic therapy does not play a role in the management of NSTE-ACS. Early assessment of left ventricular function is also important and may guide which approach is chosen [47].

The initial medical therapies used in NSTE-ACS are identical to STEMI and are aimed at relieving ischemia and reducing cardiac complications and mortality. All patients with likely or confirmed NSTE-ACS should be admitted to the hospital. Stable patients are appropriate for a step-down unit with close monitoring, whereas those with ongoing angina, hemodynamic compromise or rhythm disturbances are better served in a cardiac intensive care unit if not going directly to the catheterization laboratory for PCI [47]. Conversely, lower-risk patients without confirmed NSTE-ACS may be observed in a chest pain unit or discharged home directly from the emergency room. Accelerated protocols have been developed for evaluating patients at low risk for cardiovascular events. The presence of a normal ECG and normal troponins in these patients predicts a <1% likelihood of ACS [47].

All patients with definite or likely NSTE-ACS should be started on aspirin and a $P2Y_{12}$ inhibitor with the recommendation to continue DAPT for at least 1 year [47]. As in patients with STEMI, the use of GP IIb/IIIa inhibitors is not strongly indicated but may be considered in select patients undergoing an invasive strategy. Anticoagulation should be started on all patients regardless of the initial management strategy. Both unfractionated heparin and subcutaneous enoxaparin have shown mortality benefits in NSTE-ACS patients. However, enoxaparin is more strongly recommended as it is associated with a greater reduction in adverse cardiovascular events [49]. The dose of enoxaparin is 1 mg/kg twice daily (reduced to once daily in patients with a creatinine clearance <30 mL/min). Alternatives include bivalirudin and fondaparinux. Anticoagulation should be continued either until PCI is performed or for the duration of the hospitalization [47].

21.3.8.2 Risk Assessment

Multiple tools exist to help the clinician perform early risk assessment. The two best validated scores are the TIMI score and the Global Registry of Acute Coronary Events (GRACE) model. The TIMI score (https://www.mdcalc.com/timi-risk-score-ua-nstemi) is based on an assessment of seven risk factors on admission and predicts risk of the composite endpoint of all-cause mortality, new or recurrent MI, or severe recurrent ischemia requiring urgent revascularization within 14 days [36]. The GRACE model (https://www.mdcalc.com/grace-acs-risk-mortality-calculator) predicts all-cause in-hospital and 6-month mortalities and is applicable to all forms of ACS [36]. As the clinical status of a patient changes and evolves over time, it is important to reassess these risks throughout their hospital course.

21.3.8.3 Early Invasive Strategy

Patients at the highest risk (Table 21.2) derive the greatest benefit from an invasive strategy aimed at revascularization. An absolute risk reduction of recurrent MI or cardiovascular death of 11.1% is seen in this population, versus a <4% reduction in lower-risk patients [68]. All patients with troponin elevations are at higher risk, and greater increases in the troponin level correlate with infarct size and mortality [47, 49]. Patients with diabetes are at particular risk for poor outcomes following NSTE-ACS. The odds of mortality following NSTE-ACS are increased by 65% in the

Table 21.2 Risk factor assessment in determining treatment strategy for patients with NSTE-ACS

Immediate invasive—within 2 h	Refractory angina
	Signs or symptoms of HF or new or worsening mitral regurgitation
	Hemodynamic instability
	Recurrent angina or ischemia at rest or with low-level activities despite intensive medical therapy
	Sustained VT or VF
Ischemia-guided strategy	Low-risk score (e.g., TIMI [0 or 1], GRACE [<109])
	Low-risk Tn-negative female patients
	Patient or clinician preference in the absence of high-risk features
Delayed invasive—25–72 h	None of the above but diabetes mellitus
	Renal insufficiency (GFR <60 mL/min/1.73 m^2)
	Reduced LV systolic function (EF <0.40)
	Early postinfarction angina
	PCI within 6 months
	Prior CABG
	GRACE risk score 109–140; TIMI score ≥2
Early invasive—within 24 h	None of the above, but GRACE risk score >140
	Temporal change in Tn (Section 3.4)
	New or presumably new ST depression

HF heart failure, *VT* ventricular tachycardia, *VF* ventricular fibrillation, *Tn* troponin, *GFR* glomerular filtration rate, *LV* left ventricular, *EF* ejection fraction, *PCI* percutaneous coronary intervention, *CABG* coronary artery bypass graft

From Amsterdam EA, Wenger NK, Brindis RG, et al. 2014 AHA/ACC Guideline for the Management of Patients With Non-ST-Elevation Acute Coronary Syndromes. JACC. 2014;64(24):e139–e228

presence of diabetes, and this population faces a higher rate of restenosis after PCI. There is evidence that diabetic patients may be among the group that benefits from GP IIb/IIIa inhibitor use when undergoing PCI [49].

Outcomes for patients who develop cardiogenic shock are overall poor, but mortality is disproportionately higher in NSTE-ACS over STEMI (40.8% versus 33.1%, respectively) [69]. Although patients with NSTE-ACS in cardiogenic shock clearly benefit from aggressive intervention, they are among the least likely group to receive appropriate medical therapies or undergo revascularization. Anderson and colleagues demonstrated that only 56.5% of patients with NSTE-ACS and cardiogenic shock underwent revascularization [69]. Time to intervention was often delayed, with a median of 3.2 h to PCI and 55.9 h to CABG. In contrast, timely revascularization was performed in 95.8% of patients with STEMI and cardiogenic shock [69]. Guidelines for the management of cardiogenic shock in NSTE-ACS are not as well defined as for STEMI and permit a greater latitude for treatment based on patient and physician preference [47, 69]. This, combined with the increased morbidity of the NSTE-ACS population, likely explains the resultant differences in care for this group.

Whereas single culprit lesion PCI is recommended for patients with STEMI, multivessel PCI is often appropriate in patients with NSTE-ACS [47]. Patients with NSTE-ACS may have multiple plaque ruptures, and the risk for recurrent MI depends on the stability of all lesions present [49]. Elevated hsCRP may be able to predict those patients with multiple plaque ruptures [70]. Outcomes of PCI following NSTE-ACS are worse than for STEMI with higher rates of recurrent stenosis and MI [49]. Twenty percent of patients will have a second event within 3.4 years, frequently at the site of prior intervention [49]. Given the higher rates of multivessel disease, patients presenting with NSTE-ACS are also more likely to undergo CABG as their initial reperfusion strategy than those presenting with STEMI.

21.3.8.4 Ischemia-Guided Strategy

Patients with moderate- to low-risk profiles, including those without troponin elevations or evidence of recurrent ischemia for 12–24 h, can undergo a more conservative-based approach. There is no added mortality benefit to undertaking an early invasive approach in this population [47]. A noninvasive approach is also recommended for patients with significant comorbidities that would outweigh the risk of a revascularization procedure.

After patients have been stabilized and are ischemia-free, they should undergo noninvasive stress testing prior to hospital discharge [47]. This often starts with an exercise treadmill test. The baseline ECG abnormalities present in many ACHD patients may necessitate the use of echocardiographic imaging as opposed to evaluating for ECG changes consistent with ischemia. Patients who cannot appropriately exercise can instead undergo a pharmacologic stress test. Depressed function (EF <40%), regional wall motion abnormalities, markedly abnormal stress studies, or evidence of perfusion defects should be considered for angiography and revascularization.

Conclusions

Cardiovascular disease is at least as common in the noncyanotic ACHD population as in the general population, and most patients have at least one risk factor present. Risk assessment and treatment strategies should follow the same recommendations as in the general population. In the coming era, increasing numbers of ACHD patients will present with ACS. Total ischemic time is the most important predictor of outcome following an MI. As patients often postpone seeking medical attention after the initial onset of symptoms, minimizing delays in reperfusion is of paramount importance. Cardiac centers that routinely care for ACHD patients should be familiar with treatment guidelines and be able to rapidly assess and initiate treatment in this population.

References

1. Benjamin EJ, Blaha MJ, Chiuve SE, Cushman M, Das SR, Deo R, et al. Heart disease and stroke statistics—2017 update. Circulation. 2017;135:e1–458.
2. Pillutla P, Shetty KD, Foster E. Mortality associated with adult congenital heart disease: trends in the US population from 1979 to 2005. Am Heart J. 2009;158(5):874–9.
3. Giannakoulas G, Dimopoulos K, Engel R, Goktekin O, Kucukdurmaz Z, Vatankulu MA, et al. Burden of coronary artery disease in adults with congenital heart disease and its relation to congenital and traditional heart risk factors. Am J Cardiol. 2009;103(10):1445–50.
4. Lui GK, Fernandes S, McElhinney DB. Management of cardiovascular risk factors in adults with congenital heart disease. J Am Heart Assoc. 2014;3(6):e001076.
5. Tutarel O, Kempny A, Alonso-Gonzalez R, Jabbour R, Li W, Uebing A, et al. Congenital heart disease beyond the age of 60: emergence of a new population with high resource utilization, high morbidity, and high mortality. Eur Heart J. 2014;35(11):725–32.
6. Tutarel O. Acquired heart conditions in adults with congenital heart disease: a growing problem. Heart. 2014;100:1317–21.
7. Kannel WB, Dawber TR, Kagan A, Revotskie N, Stokes J. Factors of risk in the development of coronary heart disease-six year follow-up experience. The Framingham Study. Ann Intern Med. 1961;55:33–50.
8. Moons P, Deyk KV, Dedroog D, Troost E, Budts W. Prevalence of cardiovascular risk factors in adults with congenital heart disease. Eur J Cardiovasc Prev Rehabil. 2006;13(4):612–6.
9. Bhatt AB, Foster E, Kuehl K, Alpert J, Brabeck S, Crumb S, Davidson WR, Earing MG, Ghoshhajra BB, Karamlou T, Mital S, Ting J, Tseng ZH. Congenital heart disease in the older adult: A scientific statement from the American Heart Association. Circulation. 2015;131(21):1884–931.
10. Goff DC Jr, Lloyd-Jones DM, Bennett G, Coady S, Sean C, D'Agostino RB Sr, et al. ACC/AHA guideline on the assessment of cardiovascular risk: a report of the American College of Cardiology/American Heart Association Task Force on Practice Guidelines. J Am Coll Cardiol. 2014;63:2935–59.
11. World Health Organization. A global brief on hypertension. Geneva; 2013. p. 1–40. Report No.: WHO/DCO/WHD/2013.2.
12. Ridker PM, Libby P, Buring JE, Ridker PM, Libby P, Buring JE. Risk markers and the primary prevention of cardiovascular disease. In: Braunwald's heart disease a textbook of cardiovascular medicine. 10th ed. Philadelphia: Elsevier; 2015. p. 891–933.
13. Whelton PK, Carey RM, Aronow WS, Casey DE Jr, Collins KJ, Dennison Himmelfarb C, SM DP, Gidding S, Jamerson KA, Jones DW, MacLaughlin EJ, Muntner P, Ovbiagele B, Smith SC Jr, Spencer CC, Stafford RS, Taler SJ, Thomas RJ, Williams KA Sr, Williamson JD, Wright JT

Jr. 2017 ACC/AHA/AAPA/ABC/ACPM/AGS/APhA/ASH/ASPC/NMA/PCNA Guideline for the Prevention, Detection, Evaluation, and Management of High Blood Pressure in Adults. J Am Coll Cardiol. 2018;71(19):e127–248.
14. Cohen M, Fuster V, Steele PM, Driscoll D, McGoon DC. Coarctation of the aorta. Circulation. 1989;80:840–5.
15. Canniffe C, Ou P, Walsh K, Bonnet D, Celermajer D. Hypertension after repair of aortic coarctation—a systematic review. Int J Cardiol. 2013;167(6):2456–61.
16. Bocelli A, Favilli S, Pollini I, Bini RM, Ballo P, Chiappa E, et al. Prevalence and long-term predictors of left ventricular hypertrophy, late hypertension, and hypertensive response to exercise after successful aortic coarctation repair. Pediatr Cardiol. 2012;34(3):620–9.
17. Quennelle S, Powell AJ, Geva T, Prakash A. Persistent aortic arch hypoplasia after coarctation treatment is associated with late systemic hypertension. J Am Heart Assoc. 2015;4(7):e001978.
18. National Cholesterol Education Program (NCEP). Expert panel on detection, evaluation, and treatment of high blood cholesterol in adults (adult treatment panel III). Third report of the National Cholesterol Education Program (NCEP) expert panel on detection, evaluation, and treatment of high blood cholesterol in adults (adult treatment panel III) final report. Circulation. 2002;106(5):3143–421.
19. Cholesterol Treatment Trialists' CTT Collaboration. Efficacy and safety of more intensive lowering of LDL cholesterol: a meta-analysis of data from 170000 participants in 26 randomised trials. Lancet. 2010;376:1670–81.
20. Cholesterol Treatment Trialists' CTT Collaborators. The effects of lowering LDL cholesterol with statin therapy in people at low risk of vascular disease: meta-analysis of individual data from 27 randomised trials. Lancet. 2012;380:581–90.
21. Zomer AC, Vaartjes I, Uiterwaal CSP, van der Velde ET, Sieswerda GJT, Wajon EMC, et al. Social burden and lifestyle in adults with congenital heart disease. Am J Cardiol. 2012;109(11):1657–63.
22. Ogden CL, Carroll MD, Kit BK, Flegal KM. Prevalence of childhood and adult obesity in the United States, 2011–2012. JAMA. 2014;311(8):806–9.
23. Zaidi AN, Bauer JA, Michalsky MP, Olshove V, Boettner B, Phillips A, Cook SC. The impact of obesity on early postoperative outcomes in adults with congenital heart disease. Congenit Heart Dis. 2011;6(3):241–6.
24. World Health Organization. Global report on diabetes. Geneva; 2016. p. 1–88.
25. Wang P, Huang R, Lu S, Xia W, Sun H, Sun J, et al. HbA1c below 7% as the goal of glucose control fails to maximize the cardiovascular benefits: a meta-analysis. Cardiovasc Diabetol. 2015;14(124):1–15.
26. Boussageon R, Bejan-Angoulvant T, Saadatian-Elahi M, Lafont S, Bergeonneau C, Kassai B, et al. Effect of intensive glucose lowering treatment on all cause mortality, cardiovascular death, and microvascular events in type 2 diabetes: meta-analysis of randomised controlled trials. BMJ. 2011;343:d4169.
27. Hemmingsen B, Lund SS, Gluud C, Vaag A, Almdal TP, Wetterslev J. Targeting intensive glycaemic control versus targeting conventional glycaemic control for type 2 diabetes mellitus (Review). Cochrane Database Syst Rev. 2013;11:CD008143.
28. Savji N, Rockman CB, Skolnick AH, Guo Y, Adelman MA, Riles T, et al. Association between advanced age and vascular disease in different arterial territories. A population database of over 3.6 million subjects. J Am Coll Cardiol. 2013;61(16):1736–43.
29. Lloyd-Jones DM, Nam B-H, D'Agostino RB Sr, Levy D, Murabito JM, Wang TJ, et al. Parental cardiovascular disease as a risk factor for cardiovascular disease in middle-aged adults. JAMA. 2004;3291:2204–11.
30. Miyamoto K, Takeuchi D, Inai K, Shinohara T, Nakanishi T. Prognostic value of multiple biomarkers for cardiovascular mortality in adult congenital heart disease: comparisons of single-/two-ventricle physiology, and systemic morphologically right/left ventricles. Heart Vessel. 2016;31:1834–47.
31. Tomita H, Takamuro M, Soda W, Hatakeyama K, Tsutsumi H. Increased serum high-sensitivity C-reactive protein is related to hypoxia and brain natriuretic peptide in congenital heart disease. Pediatr Int. 2008;50:436–40.

32. Madhavan MV, Tarigopula M, Mintz GS, Maehara A, Stone GW, Généreux P. Coronary artery calcification. Pathogenesis and prognostic implications. J Am Coll Cardiol. 2014;63(17):1703–14.
33. Halpern DG, Steigner ML, Prabhu SP, Valente AM, Sanders SP. Cardiac calcifications in adults with congenital heart defects. Congenit Heart Dis. 2015;10:396–402.
34. Fox CS, Evans JC, Larson MG, Kannel WB, Levy D. Temporal trends in coronary heart disease mortality and sudden cardiac death from 1950 to 1999: the Framingham heart study. Circulation. 2004;110:522–7.
35. Sidney S, Quesenberry CP Jr, Jaffe MG, Sorel M, Nguyen-Huynh MN, Kushi LH, et al. Recent trends in cardiovascular mortality in the United States and public health goals. JAMA Cardiol. 2016;1(5):594–9.
36. Wright RS, Anderson JL, Adams CD, Bridges CR, Casey DE, Ettinger SM, et al. 2011 ACCF/AHA focused update incorporated into the ACC/AHA 2007 guidelines for the management of patients with unstable angina/non-ST-elevation myocardial infarction. J Am Coll Cardiol. 2011;57(19):e215–367.
37. O'Gara PT, Kushner FG, Ascheim DD, Casey DE, Chung MK, de Lemos JA, et al. 2013 ACCF/AHA guideline for the management of ST-elevation myocardial infarction. J Am Coll Cardiol. 2013;61(4):e78–e140.
38. Mega JL, Morrow DA. ST-elevation myocardial infarction: management. In: Braunwald's heart disease: a textbook of cardiovascular medicine. 10th ed. Philadelphia: Elsevier; 2015. p. 1095–154.
39. Anderson JL, Adams CD, Antman EM, Bridges CR, Califf RM, Casey DE Jr, et al. ACC/AHA 2007 guidelines for the management of patients with unstable angina/non-ST-elevation myocardial infarction. J Am Coll Cardiol. 2007;50(7):e1–e157.
40. Kumar A, Cannon CP. Acute coronary syndromes: diagnosis and management, Part I. Mayo Clin Proc. 2009;84(10):917–38.
41. Srikanth S, Ambrose JA. Pathophysiology of coronary thrombus formation and adverse consequences of thrombus during PCI. Curr Cardiol Rev. 2012;8:168–76.
42. Mirvis DM, Goldberger AL. Electrocardiography. In: Braunwald's heart disease: a textbook of cardiovascular medicine. 10th ed. Philadelphia: Elsevier; 2015. p. 114–54.
43. Thygesen K, Alpert JS, Jaffe AS, Simoons ML, Chaitman BR, White HD, ESC/ACCF/AHA/WHF Expert Consensus Document. Third universal definition of myocardial infarction. Circulation. 2012;126(16):2020–35.
44. Sgarbossa EB, Pinski SL, Barbagelata A, Underwood DA, Gates KB, Topol EJ, et al. Electrocardiographic diagnosis of evolving acute myocardial infarction in the presence of left bundle-branch block. N Engl J Med. 1996;334(8):481–7.
45. Smith SW, Dodd KW, Henry TD, Dvorak DM, Pearce LA. Diagnosis of ST-elevation myocardial infarction in the presence of left bundle branch block with the ST-elevation to S-wave ratio in a modified Sgarbossa rule. Ann Emerg Med. 2012;60(6):766–76.
46. Meyers HP, Limkakeng AT Jr, Jaffa EJ, Patel A, Theiling BJ, Rezaie SR, et al. Validation of the modified Sgarbossa criteria for acute coronary occlusion in the setting of left bundle branch block: a retrospective case-control study. Am Heart J. 2015;170:1255–64.
47. Amsterdam EA, Wenger NK, Brindis RG, Casey DE Jr, Ganiats TG, Holmes DR Jr, et al. 2014 AHA/ACC guideline for the management of patients with non-ST-elevation acute coronary syndromes: a report of the American College of Cardiology/American Heart Association Task Force on Practice Guidelines. J Am Coll Cardiol. 2014;64(24):e139–228.
48. Newby LK, Roe MT, Chen AY, Ohman EM, Christenson RH, Pollack CV, et al. Frequency and clinical implications of discordant creatine kinase-MB and troponin measurements in acute coronary syndromes. J Am Coll Cardiol. 2006;47:312–8.
49. Giugliano RP, Cannon CP, Braunwald E, Giugliano RP, Braunwald E. Non-ST elevation acute coronary syndromes. In: Braunwald's heart disease: a textbook of cardiovascular medicine. 10th ed. Philadelphia: Elsevier; 2015. p. 27.
50. Patti G, Cannon CP, Murphy SA, Mega S, Pasceri V, Briguori C, et al. Clinical benefit of statin pretreatment in patients undergoing percutaneous coronary intervention: a collaborative patient-level meta-analysis of 13 randomized studies. Circulation. 2011;123:1622–32.

51. Scirica BM, Morrow DA. ST-elevation myocardial infarction: pathology, pathophysiology, and clinical features. In: Braunwald's heart disease: a textbook of cardiovascular medicine. 10th ed. Philadelphia: Elsevier; 2015. p. 27.
52. Keeley EC, Hillis LD. Primary PCI for myocardial infarction with ST-segment elevation. N Engl J Med. 2007;356:47–54.
53. Pinto DS, Frederick PD, Chakrabarti AK, Kirtane AJ, Ullman E, Dejam A, et al. Benefit of transferring ST-segment-elevation myocardial infarction patients for percutaneous coronary intervention compared with administration of onsite fibrinolytic declines as delays increase. Circulation. 2011;124:2512–21.
54. Terkelsen CJ, Sorensen JT, Maeng M, Jensen LO, Tilsted H-H, Trautner S, et al. System delay and mortality among patients with STEMI treated with primary percutaneous coronary intervention. JAMA. 2010;304(7):763–71.
55. Mauri L, Bhatt DL, Mauri L, Bhatt DL. Percutaneous coronary intervention. In: Braunwald's heart disease: a textbook of cardiovascular medicine. 10th ed. Philadelphia: Elsevier; 2015. p. 24.
56. Levine GN, Bates ER, Bittl JA, Brindis RG, Fihn SD, Fleisher LA, et al. 2016 ACC/AHA guideline focused update on duration of dual antiplatelet therapy in patients with Coronary Artery Disease. J Am Coll Cardiol. 2016;68(10):1082–115.
57. Braunwald E. Unstable angina and non-ST elevation myocardial infarction. Am J Respir Crit Care Med. 2012;185(9):924–32.
58. Damman P, Woudstra P, Kuijt WJ, de Winter RJ, James SK. P2Y12 platelet inhibition in clinical practice. J Thromb Thrombolysis. 2011;33:143–53.
59. White HD, Chew DP. Acute myocardial infarction. Lancet. 2008;372:570–84.
60. Fibrinolytic Therapy Trialists' FTT Collaborative Group. Indications for fibrinolytic therapy in suspected acute myocardial infarction: collaborative overview of early mortality and major morbidity results from all randomised trials of more than 1000 patients. Lancet. 1994;343:311–22.
61. Van de Werf F. Single-bolus tenecteplase compared with front-loaded alteplase in acute myocardial infarction: the ASSENT-2 double-blind randomised trial. Lancet. 1999;354(9180):716–22.
62. Morice MC, Serruys PW, Kappetein AP, Feldman TE, Stahle E, Colombo A, et al. Five-year outcomes in patients with left main disease treated with either percutaneous coronary intervention or coronary artery bypass grafting in the synergy between percutaneous coronary intervention with taxus and cardiac surgery trial. Circulation. 2014;129(23):2388–94.
63. Sipahi I, Akay MH, Dagdelen S, Blitz A, Alhan C. Coronary artery bypass grafting vs percutaneous coronary intervention and long-term mortality and morbidity in multivessel disease. JAMA Intern Med. 2014;174(2):223–30.
64. Kutty RS, Jones N, Moorjani N. Mechanical complications of acute myocardial infarction. Cardiol Clin. 2013;31:519–31.
65. Yeh RW, Sidney S, Chandra M, Sorel M, Selby JV, Go AS. Population trends in the incidence and outcomes of acute myocardial infarction. N Engl J Med. 2010;362:2155–65.
66. Roe MT, Messenger JC, Weintraub WS, Cannon CP, Fonarow GC, Dai D, et al. Treatments, trends, and outcomes of acute myocardial infarction and percutaneous coronary intervention. J Am Coll Cardiol. 2010;56(4):254–63.
67. Vora AN, Wang TY, Hellkamp AS, Thomas L, Henry TD, Goyal A, et al. Differences in short- and long-term outcomes among older patients with ST-elevation verses non-ST-elevation myocardial infarction with angiographically proven coronary artery disease. Circ Cardiovasc Qual Outcomes. 2016;9:513–22.
68. Fox KAA, Clayton TC, Damman P, Pocock SJ, de Winter RJ, Tijssen JGP, et al. Long-term outcome of a routine versus selective invasive strategy in patients with non-ST-segment elevation acute coronary syndrome. J Am Coll Cardiol. 2010;55(22):2435–45.
69. Anderson ML, Peterson ED, Peng SA, Wang TY, Ohman EM, Bhatt DL, et al. Differences in the profile, treatment, and prognosis of patients with cardiogenic shock by myocardial infarction classification. Circ Cardiovasc Qual Outcomes. 2013;6:708–15.
70. Tanaka A, Shimada K, Sano T, Namba M, Sakamoto T, Nishida Y, et al. Multiple plaque rupture and C-reactive protein in acute myocardial infarction. J Am Coll Cardiol. 2005;45(10):1594–9.

Impact of Non-cardiac Comorbidities in Adults with Congenital Heart Disease: Management of Multisystem Complications

22

Sarah W. Goldberg, Catherine K. Allan, and Christopher P. Learn

22.1 Introduction

The prevalence and impact of non-cardiac comorbidities in adult patients with congenital heart disease increase over time, and these complications are often specifically a consequence of the long-term altered cardiovascular physiology or sequelae of previous therapies. For the ACHD patient admitted to the intensive care unit (ICU) for either surgical or medical treatment, an assessment of the burden of multisystem disease, as well as an understanding of the underlying cardiovascular pathophysiology, is essential for optimal management of these complex patients. This chapter takes an organ-system-based approach to reviewing common comorbidities in the ACHD patient, focusing on conditions that are directly related to ACHD status and may significantly impact ICU care.

22.2 Pulmonary Disease

Pulmonary disease is a common comorbidity in adult congenital heart disease (ACHD) patients. Among 1200 ACHD patients followed over 7 years, 47% had abnormal lung function, including nearly 30% with moderately to severely reduced forced vital capacity (FVC) associated with a 1.6-fold increased mortality [1]. Similarly, among 2600 ACHD patients followed over 4 years, 18.4% of those that

S. W. Goldberg (✉) · C. K. Allan
Pediatric Cardiology, Boston Children's Hospital, Boston, MA, USA
e-mail: sarah.goldberg@cardio.chboston.org

C. P. Learn
Massachusetts General Hospital, Boston, MA, USA

E. da Cruz et al. (eds.), *Intensive Care of the Adult with Congenital Heart Disease*, Congenital Heart Disease in Adolescents and Adults,
https://doi.org/10.1007/978-3-319-94171-4_22

died had lung disease versus 5% of those still living [2]. Patients with unrepaired lesions, cyanotic heart disease, single-ventricle palliation, and CHD repaired at on older age have a more significant burden of lung disease [1, 3]. Lung disease is an indication for hospital admission in 5–12% of ACHD patients and accounts for 12–14% of all postoperative readmissions [4, 5]. Furthermore, preoperative lung disease has been found to be a risk factor for longer ICU length of stay, adverse cardiovascular events, and in-hospital mortality [6–11].

22.2.1 Airway Abnormalities

Large airway abnormalities such as tracheobronchomalacia, subglottic stenosis, and airway compression, which may be congenital or acquired, can be seen in ACHD patients and may impact risk in the perioperative period or respiratory support requirements in the ICU. Tracheobronchomalacia may be associated with a syndrome such as trisomy 21 or related to chronic lung disease or prolonged mechanical ventilation requiring tracheostomy [12–14].

Tracheal or bronchus compression caused by surrounding cardiac or vascular structures can be seen in ACHD patients. For example, ventricular dilation may result in compression of the left main stem bronchus and surrounding lung tissue [13], and left atrial dilation may cause compression of the main stem bronchi [15]. Distal tracheal and right main stem compressions are frequently seen in the context of left pulmonary artery slings. Vascular rings are associated with tracheomalacia and tracheal compression [16]. Dilated vascular structures, such as pulmonary arteries in the context of severe pulmonary regurgitation or absent pulmonary valve syndrome, can cause compression of the trachea, main stem bronchi, and lung parenchyma and may be accompanied by emphysematous changes [13].

Knowledge of a patient's airway and mechanical ventilation history may suggest underlying structural airway defects and inform decisions on ventilation strategy and postoperative lung recruitment. Preoperative airway assessment by noninvasive imaging or direct laryngobronchoscopy may guide a patient's management around intubation, including choice of sedative/induction agents and available equipment and personnel resources. Additionally, structural airway abnormalities may warrant higher positive-pressure ventilation, positive end-expiratory pressure (PEEP) in particular, to maintain ventilation around functional residual capacity. Noninvasive positive-pressure ventilation and aggressive pulmonary toilet may be required after extubation. Lastly, providers should be aware of the risk of post-obstructive pneumonia.

22.2.2 Respiratory Infections

Pneumonia affects 10–20% of patients in the cardiac ICU after cardiac surgery [17, 18]. The CONCOR study, which examined 6900 ACHD patients in a Dutch national registry, revealed that 4% of deaths in ACHD patients were secondary to pneumonia, although the overall mortality rate of the population was low [19]. Risk factors for respiratory tract infections particularly relevant to ACHD patients include underlying immunodeficiency or leukocyte wasting (see section on infectious diseases), chronic malnutrition, airway abnormalities, and history of vocal cord paresis increasing aspiration risk. Malnutrition in particular results in depressed immune function and muscle wasting with consequent poor respiratory effort and atelectasis, also increasing the risk of prolonged mechanical ventilation and impaired airway clearance.

A high suspicion for respiratory infections should be maintained for ACHD patients in the ICU, and infections should be treated aggressively. In addition, preventative efforts such as optimization of nutrition, use of aspiration precautions (elevation of head of bed), and attention to oral hygiene in intubated patients should be maintained. Judicious use of gastric acid-suppression medications should be employed, as these may increase a patient's risk of airway colonization with reflux and aspiration [13, 20].

22.2.3 Restrictive Lung Disease

Sequelae of prior cardiac surgeries, including diaphragmatic paralysis, seen in up to 10% of patients with CHD after surgery [21, 22], and chest wall abnormalities, may result in restrictive lung disease. Diaphragm paralysis results in elevation of the hemidiaphragm, decreased lung excursion, and atelectasis and is an independent predictor of moderately to severely depressed FVC (odds ratio 4.64) [1]. Chest wall abnormalities due to scoliosis and prior thoracotomies also independently predict moderately to severely impaired lung function (odds ratio 3.2 and 1.9, respectively) [1]. The presence of scoliosis may result in reduced lung volumes on the side of the greater curvature, reduced number of alveoli and a proportional increase in "remnant alveolar" space closer to the spinal curvature, and abnormal development of the muscles of respiration [23, 24]. Therefore, the presence of scoliosis should factor into decisions regarding ventilation expectations and strategies to maintain adequate lung expansion. Scoliosis may complicate neck mobilization and airway visualization, possibly requiring specialized personnel and equipment for successful laryngoscopy and intubation [25–27].

22.2.4 Pulmonary Edema

Interstitial edema, a nearly ubiquitous concern with ACHD patients at some point in their clinical course, decreases lung compliance, requiring the patient to increase their work of breathing to maintain adequate minute ventilation. Pulmonary edema also disrupts the alveolar-capillary interface and impairs gas exchange, decreasing total lung capacity, impairing diffusion, and resulting in hypoxemia. The intraparenchymal airways may be compressed by edema of the peribronchial wall or vessels ("peribronchial cuffing"), leading to an obstructive pattern of lung disease [13, 28, 29].

Furthermore, chronic interstitial edema may cause fibrosis and hypertrophy of lung tissue, resulting in a restrictive lung disease pattern [1].

Pulmonary edema may result from an excess of pulmonary blood flow, as seen in intracardiac (ASD, VSD, PDA, partial anomalous pulmonary venous return) or extracardiac left-to-right shunt lesions (PDA, systemic arteriovenous malformations, aortopulmonary collateral vessels, and surgical aortopulmonary shunts). Pulmonary edema is also seen in lesions associated with high pulmonary venous pressures, including obstruction to left heart inflow (pulmonary vein stenosis or occlusive disease, cor triatriatum), obstruction to left heart outflow (mitral or aortic stenosis), and left atrial volume overload (mitral regurgitation or left ventricular systolic and diastolic dysfunction) [1, 13] requiring careful attention to diuresis and volume management in the cardiac ICU [13]. Interventions that result in pulmonary vasodilation, such as treatment with nitric oxide, sildenafil, or other vasodilators, can worsen pulmonary edema, particularly in the presence of a left-to-right shunt lesion.

Patients with elevated central venous pressures or obstruction to systemic venous drainage may also develop pulmonary edema and pleural effusions. Similarly, extracardiac abnormalities such as superior vena cava syndrome, innominate vein thrombosis, and primary lymphangiectasia may contribute to pulmonary edema and chylothoraces [13]. In addition to volume management and diuresis, these patients may require procedural interventions to alleviate their right heart or central venous obstruction or right ventricular afterload reduction strategies, including reduction of mean airway pressure during ventilation and pulmonary vasodilators, to lower central venous pressures.

Cardiopulmonary bypass also contributes to pulmonary edema in the postoperative ACHD population. The reduction in pulmonary blood flow during cardiopulmonary bypass and exposure to the artificial surfaces of the bypass circuit triggers a diffuse inflammatory response, characterized by cytokine release and pulmonary interstitial leukocyte infiltration, that results in pulmonary capillary leak and transudative edema [1, 30–34]. Attention to diuresis and ventilation strategies to minimize V/Q mismatch are therefore important in the postoperative period.

22.2.5 Other Lung Diseases

Acute respiratory distress syndrome (ARDS) is associated with significant early postoperative mortality in adults with ACHD [11]. The typical management strategies used in non-CHD patients, such as high-frequency oscillatory ventilation and high levels of PEEP, may be poorly tolerated in ACHD patients with single-ventricle physiology with passive pulmonary blood flow (Fontan circulation) or with predominantly right-sided heart disease. Strategies to minimize mean airway pressure should be employed where possible. Extracorporeal membrane oxygenation (ECMO) support may be an alternative therapy for this group of patients, although limited data are available on the outcomes of ECMO support for adult Fontan patients.

Adults with CHD may present with typical comorbid pulmonary conditions, including asthma, chronic obstructive lung disease, or emphysema, and these patients may benefit from usual treatments such as bronchodilator therapy, as well as aggressive pulmonary toilet and incentive spirometry to avoid further exacerbation of the lung disease. Other considerations for ACHD patients include pulmonary hypoplasia, a history of tobacco use, and recurrent chest infections, which may result in some degree of parenchymal lung disease.

Lastly, sleep-disordered breathing may be more prevalent in the ACHD population [35–37], related to airway abnormalities or craniofacial abnormalities, such as micrognathia, seen in genetic conditions such as 22q11.2 or Noonan syndromes. Patients with trisomy 21 may also be at increased risk of central sleep apnea [38]. Given that sleep-disordered breathing has been associated with pulmonary hypertension, ventricular dysfunction, and increased morbidity and mortality in patients with heart failure [39–41], noninvasive positive-pressure ventilation should be used in ACHD patients with known sleep-disordered breathing. Preoperative polysomnography should be considered in patients with a history suggestive of sleep-disordered breathing.

22.2.6 Pulmonary Considerations in Patients with Single-Ventricle Physiology

Notable pulmonary considerations exist for ACHD patients with single-ventricle heart disease. In a study of 52 patients with Fontan palliation over 10 years, 58% of patients demonstrated some degree of restrictive lung disease on pulmonary function testing [42]. This may be due to chest wall abnormalities due to multiple thoracotomies and scoliosis, a history of chronic pulmonary edema, recurrent infections and effusions resulting in fibrosis, and some degree of pulmonary hypoplasia due to the lack of pulsatile flow in the Fontan circulation [43].

Patients with Fontan circulation may develop progressive hypoxemia due to development of systemic to pulmonary venous collaterals related to elevated central venous pressures and venous stasis [13] and to arteriovenous malformations due to exclusion of putative hepatic factor. Chronic hypoxemia or structural pulmonary arterial disease in turn may promote development of aortopulmonary collateral vessels which may contribute to chronic pulmonary edema. Pulmonary edema is also exacerbated by activation of the renin-angiotensin-aldosterone axis in low cardiac output states as well as low oncotic pressures in those patients with protein-losing enteropathy (PLE) or malnutrition [13].

Aortopulmonary collateral vessels and arteriovenous malformations also predispose to pulmonary hemorrhage and hemoptysis. Similarly, Eisenmenger syndrome can be complicated by hemoptysis, found to be the cause of death in 11–30% of patients [44, 45]. Pulmonary embolism, due to low-flow state, venous stasis in the Fontan baffle, and baseline prothrombotic state, is also common in the single-ventricle patient population, with pulmonary embolism and chronic pulmonary embolic disease affecting 5–16% of patients [46].

Plastic bronchitis is a rare complication in the Fontan population characterized by acellular, noninflammatory casts that can result in obstructive pulmonary disease and worsening of baseline hypoxemia. It is at least in part due to elevated central venous pressures resulting in impaired lymphatic drainage and decompression into the pulmonary bed. In a study of nearly 1100 ACHD patients, 1.5% of patients were diagnosed with protein-losing enteropathy or plastic bronchitis [47]. Consultation with a pulmonologist should be considered to assist in management of casts, including aggressive pulmonary toilet in those patients who are breathing spontaneously. Treatment options in the cardiac ICU include aerosolized hypertonic saline or heparin or r-TPA nebulizer treatments to disrupt the casts and allow patients to more easily mobilize their secretions. Direct cast removal by bronchoscopy may be required in intubated patients. Beta agonists, mucolytics, expectorants, and dornase alfa administration have not shown efficacy in treating plastic bronchitis [48].

Lastly, ventilation of Fontan patients can be complicated due to competing needs of higher positive end-expiratory pressure to overcome obstructive pulmonary physiology and lower mean airway pressure to promote flow through the Fontan pathway. In the presence of a Fontan fenestration or baffle leaks, higher mean airway pressure may result in worsening of baseline hypoxia due to right-to-left shunt. Without a fenestration or baffle leak, cardiac output may be impaired due to reduced preload to the systemic ventricle. The increase in Fontan pressures due to higher positive airway pressures can lead to ascites and pleural effusions, further impairing ventilation thus requiring even higher positive airway pressures. The effects are amplified when respiratory acidosis leads to increased pulmonary vascular resistance, thereby causing further increase in Fontan pressures. Cautious drainage of ascites and pleural effusions may be beneficial in this situation.

22.2.7 Pulmonary Management Strategies

Cardiopulmonary interactions based on the underlying cardiac lesion must be considered when choosing a ventilation strategy for any ACHD patient admitted to the ICU. Patients with chronic left atrial hypertension, parenchymal lung disease, a history of smoking, frequent chest infections, chest wall deformities, or airway abnormalities may require higher positive-pressure ventilation [49]. Challenges to ventilation of single-ventricle patients, in particular those with Fontan circulation, have been covered in previous sections. Preoperative or routine outpatient pulmonary function testing and early consultation with a pulmonologist should be entertained in at-risk patients, particularly those with right ventricular disease, single-ventricle physiology, or cyanotic heart disease. Due to the myriad of possible pulmonary abnormalities in the ACHD population, all adult patients in the CICU should receive aggressive pulmonary toilet, ambulate early, and use incentive spirometry frequently.

22.3 Renal Disease

Renal dysfunction is highly prevalent in the ACHD population and can significantly impact care in the ICU. Among 1100 ACHD patients, 50% had an abnormal glomerular filtration rate (GFR) at baseline, with 9% having moderately to severely impaired GFR. For ICU patients, the presence of renal dysfunction is associated with a threefold increased risk of overall mortality and is predictive of poor postoperative outcomes [11, 50–52]. In a cohort of nearly 2600 ACHD patients over 4 years, approximately 21% of deceased patients had some degree of renal disease compared to only 3% of survivors [2]. Risk factors for renal disease include more complex congenital heart lesions, history of multiple surgical interventions, and persistent cyanosis [53]. Patients with univentricular and right ventricular disease, as well as Eisenmenger syndrome, are at a heightened risk of having moderately to severely depressed renal function, at least in part related to chronic elevation of central venous pressures [50, 51, 54].

In addition to the risk of baseline chronic renal insufficiency, ACHD patients are at increased risk of developing acute kidney injury (AKI) during hospitalizations. Estimates of any AKI in the postoperative period range from 36 to 59% [55] and of renal failure or moderate to severe AKI from 5 to 20% [55, 56]. Pre-existing renal dysfunction is a risk factor for longer length of hospitalization and postoperative readmission in ACHD patients [4, 57], though renal failure requiring renal replacement therapy is uncommon [10].

Renal dysfunction may be caused or exacerbated by several factors in the ICU. Hypothermia, hypotension, and bleeding during cardiopulmonary bypass (CPB) may all impair renal perfusion, with longer duration of CPB associated with higher risk of renal dysfunction [58]. Fluid overload may contribute to increased central venous pressure (CVP) and, therefore, decreased renal perfusion pressure. Renal dysfunction may be potentiated by factors that decrease cardiac output, including ventricular dysfunction and arrhythmias [53].

A decrease in renal perfusion pressure, the difference between the mean arterial pressure and central venous pressure, can lead to deterioration of renal function. Thus, congenital lesions with high central venous pressure, such as right ventricular lesions (e.g., tetralogy of Fallot) and single-ventricle circulation, are more commonly associated with renal dysfunction [53]. High central venous pressures may also contribute to development of ascites, causing abdominal compartment syndrome; high intra-abdominal pressures further increase CVP and therefore further reduce renal perfusion pressure. Ascites also limits downward movement of the diaphragm, necessitating higher-pressure ventilation, which further elevates right heart pressures and CVP. This increase in CVP leads to further reduction in renal perfusion pressure as well as decreased systemic venous return, potentially resulting in a low cardiac output state and further reduction in renal perfusion [59–61].

22.3.1 Renal Management Strategies

Given the morbidity and mortality associated with renal dysfunction in this patient population, preservation of renal function must be a priority. Preoperative assessment of renal function in high-risk patients by creatinine clearance calculation or renal scintigraphy allows risk stratification, anticipation of potentially nephrotoxic exposures, and employment of protective strategies when possible [53]. These strategies should include careful monitoring of a patient's hemodynamics with avoidance of hypotension and maintenance of renal perfusion pressure. Monitoring of bladder pressure has resulted in reduced incidence of abdominal compartment syndrome in non-ACHD patients and may be appropriate in those patients at highest risk for intra-abdominal hypertension [62]. Additionally, careful drainage of ascites may be appropriate in certain patients to relieve intra-abdominal hypertension, improve renal perfusion pressure, improve systemic venous return, facilitate effective positive-pressure ventilation, and maintain cardiac output [53].

Nephrotoxic agents, including iodine-based contrast, should be avoided when possible, and medications should be appropriately dose-adjusted based on either measured or estimated GFR when required. Specific considerations include dose adjustment of milrinone in patients with reduced GFR as well as avoidance of angiotensin-converting enzyme inhibitors in patients with risk of impaired renal perfusion or acute kidney injury. Medications that cause peripheral vasoconstriction and could potentially diminish renal perfusion, such as norepinephrine and vasopressin, should be avoided when possible [53]. A meta-analysis of fenoldopam administration during cardiopulmonary bypass in non-ACHD patients revealed reduced utilization of renal replacement therapy, shorter duration of stay in the intensive care unit, and decreased overall in-hospital mortality. Although there are no data on the use of fenoldopam in adults with CHD, it may be an appropriate drug to consider in those patients with baseline renal dysfunction or those at high risk of developing acute renal impairment in the cardiac ICU [63].

Contrast nephropathy prevention strategies, including the use of fenoldopam, N-acetylcysteine, and sodium bicarbonate, are controversial and insufficiently examined in the ACHD population. Studies have not demonstrated a decrease in contrast-induced nephropathy in non-ACHD patients with baseline renal dysfunction treated with fenoldopam [64]. Several studies have demonstrated reduction in contrast-induced nephropathy rates in patients treated with sodium bicarbonate and N-acetylcysteine but have failed to demonstrate a statistically significant decline in renal failure requiring renal replacement therapy [65, 66]. Despite their controversial nature, it may be reasonable to consider the use of contrast nephropathy prevention in those patients with significant baseline renal disease and those at highest risk for development of renal dysfunction in the ICU.

22.4 Infectious Disease

Infection accounts for significant morbidity and mortality in the ACHD population, with postoperative infection occurring in approximately 15% and septicemia in 7% of patients [4, 56]. Deaths of ACHD patients in the perioperative period were attributed to sepsis in 4% of cases [2]. In a study of nearly 100,000 hospitalized ACHD patients, septicemia was associated with the longest length of stay [57]. The risk of CLABSI in ACHD patients may be increased by a patient's limited venous access due to prior procedures, necessitating longer central venous catheter placement.

General infection risk may be increased by multifactorial immunodeficiency as well as prior colonization by hospital-acquired organisms, leading to nosocomial infections. First, several syndromes commonly associated with CHD, such as heterotaxy with asplenia, 22q11.2 deletion syndrome, and trisomy 21, are associated with varying degrees of immune dysfunction. Second, many adults who have undergone cardiac surgery in childhood may have undergone a complete or partial thymectomy [67], which, although associated with lower absolute T-cell numbers and T-cell subsets, is not associated with overt immunodeficiency [68]. Lastly, ACHD patients may have chronic wasting of immunoglobulins and lymphocytes due to thoracic duct injury or inadequate lymphatic drainage with resultant chylous effusions [69].

22.4.1 Immune Abnormalities in Single-Ventricle Palliations

T-cell lymphopenia and hypogammaglobulinemia may be seen in single-ventricle patients with protein-losing enteropathy (PLE). Chronic systemic venous hypertension impairs lymphatic drainage into the venous circulation, resulting in dilatation of the lymphatic channels and collateral formation to allow drainage into lower resistance reservoirs, such as the intestine [67, 70, 71]. Although patients with PLE have the most profound abnormalities, patients without overt PLE may also have some degree of lymphopenia, presumably due to a chronic low level of protein wasting [67, 72]. These abnormalities are more pronounced later after Fontan operation, with a fourfold increase in the odds of significant lymphopenia in the second decade after Fontan [67]. Depressed immunoglobulin G levels are also found in patients with PLE with an associated impaired response to the pneumococcal, diphtheria, and tetanus vaccines. Despite this, PLE is not associated with an increased risk of opportunistic infections, nor is it a risk factor for hospitalization for infection [67, 72]. Although not a risk factor in isolation, in the ICU setting, it is important to recognize the potential for baseline immunodeficiency and increased risk of infection. A low level of suspicion for infection should be maintained in these patients.

22.4.2 Endocarditis

The risk of infective endocarditis (IE) is higher in ACHD patients compared to the general population [73–78]. In a study of over 4000 ACHD patients, the incidence of IE was 3%, with the highest rates occurring in patients with unrepaired VSDs, repaired tetralogy of Fallot, and cyanotic heart disease [78]. The mortality rate of adult CHD patients with IE ranges from 4 to 8% [75]. In-hospital mortality is more likely to occur in those patients who have at least one prior cardiac surgery, patients with prosthetic material as part of their repair, patients with prior episodes of endocarditis or an intracardiac abscess, and patients of an older age [75, 76]. A specific cause of IE is identified in only 26–30% of ACHD patients [75, 79], and only 70% of patients have an identifiable source of infection by cardiac imaging [76], likely related to difficulty visualizing the intracardiac structures due to prosthetic materials and limited acoustic windows. ACHD patients may present with heart failure, embolic phenomena, or worsening valvar dysfunction as the heralding signs of IE [76]. The presence of any of these findings with associated fevers or elevated inflammatory markers, even in the absence of an identified vegetation by imaging or positive blood cultures, should raise suspicion for endocarditis. The most common organisms that cause IE in ACHD patients mirror those in the general population: streptococci and staphylococci [76]. Patients should therefore receive broad antibiotic coverage while awaiting blood culture results and speciation of organisms. Because of the potential limitations of echocardiography, PET/CTA is an emerging diagnostic modality in patients where the diagnostic suspicion is high or the identification of the site of infection may inform the decision between medical therapy and surgical intervention [76].

22.4.3 Hepatitis C

Adults who underwent surgery for congenital heart defects prior to initiation of routine screening of donor blood products for hepatitis C virus (HCV) in 1992 are at risk for hepatitis C exposure. ACHD patients have higher rates of positive HCV antibody titers, suggestive of active or past infection, than the general population, ranging from 8 to 15% of those patients who underwent surgery before 1992. However, the number of patients with active infections, indicated by the presence of HCV RNA, is lower [80, 81]. Patients with more complex congenital heart lesions are more likely to have been exposed to HCV due to higher blood product exposure [80, 82, 83]. HCV screening should occur in all patients who underwent surgery prior to 1992, and for those with exposure, hepatic function should be monitored closely during their hospitalization and hepatotoxic agents should be used with caution.

22.5 Integumentary and Musculoskeletal Considerations

Hospital-acquired pressure ulcers affect 3–34% of hospitalized patients [84]. Many of the risk factors for pressure ulcer development in the general adult population are frequently encountered in the ACHD population, including cardiac surgery, long hospital length of stay, long duration of mechanical ventilation, limited mobility, and infrequent repositioning. Chronic malnutrition contributes to decreased subcutaneous tissue, revealing more superficial pressure points, as well as hypoalbuminemia and poor wound healing. Use of vasoactive infusions is associated with pressure ulcer development due to the underlying low perfusion state as well as the medication-induced peripheral vasoconstriction [84]. Attention should be paid to frequent monitoring of adult patients for ulcer development, early treatment, repositioning of immobile patients, use of pressure-alleviating mattresses and devices on pressure points, optimization of nutritional status, and frequent ambulation when the patient is able.

ACHD patients are at risk for bone demineralization, increasing their risk of fracture in the ICU. In patients with PLE, the risk is likely even higher due to a combination of chronic protein losses and malnutrition, edema, treatment with medications such as heparin and steroids, and chronic use of loop diuretics, resulting in excess calcium losses [85]. Attention to positioning and fracture precautions should be employed in those patients with known significant bone demineralization. Lastly, chronic illness myopathy may be exaggerated in adults with CHD due to preexisting malnutrition and poor muscle tone, warranting minimization of sedation when appropriate, early ambulation, and physical therapy.

22.6 Endocrine

22.6.1 Diabetes, Insulin Resistance, and Glucose Control

Adults with CHD are at increased risk of developing type II diabetes compared to the general population (hazard ratio 1.4), and the risk is further increased in cyanotic heart disease (hazard ratio 1.9) [86]. In the ICU, improved glycemic control has been found to decrease the risk of complications in non-ACHD patients. The degree of glycemic control, however, does not have to be highly intensive. The GLUCO-CABG trial [87] demonstrated no significant difference in complications between intense target glucose range of 100–140 mg/dL and a more conservative range of 141–180 mg/dL in persons undergoing coronary artery bypass surgery. Glycemic control in the ICU setting should be achieved through the use of continuous infusions of insulin allowing more nimble control of blood glucose, as hypoglycemia is associated with poor outcomes and longer hospital stays and should be treated immediately.

22.6.2 Thyroid Disease

Thyroid disease has an increased prevalence in trisomy 21 and 22q11 deletion syndrome. Abnormal preoperative thyroid studies are predictive of increased ICU and hospital mortality [51]. Although thyroid function screening is not routinely recommended preoperatively for patients without history of thyroid dysfunction, there should be a low threshold for screening in ACHD patients with any risk factors or subclinical symptoms. Subclinical hyperthyroidism is associated with increased heart rate, atrial arrhythmias, increased left ventricular mass, impaired diastolic function, reduced exercise performance, and increased risk of cardiovascular mortality [88]. Subclinical hypothyroidism is associated with impaired systolic and diastolic function and an increased risk for atherosclerosis and myocardial infarction.

Patients with pre-existing thyroid conditions should have their thyroid status checked and medication dosages adjusted until thyroid-stimulating hormone levels are within normal limits prior to elective procedures.

Patients with moderate to severe hypothyroidism who must undergo procedures before their hypothyroidism is controlled may be at increased risk for heart failure, atrial fibrillation, and gastrointestinal and neurological complications postoperatively [89]. Those needing urgent surgery should be treated with intravenous levothyroxine prior to surgery [90]. Consider treatment with stress-dose steroids if there is concern for comorbid adrenal insufficiency.

There is a paucity of data on treatment of hyperthyroidism related to cardiac surgery. Elective surgeries should be postponed. Antithyroid medications such as thionamides (e.g., propylthiouracil and methimazole) inhibit upstream production of thyroid hormone and often take several days of treatment before having a significant clinical effect and weeks to achieve a euthyroid state. These medications should be continued postoperatively to decrease the risk of thyroid storm [91]. Beta-blockers may ameliorate many of the symptoms of hyperthyroidism in patients who require more urgent surgery. Consultation with an endocrinologist and pharmacist is recommended.

22.6.3 Metabolic Syndrome and Obesity

In a recent case-control study, metabolic syndrome (hypertension, hyperglycemia, excess body fat around the waist, and elevated cholesterol or triglyceride levels) was more prevalent in ACHD patients compared to controls [92]. Metabolic syndrome is associated with increased rates of adverse outcomes in both cardiac and non-cardiac surgery, including increased rates of stroke, deep vein thrombosis, acute kidney injury, wound infections, and increased length of stay [93]. Cardiac intensivists should recognize these increased risks and employ strategies outlined in the relevant sections of this chapter to ameliorate these specific risks.

Obesity is associated with increased risk for hypertension, diabetes, dyslipidemia, coronary artery disease, gall bladder disease, chronic kidney disease, restrictive lung changes, sleep apnea, and hypercapnia. A recent single-center review found comparable rates of being overweight and obese in ACHD patients with a somewhat lower rate of morbid obesity compared to control subjects [94]. Higher body mass index is associated with relatively better survival among adults with CHD, but this relationship likely reflects an association of cardiac cachexia with poor outcomes [95].

Obese persons in intensive care settings are at an increased risk of skin wounds, challenging vascular access, potentially difficult mask ventilation, and intubation [96, 97]. Ideal body weight should be considered when calculating nutritional goals. Furthermore, medications may need to be adjusted because of an increased volume of distribution for lipophilic medications, decreased proportionate lean body mass, and lower tissue water content compared to the general population [98]. Opioids should be used carefully given the risk of respiratory depression in obese patients, who already carry an increased risk of restrictive lung disease, sleep apnea, and hypoventilation. Given differences in the relative volume of distribution, anticoagulants often warrant adjusted dosing for obese patients. Serum monitoring (e.g., anti-X_a levels) for efficacy and avoidance of supra-therapeutic levels is warranted.

Ventilation strategies may require adjustment for obese patients. In contrast to nonobese persons, higher PEEP settings (10 cm H_2O) were associated with improved chest wall compliance, end-expiration lung volume, and increased PaO_2 in morbidly obese (BMI >40) persons [99], though the effects of increased PEEP requirements in ACHD patients with passive pulmonary blood flow (e.g., Fontan circulation) or primarily right-sided heart disease must be considered.

Practical considerations regarding bed size, limits for weight of CT/MRI platforms, and the need for team lifting/lifting assist devices should be anticipated. Anticipation of these challenges is particularly important when ACHD patients are cared for in pediatric institutions.

22.7 Hematology

As with all critically ill adult patients, ACHD patients admitted to an intensive care unit should be risk stratified for thrombosis and bleeding risks. All patients should receive interventions to reduce deep venous thrombosis (DVT) risk, including anti-embolism stockings, sequential compression devices, and early ambulation, unless contraindicated. These are particularly important in patients for whom pharmacologic DVT prophylaxis is contraindicated.

Certain congenital heart diseases increase the risk of thrombus formation, most notably the Fontan circulation. The Fontan circulation is associated with increased systemic venous stasis and alterations in circulating factors including decreased levels of antithrombin III, thrombomodulin, and α2-antiplasmin, lower protein C and protein S activity levels, and significantly higher levels of thrombin-antithrombin complex and α2-plasmin inhibitor complex [100]. A recent Japanese study found D-dimer was significantly elevated in patients with Fontan circulation and an intracardiac thrombus versus controls [101]. While an elevated D-dimer may prompt consideration of a CT pulmonary angiogram, CT-PA imaging is technically difficult in the Fontan circulation given increased venous transit time and often unbalanced streaming from the SVC and IVC to the right and left pulmonary arteries. A bolus of contrast from an upper extremity injection may stream into one lung. The absence of complete filling of the contralateral lung may raise concern for thrombus. An increased interval of time from contrast administration to image acquisition and/or simultaneous upper and lower limb injections may mitigate these technical issues [102].

Polycythemia is prevalent in patients with cyanosis but symptomatic hyperviscosity is uncommon. The optimal hemoglobin for a given saturation can be derived by the following equation: predicted hemoglobin = 57.5 − (0.444 O_{2sat}) [103]. Patients with severe, chronic hypoxemia may have a hemoglobin concentration well above the typical index range yet be functionally anemic. If patients have a hemoglobin significantly below their target concentration, transfusion should be considered for the symptomatic patient but must always be weighed against the risks of transfusion, including risk of sensitization to future blood products and potential need for organ transplantation. Iron deficiency should also be evaluated, as low iron levels may impair flexibility of erythrocytes. There should be a low threshold for long-term enteral iron replacement.

Hyperviscosity is a possible complication in chronic hypoxia, but it is rare below hematocrit levels of 70% [104]. Intravenous fluids should be considered if dehydration may be exacerbating the polycythemia. Phlebotomy should be reserved for symptomatic cases and only after appropriate hydration.

Thrombocytopenia is frequently observed in persons with the Fontan circulation, often attributed to hypersplenism. Given the increased risk for thrombus formation, platelet transfusion should be limited to patients with active bleeding or high risk of procedural bleeding. Neutropenia can also be observed in persons with the Fontan circulation or in patients with 22q11 microdeletion syndromes and trisomy 21.

22.8 Hepatic/Gastrointestinal Disease

Chronic hepatic congestion is seen in patients with Fontan circulation. Fontan-associated liver disease (FALD) can lead to increased stiffness of the liver, portal hypertension, hypervascular liver nodules, and eventual cirrhosis. Liver dysfunction has been identified as a risk factor for perioperative mortality in adults with CHD [10]. Elevated gamma-glutamyl transferase (GGT) is the most common laboratory abnormality observed in FALD [105]. In contrast to hepatobiliary disease, alkaline phosphatase is usually not elevated to the same degree as GGT. Bilirubin, predominantly unconjugated, is most commonly normal or mildly elevated. Marked hypoalbuminemia should prompt consideration of possible PLE.

Portal hypertension increases the odds of gastrointestinal bleeding via esophageal and gastric varices and portal gastropathy. Management of gastrointestinal hemorrhage in ACHD patients is more difficult in the context of therapeutic anticoagulation or acquired coagulopathy, as seen in the setting of advanced hepatic disease. Reversal of anticoagulants and administration of clotting factors and platelets may be acutely warranted but may also increase the risk of thrombosis of prosthetic valves, mechanical support devices, systemic veins, and atrial and Fontan pathways, as well as transfusion reactions and sensitization to blood products. Given the potential for catastrophic bleeding, cardiac ICUs should have well-defined pathways for treatment of acute GI hemorrhage. This requires collaboration with gastroenterology and interventional radiology teams skilled in acute interventions such as esophageal banding. Any vascular access issues (e.g., occlusion of femoral vessels from prior catheterization/surgeries) and venous abnormalities (e.g., interrupted vena cava) should be communicated to the interventional teams in advance to avoid procedural delays and complications. Access to gastroenterologists and interventional radiologists skilled in managing acute GI hemorrhage should be taken into consideration when deciding where to care for a Fontan patient with acute GI bleeding. This may be of particular relevance when deciding between a pediatric and adult center.

Hepatic encephalopathy has been reported in persons with the Fontan palliation [106]. While related to hyperammonemia, the relationship between ammonia level and degree of encephalopathy is neither linear nor exponential. However, extreme elevations (over 200 μmol per liter) can lead to cerebral edema and death. The West Haven [107] and FOUR Score [108] systems can assist with the diagnosis and grading of encephalopathy. Therapies aimed at lowering the ammonia level such as lactulose remain first-line therapies.

22.9 Neurologic Issues

22.9.1 Stroke

In a recent series, 7–9% of CHD patients suffered a stroke before age 65. Over half of adults with cyanotic CHD have evidence of prior ischemic injury on brain imaging [109]. The risk of acute thrombotic events is increased in the perioperative period and following catheter procedures. Additional risk factors include atrial arrhythmias, left-to-right shunts, and the presence of prosthetic valves. Furthermore, thrombosis of tissue valves has been increasingly recognized as a source of valve dysfunction and embolic events [110]. Infectious endocarditis can lead to embolization of infectious materials, secondary abscess formation, and vascular injury. Increasing age is also associated with atherosclerosis. Guidewires and catheters can potentially disrupt plaque and lead to an embolic event in these patients. The ICU must be vigilant for acute changes in neurological function. Focal weakness, language difficulties, and sensory impairment may more obviously raise the concern for stroke, but acute changes in level of consciousness, atypical behaviors, sudden dizziness, or changes in coordination should also be carefully evaluated.

Given the potential for significant long-term improvement with rapid reperfusion, evaluation of possible stroke must be performed in an emergent, time-efficient manner. Stroke protocols should be developed with neurology in advance to help minimize delays in diagnosis and treatment. Patients who are recovering from cardiac surgery may be ineligible for systemic thrombolytic therapy, but given advancements in catheter-based therapy, they should still be evaluated urgently by a stroke team with neuro-interventionalist involvement.

22.9.2 Therapeutic Hypothermia for In-Hospital Arrest

Hypothermia protocols for protection of neurologic injury in shock states are an area of active study. Studies have demonstrated a benefit for witnessed out-of-hospital ventricular fibrillation arrests in adults [111]. However, a recent observational study of adults [112] suggested harm, and a prospective trial in children [113] was stopped early due to futility. Pending more definitive prospective data in adults, therapeutic hypothermia cannot be routinely recommended for in-hospital arrest; however, rapid rewarming for patients who are hypothermic post cardiac arrest and hyperthermia should be avoided [114].

22.10 Psychosocial Concerns

22.10.1 Tobacco

In addition to the well-known effects of long-term smoking, nicotine withdrawal can adversely affect hospitalized patients. Nicotine withdrawal can be uncomfortable and some patients may seek to prematurely leave the hospital to smoke. Nicotine replacement therapy should be considered in patients with history of regular tobacco use. A recent meta-analysis found conflicting data about the effect of nicotine replacement therapy on agitation and delirium rates in the ICU [115]. Ideally, patients should be referred to smoking cessation programs at or prior to discharge.

22.10.2 Alcohol

Alcohol and/or frequent benzodiazepine use can lead to tolerance and dependency, which can occur without obvious social dysfunction. A thorough history regarding substance use is recommended, but patients may minimize or deny usage due to social stigma. Abrupt withdrawal of these agents can lead to tachycardia, agitation, hypertension, and delirium tremens. While withdrawal can begin as soon as 8 hours following the last use of alcohol, symptoms typically peak at 72 hours [116]. Symptoms may be delayed if benzodiazepines are used for sedation. Tolerance may increase sedation requirements and alternative agents should be considered. Expert consultation with anesthesiology is recommended in the acute setting and coordination with outpatient primary care and substance abuse specialists should be initiated prior to discharge.

22.10.3 Opiates

Opiate use and dependence are increasingly prevalent in the general population. Like patients with chronic alcohol or benzodiazepine use, opiate dependence may pose a challenge for procedural sedation. Alternative agents (e.g., propofol, ketamine, etc.) should be considered with consultation from anesthesiology. Similarly, analgesia for postoperative pain may require significant dosage adjustment and/or alternative therapies.

While postoperative pain warrants treatment, current recommendations suggest opiates should be prescribed in lower dosages and short courses with an emphasis on improving functionality rather than the elimination of discomfort. Earlier/more frequent outpatient follow-up may be warranted to help ensure that pain is well controlled while limiting the risk of developing opiate dependence.

Intravenous and subdermal opiate use increases the risk of endocarditis and teams should be vigilant for this possibility even in the absence of an obvious usage history. Patients may also potentially abuse opiates while in the inpatient setting. ICU teams should be prepared to recognize opiate intoxications and consider it in the differential of unexplained decompensation.

22.10.4 Psychiatric Care

While there are conflicting data regarding the relative prevalence of depression among adults with congenital heart disease, recent studies from Europe have suggested rates of anxiety and depression are similar or lower in ACHD patients than in matched controls [117]. Regardless of the population-based risk, depression and anxiety can have significant implications for the perioperative patient and can be provoked by cardiac surgery [118]. Depression has been associated with increased perioperative pain in coronary artery bypass graft surgery patients [119]. Screening for depression prior to surgery may help the ICU team anticipate perioperative issues of pain control, delirium, and sleep disturbance, as well as help ensure depression is properly treated postoperatively.

Serotonin-selective reuptake inhibitors (SSRI) have been associated with increased adverse perioperative event rates [120]. It is not clear to what degree the association is causal, as much of the harm may be associated with the underlying depression or other comorbid illnesses. There is conflicting data association between SSRI use and increased perioperative bleeding, possibly due to effects on platelet aggregation, with a 2010 study of CABG patients showing no significant increased bleeding risk [121]. Typically, SSRIs and serotonin-norepinephrine reuptake inhibitors (SNRI) are continued perioperatively as acute withdrawal can provoke flu-like symptoms, sleep disruption, altered sensation, changes in mood/thinking, and abnormal movements, including tardive dyskinesia. Given the potential for withdrawal phenomenon, stopping other medications which may have effects on platelet function such as NSAIDs should be considered first.

22.11 Summary

Adult patients with congenital heart disease are at significant risk for comorbidities in nearly every organ system. A thorough knowledge of how specific congenital cardiac physiology and interventions may predispose to comorbidities is essential for intensive care unit providers who are caring for this population of patients. Patients with palliated single-ventricle heart disease are at highest risk for comorbidities and proactive assessment of such patients may help providers avoid or minimize complications related to comorbidities. A strong working knowledge of Fontan physiology in particular will help ICU providers manage routine aspects of ICU care, such as mechanical ventilation, most effectively.

References

1. Alonso-Gonzalez R, Borgia F, Diller GP, et al. Abnormal lung function in adults with congenital heart disease: prevalence, relation to cardiac anatomy, and association with survival. Circulation. 2013;127:882–90.
2. Engelings CC, Helm PC, Abdul-Khaliq H, et al. Cause of death in adults with congenital heart disease—an analysis of the German National Register for Congenital Heart Defects. Int J Cardiol. 2016;211:31–6.
3. Gaultier C, Boule M, Thibert M, Leca F. Resting lung function in children after repair of tetralogy of Fallot. Chest. 1986;89:561–7.
4. Kim YY, He W, MacGillivray TE, Benavidez OJ. Readmissions after adult congenital heart surgery: frequency and risk factors. Congenit Heart Dis. 2017;12:159–65.
5. Agarwal S, Sud K, Menon V. Nationwide hospitalization trends in adult congenital heart disease across 2003–2012. J Am Heart Assoc. 2016;5:e002330.
6. Rodriguez FH, Moodie DS, Parekh DR, et al. Outcomes of heart failure-related hospitalization in adults with congenital heart disease in the United States. Congenit Heart Dis. 2013;8:513–9.
7. Engström G, Lind P, Hedblad B, et al. Lung function and cardiovascular risk: relationship with inflammation-sensitive plasma proteins. Circulation. 2002;106:2555–60.
8. Mott A, Fraser C Jr, McKenzie E, et al. Perioperative care of the adult with congenital heart disease in a free-standing tertiary pediatric facility. Pediatr Cardiol. 2002;23:624–30.
9. Dore A, Glancy DL, Stone S, Menashe VD, Somerville J. Cardiac surgery for grown-up congenital heart patients: survey of 307 consecutive operations from 1991 to 1994. Am J Cardiol. 1997;80:906–13.
10. Abarbanell GL, Goldberg CS, Devaney EJ, Ohye RG, Bove EL, Charpie JR. Early surgical morbidity and mortality in adults with congenital heart disease: the University of Michigan experience. Congenit Heart Dis. 2008;3:82–9.
11. Berdat PA, Immer F, Pfammatter J-P, Carrel T. Reoperations in adults with congenital heart disease: analysis of early outcome. Int J Cardiol. 2004;93:239–45.
12. Bertrand P, Navarro H, Caussade S, Holmgren N, Sánchez I. Airway anomalies in children with Down syndrome: endoscopic findings. Pediatr Pulmonol. 2003;36:137–41.
13. Healy F, Hanna BD, Zinman R. Pulmonary complications of congenital heart disease. Paediatr Respir Rev. 2012;13:10–5.
14. Kusak B, Cichocka-Jarosz E, Jedynak-Wasowicz U, Lis G. Types of laryngomalacia in children: interrelationship between clinical course and comorbid conditions. Eur Arch Otorhinolaryngol. 2017;274:1577–83.
15. Kussman BD, Geva T, Mcgowan FX. Cardiovascular causes of airway compression. Paediatr Anaesth. 2004;14:60–74.
16. Sebening C, Jakob H, Tochtermann U, et al. Vascular tracheobronchial compression syndromes—experience in surgical treatment and literature review. Thorac Cardiovasc Surg. 2000;48:164–74.
17. Fischer JE, Allen P, Fanconi S. Delay of extubation in neonates and children after cardiac surgery: impact of ventilator-associated pneumonia. Intensive Care Med. 2000;26:942–9.
18. Tan L, Sun X, Zhu X, Zhang Z, Li J, Shu Q. Epidemiology of nosocomial pneumonia in infants after cardiac surgery. Chest. 2004;125:410–7.
19. Verheugt CL, Uiterwaal CSPM, Van Der Velde ET, et al. Mortality in adult congenital heart disease. Eur Heart J. 2010;31:1220–9.
20. Pássaro L, Harbarth S, Landelle C. Prevention of hospital-acquired pneumonia in non-ventilated adult patients: a narrative review. Antimicrob Resist Infect Control. 2016;5:43.
21. Mok Q, Ross-Russell R, Mulvey D, Green M, Shinebourne E. Phrenic nerve injury in infants and children undergoing cardiac surgery. Br Heart J. 1991;65:287–92.
22. Joho-Arreola A, Bauersfeld U, Stauffer U, Baenziger O, Bernet V. Incidence and treatment of diaphragmatic paralysis after cardiac surgery in children. Eur J Cardiothorac Surg. 2005;27:53–7.

23. Berend N, Marlin G. Arrest of alveolar multiplication in kyphoscoliosis. Pathology. 1979;11:485–91.
24. Weber B, Smith J, Briscoe W, Friedman S, King T. Pulmonary function in asymptomatic adolescents with idiopathic scoliosis. Am Rev Respir Dis. 1975;111:389–97.
25. Day G, Upadhyay S, Ho E, Leong J, Ip M. Pulmonary functions in congenital scoliosis. Spine. 1994;19:1027–31.
26. Jones R, Kennedy J, Hasham F, Owen R, Taylor J. Mechanical inefficiency of the thoracic cage in scoliosis. Thorax. 1981;36:456–61.
27. Redding G, Song K, Inscore S, Effmann E, Campbell R. Lung function asymmetry in children with congenital and infantile scoliosis. Spine J. 2008;8:639–44.
28. Lowe K, Alvarez DF, King JA, Stevens T. Perivascular fluid cuffs decrease lung compliance by increasing tissue resistance. Crit Care Med. 2010;38:1458–66.
29. Remetz M, Cleman M, Cabin H. Pulmonary and pleural complications of cardiac disease. Clin Chest Med. 1989;10:545–92.
30. Chenoweth D, Cooper S, Hugli T, Stewart R, Blackstone E, Kirklin J. Complement activation during cardiopulmonary bypass: evidence for generation of C3a and C5a anaphylatoxins. N Engl J Med. 1981;304:497–503.
31. Kalfin R, Engelman R, Rousou J, et al. Induction of interleukin-8 expression during cardiopulmonary bypass. Circulation. 1993;88:II401–6.
32. Ng C, Wan S, Yim A, Arifi A. Pulmonary dysfunction after cardiac surgery. Chest. 2002;121:1269–77.
33. Groeneveld aBJ, Jansen EK, Verheij J. Mechanisms of pulmonary dysfunction after on-pump and off-pump cardiac surgery: a prospective cohort study. J Cardiothorac Surg. 2007;2:11.
34. Jansen P, te Velthuis H, Wildevuur W, et al. Cardiopulmonary bypass with modified fluid gelatin and heparin-coated circuits. Br J Anaesth. 1996;76:13–9.
35. Herold SE, Young TW, Ge D, Snieder H, Lovrekovic GZ. Sleep disordered breathing in pediatric patients with tetralogy of Fallot. Pediatr Cardiol. 2006;27:243–9.
36. Cotts T, Smith KR, Lu J, Dorfman AL, Norris MD. Risk for sleep-disordered breathing in adults after atrial switch repairs for d-looped transposition of the great arteries. Pediatr Cardiol. 2014;35:888–92.
37. Miles S, Ahmad W, Bailey A, Hatton R, Boyle A, Collins N. Sleep-disordered breathing in patients with pulmonary valve incompetence complicating congenital heart disease. Congenit Heart Dis. 2016;11:678–82.
38. Fan Z, Ahn M, Roth HL, Li L, Vaughn BV. Sleep apnea and hypoventilation in patients with down syndrome: analysis of 144 polysomnogram studies. Children (Basel). 2017;4:55.
39. Lanfranchi PA, Somers VK, Braghiroli A, Corra U, Eleuteri E, Giannuzzi P. Central sleep apnea in left ventricular dysfunction: prevalence and implications for arrhythmic risk. Circulation. 2003;107:727–32.
40. Javaheri S, Parker TJ, Wexler L, et al. Occult sleep-disordered breathing in stable congestive heart failure. Ann Intern Med. 1995;122:487–92.
41. Legault S, Lanfranchi P, Montplaisir J, et al. Nocturnal breathing in cyanotic congenital heart disease. Int J Cardiol. 2008;128:197–200.
42. Fredriksen PM, Therrien J, Veldtman G, et al. Lung function and aerobic capacity in adult patients following modified Fontan procedure. Heart. 2001;85:295–9.
43. Muneuchi J, Joo K, Yamamura K, et al. Exertional oscillatory ventilation during cardiopulmonary exercise test in fontan patients with total cavopulmonary connection. Pediatr Cardiol. 2009;30:452–7.
44. Dimopoulos K, Giannakoulas G, Wort SJ, Gatzoulis MA. Pulmonary arterial hypertension in adults with congenital heart disease: distinct differences from other causes of pulmonary arterial hypertension and management implications. Curr Opin Cardiol. 2008;23:545–54.
45. Engelfriet PM, Duffels MGJ, Möller T, et al. Pulmonary arterial hypertension in adults born with a heart septal defect: the Euro Heart Survey on adult congenital heart disease. Heart. 2007;93:682–7.

46. Rosenthal D, Friedman A, Kleinman C, Kopf G, Rosenfeld L, Hellenbrand W. Thromboembolic complications after Fontan operations. Circulation. 1995;92:287–93.
47. d'Udekem Y, Iyengar AJ, Galati JC, et al. Redefining expectations of long-term survival after the Fontan procedure: twenty-five years of follow-up from the entire population of Australia and New Zealand. Circulation. 2014;130:S32–S8.
48. Rubin BK. Plastic bronchitis. Clin Chest Med. 2016;37:405–8.
49. Redington A. Intensive care in the adult with congenital heart disease. Pediatr Crit Care Med. 2016;17:S377–S82.
50. Dimopoulos K, Diller G-P, Koltsida E, et al. Prevalence, predictors, and prognostic value of renal dysfunction in adults with congenital heart disease. Circulation. 2008;117:2320–8.
51. Price S, Jaggar SI, Jordan S, et al. Adult congenital heart disease: intensive care management and outcome prediction. Intensive Care Med. 2007;33:652–9.
52. Bhatt AB, Rajabali A, He W, Benavidez OJ. High resource use among adult congenital heart surgery admissions in adult hospitals: risk factors and association with death and comorbidities. Congenit Heart Dis. 2015;10:13–20.
53. Allan CK. Intensive care of the adult patient with congenital heart disease. Prog Cardiovasc Dis. 2011;53:274–80.
54. Martínez-Quintana E, Rodríguez-González F, Fábregas-Brouard M, Nieto-Lago V. Serum and 24-hour urine analysis in adult cyanotic and noncyanotic congenital heart disease patients. Congenit Heart Dis. 2009;4:147–52.
55. Kwiatkowski D, Price E, Axelrod D, et al. Incidence, risk factors, and outcomes of acute kidney injury in adults undergoing surgery for congenital heart disease. Cardiol Young. 2017;27:1068–75.
56. Nasr VG, Faraoni D, Valente AM, DiNardo JA. Outcomes and costs of cardiac surgery in adults with congenital heart disease. Pediatr Cardiol. 2017;38:1359.
57. Cedars A, Benjamin L, Burns S, Novak E, Amin A. Clinical predictors of length of stay in adults with congenital heart disease. Heart. 2017;103:1258–63.
58. Welke KF, Dearani JA, Ghanayem NS, Beland MJ, Shen I, Ebels T. Renal complications associated with the treatment of patients with congenital cardiac disease: consensus definitions from the Multi-Societal Database Committee for Pediatric and Congenital Heart Disease. Cardiol Young. 2008;18:222–5.
59. Shekerdemian LS, Bush A, Shore DF, Lincoln C, Redington AN. Cardiopulmonary interactions after Fontan operations: augmentation of cardiac output using negative pressure ventilation. Circulation. 1997;96:3934–42.
60. Malbrain MLNG, Cheatham ML, Kirkpatrick A, et al. Results from the international conference of experts on intra-abdominal hypertension and abdominal compartment syndrome. I. Definitions. Intensive Care Med. 2006;32:1722–32.
61. Williams D, Kiernan P, Metke M, Marsh H, Danielson GK. Hemodynamic response to positive end-expiratory pressure following right atrium-pulmonary artery bypass (Fontan procedure). J Thorac Cardiovasc Surg. 1984;87:856–61.
62. Cheatham ML, Malbrain MLNG, Kirkpatrick A, et al. Results from the international conference of experts on intra-abdominal hypertension and abdominal compartment syndrome. II. Recommendations. Intensive Care Med. 2007;33:951–62.
63. Landoni G, Biondi-Zoccai GGL, Marino G, et al. Fenoldopam reduces the need for renal replacement therapy and in-hospital death in cardiovascular surgery: a meta-analysis. J Cardiothorac Vasc Anesth. 2008;22:27–33.
64. Stone GW, McCullough PA, Tumlin JA, et al. Fenoldopam mesylate for the prevention of contrast-induced nephropathy. J Am Med Assoc. 2003;290:2284–91.
65. Brown JR, Block CA, Malenka DJ, O'Connor GT, Schoolwerth AC, Thompson CA. Sodium bicarbonate plus N-acetylcysteine prophylaxis. A meta-analysis. J Am Coll Cardiol Intv. 2009;2:1116–24.
66. Briguori C, Airoldi F, D'Andrea D, et al. Renal insufficiency following contrast media administration trial (REMEDIAL): a randomized comparison of 3 preventive strategies. Circulation. 2007;115:1211–7.

67. Morsheimer MM, Rychik J, Forbes L, et al. Risk factors and clinical significance of lymphopenia in survivors of the Fontan procedure for single-ventricle congenital cardiac disease. J Allergy Clin Immunol Pract. 2016;4:491–6.
68. Eysteinsdottir JH, Freysdottir J, Haraldsson A, et al. The influence of partial or total thymectomy during open heart surgery in infants on the immune function later in life. Clin Exp Immunol. 2004;136:349–55.
69. Tillipman Ladinsky H, Gillispie M, Sriaroon P, Leiding JW. Thoracic duct injury resulting in abnormal newborn screen. J Allergy Clin Immunol Pract. 2013;1:583–8.
70. Dori Y, Keller MS, Fogel MA, et al. MRI of lymphatic abnormalities after functional single-ventricle palliation surgery. Am J Roentgenol. 2014;203:426–31.
71. Lenz D, Hambsch J, Schneider P, Tárnok A. Protein-losing enteropathy after fontan surgery: is assessment of risk patients with immunological data possible? Cytometry B Clin Cytom. 2003;53:34–9.
72. Magdo HS, Stillwell TL, Greenhawt MJ, et al. Immune abnormalities in Fontan protein-losing enteropathy: a case-control study. J Pediatr. 2015;167:331–7.
73. Baumgartner H, Bonhoeffer P, De Groot NMS, et al. ESC guidelines for the management of grown-up congenital heart disease (new version 2010). Eur Heart J. 2010;31: 2915–57.
74. Verheugt CL, Uiterwaal CSPM, Van Der Velde ET, et al. Turning 18 with congenital heart disease: prediction of infective endocarditis based on a large population. Eur Heart J. 2011;32:1926–34.
75. Tutarel O, Alonso-Gonzalez R, Montanaro C, et al. Infective endocarditis in adults with congenital heart disease remains a lethal disease. Heart. 2018;104:161–5.
76. Niwa K, Nakazawa M, Tateno S, Yoshinaga M, Terai M. Infective endocarditis in congenital heart disease: Japanese national collaboration study. Heart. 2005;91:795–800.
77. Pizzi MN, Dos-Subirà L, Roque A, et al. 18 F-FDG-PET/CT angiography in the diagnosis of infective endocarditis and cardiac device infection in adult patients with congenital heart disease and prosthetic material. Int J Cardiol. 2017;248:396–402.
78. Engelfriet P, Boersma E, Oechslin E, et al. The spectrum of adult congenital heart disease in Europe: morbidity and mortality in a 5 year follow-up period—the Euro Heart Survey on adult congenital heart disease. Eur Heart J. 2005;26:2325–33.
79. Knirsch W, Haas NA, Uhlemann F, Dietz K, Lange PE. Clinical course and complications of infective endocarditis in patients growing up with congenital heart disease. Int J Cardiol. 2005;101:285–91.
80. Vogt M, Lang T, Frösner G, et al. Prevalence and clinical outcome of hepatitis C infection in children who underwent cardiac surgery before the implementation of blood-donor screening. N Engl J Med. 1999;341:866–70.
81. Wang A, Book WM, McConnell M, Lyle T, Rodby K, Mahle WT. Prevalence of hepatitis C infection in adult patients who underwent congenital heart surgery prior to screening in 1992. Am J Cardiol. 2007;100:1307–9.
82. Vogt M, Mühlbauer F, Braun SL, et al. Prevalence and risk factors of hepatitis C infection after cardiac surgery in childhood before and after blood donor screening. Infection. 2004;32:134–7.
83. Cox DA, Ginde S, Tweddell JS, Earing MG. Outcomes of a hepatitis C screening protocol in at-risk adults with prior cardiac surgery. World J Pediatr Congenit Heart Surg. 2014;5:503–6.
84. Alderden J, Rondinelli J, Pepper G, Cummins M, Whitney J. Risk factors for pressure injuries among critical care patients: a systematic review. Int J Nurs Stud. 2017;71:97–114.
85. Goldberg DJ, Dodds K, Avitabile CM, et al. Children with protein-losing enteropathy after the Fontan operation are at risk for abnormal bone mineral density. Pediatr Cardiol. 2012;33:1264–8.
86. Madsen NL, Marino BS, Woo JG, et al. Congenital heart disease with and without cyanotic potential and the long-term risk of diabetes mellitus: a population-based follow-up study. J Am Heart Assoc. 2016;5:e003076.

87. Umpierrez G, Cardona S, Pasquel F, et al. Randomized controlled trial of intensive versus conservative glucose control in patients undergoing coronary artery bypass graft surgery: GLUCO-CABG trial. Diabetes Care. 2015;38:1665–72.
88. Fazio S, Palmieri EA, Lombardi G, Biondi B. Effects of thyroid hormone on the cardiovascular system. Recent Prog Horm Res. 2004;59:31–50.
89. Ladenson PW, Levin AA, Ridgway EC, Daniels GH. Complications of surgery in hypothyroid patients. Am J Med. 1984;77:261–6.
90. Bennett-Guerrero E, Kramer DC, Schwinn DA. Effect of chronic and acute thyroid hormone reduction on perioperative outcome. Anesth Analg. 1997;85:30–6.
91. Palace MR. Perioperative management of thyroid dysfunction. Health Serv Insights. 2017;10:1178632916689677.
92. Deen JF, Krieger EV, Slee AE, et al. Metabolic syndrome in adults with congenital heart disease. J Am Heart Assoc. 2016;5:e001132.
93. Tzimas P, Petrou A, Laou E, Milionis H, Mikhailidis DP, Papadopoulos G. Impact of metabolic syndrome in surgical patients: should we bother?: table 1. Br J Anaesth. 2015;115:194–202.
94. Lerman JB, Parness IA, Shenoy RU. Body weights in adults with congenital heart disease and the obesity frequency. Am J Cardiol. 2017;119:638–42.
95. Brida M, Dimopoulos K, Kempny A, et al. Body mass index in adult congenital heart disease. Heart. 2017;103:1250–7.
96. Bajwa SJS, Sehgal V, Bajwa SK. Clinical and critical care concerns in severely ill obese patient. Indian J Endocrinol Metab. 2012;16:740–8.
97. Shashaty MGS, Stapleton RD. Physiological and management implications of obesity in critical illness. Ann Am Thorac Soc. 2014;11:1286–97.
98. Hanley MJ, Abernethy DR, Greenblatt DJ. Effect of obesity on the pharmacokinetics of drugs in humans. Clin Pharmacokinet. 2010;49:71–87.
99. Pelosi P, Croci M, Ravagnan I, Vicardi P, Gattinoni L. Total respiratory system, lung, and chest wall mechanics in sedated-paralyzed postoperative morbidly obese patients. Chest. 1996;109:144–51.
100. Tomkiewicz-Pajak L, Hoffman P, Trojnarska O, Lipczynska M, Podolec P, Undas A. Abnormalities in blood coagulation, fibrinolysis, and platelet activation in adult patients after the Fontan procedure. J Thorac Cardiovasc Surg. 2014;147:1284–90.
101. Takeuchi D, Inai K, Shinohara T, Nakanishi T, Park IS. Blood coagulation abnormalities and the usefulness of D-dimer level for detecting intracardiac thrombosis in adult Fontan patients. Int J Cardiol. 2016;224:139–44.
102. Sandler KL, Markham LW, Mah ML, Byrum EP, Williams JR. Optimizing CT angiography in patients with Fontan physiology: single-center experience of dual-site power injection. Clin Radiol. 2014;69:e562–7.
103. Broberg CS, Jayaweera AR, Diller GP, et al. Seeking optimal relation between oxygen saturation and hemoglobin concentration in adults with cyanosis from congenital heart disease. Am J Cardiol. 2011;107:595–9.
104. Oechslin E, Mebus S, Schulze-Neick I, et al. The adult patient with Eisenmenger syndrome: a medical update after dana point part III: specific management and surgical aspects. Curr Cardiol Rev. 2010;6:363–72.
105. Wu FM, Ukomadu C, Odze RD, Valente AM, Mayer JE Jr, Earing MG. Liver disease in the patient with Fontan circulation. Congenit Heart Dis. 2011;6:190–201.
106. Wijdicks EF. Hepatic encephalopathy. N Engl J Med. 2016;375:1660–70.
107. Vilstrup H, Amodio P, Bajaj J, et al. Hepatic encephalopathy in chronic liver disease: 2014 practice guideline by the American Association for the Study of Liver Diseases and the European Association for the Study of the Liver. Hepatology. 2014;60:715–35.
108. Mouri S, Tripon S, Rudler M, et al. FOUR score, a reliable score for assessing overt hepatic encephalopathy in cirrhotic patients. Neurocrit Care. 2015;22:251–7.
109. Jensen AS, Idorn L, Thomsen C, et al. Prevalence of cerebral and pulmonary thrombosis in patients with cyanotic congenital heart disease. Heart. 2015;101:1540–6.

110. Puri R, Auffret V, Rodés-Cabau J. Bioprosthetic valve thrombosis. J Am Coll Cardiol. 2017;69:2193–211.
111. Arrich J, Holzer M, Havel C, Warenits AM, Herkner H. Pre-hospital versus in-hospital initiation of cooling for survival and neuroprotection after out-of-hospital cardiac arrest. Cochrane Database Syst Rev. 2016;3:CD010570.
112. Chan PS, Berg RA, Tang Y, Curtis LH, Spertus JA. Association between therapeutic hypothermia and survival after in-hospital cardiac arrest. JAMA. 2016;316:1375.
113. Moler FW, Silverstein FS, Holubkov R, et al. Therapeutic hypothermia after in-hospital cardiac arrest in children. N Engl J Med. 2017;376:318–29.
114. Callaway CW, Donnino MW, Fink EL, et al. Part 8: post-cardiac arrest care: 2015 American Heart Association guidelines update for cardiopulmonary resuscitation and emergency cardiovascular care. Circulation. 2015;132:S465–82.
115. Kowalski M, Udy AA, McRobbie HJ, Dooley MJ. Nicotine replacement therapy for agitation and delirium management in the intensive care unit: a systematic review of the literature. J Intensive Care. 2016;4:69.
116. Schuckit MA. Recognition and management of withdrawal delirium (delirium tremens). N Engl J Med. 2014;371:2109–13.
117. Moons P, Kovacs AH, Luyckx K, et al. Patient-reported outcomes in adults with congenital heart disease: inter-country variation, standard of living and healthcare system factors. Int J Cardiol. 2018;251:34–41.
118. Ghoneim MM, O'Hara MW. Depression and postoperative complications: an overview. BMC Surg. 2016;16:5.
119. Morone NE, Weiner DK, Herbeck Belnap B, et al. The impact of pain and depression on recovery after coronary artery bypass grafting. Psychosom Med. 2010;72:620–5.
120. Auerbach AD, Vittinghoff E, Maselli J, Pekow PS, Young JQ, Lindenauer PK. Perioperative use of selective serotonin reuptake inhibitors and risks for adverse outcomes of surgery. JAMA Intern Med. 2013;173:1075–81.
121. Xiong GL, Jiang W, Clare RM, et al. Safety of selective serotonin reuptake inhibitor use prior to coronary artery bypass grafting. Clin Cardiol. 2010;33:E94–8.

Critical Care Nursing of the Adult with Congenital Heart Disease

23

Christine Peyton, Deborah Bedard, Meghan Williams, and Molly Wallrich

23.1 Introduction

Congenital heart defects (CHD) affect about 1% or 40,000 births per year making CHD the most common type of birth defect in the USA [1]. Children born with a CHD are living longer and surviving into adulthood due to the advancements in cardiac medicine and the evolution of cardiac surgery. Given the complexities of these patients, they require lifelong follow-up, and controversy exists as to whether the adult congenital patient should be cared for in pediatric hospital setting or in adult hospital setting [2]. Currently, the most common model used in large cardiac centers is for the ACHD patients to be treated at a children's hospital. In-hospital death rates are lower for adults with congenital heart disease when surgery is performed by a pediatric congenital heart surgeon [3]. Furthermore, in-hospital mortality for adults with congenital heart disease is reported at its lowest when their operations are performed in a children's hospital and by a congenital heart surgeon [4]. Despite the controversy, the postoperative adult patient with congenital heart disease should be cared for in an intensive care environment where the staff is adequately trained in the care and hemodynamic management of adults with congenital heart disease.

With the nearly 1.4 million adults now living with congenital heart disease in the USA [5], pediatric cardiology has seen an evolution of a new subspecialty to care for these patients as they age. ACHD specialists are tasked with challenges never before seen in this population. Additional challenges exist when adult patients are admitted to a pediatric cardiac intensive care unit (CICU). There are differences in management of the adult patient as compared to the pediatric patient related to fluid administration, medication dosing, developmental needs, comorbidities, and

C. Peyton (✉) · D. Bedard · M. Williams · M. Wallrich
Department of Pediatrics, The Heart Institute, Children's Hospital Colorado, Aurora, CO, USA
e-mail: Christine.peyton@childrenscolorado.org

E. da Cruz et al. (eds.), *Intensive Care of the Adult with Congenital Heart Disease*, Congenital Heart Disease in Adolescents and Adults,
https://doi.org/10.1007/978-3-319-94171-4_23

coordination of care [1]. Consideration of these differences can make the pediatric nurse uncomfortable. Conversely, the adult critical care nurse and adult cardiac surgeons who do not have further specialization with the complexities of congenital heart disease can feel uncomfortable as well when dealing with these patients. Care of the adult congenital patient in any setting requires that the nursing staff is trained to adequately care for the adult patient as well as the congenital heart disease, with a goal to improve outcomes through evidenced-based care.

23.2 Perioperative Preparation for the ACHD Patient

Adult congenital patients undergoing surgical repair have either been operated in early childhood or may be newly diagnosed with a congenital heart defect. A comprehensive physical, psychosocial, and financial history of the patient should be performed prior to admission to the intensive care unit following a surgical repair or interventional procedure or for medical reasons. Nurses need to be aware that the two most common perioperative complications for ACHD patients are heart failure and atrial dysrhythmias [6]. Etiology of heart failure for these patients is either systolic dysfunction from primary pump failure, diastolic dysfunction from hypertrophy, or a combination of both. Patients who present with a pressure-loaded systemic right ventricle or a functional single ventricle are at the highest risk for heart failure. Right heart failure can also be found in patients with Ebstein's anomaly of the tricuspid valve and tetralogy of Fallot (TOF) with corrective repair but varying degrees of pulmonary insufficiency [6]. Left heart failure can result from chronic aortic and mitral insufficiency. Nursing assessment should consider changes in lung and heart auscultation findings, blood pressure measurements, or worsening signs of heart failure.

Atrial arrhythmias are the most common dysrhythmia in ACHD patients. Atrial fibrillation, atrial flutter, and atrial tachycardia are the most common among these. Atrial arrhythmias may be notoriously resistant to antiarrhythmic pharmacological therapy and can be associated with rapid hemodynamic deterioration [7, 8]. The onset of arrhythmias may be a signal of hemodynamic decompensation; therefore ACHD patients should have a preoperative assessment of arrhythmia risk, as anticipation matters. All ACHD patients should be monitored with pulse oximetry along with obtaining an electrocardiogram (ECG). The nurse should be aware of diagnostic tests such as Holter monitoring, event recorders, and electrophysiology testing that have been performed to determine arrhythmia risk prior to surgical repair or cardiac intervention. A full diagnostic work-up of arrhythmias allows the nurse to be prepared for optimal pacing strategies with a temporary pacemaker or medical management in the postoperative period.

23.3 Diagnostic Testing

The critical care nurse should be familiar with both invasive and noninvasive diagnostic testing for the ACHD patient, as diagnostic tools will help determine timing and planning of surgery or intervention. A preoperative echocardiography is helpful to determining the following: cardiac anatomy, morphology of cardiac chambers, ventricular function, function of heart valves, estimation of pulmonary pressures, and evaluation of shunt lesions. Other essential noninvasive diagnostic tests to evaluate anatomy and physiology of congenital heart defects are cardiovascular magnetic resonance (CMR) and computed tomography (CT). CMR is helpful for evaluating volumetric measurements, assessment of the great vessels, and detection of myocardial fibrosis [9]. CT imaging is useful to evaluate the coronary arteries, any existing collateral arteries, and parenchymal lung disease [9]. Cardiac catheterization may be necessary in some patients to confirm anatomy and physiology of CHD when noninvasive tests are inconclusive. Pulmonary vascular resistance (PVR), LV and RV diastolic function, pressure gradients, and shunt quantification can be obtained during cardiac catheterization. The degree of pulmonary hypertension can be determined as well, which can allow the nurse to prepare for medical management of pulmonary hypertension in the postoperative period.

23.4 Neurodevelopmental and Psychosocial Issues

One of the largest areas currently being studied in CHD patients is neurodevelopment and quality of life issues. Developmental needs in this group of patients stretch beyond finishing high school, making friends, and playing sports. ACHD patients are thriving, maintaining employment, having families, and leading normal lives. Fifty percent of patients with congenital heart disease meet diagnostic criteria for at least one lifetime mood or anxiety disorder [10]. Surgery, hospital admission, invasive medical procedures, and even routine appointments may trigger emotional distress, especially in individuals with a pre-existing emotional disorder. The type of congenital defect and intervention that has been done is important in determining factors that can impact psychosocial issues for ACHD patients. ACHD patients that have cyanosis from an uncorrected repair, undergone cardiopulmonary bypass, and have genetic or chromosomal syndromes may account for neurologic motor and developmental deficits [11]. The nurse's psychosocial assessment should include screening for negative body image due to surgical scars, clubbing of digits from cyanotic heart disease, or short stature from failure to thrive as an infant or child. Adult Fontan patients are more at risk of abnormal growth parameters due to gastrointestinal malabsorption syndrome related to chronically elevated central venous pressures, protein losing enteropathy and low cardiac output [12]. Adults with complex congenital conditions should be considered as well for abnormal growth parameters. Patients may have dysmorphic facial features from genetic or chromosomal syndromes [11].

Screening tools for substance abuse should be completed by the nurse for alcohol, tobacco, recreational drugs, and chronic opioid use. Perceptions of pain and history of chronic pain are vital data to elaborate a successful pain management plan in the postoperative period. ACHD patients undergoing open heart surgery are more likely to experience stress, feelings of fear, anxiety, uncertainty, loss of control, and other emotional problems [13]. The critical care nurse needs to assess the patient to determine who has had previous experiences recovering from open heart surgery as a pediatric patient versus an adult patient who may be experiencing recovery in the

CICU for the first time. ACHD patients that have been newly diagnosed may have no prior exposure to the hospital environment or understand the progression of being critically ill to discharging back to home. Multiple studies have demonstrated that the psychological stress an ACHD patient experiences can impact recovery [14–17].

Women with complex congenital heart disease are having children of their own. One unique consideration in this population is whether the ACHD patient is a parent and the impact of hospitalization on family dynamics. Many ICUs have strict visitation policies for children. It is imperative that attention is brought to the patient's need to see their family and children. Patient satisfaction has been shown to be higher when an ACHD patient can meet with an adult congenital nurse to counsel and provide information to the patient prior to surgical repair [14]. Financial concerns and lack of appropriate health insurance may be additional stressors for the patient and family. ACHD patients who have been admitted urgently to the CICU may be burdened by financial concerns or lack of appropriate health insurance.

Education level also needs to be assessed as many ACHD patients may have had extended hospitalizations as a child and/or have neurodevelopmental disturbances that may have interfered with completing secondary education. Learning readiness assessment is necessary for all ACHD patients to determine the appropriate education techniques to promote success upon discharge to home. ACHD patients are more likely to continue dependent lifestyles compared to their healthy peers, which can allow their parents to heavily influence their health-care decisions [18]. Previous studies have revealed that young adults lack knowledge about which type of cardiac defect they have, its treatment, risk of complications, and the importance of continued medical follow-up [19]. Years of hypervigilant behavior by parents can lead to inhibiting the patient's ability to mature and promote independent decision-making. Parents have often been the primary decision-makers and have difficulty relinquishing care, even as patients become adults. Patients may experience despair due to their awareness of residual morbidities and the knowledge of possible or probable early mortality or limitations in their social lives and educational or occupational attainment [20]. These patients should be screened for depression and social isolation as these issues can extend hospitalization.

Every patient 18 years of age and older should be asked about an advanced directive prior to admission to the hospital for surgical repair or cardiac intervention. The advance directive should be part of the medical record and easy to access for all staff. Nursing staff need to be aware of the patient's desire to have artificial life-sustaining therapies and if a do not resuscitate (DNR) order needs to be obtained. Most adult and children's hospitals have palliative care and social work teams that can assist the medical and nursing team with these discussions if they have not occurred with the ACHD patient. It is also important to identify if the ACHD patient with developmental delays can make decisions or if a parent/guardian is making health-care decisions via health-care proxy.

23.5 Postoperative Care of the ACHD Patient

When the ACHD patient is admitted to a pediatric CICU postsurgery, there are many considerations that need to occur for the pediatric nurse. Standard dosing for medications versus weight-based medication dosing in the pediatric patient as well as standard output measurements in the adult patient may not be well known. There are also considerations for standardly used medications in the adult population that are not FDA approved in pediatrics. Some examples include pain and anticoagulation medications [1].

Although critical care nurses should always have an understanding of a patient's condition prior to entering the operating room, the ACHD patient poses a unique challenge. Pediatric nurses may not be familiar with the implications of the multiple comorbidities ACHD patients are at risk for and how they relate to their postoperative care. Furthermore, pediatric nurses report discomfort with the monitoring and interventions required as a result of the adult comorbidities [1]. Common comorbidities include renal failure, hepatic failure, gastrointestinal complications, Eisenmenger's syndrome, pulmonary hypertension, heart failure, endocarditis, diabetes, thromboembolism, arrhythmias, chronic pain, and substance abuse.

23.6 Hemodynamic Monitoring

Management of hemodynamic status of the ACHD patient in the intensive care unit and most importantly in the early postoperative period is critical. Management strategies to optimize preload, afterload, and contractility are important to maintain hemodynamic stability with an overarching goal of providing adequate oxygen delivery and maintaining adequate organ perfusion [21]. Routine monitoring for these patients includes continuous ECG monitoring on a cardiorespiratory monitor, continuous pulse oximetry, continuous arterial blood pressure monitoring, as well as continuous central venous pressure (CVP) monitoring. More invasive monitoring includes a pulmonary artery catheter. Continuous monitoring of the pulmonary artery pressure can be important in the adult congenital population as the development of pulmonary artery hypertension can be contributory of congenital heart disease [22]. However, continuous pulmonary artery catheters have been shown to increase morbidity in adult patients without showing a contribution to improved clinical outcome [6]. Hemodynamic monitoring with pulmonary artery catheters may not be possible in this population due to the heart anatomy and pathophysiology or to the presence of intracardiac shunts [6].

Prompt recognition and treatment of hemodynamic instability of the ACHD patient in the ICU is critical. There are many nursing considerations, and as the complexity of the patient increases, they can become more difficult to manage. This is true of the ACHD patient with complex congenital heart disease and multiple comorbidities. Changes in cardiac output directly affect delivery of oxygen. Low cardiac output interventions should include the assessment of heart rate and stroke volume, which includes rhythm, preload, afterload, and contractility. Other data to assess for good perfusion include warm extremities, good pulses, adequate urine output, acid-base balance, and, more objectively, lactate analysis. Concurrent assessment of all variables is necessary [21].

Central venous catheters are a necessary requirement for not only hemodynamic monitoring but for blood sampling and medication infusions. Central venous catheters offer more stable access for continuous vasoactive infusions that are critical to the hemodynamic stability of the patient. The central venous catheter is not, however, without its risks. It is estimated that there are 41,000 central line-associated bloodstream infections that occur per year in hospitals in the USA [23]. With the added increase of morbidity and risks of mortality of central lines, nursing care for all patients in the ICU should include prevention of central line-associated bloodstream infections and quick removal of the line.

23.7 Fluid Resuscitation and Bleeding

Intravascular volume depletion is very common following cardiac surgery, and the need for aggressive fluid resuscitation may be required due to bleeding, third spacing from cardiopulmonary bypass inflammatory response, and increased preload reload requirements [21]. Fluid management in the adult is very different as compared to the pediatric patient, and pediatric nurses are often uncomfortable giving large volumes of fluid to their patient even when warranted. When giving fluids, special consideration should be given to the type of fluid infusing, how much, how fast, and the patient's hemodynamic response to the fluid, all of which varies from patient to patient [24].

Bleeding is another common complication post cardiac surgery with risk factors including age, gender (male predominant), complexity of surgery, emergent vs. elective surgery, presence of anemia preoperatively, long or multiple cardiopulmonary bypass time, suppressed cardiac function, low body mass, and surgeon-specific factors [21]. Excessive bleeding in the postoperative period requires prompt intervention from the nurse. It is important to manage the blood pressure. Higher blood pressures can actually increase bleeding. Therefore, it is prudent to provide interventions to decrease the patient's blood pressure. Continuous infusions of vasodilatory medications can be used to manage the blood pressure. In addition, close monitoring of hematocrit and coagulation laboratory values (i.e. PT, PTT, platelets, fibrinogen) can help the team determine if blood products need to be administered. Thromboelastograms (TEG) can be useful as well in the postoperative period. TEGs can more specifically identify what blood product the patient needs thereby decreasing the amount of bleeding and reducing unnecessary blood product administration [21, 25].

Management of chest tubes is important when the patient is bleeding. It is the nurse's responsibility to maintain patency of the chest tubes and keep track of the output. Determining excessive chest tube drainage for the adult patient is different than the pediatric patient. In pediatric settings, excessive bleeding is calculated in mL/kg/hour. In adult settings, excessive bleeding varies. The most common definition of excessive bleeding in the adult population is no more than 200 mL/h in the first hour or 1000 mL in the first 24 h [26]. It is important for the pediatric nurse to know and understand the difference.

In the presence of pulmonary edema, diuretics should be used carefully, and in Fontan-palliated patients whose pulmonary blood flow is dependent upon adequate preload, diuretics should be very carefully considered [6]. Nursing should be attentive to the patient's response to diuretics and monitor closely for decreased preload, particularly in the single ventricle patient for this reason.

23.8 Pulmonary Dysfunction

As discussed previously, ACHD patients with single ventricle physiology often present with failure of the systemic ventricle and subsequently are at incredible risk for pulmonary dysfunction. Of particular risk in ACHD patients are parenchymal insults from years of elevated left atrial pressures due to ventricular dysfunction, possible smoking, chest infections, and multiple sternotomies or thoracotomies. In the postoperative period, these risks may require higher mean airway and positive end-expiratory pressure (PEEP) to effectively ventilate. However, it must be understood that high PEEP can also be detrimental in the setting of RV failure and in patients with single ventricle physiology by decreasing preload. It is possible that the use of airway pressure release ventilation may be useful in ACHD patients, but it has not been studied [27].

Pulmonary hypertension in the adult patient is defined as pulmonary arterial pressure (PAP) >25 mm HG at rest with a normal pulmonary capillary wedge pressure (<15 mmHg). Cardiac or thoracic surgery, acute LV dysfunction, and ARDS are all causes of pulmonary hypertension. It is important for nurses to understand which ACHD patients are at risk for postoperative PHT based on their anatomy and physiology. Patients with lesions that increase pulmonary blood or obstruct pulmonary outflow are at risk along with those patients with systemic ventricular dysfunction, palliative aortopulmonary shunts, or residual PHT despite congenital correction of the defect. Patients who have Glenn or Fontan physiology require low PVR and must be managed accordingly in the postoperative period. Even a moderate increase in PVR or PAP can be critical for this physiology resulting in a low cardiac output state. Nurses play an essential role in the prevention of events that may trigger PHT during the postoperative period. Thorough assessment and evaluation of these patients is critical to early intervention and outcomes. Nurses must be aware of the fragility of these patients and have a healthy fear of an acute PHT "crisis" that can result in cardiovascular collapse and death. Hypoxia, acidosis, respiratory infections, and suctioning are all detrimental to outcomes and can be avoided or detected early with attentive nursing care. The overall goals of PHT care include lowering PAP, PVR, and RV afterload with pulmonary vasodilators such as oxygen and nitric oxide if necessary and maximizing RV function to improve cardiac output, which may include vasopressor and inotropic support. A CVP is useful in assessing volume status and RV function. A high CVP may indicate an acute rise in PA pressure. Jugular venous distention on assessment also indicates an elevated CVP and can reflect RV dysfunction. If a direct line in the left atrium is present, it is important to note that a low left atrial pressure (LAP) may indicate decreased pulmonary venous return, which indicates a PHT crisis and requires intervention. During a crisis, intervention focuses on elimination of the cause: pain (sedation/pain medications), hypoxia (oxygen administration) or acidosis (permissive hypocarbia) and treatments that promote pulmonary vasodilation and reduce PVR with pulmonary vasodilators such as nitric oxide and sildenafil. General nursing management to avoid PHT crisis includes hyper oxygenating prior to and during suctioning, adequate sedation and pain control with considerations for sedation prior to any noxious stimuli, avoiding hypoxia, ensuring adequate fluid balance through close monitoring of the CVP to optimize preload, close monitoring for arrhythmias that may compromise cardiac output, and utilizing low tidal volumes and PEEP on the ventilator. Additional therapies such as bosentan, an endothelin-receptor antagonist and sildenafil, a phosphodiesterase inhibitor are still being trialed for heart failure [6, 22].

23.9 Arrhythmia Management

Early recognition of tachycardia with a heart rate above 100 should raise suspicion for the intensive care nurse. A heart rate above 100 beats per minute for the ACHD patient potentially reflects an underlying sustained arrhythmia [6]. Supraventricular tachycardia (SVT) needs to be treated in the ACHD patient to prevent hemodynamic instability. Adult patients with SVT or atrial tachycardia also exhibit a fixed heart rate despite changes in fluid status, ventilatory management, or inotropic support. A CVP reading with cannon waves present may also indicate a tachyarrhythmia that requires treatment. A 12- or 15-lead ECG should be obtained by the nurse. When a bedside monitor or full ECG recording is still inconclusive, a simple method to diagnose atrial tachyarrhythmias is the use of temporary pacing wires to record an atrial ECG [6]. Rapid administration of adenosine can treat SVT or atrial tachycardia and facilitate a specific diagnosis. Adenosine can be administered through an intravenous line, but it must be followed by a rapid saline flush due to the short half-life of the drug. The nurse should perform a running ECG rhythm strip during adenosine administration, which assists with the diagnosis of SVT or atrial tachycardia. A defibrillator should be available at the bedside in the unlikely event that the patient converts to a lethal arrhythmia following adenosine administration.

Once the diagnosis of atrial tachycardia has been made and if the rate or cycle length of tachycardia is stable, it is most likely a reentry mechanism of atrial tachycardia [6]. The bedside nurse should prepare for overdrive pacing with pacing wires and a temporary pacemaker. The nurse in conjunction with a licensed provider should select rapid atrial pacing and attempt to adjust the rate at 20–30 beats per minute (bpm) faster than the atrial tachycardia. The patient should be on a continuous ECG and bedside monitor during overdrive pacing. The nurse needs to be familiar with temporary pacing procedures, as the atrial wires should only be capturing the atrium and not the ventricle. The nurse can test pacing at higher output at a rate just above the ventricular rate to determine that only the atrium is being paced prior to initiating rapid atrial pacing [6]. Atrial fibrillation can be a consequence of overdrive pacing. The nurse will need to recognize if sustained atrial fibrillation is causing hemodynamic instability. Synchronized cardioversion may need to be performed for hemodynamic instability from sustained atrial fibrillation, and therefore a defibrillator should be available when overdrive pacing is being attempted. The defibrillator should be set in synchronized shock, and initial shock delivered should be 100 joules [28]. Overdrive pacing succeeds in up to ¾ of cases of postoperative reentry atrial tachycardia, but it can occur immediately, so medical management should be considered [6].

Medical management of atrial tachycardia, such as atrial fibrillation, should focus on arrhythmia termination and not rate control, which is the goal of many adult cardiac units treating adults with atrial fibrillation [6]. Intravenous amiodarone can be administered to treat atrial tachycardias. It is preferable to administer amiodarone through a central line, but it can be administered through a peripheral intravenous line. A bolus of 300 mg over 30 min should be administered first followed by a continuous infusion of 50–100 mg/h [28]. Nursing considerations include incompatibility with many other intravenous drugs, and amiodarone does require special tubing to prevent the drug from being a plasticizer. Rapid push administration of amiodarone can induce lethal arrhythmias and possible cardiac arrest. Procainamide is another option for treating atrial tachycardias. An initial bolus dose of 7–10 mg/kg over 30–40 min followed by an intravenous infusion 40 mcg/kg/min [28]. Nursing considerations include obtaining serum procainamide and n-acetylprocainamide (NAPA) levels 4 h after start of intravenous administration [6]. NAPA is the hepatic metabolite of procainamide, so both levels should be monitored by the nurse.

Lethal arrhythmias can occur anytime in the postoperative period. A defibrillator should be available, and all nursing staff needs to be knowledgeable on how to operate the defibrillator. Furthermore, to improve outcomes for the ACHD patient that experiences cardiopulmonary arrest, all pediatric nurses need to be familiar with advanced cardiovascular life support (ACLS) protocols. Early recognition and intervention for shockable lethal arrhythmias is essential to outcomes.

23.10 Postoperative Glycemic Control

In contrast to care for the pediatric patient, moderately tight glycemic control is recommended for all adult patients intraoperatively and postoperatively. In the pediatric population, there is an increased risk of hypoglycemia with no significant evidence of decreasing infection, mortality, length of stay, or organ failure when keeping tight glycemic control. However, for the adult patient, increased glucose levels increase the risk of complications and death tenfold. Additionally, in the adult cardiac patient, utilizing insulin therapy to keep glucose levels below 180 mg/dL reduces the risk of deep sternal wound infections and sepsis, decreases length of stay, and enhances long-term survival [21]. Typical treatment includes insulin therapy for the first 12–24 h postoperatively with transition to subcutaneous insulin prior to discontinuation of the insulin infusion. It is essential for specific protocols and order sets to be in place to ensure effective management based on blood glucose evaluation [29], and special considerations should be given to patients with insulin resistance and diabetes to avoid hyperglycemia in addition to hypoglycemia [21].

23.11 Pain and Comfort

Adequate pain and sedation is an important variable in postoperative care for the adult congenital patient. Sedation should be minimized once the neuromuscular blockades from the operating room have worn off in attempts to extubate quickly, decrease delirium, and initiate ambulation and rehabilitation. Benzodiazepines should be used with caution in the ACHD patients due to risk of delirium; however, benzodiazepines are the drug of choice for patients experiencing alcohol withdrawal. Propofol is often used for sedation in conjunction with a narcotic agent, but dexmedetomidine may be a good substitute for both its analgesic and sedating effects. Nursing pain assessment should include an approved pain screening tool, individual pain goal, and screening for delirium. Adequate pain management enhances patient satisfaction while decreasing delirium and improving pulmonary function [21]. Patient-controlled analgesia (PCA) should be considered when extubation occurs with transition to an oral regimen once the patient can tolerate oral intake. In the early postoperative period, opioids delivered through a PCA provide better analgesia than conventional parenteral opioid regimens and also result in better patient satisfaction [30]. Nonsteroidal anti-inflammatory medications are used judiciously due to the risk of bleeding and delayed bone healing. Nonpharmacologic methodology should be used in conjunction with pharmacologic treatment [21].

Pain assessment should also include neuropathic and chronic pain especially if adult patients may not respond well to acute pain management with opioids. In assessing acute pain after surgery, acute neuropathic pain is often overlooked or its severity underestimated [30]. Neuropathic pain does not respond to many opioids or analgesics and requires specific therapeutic approaches [30]. Ketamine and gabapentin have a rapid onset and are preferred treatment options for ACHD patients experiencing neuropathic pain. Untreated neuropathic pain can lead to the development of chronic pain. Risk factors for development of chronic pain include severity of preoperative chronic pain, severity of postoperative acute pain, and intra-operative nerve injury. Chronic pain after surgical repair is becoming more prevalent and can lead to significant disability or impair the rehabilitation process.

23.12 Rehabilitation

Cardiac rehabilitation is one of the most important components of postoperative care to improve long-term outcomes and transition to home. It is important that nurses understand the implications for early rehabilitation and ambulation and advocate for early coordination of the multidisciplinary team, particularly if in a pediatric setting where resources and familiarity may vary. Patients with ventricular assist devices or undergoing extracorporeal membrane oxygenation (ECMO) can and should begin rehabilitation if stable. This early rehabilitation decreases risk of deconditioning and improves outcomes [1].

References

1. Kogon BE, Plattner C, Leong T, Kirshbom PM, Kanter KR, McConnell M, Book W, et al. Adult congenital heart surgery: adult or pediatric facility? Adult or pediatric surgeon? Ann Thorac Surg. 2009;87:833–40.
2. Karamlou T, Diggs BS, Person T, Ungerleider RM, Welke KF, et al. National practice patterns for management of adult congenital heart disease: operation by pediatric heart surgeons decreases in-hospital death. Circulation. 2008;118:2345–53.
3. Karamlou T, Diggs BS, Person T, Ungerleider RM, Welke KF, et al. Adults or big kids: what is the ideal clinical environment for management of grown-up patients with congenital heart disease? Ann Thorac Surg. 2010;90:573–9.
4. Centers for Disease Control and Prevention. 2016. https://www.cdc.gov/ncbddd/heartdefects/data.html. Accessed 8 July 2017.
5. Anton K. Challenges caring for adults with congenital heart disease in pediatric settings: how nurses can aid the transition. Crit Care Nurse. 2016;36:1–8.
6. Perry J, Lanzberg M, Franklin W, Webb G, Chang AC, et al. Cardiac intensive care of the adult with congenital heart disease: basic principles in the management of common problems. World J Pediatr Congenit Heart Surg. 2011;2:430–44. https://doi.org/10.1177/2150135111407936.
7. Kahairy P, Poirer N, Mercier LA. Univentricular heart. Circulation. 2007;115:800–12.
8. Kamphuis M, Ottenkamp J, Vliegen HW, et al. Health related quality of life and health status in adult survivors with previously operated complex congenital heart disease. Heart. 2002;87:356–62.
9. Baumgartner H, Bonhoeffer P, De Groot N, et al. ESC guidelines for the management of grown up congenital heart disease: the task force on the management of grown-up congenital heart disease of the European Society of Cardiology (ESC). Eur Heart J. 2010;31:2915–57.
10. Kovacs AH, Saidi AS, Kuhl EA, al e. Depression and anxiety in adult congenital heart disease: predictors and prevalence. Int J Cardiol. 2009;137:158–64.
11. Richards NM. Outcomes in special populations undergoing cardiac surgery: octogenarians, woman and adults with congenital heart disease. Crit Care Nurs Clin North Am. 2007;19:467–85.
12. Pike NA, Evangelist L, Doering LV, Koniak-Griffin D, Lewis AB, Child JS. Clinical profile of the adolescent/adult fontan survivor. Congenit Heart Dis. 2011;6:9–17.

13. Asiloglu K, Celik SS. The effect of preoperative education on anxiety of open cardiac surgery patients. Patient Educ Couns. 2004;53:65–70.
14. Schoormans D, Smets EM, Zwart R, Sprangers MG, et al. Peri-operative care in adults with congenital heart disease: room for improvement in after care. Cardiol Young. 2013;23:540–5.
15. Cserep Z, Balog P, Szekely J, et al. Psychosocial factors and major adverse cardiac and cerebrovascular events after cardiac surgery. Interact Cardiovasc Thorac Surg. 2010;11:567–72.
16. Contrada RJ, Goyal TM, Cather C, Rafalson L, Idler EL, Krause TJ. Psychosocial factors in outcomes of heart surgery: the impact of religious involvement and depressive symptoms. Health Psychol. 2004;23:227–38.
17. Mavros MN, Athanasiou S, Gkegkes ID, Polyzos KA, Peppas G, Falagas ME. Do psychological variables affect early surgical recovery? PLoS One. 2011;6:e20306.
18. Horner T, Liberthson R, Jelinek MS. Psychosocial profile of adults with complex congenital heart disease. Mayo Clin Proc. 2000;75(1):31–6.
19. Asp A, Bratt EL, Bramhagen AC. Transfer to adult care-experiences of young adults with congenital heart disease. J Pediatr Nurs. 2015;30:e3–e10.
20. Foster E, Graham T, Driscoll D, et al. Task force 2: special health care needs of adults with congenital heart disease. J Am Coll Cardiol. 2001;37:1176–83.
21. Stephens RS, Whitman GJR. Postoperative critical care of the adult cardiac surgical patient. Part I: routine postoperative care. Crit Care Med. 2015;43:1477–97.
22. Nieves J, Haynes A. Pulmonary hypertension in the adult with congenital heart disease. The Society of Pediatric Cardiovascular Nurse. October 2015. http://www.spcnonline.com/download/guidelines/adult_chd_care_problems/PulmonaryHypertensioninAdultswithCongenitalHeartDisease-Final2015.pdf. Accessed 10 June 2017.
23. Wallace MC, Macy DL. Reduction of central line-associated bloodstream infection rates in patients in the adult intensive care unit. J Infus Nurs. 2016;39:47–55.
24. Myburgh JA, Mythen MG. Resuscitation fluids. N Engl J Med. 2013;369:2462–3.
25. Yildirim F, Tuncer B, Ozbakkaloglu A, Kurda AT, Ozurk T, Iskesen I, et al. Thromboelastogram reduces blood use by inspecting coagulation in heart surgery. Asian Cardiovasc Thorac Ann. 2016;24:441–4.
26. Stephens RS, Whitman GJR. Postoperative critical care of the adult cardiac surgical patient. Part II: procedure specific considerations, management of complications, and quality improvement. Crit Care Med. 2015;43:1995–2014.
27. Redington A. Intensive care in the adult with congenital heart disease. Pediatr Crit Care Med. 2016;17:S377–82. https://doi.org/10.1097/pcc.0000000000000782.
28. American Heart Association. http://cpr.heart.org/AHAECC/CPRAndECC/Training/HealthcareProfessional/AdvancedCardiovascularLifeSupportACLS/UCM_473186_Advanced-Cardiovascular-Life-Support-ACLS.jsp. Accessed 11 July 2017.
29. Rummell M. Postoperative glycemic control in adults with CHD. The Society of Pediatric Cardiovascular Nurse. September 2015. http://www.spcnonline.com/download/guidelines/adult_chd_care_problems/PostoperativeGlycemic_Control-Final2015.pdf. Accessed 10 June 2017.
30. Schug SA, Plamer GM, Scott DA, Halliwell R, Trinca J, et al. Acute pain management scientific evidence, fourth edition, 2015. Med J Aust. 2016;204(8):315–7.

24 Nutrition of the Critically Ill Adult with Congenital Heart Disease and Nutritional Rehabilitation

Stephen J. Dolgner and Jason F. Deen

24.1 Introduction

Critically ill adults with congenital heart disease (ACHD) need meticulous nutritional management in attempts to attenuate the catabolic state inherent to an intensive care unit (ICU) stay. Catabolism and anorexia are common components of the physiologic response to critical illness and are common findings among ICU patients, even among patients with good baseline nutritional status. While ACHD patients may be admitted to an ICU for a variety of reasons, both related and unrelated to their heart disease, the most common indication is elective admission after scheduled cardiac surgery [1]. Therefore, avoiding the morbid complications commonly associated with malnutrition, such as poor wound healing, infections, and pneumonia, is paramount to decreasing mortality and ICU length of stay. Because of these issues, there has been interest in aggressive early nutrition to help combat skeletal muscle wasting and weakness associated with prolonged ICU stays. To pursue this, there have been multiple well-designed, randomized, controlled studies in general ICU populations over the last 10 years, some of which specifically evaluated cardiac surgery patients, though these are usually included as a subgroup analysis. While there is minimal directly applicable data for ACHD patients who are hospitalized in the ICU, effective methods to provide them proper nutrition to allow recovery from their critical illness are extrapolated from other subsets of patients as available. The following review will discuss optimal approaches to nutritional

S. J. Dolgner (✉) · J. F. Deen
Division of Cardiology, Seattle Children's Hospital, University of Washington, Seattle, WA, USA

Division of Cardiology, Department of Medicine, University of Washington Medical Center, Seattle, WA, USA
e-mail: Stephen.Dolgner@seattlechildrens.org

E. da Cruz et al. (eds.), *Intensive Care of the Adult with Congenital Heart Disease*, Congenital Heart Disease in Adolescents and Adults,
https://doi.org/10.1007/978-3-319-94171-4_24

management including nutritional assessment, timing and route of nutrient administration, and disease-specific recommendations.

24.2 Nutritional Assessment

Adults with congenital heart disease are at risk for nutritional deficits for a variety of reasons, some of which may be unique to the disease state. Depending on the specific criteria used to define it, malnutrition is estimated in 9–15% of typical adult patients undergoing non-congenital cardiac surgery [2–4]. Preoperative markers of malnutrition such as weight loss before surgery, low BMI, and low fat-free mass index should be assessed, because these factors have been associated with adverse outcomes after surgery including longer stays in the ICU and increased incidence of infections [3, 4]. There are multiple screening methods available to assess for undernutrition, including laboratory tests, measurement of body mass index (BMI), and simple surveys [5]. When this information is available, these factors can help identify patients who are particularly at risk for nutritional deficits after surgery, potentially leading to earlier nutritional intervention. However, all of these methods of assessment are fraught with confounding factors, making them difficult to apply broadly across a heterogeneous population.

Laboratory assessment of malnutrition involves assessment of a variety of hepatic proteins, such as albumin, prealbumin, and transferrin. Low albumin levels have been associated with increased mortality, length of stay, renal failure, bleeding, and need for prolonged ventilator support after cardiac surgery, and low prealbumin levels have also been associated with increased postoperative infections and a need for longer mechanical ventilation after cardiac surgery in a small study of 69 patients [2, 6]. There also appears to be a complex interaction between prealbumin level and the consequences of permissive underfeeding. In a recent post hoc analysis of the Permissive Underfeeding versus Target Enteral Feeding in Critically Ill Patients (PermiT) trial, the effect of permissive underfeeding varied by prealbumin level—those with a lower prealbumin had less 90-day mortality with permissive underfeeding when compared to standard feeding [7]. In spite of the association with outcomes as described above, it is worth to mention that many factors affect hepatic protein levels, and these are not always specific for malnutrition or a recent acute change in nutrition status. Similarly, there have not been large trials evaluating the impact of low preoperative albumin, specifically with regard to acting upon abnormal lab values, in this high-risk population.

Given the high incidence of obesity in the population as a whole, there have been several studies evaluating the role obesity plays in predicting outcomes, both for ACHD patients and for cardiac surgery patients overall. Brida and colleagues recently evaluated the association between BMI and mortality in ACHD patients and found that overweight and obese patients had increased survival in comparison with normal weight patients in both univariate and multivariate analysis, with the lowest mortality found at a BMI of 34.1 kg/m^2 [8]. Patients with complex congenital heart defects in that study were noted to have worse survival if they experienced weight loss during follow-up than if they had a stable weight or weight gain. In general cardiac surgery patients, BMI < 20 kg/m^2 has been independently associated with increased mortality after cardiopulmonary bypass [2]. Additionally, in a different series, BMI < 24 kg/m^2 was associated with worse 10-year survival after adult cardiac valvar surgery when compared to either BMI 25–35 kg/m^2 or BMI >35 kg/m^2 (53.5% survival vs. 63.4% and 62.2%, respectively, $p < 0.001$) [9]. A recent large retrospective analysis of >400,000 adult cardiac surgery patients confirmed this paradoxical association with BMI and mortality after cardiac surgery, with the highest incident mortality of 8.5% in patients with a BMI <18.5 kg/m^2, a mortality rate of 4.4% in normal weight patients, and an incident mortality of 2.7–3.7% seen in overweight and obese patients [10]. These differences persisted after adjustments for multiple confounders. A similar analysis of 13,637 general adult cardiac surgery patients noted lowest mortality at a BMI of 30 kg/m^2 [11]. This BMI-mortality paradox is not consistent, however, at higher BMI measurements; this study detailed exaggerated mortality in morbidly obese patients when compared to normal/overweight patients and obese cohort (4.6% vs. 2.9% and 2.3%, respectively). Additionally, both obesity and morbid obesity were associated with higher rates of overall major morbidity in comparison with normal and overweight status. Specifically, the obese patients had higher rates of wound infection, renal failure, and prolonged ventilation. This analysis substantiated an earlier analysis of patients after general cardiac surgery where BMI > 30 kg/m^2 was associated with increased infection risk, both at the sternal site and the site of saphenous vein harvest [2].

Overall, the relationship between BMI and mortality after cardiac surgery displays a U-shaped curve with highest risks in severely underweight patients, lower risks in normal weight, overweight and modestly obese patients, and increased risks in morbidly obese patients. The precise etiology for better outcomes in heavier patients has not been fully elucidated, but it may be related to better underlying nutritional status in those patients. Additionally, most of these studies are cross-sectional in nature, so it is difficult to assess the trend of BMI in an individual patient. Patients who experience a significant decrease in BMI may have a concurrent concerning underlying disease processes (either cardiac or noncardiac), though this would not be captured by the studies described above.

24.3 Enteral vs. Parenteral Nutrition

Enteral nutrition (EN) is not only more physiologic and less expensive than parenteral nutrition (PN) but also maintains optimal gut function and has been associated with decreased risk of infection and ICU length of stay [12]. Additionally, theoretical benefits of EN over PN include maintenance of the integrity of the intestinal mucosal tissue, improved immune function, and less systemic inflammation. Therefore, in general, the enteral route is preferred over the parenteral route for patients who require supplemental nutritional support and is accomplished via oral, gastric, or small bowel routes.

While PN may be useful in those patients who have gastrointestinal issues such as short gut syndrome or in those who do not tolerate oral feeding, older studies showed that PN was associated with increased risk of both infectious and noninfectious complications as well as length of stay. However, there was no demonstrable effect on mortality in a 2005 meta-analysis of 30 studies evaluating EN vs. PN [13]. Given the heterogeneity and lack of clarity in the data, however, it was somewhat difficult for the authors to make definitive recommendations for nutritional management. As a result, multiple subsequent trials attempted to clarify the benefits and risks of use of EN vs. PN. In spite of the data currently available from multiple trials, multiple questions persist about the optimal management of early nutrition in the ICU patient. Recent guidelines from both the Society of Critical Care Medicine/ American Society for Parenteral and Enteral Nutrition and the European Society of Intensive Care Medicine recommend starting EN over PN in critically ill patients who require nutritional support [14, 15], but both state that the data supporting these recommendations are limited. Salient data are summarized below.

The Impact of Early Parenteral Nutrition Completing Enteral Nutrition in Adult Critically Ill Patients (EPaNIC) trial enrolled 4640 adults admitted to an ICU who were assessed to be nutritionally "at risk" by nutrition screening and randomized them to early or late initiation of parenteral nutrition [16]. In the early-initiation group, parenteral nutrition was instituted within 48 h of ICU admission, while parenteral nutrition was not instituted before day 8 of hospitalization in the delayed initiation group. Both groups followed an early enteral nutrition initiation protocol, and the amount of parenteral nutrition needed in the intervention group was calculated as the difference between caloric goal and calories provided by enteral nutrition. The primary outcome was ICU length of stay, which was found to be shorter in the late-initiation group than in the early-initiation group (median 3 days, IQR 2–7 days vs. median 4 days, IQR 2–9 days, $p = 0.02$). Patients in the late-initiation group were more likely to be discharged alive from the ICU within 8 days (75.2% vs 71.7%, $p = 0.007$). Additionally, fewer patients developed a new infection in the ICU in the late-initiation group (22.8% vs. 26.2%, $p = 0.008$), and the hospital length of stay was shorter in the late-initiation group than the early-initiation group (median 14 days, IQR 9–27 days vs. median 16 days, IQR 9–29 days, $p = 0.004$). A prospectively planned sub-analysis of the EPaNIC data showed that, among 600 total patients, fewer patients had weakness on initial physical therapy assessment in the late-initiation group than the early-initiation group (34% vs. 43%, $p = 0.03$) [17]. Additionally, patients in the late-initiation group had faster recovery from their weakness than those in the early-initiation group.

The Early Nutritional Support in the Critically Ill (CALORIES) trial enrolled 2400 patients admitted to an intensive care unit and randomized them to either enteral or parenteral nutrition for up to 5 days after admission [18]. The primary outcome of all-cause mortality was assessed at 30 days, and there was no difference noted between the two groups (mortality rate 33.1% vs. 34.2%, $p = 0.57$). Both groups achieved similar caloric intake, though neither achieved the study's prespecified goal. The parenteral nutrition group had lower rates of hypoglycemia (3.7% vs. 6.2%, $p = 0.006$) and emesis (8.4% vs. 16.2%, $p < 0.001$). There were no significant differences noted in the other 16 secondary outcomes, including mean number of infectious complications and 90-day mortality. However, a systematic review published in 2016 that included the results from the CALORIES study found no difference in overall mortality but a decreased number of infectious complications and a decrease in ICU length of stay in the EN group [19]. Overall length of stay and days of mechanical ventilation were similar between groups. This systematic review also performed a sub-analysis looking at risk of infection by caloric intake. In studies in which the EN and PN arms received a similar number of calories, the rate of infectious complications was not increased. However, the rate of infectious complications was increased in studies where the PN group had higher caloric intake than the EN group.

The Early Parenteral Nutrition (Early PN) trial randomized 1462 patients with relative contraindications to starting early EN to either standard of care or early parenteral nutrition within 24 h of ICU admission with a primary outcome of 60-day mortality [20]. While there was no difference in 60-day mortality, the intervention group had fewer days of invasive ventilation. ICU and overall length of stay were similar. Additionally, all of the assessments of the numbers of new infections during the study, including catheter-associated infections, bloodstream infections, and pneumonia, were similar between groups.

Additionally, in a single-center, randomized trial of 305 adults, Heidegger and colleagues found that optimized nutrition with supplemental PN between days 4 and 8 of ICU admission was associated with lower rates of nosocomial infections between days 9 and 28 (their pre-specified primary endpoint) than EN alone (27% vs. 38%, HR 0.65, 95% CI 0.43–0.97) [21]. But, they did not include all infections during the intervention in the analysis, which potentially could have changed the outcome.

Despite earlier research and the EPaNIC study showing PN to be associated with more infectious risk, later studies such as the CALORIES and the Early PN trials did not find an increased risk for infection. The reason for the discrepancy between studies is not clear, but this data does suggest that the infectious risk of PN in the modern era may be lower than previously reported, particularly with improved central line care.

24.4 Timing of Nutritional Support

Nutritional assessment markers change over the course of a patient's critical illness and are unreliable for determining the optimal time to start nutritional support; therefore, clinical judgment must be used. Timing of nutritional support is a controversial topic, and there is conflicting data regarding when to begin nutritional therapy after ICU admission. The Early Versus Delayed Enteral Feeding (EDEN) trial enrolled 1000 adult patients requiring ICU admission for acute lung injury and randomized them to receive either trophic or full enteral feeding for the first 6 days of hospitalization [22]. The primary outcome was ventilator-free days before study day 28, and there were no differences between the two groups. Additionally, there were no differences in mortality or infectious complications, though the full-feed group did experience more emesis (2.2% vs. 1.7% of feeding days, $p = 0.05$). Additionally, long-term functional outcomes at 1 year were similar between groups [23].

The Permissive Underfeeding Versus Target Enteral Feeding in Adult Critically Ill Patients (PermiT) trial enrolled 894 adults admitted to an ICU and randomized them to permissive underfeeding versus standard enteral feeding, with goal caloric intake of 40–60% of expected caloric needs in the underfeeding group and 70–100% of expected caloric needs in the standard group [24]. Despite the difference in caloric goals, both groups received a similar number of calories from protein that were adequate to supply their full daily protein requirement. The primary outcome of 90-day mortality revealed no difference between the groups (27.2% in the intervention group vs. 28.9% in the control group, $p = 0.58$). The intervention group received significantly fewer calories than the standard group, but both groups had similar protein intake, per the trial design. There was a slightly higher rate of renal replacement therapy in the standard feeding group (11.4% vs. 7.1%, $p = 0.04$), but there were no other differences between groups in secondary outcomes including mortality at time points up to 180 days, duration of mechanical ventilation, ICU and hospital length of stay, and infection risk.

In general, the medical literature supports early appropriate nutritional support for those with critical illness. This is born out in two recent meta-analyses which evaluated the available data regarding the timing of enteral nutrition support. In the first study, they found that there was no survival benefit comparing early EN vs. delayed EN, but they did find that early EN was associated with a decreased risk of infection in comparison with delayed EN [15]. Based on this data, the authors recommended using early EN as opposed to delayed nutrition in critically ill adult patients. The second study found that early EN was associated with lower mortality as well as infectious morbidity; consequently, they also recommended early EN within 24–48 h of admission to the ICU [14].

24.5 Macronutrients

It is estimated that critically ill patients use approximately 25–35 kcal/kg/day, and of these total daily calories, it is recommended to have 50% carbohydrates, 20% protein, and 30% lipids. Usually the lower end of that scale is administered and meets the energy requirements in ICU patients. Exceeding this recommendation risks hyperglycemia, which exacerbates infectious risk, leading to undue morbidity, though diligent glycemic control through the use of insulin attenuates this risk.

24.5.1 Carbohydrates

Glucose remains a good source of energy that aids in protein utilization. While attention should be paid to the amount of carbohydrate supplied in any proposed nutritional regimen to avoid hyperglycemia, one must not discount the normal endogenous production of hepatic glucose, which is estimated at approximately

200 g per day [25]. The appropriate amount of glucose, therefore, needs to fulfill the obligate needs of dependent tissues, but must also serve to replenish glycogen stores, which are rapidly depleted with metabolic stress [26].

24.5.2 Protein

Multiple recent studies have found that providing adequate protein is important to ensure adequate nutrition in the ICU. The PermiT study, which evaluated permissive underfeeding in critical illness, aimed to provide patients in both groups with 1.2–1.5 g/kg of protein per day; similarly, the 2016 American Society for Parenteral and Enteral Nutrition/Society of Critical Care Medicine guidelines recommended 1.2–2.0 g/kg/day [14, 24]. In support of these recommendations, a 2014 observational study found lower mortality in critically ill, non-septic patients with more than 1.2 g/kg/day of protein intake compared to those with less protein intake [27]. Certain nonessential amino acids become essential during critical illness. Glutamine is critical for immune function, and low glutamine levels have been associated with poor outcomes in critical illness [28], and the REducing Deaths due to Oxidative Stress (REDOXS) trial evaluated the effect of glutamine supplementation in the ICU. REDOXS was a factorial 2 × 2 trial that assigned 1223 ICU patients with multiorgan failure and who were receiving mechanical ventilation to receive supplementation with glutamine, antioxidants, both, or placebo with a primary outcome of 28-day mortality [29]. This trial used a relatively high dose of glutamine (0.6–0.8 g/kg/day). There was a trend toward increased 28-day mortality in the glutamine group (aOR 1.28, 95% CI 1.00–1.64, $p = 0.05$). Both in-hospital mortality and 6-month mortality were higher among the patients in the glutamine group (37.2% vs. 31% for in-hospital, $p = 0.02$; 43.7% vs. 37.2% for 6 months, $p = 0.02$). Additionally, the Scottish Intensive care Glutamine or seleNium Evaluative Trial (SIGNET) randomized 502 ICU patients to receive parenteral glutamine, selenium, both, or neither with a primary outcome of new infections in the first 14 days and mortality [30]. This study used a significantly lower dose of glutamine of 0.1–0.2 g/kg/day. There were no differences in the intent-to-treat population between any of the groups in either number of new infections or mortality. Additionally, the MetaPlus trial randomized 301 patients to receive high-protein enteral nutrition enhanced with glutamine, omega-3 fatty acids, and antioxidants versus normal high-protein enteral nutrition with a primary endpoint of new infections [31]. There were no differences overall or in any subgroups between the intervention and control groups in the incidence of new infections; however, there was an increased 6-month mortality hazard ratio in the intervention group (HR 1.57, 95% CI 1.03–2.39, $p = 0.04$).

24.5.3 Lipids

In addition to protein, the type of lipid used for nutritional supplementation has also been reevaluated due to the finding that different types of long-chain fatty acids have different inflammatory effects. Specifically, n-3 fatty acids have previously been found to have an anti-inflammatory effect, while n-6 fatty acids have a pro-inflammatory effect and the n-9 fatty acids a neutral effect. Initial studies showed decreased mortality and less incident organ failure using an altered lipid formulation with a higher ratio of n-3 fatty acids to n-6 fatty acids in comparison with a more typical ratio [32]. In order to evaluate this further, the OMEGA trial randomized 272 adults with acute lung injury to enteral feeding including supplementation with omega-3 fatty acids, γ-linolenic acid, and antioxidants versus control feeds with the same number of calories [33]. The primary endpoint was ventilator-free days before study day 28, and the trial was stopped at the first interim data analysis due to lack of efficacy and concern for harm. The patients in the intervention group had fewer ventilator-free days and fewer ICU-free days than the control group. Adjusted mortality was similar between groups, though there was a trend toward increased 60-day mortality in the intervention group (25.1% vs. 17.6%, $p = 0.11$). Based on the lack of improvement and some evidence of harm with either glutamine supplementation or an altered ratio of fatty acids, neither is currently recommended for ICU patients, and they should not be routinely considered in ACHD patients in the ICU.

24.6 Micronutrients

In addition to ensuring an appropriate number of calories, it is also important to ensure that patients receive appropriate micronutrients to prevent nutritional deficiencies. While electrolytes such as sodium, potassium, calcium, phosphate, and magnesium are usually present in acceptable amounts in enteral feeding regimens, they must be supplemented to maintain normal serum levels with parenteral nutrition. Although daily requirements of vitamins and trace elements have not been established, nutritional deficiencies may be worsened by poor nutritional intake while hospitalized in the intensive care unit. Given this and the potential complications of vitamin deficiencies if untreated, serum assessment with subsequent administration (if needed) of these micronutrients is recommended until they are provided by enteral route [34].

There has also been interest in specific micronutrients due to their proposed anti-oxidative and anti-inflammatory effects. As discussed above, the SIGNET trial evaluated the effect of selenium supplementation in a randomized trial of 502 patients [30]. Supplemental selenium did not alter the number of patients who developed a new infection in the intention to treat analysis, but those patients who received at least 5 days of selenium supplementation did have lower odds of developing a new infection (OR 0.53, 95% CI 0.30–0.93, $p = 0.03$). Mortality was the same between the two groups. Due to concern for oxidative stress in multiple disease states in ICU patients, including postoperative atrial fibrillation, investigators have evaluated possible mechanisms to alter antioxidant balance. While omega-3 fatty acids alone have not been shown to prevent postoperative atrial fibrillation in postoperative cardiac surgery patients based on the OPERA trial [35], the addition of vitamin C and vitamin E to the regimen resulted in a decreased rate of postoperative atrial fibrillation in a randomized trial of 203 patients who underwent on-pump cardiac surgery (9.7% vs. 32%, $p < 0.001$) [36].

24.7 Issues Specific to Certain Patient Populations

Certain populations are predisposed to worse underlying nutritional status than other patients. Among patients with congenital heart disease, one of the highest-risk groups relates to patients who have undergone the Fontan palliation. It is known that children and young adults with Fontan circulation have decreased lean mass as well as shorter stature in comparison with the general population [37]. Furthermore, patients with failing Fontan circulation most frequently are underweight; cardiac cachexia often portends a grave prognosis. Compatible with this, a recent paper by Brida and colleagues showed that interval weight loss in ACHD patients is associated with increased mortality in comparison with patients whose weight is stable or who gain weight [8]. In addition to overall cardiac cachexia, patients with Fontan physiology are also at increased risk of protein losing enteropathy, which can lead to significant nitrogen malnutrition due to associated protein wasting [38].

References

1. Price S, Jaggar SI, Jordan S, Trenfield S, Khan M, Sethia B, et al. Adult congenital heart disease: intensive care management and outcome prediction. Intensive Care Med. 2007;33(4):652–9.
2. Engelman DT, Adams DH, Byrne JG, Aranki SF, Collins JJ Jr, Couper GS, et al. Impact of body mass index and albumin on morbidity and mortality after cardiac surgery. J Thorac Cardiovasc Surg. 1999;118(5):866–73.
3. van Venrooij LM, de Vos R, Borgmeijer-Hoelen MM, Haaring C, de Mol BA. Preoperative unintended weight loss and low body mass index in relation to complications and length of stay after cardiac surgery. Am J Clin Nutr. 2008;87(6):1656–61.
4. van Venrooij LM, de Vos R, Zijlstra E, Borgmeijer-Hoelen MM, van Leeuwen PA, de Mol BA. The impact of low preoperative fat-free body mass on infections and length of stay after cardiac surgery: a prospective cohort study. J Thorac Cardiovasc Surg. 2011;142(5):1263–9.
5. van Venrooij LM, van Leeuwen PA, Hopmans W, Borgmeijer-Hoelen MM, de Vos R, De Mol BA. Accuracy of quick and easy undernutrition screening tools--short nutritional assessment questionnaire, malnutrition universal screening tool, and modified malnutrition universal screening tool--in patients undergoing cardiac surgery. J Am Diet Assoc. 2011;111(12):1924–30.
6. Yu PJ, Cassiere HA, Dellis SL, Manetta F, Kohn N, Hartman AR. Impact of preoperative Prealbumin on outcomes after cardiac surgery. JPEN J Parenter Enteral Nutr. 2015;39(7):870–4.
7. Arabi YM, Aldawood AS, Al-Dorzi HM, Tamim HM, Haddad SH, Jones G, et al. Permissive underfeeding or standard enteral feeding in high- and low-nutritional-risk critically ill adults. Post hoc analysis of the PermiT trial. Am J Respir Crit Care Med. 2017;195(5):652–62.
8. Brida M, Dimopoulos K, Kempny A, Liodakis E, Alonso-Gonzalez R, Swan L, et al. Body mass index in adult congenital heart disease. Heart. 2017;103:1250.
9. Thourani VH, Keeling WB, Kilgo PD, Puskas JD, Lattouf OM, Chen EP, et al. The impact of body mass index on morbidity and short- and long-term mortality in cardiac valvular surgery. J Thorac Cardiovasc Surg. 2011;142(5):1052–61.
10. Mariscalco G, Wozniak MJ, Dawson AG, Serraino GF, Porter R, Nath M, et al. Body mass index and mortality among adults undergoing cardiac surgery: a Nationwide study with a systematic review and meta-analysis. Circulation. 2017;135(9):850–63.
11. Ghanta RK, LaPar DJ, Zhang Q, Devarkonda V, Isbell JM, Yarboro LT, et al. Obesity increases risk-adjusted morbidity, mortality, and cost following cardiac surgery. J Am Heart Assoc. 2017;6(3):e003831.
12. Seres DS, Valcarcel M, Guillaume A. Advantages of enteral nutrition over parenteral nutrition. Therap Adv Gastroenterol. 2013;6(2):157–67.

13. Peter JV, Moran JL, Phillips-Hughes J. A metaanalysis of treatment outcomes of early enteral versus early parenteral nutrition in hospitalized patients. Crit Care Med. 2005;33(1):213–20. discussion 60-1
14. Taylor BE, McClave SA, Martindale RG, Warren MM, Johnson DR, Braunschweig C, et al. Guidelines for the provision and assessment of nutrition support therapy in the adult critically ill patient: Society of Critical Care Medicine (SCCM) and American Society for Parenteral and Enteral Nutrition (ASPEN). Crit Care Med. 2016;44(2):390–438.
15. Reintam Blaser A, Starkopf J, Alhazzani W, Berger MM, Casaer MP, Deane AM, et al. Early enteral nutrition in critically ill patients: ESICM clinical practice guidelines. Intensive Care Med. 2017;43(3):380–98.
16. Casaer MP, Mesotten D, Hermans G, Wouters PJ, Schetz M, Meyfroidt G, et al. Early versus late parenteral nutrition in critically ill adults. N Engl J Med. 2011;365(6):506–17.
17. Hermans G, Casaer MP, Clerckx B, Guiza F, Vanhullebusch T, Derde S, et al. Effect of tolerating macronutrient deficit on the development of intensive-care unit acquired weakness: a subanalysis of the EPaNIC trial. Lancet Respir Med. 2013;1(8):621–9.
18. Harvey SE, Parrott F, Harrison DA, Bear DE, Segaran E, Beale R, et al. Trial of the route of early nutritional support in critically ill adults. N Engl J Med. 2014;371(18):1673–84.
19. Elke G, van Zanten AR, Lemieux M, McCall M, Jeejeebhoy KN, Kott M, et al. Enteral versus parenteral nutrition in critically ill patients: an updated systematic review and meta-analysis of randomized controlled trials. Crit Care. 2016;20(1):117.
20. Doig GS, Simpson F, Sweetman EA, Finfer SR, Cooper DJ, Heighes PT, et al. Early parenteral nutrition in critically ill patients with short-term relative contraindications to early enteral nutrition: a randomized controlled trial. JAMA. 2013;309(20):2130–8.
21. Heidegger CP, Berger MM, Graf S, Zingg W, Darmon P, Costanza MC, et al. Optimisation of energy provision with supplemental parenteral nutrition in critically ill patients: a randomised controlled clinical trial. Lancet. 2013;381(9864):385–93.
22. National Heart. L, blood institute acute respiratory distress syndrome clinical trials N, Rice TW, wheeler AP, Thompson BT, Steingrub J, et al. initial trophic vs full enteral feeding in patients with acute lung injury: the EDEN randomized trial. JAMA. 2012;307(8):795–803.
23. Needham DM, Dinglas VD, Morris PE, Jackson JC, Hough CL, Mendez-Tellez PA, et al. Physical and cognitive performance of patients with acute lung injury 1 year after initial trophic versus full enteral feeding. EDEN trial follow-up. Am J Respir Crit Care Med. 2013;188(5):567–76.
24. Arabi YM, Aldawood AS, Haddad SH, Al-Dorzi HM, Tamim HM, Jones G, et al. Permissive underfeeding or standard enteral feeding in critically ill adults. N Engl J Med. 2015;372(25):2398–408.
25. Cahill GF Jr. Starvation in man. N Engl J Med. 1970;282(12):668–75.
26. Wolfe RR. Carbohydrate metabolism in the critically ill patient. Implications for nutritional support Crit Care Clin. 1987;3(1):11–24.
27. Weijs PJ, Looijaard WG, Beishuizen A, Girbes AR, Oudemans-van Straaten HM. Early high protein intake is associated with low mortality and energy overfeeding with high mortality in non-septic mechanically ventilated critically ill patients. Crit Care. 2014;18(6):701.
28. Novak F, Heyland DK, Avenell A, Drover JW, Su X. Glutamine supplementation in serious illness: a systematic review of the evidence. Crit Care Med. 2002;30(9):2022–9.
29. Heyland D, Muscedere J, Wischmeyer PE, Cook D, Jones G, Albert M, et al. A randomized trial of glutamine and antioxidants in critically ill patients. N Engl J Med. 2013;368(16):1489–97.
30. Andrews PJ, Avenell A, Noble DW, Campbell MK, Croal BL, Simpson WG, et al. Randomised trial of glutamine, selenium, or both, to supplement parenteral nutrition for critically ill patients. BMJ. 2011;342:d1542.
31. van Zanten AR, Sztark F, Kaisers UX, Zielmann S, Felbinger TW, Sablotzki AR, et al. High-protein enteral nutrition enriched with immune-modulating nutrients vs standard high-protein enteral nutrition and nosocomial infections in the ICU: a randomized clinical trial. JAMA. 2014;312(5):514–24.

32. Pontes-Arruda A, Demichele S, Seth A, Singer P. The use of an inflammation-modulating diet in patients with acute lung injury or acute respiratory distress syndrome: a meta-analysis of outcome data. JPEN J Parenter Enteral Nutr. 2008;32(6):596–605.
33. Rice TW, Wheeler AP, Thompson BT, deBoisblanc BP, Steingrub J, Rock P, et al. Enteral omega-3 fatty acid, gamma-linolenic acid, and antioxidant supplementation in acute lung injury. JAMA. 2011;306(14):1574–81.
34. Casaer MP, Van den Berghe G. Nutrition in the acute phase of critical illness. N Engl J Med. 2014;370(13):1227–36.
35. Mozaffarian D, Marchioli R, Macchia A, Silletta MG, Ferrazzi P, Gardner TJ, et al. Fish oil and postoperative atrial fibrillation: the Omega-3 fatty acids for prevention of post-operative atrial fibrillation (OPERA) randomized trial. JAMA. 2012;308(19):2001–11.
36. Rodrigo R, Korantzopoulos P, Cereceda M, Asenjo R, Zamorano J, Villalabeitia E, et al. A randomized controlled trial to prevent post-operative atrial fibrillation by antioxidant reinforcement. J Am Coll Cardiol. 2013;62(16):1457–65.
37. Avitabile CM, Leonard MB, Zemel BS, Brodsky JL, Lee D, Dodds K, et al. Lean mass deficits, vitamin D status and exercise capacity in children and young adults after Fontan palliation. Heart. 2014;100(21):1702–7.
38. Umar SB, DiBaise JK. Protein-losing enteropathy: case illustrations and clinical review. Am J Gastroenterol. 2010;105(1):43–9. quiz 50

Cardiac Rehabilitation in Adults with Congenital Heart Disease

25

John Willner, Robert Haennel, Ailar Ramadi, Isabelle Vonder Muhll, and Andrew Mackie

25.1 Introduction

Adults with congenital heart disease (CHD) represent a small but growing population of patients presenting for cardiac rehabilitation (CR). In fact, surgery for adult CHD (ACHD) is one of the major growth areas in cardiac surgery. While some patients are referred to CR after cardiac surgery, others are referred for CR because of acute or chronic deconditioning. Furthermore, as this population ages, their risk of developing comorbidities such as obesity, diabetes, and coronary artery disease (CAD) increases their need for CR services [1].

As a group, ACHD patients are challenging for CR programs in several ways (Table 25.1). Unlike coronary artery disease, CHD is pathologically diverse encompassing many different cardiac lesions with varying pathophysiology. ACHD patients may be cyanotic and are typically younger than the traditional CR population, and exercise testing and training protocols are not well established for ACHD patients. Nevertheless, compared to elderly patients with acquired heart disease, ACHD patients may be more adaptable and may easily acquire exercise skills and knowledge in CR. A growing body of evidence is emerging demonstrating the benefits of CR on both quality of life and aerobic capacity in ACHD patients [2–4]. This chapter will provide an overview of general principles of CR and review the evidence for CR in ACHD patients including patient assessment and recommendations for exercise training and physical activity.

J. Willner · R. Haennel · A. Ramadi
Faculty of Rehabilitation Medicine, University of Alberta, Edmonton, AB, Canada

I. V. Muhll
Faculty of Medicine & Dentistry, University of Alberta, Edmonton, AB, Canada

A. Mackie (✉)
Stollery Children's Hospital, Edmonton, AB, Canada
e-mail: Andrew.mackie@ualberta.ca

E. da Cruz et al. (eds.), *Intensive Care of the Adult with Congenital Heart Disease*, Congenital Heart Disease in Adolescents and Adults,
https://doi.org/10.1007/978-3-319-94171-4_25

Table 25.1 Comparison of typical cardiac rehabilitation population versus adult congenital heart disease population

Factor	Usual cardiac rehabilitation population	ACHD population
Age	Older	Younger
Underlying heart disease	Coronary artery disease	Congenital heart disease; variable lesions
Circulation	Biventricular	Biventricular or univentricular
Ventricular function	Left ventricular dysfunction predominant Left ventricle is systemic	Right ventricular dysfunction predominant Right ventricle might be systemic
Valvular function	Often normal; mitral and aortic valve disease predominant	Often abnormal: tricuspid and pulmonary regurgitation predominant
Prosthetic valve	Uncommon	Common: may include right ventricular to pulmonary artery conduits, valve repairs, aortic or mitral valve prosthesis, depending on lesion
Oxygen saturation	Normal	Normal in most repaired patients. Expected to be abnormal in: Fontan—mild cyanosis Unrepaired lesions, Eisenmenger—moderate cyanosis (O_2 Sats ≥70%) that worsens with exercise
Comorbidities	Vascular risk factors: hypertension, dyslipidemia, obesity, smoking	Genetic syndromes: Down's, DiGeorge, Noonan's, Marfan Neurodevelopmental delay

25.2 Patient Assessment

25.2.1 Clinical Evaluation

CHD is pathologically diverse encompassing many different cardiac lesions with varying pathophysiology. Hence each patient is unique: ACHD patients may have a biventricular or univentricular circulation; they may be surgically repaired or uncorrected; they may have normal oxygen saturations or be cyanotic. They may have normal intellectual and psychosocial development or have neurodevelopmental delay. They may also have an associated genetic syndrome. Hence, understanding the patient's cardiac history, residual hemodynamic burden, and the potential electrophysiological complications, which may occur during exercise, is essential prior to making exercise recommendations.

Elements of the clinical evaluation include:

(a) History, including a focus on the patient's current functional status and eliciting any cardiac symptoms, particularly those associated with exertion (e.g., chest pain, palpitations, syncope)
(b) Physical examination of the cardiovascular and respiratory system with measurement of oxygen saturation with the intent of eliciting any findings consistent with residual hemodynamic lesions, cyanosis, congestive heart failure, etc.

(c) Review of all prior cardiac interventions, both operative notes and cardiac catheterization reports
(d) Assessment of ventricular size, systolic and diastolic function, valve morphology and function, aortic dimensions, and potential residual lesions through imaging of the heart (echocardiography, cardiac MRI) with interpretation by an expert in ACHD
(e) Assessment of the 12-lead ECG, to monitor for resting bradycardia, atrial arrhythmia, and pacemaker response as well as to document the baseline QRS and ST segment morphology

Direct communication between the CR program and the CHD team may be helpful. A case conference to review the specifics of each case may serve both to educate the CR team about CHD and to better prepare the CR team to design a program appropriate for that patient. The use of a diagram outlining the patient's anatomy and previous interventions can be instructive. The location of suture lines from previous cardiac surgery is predictive of the type of hemodynamic complications and arrhythmia. For example, those with previous atrial surgery are at greater risk for atrial arrhythmias and sinus node dysfunction, while ventricular outflow tract patches and wide QRS are risk factors for ventricular tachycardia [5, 6].

25.2.2 Assessment of Aerobic Capacity

Prior to starting formal CR programs, a baseline aerobic exercise test is recommended to serve as documentation of the patient's aerobic capacity and to guide the exercise prescription [7]. Aerobic exercise testing is also useful in return to work evaluation and disability assessment and to help estimate prognosis [8]. There is no consensus as to the best form of aerobic exercise testing. Assessment can be laboratory based, such as symptom-limited graded exercise test (SL-GXT) using a cycle ergometer or treadmill, or field-based such as the 6-minute walk test (6MWT), which is often used in those with very limited physical capacity.

For laboratory-based exercise testing, the most commonly used modalities are treadmills and cycle ergometers. Treadmills utilize walking and accommodate a wide spectrum of fitness levels [8]. For treadmill-based exercise testing, the Bruce protocol is commonly conducted, using endurance time as an index of aerobic capacity [9, 10]. The Bruce protocol increases in intensity in relatively large increments of 2–3 METs per stage (i.e., every 3 min) [8]. As a result of the large MET increments/stage, aerobic capacity may be markedly overestimated when it is predicted from exercise time or workload. SL-GXTs using the Bruce protocol are better suited for younger and/or physically active individuals [8]. By contrast, it has been proposed that protocols such as Naughton or Balke-Ware (i.e., $\leq$1 MET increase per stage) may be better suited for the elderly and patients with chronic disease [8].

Unfortunately, treadmills are expensive and not easily transportable, and monitoring physiological responses during exercise is difficult. Alternatively, cycle ergometers provide a non-weight-bearing test modality with easily adjusted work rates to determine aerobic capacity [8]. Cycle ergometers are relatively inexpensive and easily transportable and minimize artifacts that can impact physiological monitoring. The main disadvantage to the cycle ergometer is most participants are less experienced in cycling, which may result in localized leg fatigue [8].

Ramp protocols provide an alternate approach to aerobic exercise testing. Whether on a treadmill or a cycle ergometer, ramp protocols increase exercise intensity/work rate every minute in a constant and continuous manner [8]. Advantages to ramp protocols include reduced testing time, avoidance of large and unequal increments in workload, uniform increase in hemodynamic and physiologic responses, and more accurate estimates of exercise capacity [8].

Prior to entering a hospital-based CR program, a SL-GXT with continuous ECG monitoring is usually performed on incoming patients. At a minimum, the exercise test should include continuous measurement of heart rate (HR) via a 12-lead ECG, blood pressure assessment at each stage of the SL-GXT, and the patient's rating of perceived exertion at rest, during exercise, and during the immediate post-exercise recovery period (e.g., the first 5 min of recovery) [8]. Exercise testing with ECG monitoring is useful for detecting exercise-induced arrhythmias and ST changes [9].

During a SL-GXT, HR should increase linearly with increments in workload from baseline to HR_{peak} [7–9]. Age-predicted HR_{max} may be estimated from the equation, $HR_{max} = 220 - \text{age (years)}$, provided the patient is not on medication that impacts HR (e.g., beta-blockers) [8]. The inability to appropriately increase HR during progressive exercise (i.e., chronotropic incompetence; <85% age-predicted HR_{max}) is associated with the presence of heart disease and increased mortality [8, 11] and is commonly observed in patients after CHD surgery [9]. Chronotropic incompetence may be due to conduction system malfunction due to injury to the SA node secondary to intervention, by drug therapy or chronic pacing [10]. As such, HR reserve (HRR) and chronotropic index should be assessed in ACHD patients [12]. The HRR, defined as $HR_{peak} - HR_{rest}$, may be a predictor of mortality in patients with CHD [13]. The chronotropic index, used to predict a normal HR response to submaximal exercise, is calculated as $HRR/[(220\text{-age}) - HR_{rest}]$ and is independent of age, resting HR, and functional state [11].

Blood pressure (BP) should be monitored throughout the SL-GXT (pre-, during each exercise stage, and immediately post-exercise). Systolic BP (SBP) should increase with each increment in workload, and little to no change in diastolic blood pressure (DBP) is expected [8]. If SBP appears to be decreasing with increments in exercise intensity, it should be reassessed immediately. If a drop in SBP > 10 mmHg occurs with an increase in exercise intensity, or if it drops below the value obtained in the same position prior to the SL-GXT, the test should be stopped, particularly if accompanied by adverse signs and symptoms. The SL-GXT should also be terminated if a hypertensive response is observed (SBP >250 mmHg and/or DBP >115 mmHg). The BP response to exercise is variably attenuated in patients on vasodilators, calcium channel blockers, angiotensin-converting enzyme inhibitors, and alpha- and beta-adrenergic blockers [8]. An important indicator of myocardial oxygen demand may be derived from the rate pressure product which is defined as

SBP x HR [8]. Signs and symptoms of ischemia generally occur at a reproducible rate pressure product [8].

Pulse oximetry should be employed to assess arterial oxygen saturation during exercise testing in ACHD [9, 14]. Normal resting pulse oximetry values are ~98% [15]. A decrease in arterial oxygen saturation of >5% during SL-GXT is suggestive of abnormal exercise-induced arterial hypoxemia [14, 15]. Exercise-induced arterial hypoxemia may be defined as mild (O_2 Sat. of 93–95%), moderate (O_2 Sat. 88–93%), and severe (O_2 Sat. <88%) [15], and exercise testing should be discontinued if arterial oxygen saturation falls to <85% in patients who have normal resting oxygen saturation [14]. Many ACHD patients, especially those with the Fontan circulation, are mild to moderately desaturated at rest and drop their oxygen saturation further with exercise. Rather than an absolute threshold of <85%, the clinician may use a drop in oxygen saturation of 10–20% or rely on patient symptoms as a guide to terminating exercise.

In cardiopulmonary exercise testing, oxygen uptake and related respiratory parameters may also be measured during the SL-GXT. Physiologic parameters which may be measured during a SL-GXT with concurrent ventilator gas analysis include the measurement of oxygen uptake (VO_2), carbon dioxide production (VCO_2), and minute ventilation (VE). These measures are used to determine maximum oxygen uptake (VO_{2max}), aerobic exercise capacity (VO_{2peak}), ventilatory threshold (VT), and the ventilatory equivalents (i.e., VE/VO_2, VE/VCO_2). The measurement of these parameters provides a more detailed physiologic understanding of the underlying mechanisms of exercise impairment and subsequent improvement with training.

Maximum oxygen uptake (VO_{2max}): reflects the integrated ability of an individual to transport oxygen from the atmosphere to the mitochondria to perform physical work [16]. As such, VO_{2max} encompasses a chain of processes that include gas exchange in the lungs, right and left ventricular cardiac output, transport of oxygen in the blood through the vascular system, as well as peripheral factors that include the metabolic efficiency and vascularization of skeletal muscles [16]. VO_{2max} is defined as the plateau in VO_2 despite increasing workload (Fig. 25.1a), and it is effort-dependent and is verified by the respiratory exchange ratio (VCO_2/VO_2) which will exceed 1.1 [14].

The assessment of VO_{2max} is considered the gold standard for measuring aerobic capacity and the overall health of the cardiorespiratory system. It has been shown to be an important predictor of health outcome and survival in diverse groups of cardiac patients [16] including ACHD [12, 17–21].

Peak VO_2 (VO_{2peak}): Because VO_{2max} is effort-dependent and is not always reached by ACHD patients during a SL-GXT, VO_{2peak} is often used as a surrogate for VO_{2max}. The inability to achieve VO_{2max} during a SL-GXT may be attributed to the caution employed during the testing and/or the fact that patients experience volitional fatigue before achieving the physiological markers associated with VO_{2max} (Fig. 25.2). In these tests, the highest VO_2 observed during the test, termed VO_{2peak}, is reported [22, 23]. The intensity of an exercise prescription can then be set at a workload corresponding to 50–70% of VO_{2peak}. Like VO_{2max}, VO_{2peak} also has prognostic significance for ACHD. A VO_{2peak} of <15 mL/kg/min has been shown to be an independent predictor of hospitalization and increased mortality [13, 17].

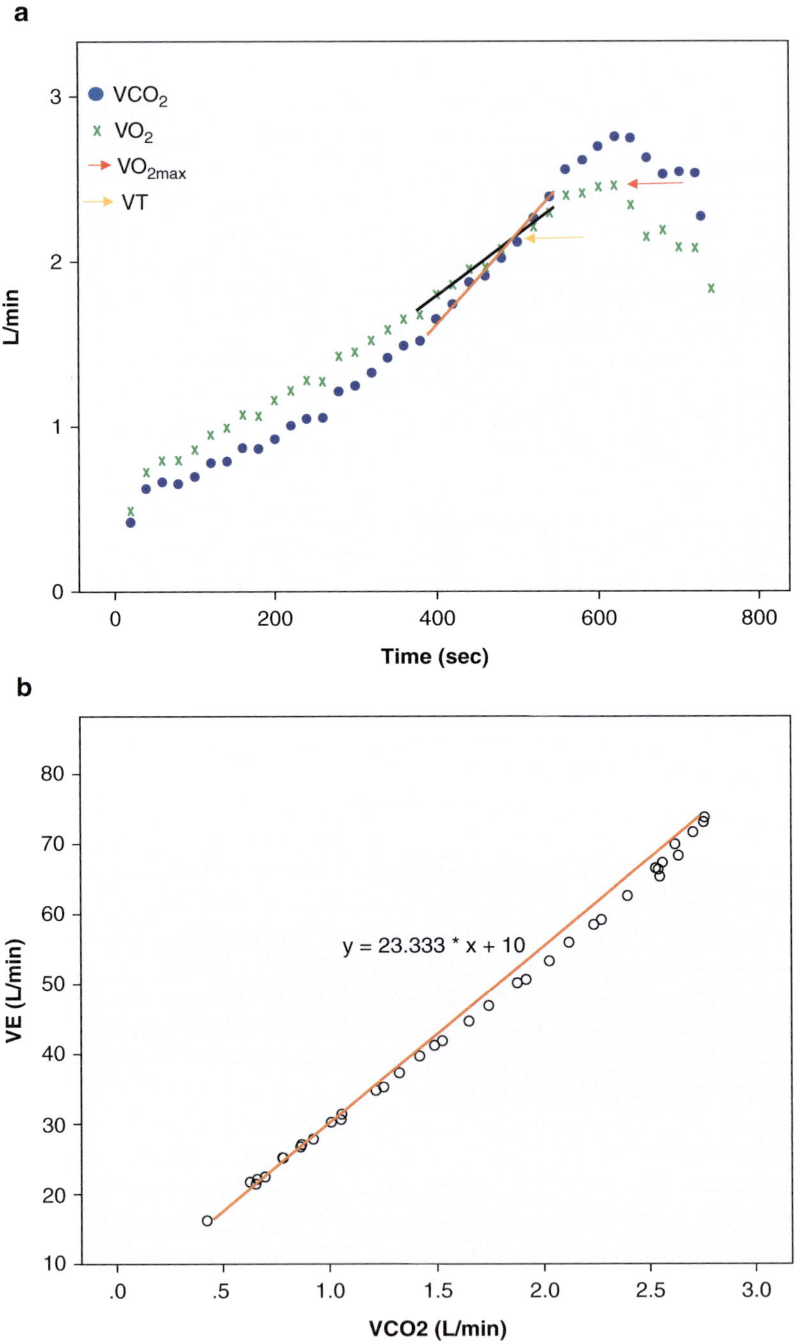

Fig. 25.1 Clinical exam of a SL-GXT with physiological monitoring where patient achieved VO_{2max}, (**a**) respiratory gas analysis as a function of time/exercise workload. VO_{2max}, shown by red arrow, represents plateau of VO_2 just before volitional fatigue. The ventilatory threshold (VT) represents the point at which CO_2 production exceeds O_2 consumption. (**b**) VE/VCO_2 slope is calculated from respiratory gas analysis as the slope of the line of minute ventilation related to CO_2 production

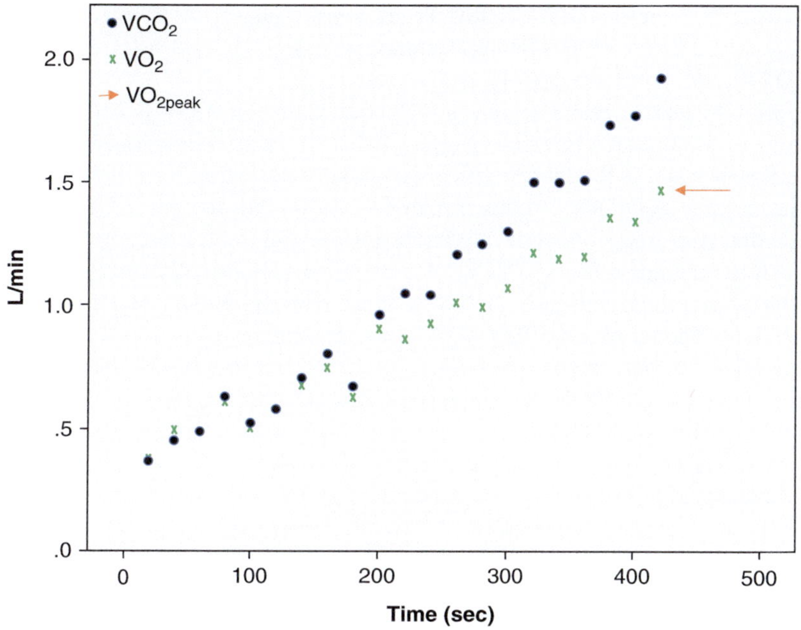

Fig. 25.2 Clinical exam of a SL-GXT with physiological monitoring where patient did not achieve VO_{2max}. Note the lack of a plateau in VO_2. In this example, the maximum VO_2 consumption represents VO_{2peak}

While an assessment of VO_{2peak} provides an index of aerobic capacity, respiratory parameters such as ventilatory threshold (VT) and ventilatory equivalent (e.g., VE/VCO_2 slope) may also be assessed during submaximal exercise and are valuable in the assessment of cardiorespiratory fitness and in prescribing aerobic exercise [22, 24].

Ventilatory threshold (VT): reflects the point at which aerobic metabolism is substantially supplemented by anaerobic processes [10]. During a SL-GXT, the ratio of ventilation to CO_2 production (VE/VCO_2) remains relatively stable with increasing workloads, whereas the ratio of ventilation to VO_2 (VE/VO_2) starts to increase. The VT is defined as the workload at which there is an increase in VE/VO_2 and no change in VE/VCO_2. The regression analysis of the VCO_2 and VO_2 slopes (the so-called V-slope method) indicating the beginning of excess VCO_2 as a means of buffering excess [H^+] (Fig. 25.1a) is used to determine the VT [25]. The VT is not affected by patient effort or motivation and may be determined on a submaximal exercise test; thus, VT is considered an excellent index of the cardiovascular system's capacity to support the hemodynamic demands of exercise [10]. Often described as a percentage of VO_{2peak}, VT is useful for predicting the ability of the patient to sustain a given work rate for a prolonged period of time [26]. Using the VT as a basis for prescription allows for matching the unique physiological responses of different exercise intensities to the individual pathology and clinical status [27]. As such, using the VT for exercise prescription may maximize the benefits obtainable from aerobic exercise training in CR [27]. In healthy untrained populations, the VT typically occurs at a workload of approximately 50–60% of VO_{2peak}. However in the presence of cardiovascular disease, the VT lowers to approximately 40% of VO_{2peak} [10]. Additionally, a lower VT has been associated with an increased risk for mortality in ACHD [10, 13].

Ventilatory equivalent: The ventilatory equivalent (for CO_2) is calculated from the slope of the line of VE/VCO_2 (Fig. 25.1b). This slope is an indicator of ventilatory efficiency and is thought to reflect pulmonary perfusion, ventilation/perfusion mismatch, and ventilatory reflex sensitivity [28]. Advantages of this measure include that it is independent of maximal exertion and there is a large body of data linking it to outcomes. The VE/VCO_2 slope becomes abnormally elevated in cardiovascular or pulmonary disease, including those with pulmonary hypertension [16]. Studies have shown that the VE/VCO_2 slope exhibits a high prognostic value for cardiac-related events in patients with coronary artery disease and the risk of mortality increases as the VE/VCO_2 slope rises. For example, Arena et al. [29] reported that the quartiles of VE/VCO_2 slope in heart failure patients can predict cardiac outcomes, where <30 implies negligible risk of a major cardiac event; 30–35, a low risk of major cardiac event; 36–44, moderate risk of major cardiac event; and ≥45, high risk of major cardiac event.

The VE/VCO_2 slope has been shown to be higher in adults with d-transposition of the great arteries (32 ± 14) and tetralogy of Fallot (26 ± 6) than in healthy controls (25 ± 4) [22, 30]. Even young ACHD patients have been observed to have VE/VCO_2 slopes >30 [10]. A linear relationship has been suggested between VE/VCO_2 and New York Heart Association (NYHA) classification, suggesting a link between ventilatory responses to exercise and the occurrence of symptoms [28]. Similar to the findings of Arena et al. [29], Dimopoulos et al. [28] noted a VE/VCO_2 slope of >38 was a prognostic marker associated with a tenfold increase in the risk of death within 2 years. Interestingly, Inuzuka et al. [13] found no predictive value in cyanotic patients; however, non-cyanotic patients had an increased risk of death with a slope >39, concluding a slope of 39 as an optimal cutoff value based on the authors' time-dependent Receiver Operating Characteristics (ROC) analysis. Moreover, since one of the most important pathophysiological processes affecting VE/VCO_2 slope is maldistribution of pulmonary blood flow causing ventilation/perfusion mismatch, it is not surprising that patients with repaired tetralogy of Fallot, who often have pulmonary artery stenosis, have been found to have elevated VE/VCO_2 slope attributable to pulmonary blood flow maldistribution [10, 18, 30–32].

6-minute walk test (6MWT): is a simple means of objectively assessing aerobic capacity and is suitable as an alternative to treadmill or bicycle exercise testing in patients with limited exercise ability [33], such as those with moderate to severe heart or lung disease; however, it should not be used in mildly impaired or asymptomatic patients due to a "ceiling effect" which may mask improvements after interventions [34]. The advantages of the 6MWT include it is easy to administer, is inexpensive, does not require physician supervision, and mimics activities of daily living [9, 33]. In patients with heart failure, mean distances of 310–427 m have been observed, with distance being inversely correlated with NYHA functional class [35]. The 6MWT has been determined to be a reliable form of functional assessment for ACHD patients who walk less than 400 m [9].

25.2.3 Assessment of Muscular Strength and Endurance

Performing muscular strength and endurance tests is recommended prior to exercise training and can provide valuable information on the patient's baseline fitness level [8]. Muscular strength and endurance tests may identify muscular weaknesses or imbalances that could be targeted in an exercise training program [8]. Additionally, muscular strength and endurance tests are useful in showing patients' progressive improvement, which may promote long-term exercise adherence [8]. Unfortunately, muscular strength and endurance tests are specific to the procedures used, and no single test evaluates total-body muscular strength or endurance. As well, normative data may not include a representative ACHD sample; thus, interpretation of results is difficult [8].

Muscular Strength. Muscular strength is the external force that can be generated by a specific muscle or muscle group [8]. Muscular strength can be assessed statically (i.e., no excessive muscular or limb movement) or dynamically (i.e., movement of an external load or body part, in which the muscle changes length) [8]. Peak force development is measured and referred to as maximum voluntary contraction (MVC) as a representation of muscular strength. Static strength may be evaluated using a variety of devices such as a handgrip dynamometer. However, static strength measurements are suboptimal because the test is specific to both the muscle group and joint angle involved in testing, limiting the evaluation of total-body muscular strength [8]. In healthy populations, traditional dynamic muscular strength tests evaluate the participants' one-repetition max (1RM), the greatest resistance that can be moved through the full range of motion in a controlled manner [8]. At high levels of muscle tension to lift or otherwise move a heavy weight, there is a potential risk of eliciting the Valsalva maneuver (forced expiration invoked against a closed glottis). The Valsalva maneuver increases intrathoracic pressure potentially leading to a decrease in venous return and cardiac output [36, 37]. Thus, 1RM muscular strength testing may not be suitable for some ACHD patients. Alternatively, 4- or 8RM may be used as a measure of muscular strength as an index of how strength changes over time, independent of 1RM [8].

Muscular Endurance. Despite concerns that resistance exercise elicits abnormal cardiovascular pressor responses in coronary artery disease patients, studies have found muscular endurance testing elicits HR and BP responses within acceptable clinic limits [36]. Muscular endurance is the ability of a muscle group to complete repeated contractions over a period of time, sufficient to cause muscular fatigue, or to maintain a specific percentage of MVC for a prolonged period of time [8]. Participants are scored by the number of successful repetitions completed. Absolute muscular endurance is the total number of repetitions measured at a given amount of resistance, whereas relative muscular endurance is the total repetitions completed at a percentage of 1RM [8]. For example, field tests to evaluate upper body muscular endurance include the push-up test (i.e., absolute muscular endurance test) where the participant must complete as many successful repetitions as possible [8] and the YMCA bench press test (i.e., relative muscular endurance test), in which the participant must complete as many successful reps as possible at 80 lb for men and 35 lb for women at a rate of 30 repetitions/min [38].

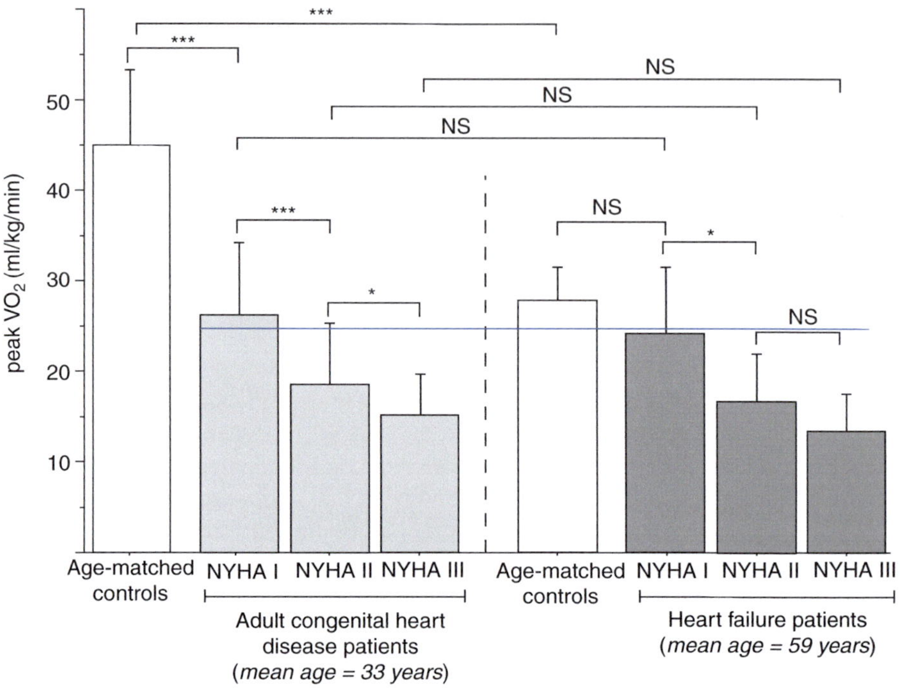

Fig. 25.3 Observed VO_{2peak} in patients with CHD vs. HF. *Source*: Diller G, et al. [17]. Used with permission from *Circulation*

25.3 Aerobic Exercise Capacity in Adults with CHD

Although muscular strength and endurance is important to ACHD patients' overall exercise capacity, most research has focused on aerobic exercise capacity and aerobic training in ACHD patients.

25.3.1 General Findings

As a group, asymptomatic CHD patients have a significantly reduced VO_{2peak} (average 22 ± 8 mL/kg/min) compared to aged-matched healthy controls (45 ± 9 mL/kg/min) [17]. Indeed, ACHD patients have a VO_{2peak} comparable to that seen in elderly patients with heart failure (HF) (Fig. 25.3). It has been widely reported that ACHD patients have a reduced aerobic capacity that spans all diagnostic groups [17, 39]. The diminished VO_{2peak} in ACHD had been reported in patients with simple lesions such as pulmonary stenosis [40], aortic stenosis, and ventricular septal defects [41, 42]. Moreover, those with more complex anatomical features, such as Eisenmenger,

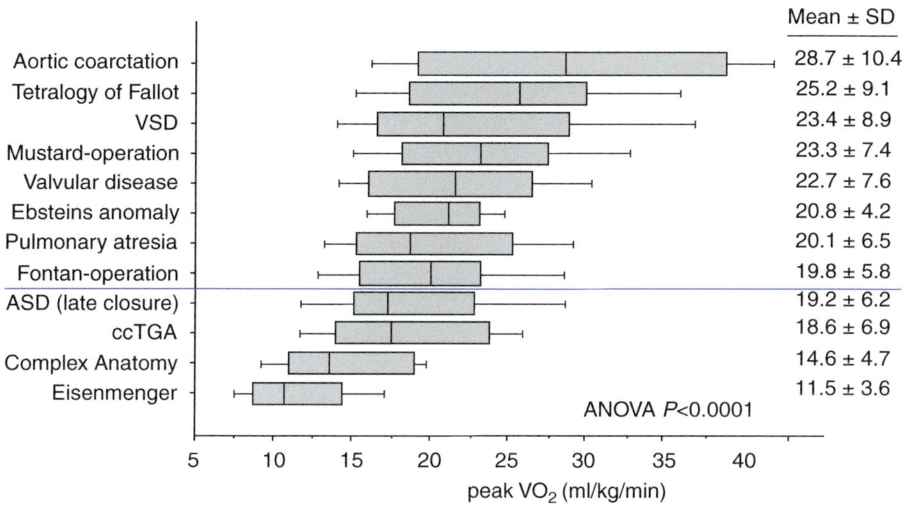

Fig. 25.4 Average VO_{2peak} in CHD by lesion type. *Source*: Diller G, et al. [17]. *VSD* Ventricular septal defect, *ASD* Atrial septal defect, *ccTGA* congenitally corrected Transposition. Used with permission from *Circulation*

congenitally corrected transposition (ccTGA), Fontan, or Ebstein's malformation of the tricuspid valve, typically have the lowest VO_{2peak} (Fig. 25.4) [12, 17, 22, 43–45].

The mechanisms underlying low aerobic capacity seen in ACHD are multifactorial. ACHD patients may be unable to adequately increase cardiac output (e.g., cyanotic CHD patients) during exercise due to systolic or diastolic dysfunction, valvular stenosis or regurgitation, chronotropic incompetence, arrhythmias, residual intracardiac shunts, or pericardial disease [10]. Approximately 60% of ACHD patients experience chronotropic incompetence during exercise, which may be attributed to intrinsic malfunction of the conduction system, inadvertent injury to the sinus or atrioventricular nodes, drug therapy, or chronic pacing [10, 17].

Reduced aerobic capacity in ACHD may also be attributed to an abnormal ventilatory response to exercise. It has been reported that ACHD patients with complex lesions have a severely elevated ventilatory response to exercise (i.e., VE) as compared to healthy controls [28, 46]. The presence of cyanosis is a powerful predictor of an abnormal ventilatory response to exercise, postulated to be due to the shunting of deoxygenated blood to the systemic circulation being a strong stimulus for ventilation [28]. Other important contributors to an abnormal ventilatory response include the presence of lung disease [47], pulmonary vascular disease, systemic vascular disease, skeletal muscle dysfunction/deconditioning, anemia, and iron deficiency [10].

Finally, peripheral oxygen extraction may play a significant role in the reduced aerobic capacity seen in ACHD. Skeletal muscles may be deconditioned [48], or in rare cases there may be glycogen storage disease or other metabolic disorders that affect peripheral oxygen extraction.

25.3.2 Tetralogy of Fallot

Like most congenital heart lesions, adults with repaired tetralogy of Fallot (ToF) have a reduced VO_{2peak} compared to healthy controls (average VO_{2peak} 26 ± 7 mL/kg/min) [18]. Moreover, similar to HF patients, ToF patients experience an increase in oxygen debt and prolonged recovery (e.g., VO_2 and VE) postexercise [49]. Due to pulmonary valvotomy and reconstruction of the right ventricular (RV) outflow tract during primary repair of ToF, the dominant residual lesion in adult ToF patients is pulmonary regurgitation. Significant pulmonary regurgitation may limit augmentation of cardiac output during exercise and may prolong the recovery phase post-exercise. Indeed more severe pulmonary regurgitation is associated with a diminished aerobic exercise capacity in adults with ToF [49]. However the findings of Mercer-Rosa et al. [50] suggest that pulmonary regurgitation alone does not explain the impaired aerobic capacity. These authors compared ToF patients to valvular pulmonary stenosis patients post-valvotomy and found lower aerobic capacity, higher RV mass, and lower RV ejection fraction in ToF patients despite similar degrees of pulmonary regurgitation. Based on these findings, they postulated that ToF patients may have an intrinsic RV cardiomyopathy from prior cyanosis and abnormalities of the distal pulmonary arterial tree or as a consequence of transannular patching and surgical repair that alters the RV performance during exercise.

Pulmonary valve replacement is commonly performed in adults with repaired ToF who have symptomatic pulmonary regurgitation or objective evidence of severe RV dilatation or progressive RV dysfunction. Interestingly, elimination of the pulmonary regurgitation by surgical or transcatheter implantation of a prosthesis is not associated with an improvement in aerobic exercise capacity [51]. Some investigators have implicated a pre-existing impairment of lung function may cause a ventilation limitation to VO_{2peak} in ACHD patients with pulmonary valve replacements [47].

25.3.3 Systemic Right Ventricle: Transposition of the Great Arteries

Patients with a systemic right ventricle represent a relatively small subset of ACHD patients. However, their aerobic capacity is significantly reduced. Patients with transposition of the great arteries who have undergone an atrial redirection procedure (Senning or Mustard operation) have an average VO_{2peak} of 24 ± 7 mL/kg/min compared to those with congenitally corrected transposition (ccTGA) whose average VO_{2peak} is 21 ± 7 mL/kg/min [12]. The reduced aerobic capacity in the ccTGA group likely reflects the presence of multiple associated lesions [12].

Mechanisms underlying reduced aerobic capacity in patients with a systemic right ventricle are varied and differ from patients with ToF. Noncompliant systemic venous return after the atrial redirection procedure limits augmentation of cardiac output during exercise [52]. Moreover, abnormal systemic right ventricle function, tricuspid regurgitation, atrial arrhythmias, AV conduction disturbances, and chronotropic incompetence also contribute to impaired aerobic capacity [53].

25.3.4 Fontan Procedure

Patients with single-ventricle physiology (e.g., tricuspid atresia, double-inlet ventricle, and hypoplastic left heart syndrome) who have undergone the Fontan procedure represent some of the most complex ACHD patients with markedly altered anatomy and physiology that ultimately affect aerobic capacity. While the Fontan procedure reduces right-to-left shunt and systemic ventricular volume overload, thus improving VO_{2peak} immediately following the Fontan procedure [54], patients still have an aerobic capacity well below that of healthy controls [12, 17, 55]. The large Pediatric Heart Network cohort of 402 Fontan children found a VO_{2peak} of 26 ± 7 mL/kg/min, which was approximately 65% predicted VO_{2peak} for those whose average age was 12 years [56].

One of the most important mechanisms underlying reduced aerobic capacity in Fontan patients is diminished stroke volume due to reduced pulmonary venous diastolic return during exercise due to the lack of a sub-pulmonary ventricle [55]. Other mechanisms contributing to the diminished aerobic capacity include chronotropic incompetence, chronic ventricular volume overload which may result in ventricular hypertrophy, impaired ventricular systolic contractile function, altered pulmonary blood flow, and impaired respiratory gas exchange [55]. Moreover it is increasingly recognized that decreased skeletal muscle mass is associated with lower VO_{2peak}, underscoring the importance of peripheral muscle determining VO_{2peak} in these patients [57].

25.4 Cardiac Rehabilitation Interventions

25.4.1 Moderate Continuous Aerobic Training

Traditionally, most CR programs utilize a medically supervised exercise program which focuses on moderate continuous aerobic training (MCAT) in addition to physical activity (PA) counseling. In general, exercise prescription for ACHD patients follows the same basic FITT (i.e., frequency, intensity, time, type) principles used in healthy populations (Table 25.2).

Frequency: While the goal for most patients is to perform moderate to vigorous PA (MVPA) 5 days of the week, the frequency of exercise training sessions at a formal CR program is usually less than this due to resource considerations. Most CR programs offer exercise training between two to three times weekly for an 8–12-week period. Hence patients are encouraged to supplement the CR program with two to three additional exercise sessions on their own each week.

Intensity: In MCAT, the exercise intensity is typically set at 50–70% VO_{2peak} [19] or 60–80% of HR_{peak} observed in a SL-GXT [33, 58–61]. For those with chronotropic incompetence or atrial fibrillation or for whom HR_{peak} is inappropriate for determining an exercise prescription, exercise intensity may be prescribed based on maximal workload achieved or the VT [62].

To gauge the patient's perception of exercise intensity during training, the Borg scale for rating of perceived exertion (RPE) is often used (Table 25.3). The Borg

Table 25.2 Exercise Prescription Guidelines for adults with Congenital heart disease (ACHD)

Appropriate for:	Moderate continuous aerobic training	High-intensity interval training	Resistance training	Special concerns
Tetralogy of Fallot	F: 3–5 times/week	F: 3 times/week	F: 2–3 times/week	Significant pulmonary or tricuspid valve regurgitation: Recommendations should fall to low-to-moderate intensity if right ventricular dysfunction is present
	I: 40–85% VO_{2peak}	I: 3–5 min 30–60% VO_{2peak} + 1–3 min >85% VO_{2peak}	I: 50–70% MVC	
	T: 150 min/week, 30–60 min/day	T: 6–8 sets/day, 30–60 min/day	T: 8–12 reps/exercise, 1–2 sets/exercise, >30 min/day	
	T: Walking, jogging, cycling, swimming	T: Walking, jogging, cycling, swimming	T: Body weight (push-ups, pull-ups, squats), free weights, machine weights, martial arts	
Systemic RV and Fontan circulation	F: 3–5 times/week	F: 3 times/week	F: 2–3 times/week	ICD/pacemaker: avoid activities with risk of contacting device or leads
	I: 30–60% VO_{2peak}	I: 3–5 min 30–40% VO_{2peak} + 1–3 min 60–85% VO_{2peak}	I: 30–60% MVC	
	T: 150 min/week, 30–60 min/day	T: 3–5 sets/day, 20–60 min/day	T: 10–15 reps/exercise, 1–2 sets/exercise, ≥30 min/day	
	T: Walking, jogging, cycling	T: Walking, jogging, cycling	T: Body weight (modified push-ups, pull-ups, squats), free weights, machine weights	

F Frequency, *I* intensity, *T* time/type, *MVC* maximum voluntary contraction. SL-GXT recommended: Document cardiac response to exertion. Individualized exercise prescription based on clinical status and response to SL-GXT

Modified from Takken et al. [17]. Used with permission

Table 25.3 The relation between rate of perceived exertion (Borg scale), % HR_{max}, and %VO_{2peak}

Intensity	% of HR_{max}	%VO_{2peak}	RPE
Very light	<35	<20	<10
Light	35–54	20–39	10–11
Moderate	55–69	40–59	12–13
Hard	70–89	60–84	14–16
Very hard	≥90	≥85	17–19

%VO_{2peak} percent VO_{2peak}, *RPE* rate of perceived exertion, *%HR_{max}* percent maximal heart rate achieved during SL-GXT

Modified from the *ACSM Guidelines for Exercise Testing and Prescription* [8]. Used with permission

scale is a practical and valid tool for monitoring exercise intensity that is independent of gender, age, and function status [63]. The American College of Sports Medicine (ACSM) has suggested that RPE adds precision to HR in monitoring exercise intensity [63]. It has been suggested that a strong relationship between RPE and heart rate exists during exercise, whereby 1 RPE point equates to roughly 10 bpm [63]. Exercising at an RPE of 11–15 ("light"—"moderate/hard") has been recommended for patients with CHD [53, 63].

Time: Experience with exercise training demonstrates that it is safe for most ACHD patients to participate in aerobic exercise for 15–30 min and gradually increase exercise duration to 20–45 min (as tolerated) [55, 64, 65]. These exercise sessions should also include a 10-min warm-up to prevent muscular strains and cardiac arrhythmias that might result from sudden exertion [64–70]. Sessions should conclude with a 10-min cool-down period of light exercise to prevent venous pooling [70].

Type: Between warm-up and cool-down, the type of exercise training provided will vary depending on equipment available but typically consists of a circuit of bicycle ergometer, treadmill, and other equipment that will allow involvement of a large percentage of the participant's muscle mass [33, 58, 60].

25.4.2 High-Intensity Interval Aerobic Training

While MCAT has been the mainstay of CR exercise prescription, outside the CR environment, interest in interval training has grown. High-intensity interval training (HIIT) results in greater cardiovascular stress and hence promotes greater training adaptation resulting in superior effects on aerobic capacity [71]. HIIT consists of alternating high-intensity work bouts (i.e., 90–100% VO_{2peak}, HR_{peak}, or peak power output [PPO]) with periods of rest or active recovery at relative low intensities (i.e., 30–60% VO_{2peak}, HR_{peak}, or PPO). Studies in healthy individuals found HIIT increased VO_{2peak}, O_2 pulse (i.e., VO_{2peak}/HR_{peak}), and post-training PPO [72].

HIIT may be more tolerable than MCAT. In healthy participants, short work periods at a higher intensity also result in a reduction in the ventilatory response and dyspnea. This has been shown to be of particular benefit to patients with chronic lung disease where dyspnea may limit exercise [73]. Guiraud et al. [71] reported that heart failure patients with severely reduced VO_{2peak} were able to spend a considerably longer period of time at 85% VO_{2peak} during 30 sec bouts of HIIT. These authors added that HIIT is better tolerated and allows patients to increase their total exercise time compared to longer exercise intervals [71].

HIIT allows for more intense exercise stimuli on peripheral muscles with less cardiac strain than MCAT [71]. Guiraud et al. [71] evaluated PPO (i.e., watts produced) and cardiac stress (i.e., rate pressure product) in HF patients during the last minute of interval exercise compared to MCAT and found that HIIT produced more than double the total PPO, while cardiac stress was 14% lower than during MCAT [74].

HIIT elicits positive adaptations compared to MCAT in healthy, CAD and HF participants [72, 75, 76]. Therefore, exploring the beneficial effects of HIIT in patients with CHD appears warranted.

Unfortunately, there is significant study-to-study variation in HIIT protocols, altering time spent at high intensities and time to exhaustion [71]. As such, there is no consensus on the appropriate HIIT protocol for clinical populations [71]. At present the role of HIIT is established in HF [75] and coronary artery disease patients [77], but data is lacking in the ACHD population.

25.4.3 Resistance Training

Resistance training (RT) specifically aims to increase muscular strength by targeted resistance exercises. Physical strength is important for functional capacity and activities of daily living. For healthy populations, the World Health Organization (W.H.O.) recommends strengthening exercises be performed 2–3 days/week, >30 min per session [78]. RT not only increases muscular strength but has been shown to increase aerobic capacity [79–81]. Some evidence indicates that RT independently improves both aerobic and anaerobic skeletal muscle performance in patients with CAD [82]. Feiereisen et al. [81] conducted a study in patients with HF utilizing RT (40 sessions; 3× per week for 45 min per day, consisting of 4 sets of 10 repetitions at 60–70% 1 repetition max (RM) of upper body, lower body, and trunk exercises). Their results showed an increase in VO_{2peak} by 16% versus 11% for MCAT (40 min at 60–75% VO_{2peak}) [81]. Ejection fraction was also shown to improve with RT over an 8-week and 12-week intervention (13% and 18% respectively) [81, 83]. Skeletal muscle function may be particularly important in those with Fontan circulation who lack a sub-pulmonary ventricle. Resistance training in this population has been shown to improve cardiac filling and cardiac output at rest, aerobic capacity, and a reduced dependence on respiration for venous return to the heart [57].

In training studies by McCall and Humphrey [58] and Rhodes et al. [66], light resistance exercises (e.g., 12–15 repetitions of 3–5 lbs barbells or elastic bands) were incorporated; however, neither group reported the impact of such training on muscular strength or endurance in patients with CHD. Thus, the additive effect of RT in ACHD patients remains unclear.

25.5 Benefits of Exercise Training for Adults with CHD

25.5.1 Overview

Because ACHD patients have a reduced aerobic capacity, an obvious question is whether exercise training can reduce symptoms and improve exercise tolerance. A growing body of evidence supports the efficacy of CR programs in improving aerobic capacity in ACHD patients [21]. In a report from Norway of 55 children and adolescents (mean age of 12 years) with CHD, a 5-month sport and recreation intervention performed at 60–85% HR_{peak} yielded slight improvements in exercise duration and VO_{2peak} [84]. In a similar study involving 61 ACHD participants (mean age of 32 years), Dua et al. [85] used a 10-week home-based walking program and demonstrated significantly increased walking time and VO_{2peak}. This implies that regular PA can improve aerobic capacity in patients with CHD. Several studies have reported that ACHD patients who had lower PA scores also recorded a lower VO_{2peak} [86, 87]. A systematic review by Duppen et al. [21] on the impact of CR in ACHD patients noted an average increase in VO_{2peak} of 2.6 mL/kg/min.

Improved aerobic capacity plays an integral part in activities of daily living; hence, it is considered an important health marker that may predict risk for morbidity and mortality [2]. Several studies have shown the associations between PA and aerobic capacity in healthy participants [88–90], and in addition to the physical benefits of MCAT, studies have shown improvements in mental health, self-esteem, resilience to stress, and sleep patterns and reduced anxiety and depression [21, 91].

25.5.2 Tetralogy of Fallot

CR for patients with ToF has been studied in two randomized controlled trials which demonstrated an improvement in aerobic capacity post-training. In a small study of 18 ToF adults, Therrien and colleagues [91] randomized patients to 12 weeks of MCAT versus usual care. They found a 2 mL/kg/min improvement in VO_{2peak} in the training group. Duppen et al. [92] conducted a randomized trial of 12 weeks of MCAT versus usual care in 47 young adults with ToF (mean age of 15 years). Their results supported the findings of Therrien and colleagues [91] as MCAT produced a 3 ml/kg/min improvement in VO_{2peak} compared to controls [92].

25.5.3 Systemic Right Ventricle: Transposition of the Great Arteries

Like patients with ToF who are at risk for sub-pulmonary right ventricular dysfunction, MCAT has been shown to be beneficial to patients with a systemic RV [43, 93]. Westhoff-Bleck et al. [93] evaluated 48 patients after an atrial redirection procedure (Mustard/Senning for TGA, mean age of 29 years) and showed a 24-week MCAT protocol at an intensity corresponding to 50% VO_{2peak} resulted in an ~8% increase in VO_{2peak} (3.8 mL/kg/min) compared to the control group, whose VO_{2peak} declined by 7.5%. Cardiac MRI performed before and after the MCAT program showed no adverse effect of training on systemic RV volume and function [93]. Similarly, Winter et al. [43] performed a randomized controlled trial of exercise training in 46 patients with a systemic RV (including both Mustard/Senning patients and ccTGA). They used a 10-week home-based, step aerobics interval training program (i.e., 5 sets of 4 min at 75–90% HR_{max} alternated with 4 sets of 3 min at 60% HR_{max}) and found an average increase in VO_{2peak} of 2.2 mL/kg/min in the exercise group [43].

25.5.4 Fontan Procedure

Multiple studies of MCAT in small numbers of Fontan patients have been performed across different centers, encompassing about 200 Fontan patients to date [94]. Longmuir et al. [95] published a cohort of 61 Fontan patients undergoing a 12-month home-based, "play-based" intervention intended to increase daily PA, without a specific intensity. These authors show an improvement of 2.3 mL/kg/min in VO_{2peak} and motor skill by 49% post-intervention [95]. Cordina et al. [57] conducted a novel study in 11 Fontan patients with an exercise intervention consisting of 20 weeks of high-intensity, total-body RT without an additional aerobic component. Significant increases in muscle mass, muscle strength, and VO_{2peak} and MRI-measured stroke volume and cardiac output were observed [51]. These findings underscore the potential importance of resistance training in the Fontan population.

25.6 Beyond Cardiac Rehabilitation: Recommendations for Physical Activity in ACHD

One of the desired outcomes of CR programs is that patients assume the responsibility to maintain their own PA once the CR program is completed. Unfortunately, there is ample data suggesting that by 1 year post-CR, many patients discontinue structured exercise training [96–98]. Since even simple unstructured activities at modest intensity may elicit significant health benefits [99], ACHD patients should be encouraged to engage in a physically active lifestyle, which includes both structured exercise and unstructured PA such as walking, cycling, or other leisure activities that involve continuous movement of large muscle groups [99].

According to the W.H.O, adults (aged 18–64 years) should accumulate 150 min of moderate-vigorous PA (i.e., ≥3.0 METs) each week, and the activities should be performed in bouts of ≥10 min [78, 86]. Sandberg et al. [100] reported that approximately half of ACHD patients did not achieve this W.H.O recommendation. Dua et al. [85] noted that while ACHD patients in New York Heart Association (NYHA) Class I were more active than NYHA Class II or III patients, overall only a small percentage of participants met the current W.H.O PA recommendation. While most ACHD patients are less active than their healthy peers, even those with complex lesions may still safely achieve daily activity recommendations [101].

One way to monitor and encourage ACHD patients to complete daily unstructured PA is through the use of accelerometers, which can assess daily step counts. Tudor-Locke et al. [102] suggested that, for optimal health benefits from PA, healthy young adults should achieve ≥10,000 steps per day. Several reports have documented that ACHD patients typically do not achieve this step goal [87, 100, 103]. HF patients, who have a similar aerobic capacity to ACHD patients, have a goal of ≥7,500 steps/day [87, 104].

Sedentary behavior (defined as <5,000 steps per day) is known to be increased in ACHD patients and is linked to reduced aerobic capacity [22, 101, 105–107]. Since there is evidence indicating that sedentary behavior is often replaced with light PA rather than more vigorous PA [108], CR staff may wish to encourage ACHD patients to reduce their sedentary behavior by increasing their time spent in light PA [108–111]. In fact more frequent breaks in sedentary time may result in greater engagement in light PA, which may be an important step toward a more active lifestyle [112]. Indeed, Manns et al. [111] have suggested that focusing on reducing sedentary behavior and increasing light PA may be a more feasible first step in PA behavior change and may lead to more successful and sustainable behavior change. PA counseling and ensuring good communication between clinician, therapist, and caregivers regarding PA recommendations should be emphasized [19].

25.7 Summary

Adults with CHD represent a unique and diverse group of patients presenting for cardiac rehabilitation. Understanding the specific congenital heart lesion, its hemodynamic sequelae, and long-term complications is important in designing an appropriate CR program. Aerobic capacity is reduced in ACHD and comparable to the elderly and HF patients. Assessment of exercise parameters with respiratory gas analysis yields several variables that are of prognostic value. Exercise prescription should be done after a baseline assessment of exercise capacity and adhere to exercise prescription guidelines. Exercise training, using MCAT, HIIT, and/or RT, has been shown to improve aerobic capacity in ACHD.

ACHD patients remain less physically active than their healthy peers. Regardless of the complexity of their cardiac lesions, ACHD should be encouraged to maintain an active lifestyle by participating in exercise that is interesting and enjoyable to them and to reduce sedentary behavior. By engaging in a physically active lifestyle, ACHD patients may lower their risk of developing CAD and adverse events related to their congenital defect, as well as experience an improvement in overall functional ability and quality of life.

References

1. Pinto NM, Marino BS, Wernovsky G, de Ferranti SD, Walsh AZ, Laronde M, et al. Obesity is a common comorbidity in children with congenital and acquired heart disease. Pediatrics. 2007;120(5):e1157–e64.
2. Lunt D, Briffa T, Briffa NK, Ramsay J. Physical activity levels of adolescents with congenital heart disease. Aust J Physiother. 2003;49(1):43–50.
3. Reybrouck T, Mertens L. Physical performance and physical activity in grown-up congenital heart disease. Eur J Cardiovasc Prev Rehabil. 2005;12(5):498–502.
4. Duppen N, Etnel JR, Spaans L, Takken T, van den Berg-Emons RJ, Boersma E, et al. Does exercise training improve cardiopulmonary fitness and daily physical activity in children and young adults with corrected tetralogy of Fallot or Fontan circulation? A randomized controlled trial. Am Heart J. 2015;170(3):606–14.
5. Gatzoulis M, Balaji S, Webber S, Siu S, Hokanson J, Poile C, et al. Risk factors for arrhythmia and sudden cardiac death late after repair of tetralogy of Fallot: a multicentre study. Lancet. 2000;356:975–81.

6. Baumgartner H, Bonhoeffer P, De Groot NM, de Haan F, Deanfield JE, Galie N, et al. ESC Guidelines for the management of grown-up congenital heart disease (new version 2010). Eur Heart J. 2010;31(23):2915–57.
7. Thompson PD, Arena R, Riebe D, Pescatello LS. ACSM's new preparticipation health screening recommendations from ACSM's guidelines for exercise testing and prescription. Curr Sports Med Rep. 2013;12(4):215–7.
8. American College of Sports Medicine. ACSM's guidelines for exercise testing and prescription. 10th ed. Philadelphia: Lippincott Williams & Wilkins; 2017.
9. Rhodes J, Tikkanen AU, Jenkins KJ. Exercise testing and training in children with congenital heart disease. Circulation. 2010;122(19):1957–67.
10. Buber J, Rhodes J. Exercise physiology and testing in adult patients with congenital heart disease. Heart Fail Clin. 2014;10(1):23–33.
11. Diller G-P, Dimopoulos K, Okonko D, Uebing A, Broberg CS, Babu-Narayan S, et al. Heart rate response during exercise predicts survival in adults with congenital heart disease. J Am Coll Cardiol. 2006;48(6):1250–6.
12. Kempny A, Dimopoulos K, Uebing A, Moceri P, Swan L, Gatzoulis MA, et al. Reference values for exercise limitations among adults with congenital heart disease. Relation to activities of daily life—single centre experience and review of published data. Eur Heart J. 2011;33(11):1386–96.
13. Inuzuka R, Diller G-P, Borgia F, Benson L, Tay EL, Alonso-Gonzalez R, et al. Comprehensive use of cardiopulmonary exercise testing identifies adults with congenital heart disease at increased mortality risk in the medium term. Circulation. 2012;125(2):250–9.
14. Balady GJ, Arena R, Sietsema K, Myers J, Coke L, Fletcher GF, et al. Clinician's guide to cardiopulmonary exercise testing in adults. Circulation. 2010;122(2):191–225.
15. Dempsey JA, Wagner PD. Exercise-induced arterial hypoxemia. J Appl Physiol. 1999;87(6):1997–2006.
16. Ross R, Blair SN, Arena R, Church TS, Després J-P, Franklin BA, et al. Importance of assessing cardiorespiratory fitness in clinical practice: a case for fitness as a clinical vital sign: a scientific statement from the American Heart Association. Circulation. 2016;134:e653.
17. Diller G, Dimopoulus K, Okonko D, Li W, Babu-Narayan S, Broberg C, et al. Exercise intolerance in adult congenital heart disease: comparative severity, correlates, and prognostic implication. Circulation. 2005;112:828–35.
18. Giardini A, Specchia S, Tacy TA, Coutsoumbas G, Gargiulo G, Donti A, et al. Usefulness of cardiopulmonary exercise to predict long-term prognosis in adults with repaired tetralogy of Fallot. Am J Cardiol. 2007;99(10):1462–7.
19. Takken T, Giardini A, Reybrouck T, Gewillig M, Hövels-Gürich H, Longmuir P, et al. Recommendations for physical activity, recreation sport, and exercise training in paediatric patients with congenital heart disease: a report from the Exercise, Basic & Translational Research Section of the European Association of Cardiovascular Prevention and Rehabilitation, the European Congenital Heart and Lung Exercise Group, and the Association for European Paediatric Cardiology. Eur J Prev Cardiol. 2012;19(5):1034–65.
20. Rhodes J. Serial exercise testing in patients with congenital heart disease. J Cardiol Ther. 2015;2(1):250–4.
21. Duppen N, Takken T, Hopman M, At H, Dulfer K, Utens E, et al. Systemic review of the effects of physical exercise training programmes in children and young adults with congenital heart disease. Int J Cardiol. 2013;168:1779–87.
22. Buys R, Cornelissen V, Van De Bruaene A, Stevens A, Coeckelberghs E, Onkelinx S, et al. Measures of exercise capacity in adults with congenital heart disease. Int J Cardiol. 2011;153(1):26–30.
23. Johnson JT, Yetman AT. Cardiopulmonary exercise testing in adults with congenital heart disease. Prog Pediatr Cardiol. 2012;34(1):47–52.
24. Müller J, Böhm B, Semsch S, Oberhoffer R, Hess J, Hager A. Currently, children with congenital heart disease are not limited in their submaximal exercise performance. Eur J Cardiothorac Surg. 2013;43(6):1096–100.

25. Beaver WL, Wasserman K, Whipp BJ. A new method for detecting anaerobic threshold by gas exchange. J Appl Physiol. 1986;60(6):2020–7.
26. Wasserman K. The anaerobic threshold measurement to evaluate exercise performance 1, 2. Am Rev Respir Dis. 1984;129(2P2):S35–40.
27. Mezzani A, Hamm LF, Jones AM, McBride PE, Moholdt T, Stone JA, et al. Aerobic exercise intensity assessment and prescription in cardiac rehabilitation: a joint position statement of the European Association for Cardiovascular Prevention and Rehabilitation, the American Association of Cardiovascular and Pulmonary Rehabilitation and the Canadian Association of Cardiac Rehabilitation. Eur J Prev Cardiol. 2013;20(3):442–67.
28. Dimopoulos K, Okonko DO, Diller GP, Broberg CS, Salukhe TV, Babu-Narayan SV, et al. Abnormal ventilatory response to exercise in adults with congenital heart disease relates to cyanosis and predicts survival. Circulation. 2006;113(24):2796–802.
29. Arena R, Myers J, Williams MA, Gulati M, Kligfield P, Balady GJ, et al. Assessment of functional capacity in clinical and research settings: a scientific statement from the American Heart Association Committee on Exercise, Rehabilitation, and Prevention of the Council on Clinical Cardiology and the Council on Cardiovascular Nursing. Circulation. 2007;116(3):329–43.
30. Clark AL, Gatzoulis MA, Redington AN. Ventilatory responses to exercise in adults after repair of tetralogy of Fallot. Br Heart J. 1995;73(5):445–9.
31. Fletcher GF, Ades PA, Kligfield P, Arena R, Balady GJ, Bittner VA, et al. Exercise standards for testing and training a scientific statement from the American Heart Association. Circulation. 2013;128(8):873–934.
32. Sutton NJ, Peng L, Lock JE, Lang P, Marx GR, Curran TJ, O'Neill JA, Picard ST, Rhodes J. Effect of pulmonary artery angioplasty on exercise function after repair of tetralogy of Fallot. Am Heart J. 2008;155(1):182–6.
33. Moalla W, Gauthier R, Maingourd Y, Ahmaidi S. Six-minute walking test to assess exercise tolerance and cardiorespiratory responses during training program in children with congenital heart disease. Int J Sports Med. 2005;26(9):756–62.
34. American Thoracic Society. ATS statement: guidelines for the six minute walk test. Am J Crit Care Med. 2002;166:111–7.
35. Rasekaba T, Lee A, Naughton M, Williams T, Holland A. The six-minute walk test: a useful metric for the cardiopulmonary patient. Intern Med J. 2009;39(8):495–501.
36. Williams MA, Haskell WL, Ades PA, Amsterdam EA, Bittner V, Franklin BA, et al. Resistance exercise in individuals with and without cardiovascular disease: 2007 update: a scientific statement from the American Heart Association Council on Clinical Cardiology and Council on Nutrition, Physical Activity, and Metabolism. Circulation. 2007;116(5):572–84.
37. Van De Bruaene A, Claessen G, La Gerche A, Kung E, Marsden A, De Meester P, et al. Effect of respiration on cardiac filling at rest and during exercise in Fontan patients: a clinical and computational modeling study. Int J Cardiol Heart Vasc. 2015;9:100–8.
38. Kim PS, Mayhew JL, Peterson DF. A modified YMCA bench press test as a predictor of 1 repetition maximum bench press strength. J Strength Cond Res. 2002;16(3):440–5.
39. Fredriksen PM, Veldtman G, Hechter S, Therrien J, Chen A, Warsi MA, et al. Aerobic capacity in adults with various congenital heart diseases. Am J Cardiol. 2001;87(3):310–4.
40. Foster E, Graham TP Jr, Driscoll DJ, Reid GJ, Reiss JG, Russell IA, et al. Task force 2: special health care needs of adults with congenital heart disease. J Am Coll Cardiol. 2001;37(5):1176–83.
41. Deanfield J, Thaulow E, Warnes C, Webb G, Kolbel F, Hoffman A, et al. Management of grown up congenital heart disease. Eur Heart J. 2003;24(11):1035–84.
42. Reybrouck T, Bisschop A, Dumoulin M, van der Hauwaert LG. Cardiorespiratory exercise capacity after surgical closure of atrial septal defect is influenced by the age at surgery. Am Heart J. 1991;122(4 Pt 1):1073–8.
43. Winter MM, van der Bom T, de Vries LCS, Balducci A, Bouma BJ, Pieper PG, et al. Exercise training improves exercise capacity in adult patients with a systemic right ventricle: a randomized clinical trial. Eur Heart J. 2012;33(11):1378–85.

44. Driscoll DJ, Staats BA, Heise CT, Rice MJ, Puga FJ, Danielson GK, et al. Functional single ventricle: cardiorespiratory response to exercise. J Am Coll Cardiol. 1984;4(2):337–42.
45. Driscoll DJ, Durongpisitkul K. Exercise testing after the Fontan operation. Pediatr Cardiol. 1999;20(1):57–9; discussion 60.
46. Sietsema KE, Cooper D, Perloff JK, Rosove M, Child J, Canobbio M, et al. Dynamics of oxygen uptake during exercise in adults with cyanotic congenital heart disease. Circulation. 1986;73(6):1137–44.
47. Sterrett LE, Ebenroth ES, Query C, Ho J, Montgomery GS, Hurwitz RA, et al. Why exercise capacity does not improve after pulmonary valve replacement. Pediatr Cardiol. 2014;35(8):1395–402.
48. Greutmann M, Le TL, Tobler D, Biaggi P, Oechslin EN, Silversides CK, et al. Generalised muscle weakness in young adults with congenital heart disease. Heart. 2011;97(14):1164–8.
49. Giardini A, Specchia S, Coutsoumbas G, Donti A, Formigari R, Fattori R, et al. Impact of pulmonary regurgitation and right ventricular dysfunction on oxygen uptake recovery kinetics in repaired tetralogy of Fallot. Eur J Heart Fail. 2006;8(7):736–43.
50. Mercer-Rosa L, Ingall E, Zhang X, McBride M, Kawut S, Fogel M, et al. The impact of pulmonary insufficiency on the right ventricle: a comparison of isolated valvar pulmonary stenosis and tetralogy of Fallot. Pediatr Cardiol. 2015;36(4):796–801.
51. Sabate Rotes A, Johnson JN, Burkhart HM, Eidem BW, Allison TG, Driscoll DJ. Cardiorespiratory response to exercise before and after pulmonary valve replacement in patients with repaired tetralogy of Fallot: a retrospective study and systematic review of the literature. Congenit Heart Dis. 2015;10(3):263–70.
52. Derrick GP, Narang I, White PA, Kelleher A, Bush A, Penny DJ, et al. Failure of stroke volume augmentation during exercise and dobutamine stress is unrelated to load-independent indexes of right ventricular performance after the Mustard operation. Circulation. 2000;102(Suppl 3):Iii-154–9.
53. Graham TP Jr, Driscoll DJ, Gersony WM, Newburger JW, Rocchini A, Towbin JA. Task force 2: congenital heart disease. J Am Coll Cardiol. 2005;45(8):1326–33.
54. Driscoll DJ, Danielson GK, Puga FJ, Schaff HV, Heise CT, Staats BA. Exercise tolerance and cardiorespiratory response to exercise after the Fontan operation for tricuspid atresia or functional single ventricle. J Am Coll Cardiol. 1986;7(5):1087–94.
55. Takken T, Tacken MH, Blank AC, Hulzebos EH, Strengers JL, Helders PJ. Exercise limitation in patients with Fontan circulation: a review. J Cardiovasc Med (Hagerstown). 2007;8(10):775–81.
56. Paridon SM, Mitchell PD, Colan SD, Williams RV, Blaufox A, Li JS, et al. A cross-sectional study of exercise performance during the first 2 decades of life after the Fontan operation. J Am Coll Cardiol. 2008;52(2):99–107.
57. Cordina RL, O'Meagher S, Karmali A, Rae CL, Liess C, Kemp GJ, et al. Resistance training improves cardiac output, exercise capacity and tolerance to positive airway pressure in Fontan physiology. Int J Cardiol. 2013;168(2):780–8.
58. McCall R, Humphrey R. Exercise training in a young adult late after a fontan procedure to repair single ventricle physiology. J Cardpulm Rehabil. 2001;21(4):227–30.
59. Minamisawa S, Nakazawa M, Momma K, Imai Y, Satomi G. Effect of aerobic training on exercise performance in patients after the Fontan operation. Am J Cardiol. 2001;88(6):695–8.
60. Moalla W, Maingourd Y, Gauthier R, Cahalin LP, Tabka Z, Ahmaidi S. Effect of exercise training on respiratory muscle oxygenation in children with congenital heart disease. Eur J Cardiovasc Prev Rehabil. 2006;13(4):604–11.
61. Opocher F, Varnier M, Sanders SP, Tosoni A, Zaccaria M, Stellin G, et al. Effects of aerobic exercise training in children after the Fontan operation. Am J Cardiol. 2005;95(1):150–2.
62. Budts W, Börjesson M, Chessa M, van Buuren F, Trindade PT, Corrado D, et al. Physical activity in adolescents and adults with congenital heart defects: individualized exercise prescription. Eur Heart J. 2013;34(47):3669–74.
63. Scherr J, Wolfarth B, Christle JW, Pressler A, Wagenpfeil S, Halle M. Associations between Borg's rating of perceived exertion and physiological measures of exercise intensity. Eur J Appl Physiol. 2013;113(1):147–55.

64. Tomassoni TL, Galioto P, Vaccaro P, Vaccaro J. Effects of exercise training on exercise tolerance and cardiac output in children after repair of congenital heart disease. Sports Train Med Rehab. 1990;2:57–62.
65. Tomassoni TL. Role of exercise in the management of cardiovascular disease in children and youth. Med Sci Sports Exerc. 1996;28(4):406–13.
66. Rhodes J, Curran TJ, Camil L, Rabideau N, Fulton DR, Gauthier NS, et al. Impact of cardiac rehabilitation on the exercise function of children with serious congenital heart disease. Pediatrics. 2005;116(6):1339–45.
67. Bradley LM, Galioto FM Jr, Vaccaro P, Hansen DA, Vaccaro J. Effect of intense aerobic training on exercise performance in children after surgical repair of tetralogy of Fallot or complete transposition of the great arteries. Am J Cardiol. 1985;56(12):816–8.
68. Calzolari A, Turchetta A, Biondi G, Drago F, De Ranieri C, Gagliardi G, et al. Rehabilitation of children after total correction of tetralogy of Fallot. Int J Cardiol. 1990;28(2):151–8.
69. Galioto F, Romassoni T. Cardiac rehabilitation for children with heart disease. Med Exerc Nutr Health. 1992;1:272–80.
70. Galioto F, Tomassoni T. Exercise rehabilitation in congenital heart disease. Prog Pediatr Cardiol. 1993;2(3):50–4.
71. Guiraud T, Nigam A, Gremeaux V, Meyer P, Juneau M, Bosquet L. High-intensity interval training in cardiac rehabilitation. Sports Med. 2012;42(7):587–605.
72. Astorino TA, Allen RP, Roberson DW, Jurancich M. Effect of high-intensity interval training on cardiovascular function, VO2max, and muscular force. J Strength Condit Res. 2012;26(1):138–45.
73. Beauchamp MK, Nonoyama M, Goldstein RS, Hill K, Dolmage TE, Mathur S, et al. Interval versus continuous training in individuals with chronic obstructive pulmonary disease—a systematic review. Thorax. 2010;65(2):157–64.
74. Meyer K, Samek L, Schwaibold M, Westbrook S, Hajric R, Beneke R, et al. Interval training in patients with severe chronic heart failure: analysis and recommendations for exercise procedures. Med Sci Sports Exerc. 1997;29(3):306–12.
75. Wisloff U, Stoylen A, Loennechen JP, Bruvold M, Rognmo O, Haram PM, et al. Superior cardiovascular effect of aerobic interval training versus moderate continuous training in heart failure patients: a randomized study. Circulation. 2007;115(24):3086–94.
76. Moholdt T, Aamot IL, Granoien I, Gjerde L, Myklebust G, Walderhaug L, et al. Long-term follow-up after cardiac rehabilitation: a randomized study of usual care exercise training versus aerobic interval training after myocardial infarction. Int J Cardiol. 2011;152(3):388–90.
77. Elliott AD, Rajopadhyaya K, Bentley DJ, Beltrame JF, Aromataris EC. Interval training versus continuous exercise in patients with coronary artery disease: a meta-analysis. Heart Lung Circ. 2015;24(2):149–57.
78. World Health Organization. Global recommendations on physical activity for health. Geneva: World Health Organization; 2010.
79. Kiilavuori K, Sovijärvi A, Näveri H, Ikonen T, Leinonen H. Effect of physical training on exercise capacity and gas exchange in patients with chronic heart failure. Chest. 1996;110(4):985–91.
80. Edelmann F, Gelbrich G, Düngen H-D, Fröhling S, Wachter R. Stahrenberg R, et al. In: Exercise training improves exercise capacity and diastolic function in patients with heart failure with preserved ejection fraction results of the ex-DHF (exercise training in diastolic heart failure) pilot study; 2015.
81. Feiereisen P, Delagardelle C, Vaillant M, Lasar Y, Beissel J. Is strength training the more efficient training modality in chronic heart failure? Med Sci Sports Exerc. 2007;39(11):1910–7.
82. Marzolini S, Oh PI, Thomas SG, Goodman JM. Aerobic and resistance training in coronary disease: single versus multiple sets. Med Sci Sports Exerc. 2008;40(9):1557–64.
83. Levinger I, Bronks R, Cody DV, Linton I, Davie A. The effect of resistance training on left ventricular function and structure of patients with chronic heart failure. Int J Cardiol. 2005;105(2):159–63.
84. Fredriksen PM, Kahrs N, Blaasvaer S, Sigurdsen E, Gundersen O, Roeksund O, et al. Effect of physical training in children and adolescents with congenital heart disease. Cardiol Young. 2000;10(2):107–14.

85. Dua JS, Cooper AR, Fox KR, Stuart AG. Exercise training in adults with congenital heart disease: feasibility and benefits. Int J Cardiol. 2010;138(2):196–205.
86. Haskell WL, Lee I-M, Pate RR, Powell KE, Blair SN, Franklin BA, et al. Physical activity and public health. Updated recommendation for adults from the American College of Sports Medicine and the American Heart Association Circulation. Med Sci Sports Exerc. 2007;39(8):1423–34.
87. Tudor-Locke C, Craig CL, Brown WJ, Clemes SA, De Cocker K, Giles-Corti B, et al. How many steps/day are enough? For adults. Int J Behav Nutr Phys Act. 2011;8:79.
88. Rognmo O, Moholdt T, Bakken H, Hole T, Molstad P, Myhr N, et al. Cardiovascular risk of high- versus moderate- intensity aerobic exercise in coronary heart disease patients. Circulation. 2012;126:1436–40.
89. Thorp AA, Owen N, Neuhaus M, Dunstan DW. Sedentary behaviors and subsequent health outcomes in adults: a systematic review of longitudinal studies, 1996–2011. Am J Prev Med. 2011;41(2):207–15.
90. Pate RR, Pratt M, Blair SN, Haskell WL, Macera CA, Bouchard C, et al. Physical activity and public health. A recommendation from the Centers for Disease Control and Prevention and the American College of Sports Medicine. JAMA. 1995;273(5):402–7.
91. Therrien J, Fredriksen P, Walker M, Granton J, Reid GJ, Webb G. A pilot study of exercise training in adult patients with repaired tetralogy of Fallot. Can J Cardiol. 2003;19(6):685–9.
92. Duppen N, Kapusta L, de Rijke Y, Snoeren M, Kuipers I, Koopman L, et al. The effect of exercise training on cardiac remodelling in children and young adults with corrected tetralogy of Fallot or Fontan circulation: a randomized controlled trial. Int J Cardiol. 2015;179:97–104.
93. Westhoff-Bleck M, Schieffer B, Tegtbur U, Meyer GP, Hoy L, Schaefer A, et al. Aerobic training in adults after atrial switch procedure for transposition of the great arteries improves exercise capacity without impairing systemic right ventricular function. Int J Cardiol. 2013;170(1):24–9.
94. Sutherland N, Jones B, d'Udekem Y. Should we recommend exercise after the Fontan procedure? Heart Lung Circ. 2015;24(8):753–68.
95. Longmuir PE, Tyrrell PN, Corey M, Faulkner G, Russell JL, McCrindle BW. Home-based rehabilitation enhances daily physical activity and motor skill in children who have undergone the Fontan procedure. Pediatr Cardiol. 2013;34(5):1130–51.
96. Moore SM, Charvat JM, Gordon NH, Roberts BL, Pashkow F, Ribisl P, et al. Effects of a CHANGE intervention to increase exercise maintenance following cardiac events. Ann Behav Med. 2006;31(1):53–62.
97. Bock BC, Carmona-Barros RE, Esler JL, Tilkemeier PL. Program participation and physical activity maintenance after cardiac rehabilitation. Behav Modif. 2003;27(1):37–53.
98. Stone JA, Arena R, Hauer T, Martin BJ, Austford LD, Aggarwal S. Long-term retention of aerobic fitness improvements following participation in cardiac rehabilitation. Int J Cardiol. 2011;150(3):355–6.
99. Longmuir PE, Brothers JA, de Ferranti SD, Hayman LL, Van Hare GF, Matherne GP, et al. Promotion of physical activity for children and adults with congenital heart disease a scientific statement from the American Heart Association. Circulation. 2013;127(21):2147–59.
100. Sandberg C, Pomeroy J, Thilén U, Gradmark A, Wadell K, Johansson B. Habitual physical activity in adults with congenital heart disease compared to age and gender matched controls. Can J Cardiol. 2016;32(4):547–53.
101. Müller J, Hess J, Hager A. Daily physical activity in adults with congenital heart disease is positively correlated with exercise capacity but not with quality of life. Clin Res Cardiol. 2012;101(1):55–61.
102. Tudor-Locke C, Bassett DR Jr. How many steps/day are enough? Preliminary pedometer indices for public health. Sports Med. 2004;34(1):1–8.
103. Dua JS, Cooper AR, Fox KR. Physical activity levels in adults with congenital heart disease. Eur J Cardiovasc Prev Rehabil. 2007;14(2):287–93.
104. Dontje ML, van der Wal MH, Stolk RP, Brugemann J, Jaarsma T, Wijtvliet PE, et al. Daily physical activity in stable heart failure patients. J Cardiovasc Nurs. 2014;29(3):218–26.

105. Buys R, Budts W, Delecluse C, Vanhees L. Determinants of physical activity in young adults with tetralogy of Fallot. Cardiol Young. 2014;24(1):20–6.
106. Lawler PR, Filion KB, Eisenberg MJ. Efficacy of exercise-based cardiac rehabilitation post-myocardial infarction: a systematic review and meta-analysis of randomized controlled trials. Am Heart J. 2011;162(4):571–84.e2.
107. Bassareo P, Saba L, Solla P, Barbanti C, Marras A, Mercuro G. Factors influencing adaptation and performance at physical exercise in complex congenital heart diseases after surgical repair. Biomed Res Int. 2014;2014:1.
108. Healy GN, Dunstan DW, Salmon J, Cerin E, Shaw JE, Zimmet PZ, et al. Breaks in sedentary time: beneficial associations with metabolic risk. Diabetes Care. 2008;31(4):661–6.
109. Tremblay MS, Warburton DE, Janssen I, Paterson DH, Latimer AE, Rhodes RE, et al. New Canadian physical activity guidelines. Appl Physiol Nutr Metab. 2011;36(1):36–46, 47–58.
110. Owen N, Healy GN, Matthews CE, Dunstan DW. Too much sitting: the population health science of sedentary behavior. Exerc Sport Sci Rev. 2010;38(3):105–13.
111. Manns PJ, Dunstan DW, Owen N, Healy GN. Addressing the nonexercise part of the activity continuum: a more realistic and achievable approach to activity programming for adults with mobility disability? Phys Ther. 2012;92(4):614–25.
112. Jakicic JM, Rickman AD, Lang W, Davis KK, Gibbs BB, Neiberg R, et al. Time-based physical activity interventions for weight loss: a randomized trial. Med Sci Sports Exerc. 2015;47(5):1061.

Neuropsychological Outcomes and Posttraumatic Stress Disorder in Adults with Congenital Heart Disease

26

Adrienne H. Kovacs

26.1 Introduction

It is well established that most infants born with congenital heart disease (CHD) now reach adulthood and are living longer lives than ever before. However, patients with moderate or complex CHD are not cured and require lifelong follow-up to effectively manage adult-onset medical sequelae. Examples include heart failure, arrhythmias, endocarditis, and additional surgeries and/or catheter interventions. Such complications often require hospital admissions and management in an intensive care unit (ICU). Patient needs in the inpatient setting, however, are not restricted to the physical domain and often carry psychosocial implications. Consider the two following cases:

Peter is a 52-year-old with bicuspid aortic valve stenosis who underwent mechanical aortic valve replacement yesterday. Leading up to this surgery, he had attended all clinic appointments on his own and expressed understanding and agreement with the decision to proceed with surgery and then initiate anticoagulation therapy. In the surgical ICU today, his elderly parents, with whom he lives, learn about warfarin treatment for the first time and express significant concern to the medical team about Peter's ability to take this on a daily basis and undergo regular monitoring. They explain that he has not succeeded with multiple previous attempts to oversee his medication regimen and schedule appointments; he relies on his parents for daily reminders. His parents are also concerned because Peter has recently seemed withdrawn and has less interest in usual hobbies. Peter's parents ask you to help them with a plan.

A. H. Kovacs
Knight Cardiovascular Institute, Oregon Health and Science University, Portland, OR, USA
e-mail: kovacs@ohsu.edu

E. da Cruz et al. (eds.), *Intensive Care of the Adult with Congenital Heart Disease*, Congenital Heart Disease in Adolescents and Adults,
https://doi.org/10.1007/978-3-319-94171-4_26

Maria is a 34-year-old who underwent Fontan revision 2 days ago. Since waking in the ICU, she has been visibly anxious and unable to sleep. Her husband explains that a psychiatrist recently diagnosed her with posttraumatic stress disorder (PTSD) associated with memories of pediatric cardiac surgery. She has very vivid recollections of feeling helpless during the recovery period. Maria's husband explains that Maria was concerned that if she had shared this information with the medical team prior to surgery, they would have been reluctant to proceed. He said that she now wants to be discharged from hospital and return to her home environment as soon as possible.

These two cases highlight the association between physical and psychosocial factors, which demands that we attend to both in order to optimize patient outcomes. In Peter's case, his limited self-management skills call into question his ability to remain adherent with postsurgical medication management (particularly when his parents become unable to care for him). For Maria, anxiety and sleep deprivation negatively impact quality of life and may interfere with surgical recovery. This bidirectional relationship between physical and psychosocial factors in the inpatient setting informs the overarching aims of this chapter. First, we hope to improve the awareness of adult CHD (ACHD) providers regarding the psychosocial challenges faced by many hospitalized adults with CHD, with a particular emphasis on neuropsychological outcomes and trauma experiences. Second, we aim to improve providers' abilities to more effectively recognize and address these challenges in the inpatient setting.

26.2 Neuropsychological Outcomes

26.2.1 Neurocognitive Functioning

Authors of an American Heart Association Scientific Statement on neurodevelopmental outcomes in children with CHD stated the following: "Among pediatric patients with complex CHD, there is a distinctive pattern of neurodevelopmental and behavioral impairment characterized by mild cognitive impairment, impaired social interaction, and impairments in core communication skills, including pragmatic language, as well as inattention, impulsive behavior, and impaired executive function" [1]. The risk and severity of neurodevelopmental impairment increase with defect complexity due to the contribution and interrelationships between multiple factors [1]. Although these are beyond the scope of this chapter, what is most relevant for ACHD providers is knowing that these problems do not vanish when a patient turns 18 and that the impact of neurocognitive deficits might become even more pronounced in adulthood [2].

Although neurodevelopmental deficits and disabilities are relatively understood in the pediatric setting, there have been far fewer studies examining neurocognitive outcomes among adults with CHD. In one of the earliest studies, published in 1994, Utens and colleagues compared the intellectual functioning of over 200 young adults (aged 18–35 years) with operated CHD to reference groups [3]. Overall, intellectual functioning was slightly higher than the reference group although 17% had scores indicative of borderline functioning or mental retardation. A subsequent study of 133 patients with Fontan physiology (including 33 adults ≥18 years) determined that the mean full-scale intelligence quotient (IQ) was 96, thus within the normal range, though still significantly lower than the general population [4]. These two studies suggested that, as a group, patients with CHD achieve IQ scores comparable to peers. However, in a study of 54 adults with tetralogy of Fallot (mean age of 32 years) who underwent neurocognitive testing in multiple domains, it was observed that difficulties with problem-solving, planning, and executive functions were more prevalent [5].

Studies from the past couple of years, with samples ranging from 18 to 310 patients, have shed further light on neurocognitive outcomes in adults with CHD [6–9]. In studies that enrolled patients with various forms of CHD, neuropsychological testing revealed deficits in the domains of visuospatial skills, working memory, divided attention, and executive functioning [6, 7]. Further, greater disease severity was associated with poorer outcomes [6–8]. A recent study compared adolescents and young adults with tetralogy of Fallot and d-transposition of the great arteries to reference norms as well as healthy, unaffected siblings [9]. The researchers observed that patients with CHD performed poorer than one or both comparison groups in terms of intelligence, processing speed, perceptual reasoning, and attention. In summary, particularly when assessment goes beyond IQ testing, neurocognitive deficits are more common among adults with CHD patients than their healthy peers.

Executive functions is a broad term that encompasses several abilities including inhibition, working memory, and cognitive flexibility [10]. Readers are referred to Diamond (2013) for an excellent review that includes a summary of ways in which executive function impairments impact "just about every aspect of life" including mental and physical health, quality of life, school readiness and success, employment success, marital satisfaction, and public safety [10]. There are modifiable factors that impact executive functions (e.g., stress, sleep, loneliness, physical inactivity) and known interventions to improve executive functions, including computer-based training, school curriculum-based strategies, mindfulness training, and physical activity [10, 11].

Deficits in executive functions are common in youth with CHD and create potential challenges with planning, problem-solving, and regulating one's behaviors [11–13], all of which are key for health-care oversight. As adolescents with CHD transition into adulthood and transfer to adult care, it is hoped (and often expected) that they will attain the knowledge and self-management skills in order to gradually assume responsibility for their health-care oversight and avoid lapses in care [14–16]. Examples of transition-related tasks include speaking independently with health providers, attending medical appointments, adhering with medications and other health behaviors, and recognizing situations in which urgent health care is indicated. The achievement of these tasks will certainly be more challenging for patients with deficits in cognitive skills, particularly executive function impairment. Among youth with type 1 diabetes, for example, an association between adherence, glycemic control, and executive functions has been observed [17].

Many adolescents with moderate and complex forms of CHD receive tutoring, occupational intervention, or special education [18, 19]. Adults with CHD, especially those with more complex disease, have historically been less likely to achieve higher education and employment [20–22]. Poorer executive functions have been associated with receiving disability [6]. In addition, many patients have difficulties with social cognition [23, 24], and social anxiety and loneliness have been associated with depressive and anxiety symptoms [25]. Factors indicative of better social functioning and executive functions (e.g., independent living, higher education, employment, and marriage) have been linked with superior quality of life [26, 27]. Thus, there is a relationship between neurocognitive outcomes and psychosocial well-being and quality of life that must be recognized.

Adult neurocognitive function is not solely predicted by fetal or pediatric-onset neurodevelopmental delays, deficits, and disorders. It has been suggested that patients with CHD are "vulnerably hosts" who face additional cognitive risks in adulthood [2]. Neurocognitive deficits may become more evident in early adulthood, a time in which individuals typically have less structured environments at school and home and face expectations of independent decision-making [2]. A lifelong perspective is necessary in order to understand the "cumulative burden of injury" [28]. Adult-onset factors include the risk of stroke, acquired cardiovascular disease, end-stage heart failure, atrial fibrillation, cardiac surgery, and critical illness [29–41].

26.2.2 Psychological Functioning

A meta-analysis of 22 studies revealed no consistent evidence of increased psychological distress among adults with CHD, although significant heterogeneity in methodology (e.g., patient samples, measures of distress) was noted and 2 of 3 American samples were indicative of elevated distress among patients [42]. Although the research remains equivocal from a global perspective, North American studies that employed diagnostic clinical interviews suggested that approximately one-third face significant depression and/or anxiety [25, 43, 44]. What are most concerning regarding psychosocial outcomes of adults with CHD are two sets of findings. First, few adults with CHD and mood or anxiety disorders receive psychological care [25, 43, 44]. The reasons for this are certainly multifactorial and likely reflect under-recognition by health-care providers, under-disclosure by patients to providers, and challenges accessing suitable mental health-care providers. Second, among adults with CHD, psychological symptoms have been linked with nonadherence, increased morbidity and mortality, and higher resource use [45–47].

Screening for depression has been recommended in both congenital and acquired heart disease [48, 49]. However, this recommendation is not without its detractors who emphasize that routine screening for depression is a resource-intensive process that has not been proven to consistently improve mood or cardiac outcomes [50]. Further, screening that is limited to depression would not identify patients with other psychiatric disorders (e.g., anxiety, trauma-related conditions, and substance use) or neurocognitive deficits. In a retrospective study of 100 adults with CHD who presented for psychological services, anxiety concerns were observed to be more prominent than mood disturbance [51]. In summary, effective and efficient strategies to identify patients with clinically significant neurocognitive and/or psychosocial challenges in the outpatient setting are currently unknown.

As a group, adults with CHD value access to mental health care. In a study of over 150 patients, half reported high interest in psychological treatment, most often coping with a cardiac condition and/or stress management [52]. Qualitative research has also supported patients' desire for counseling and opportunities for peer interaction [53]. Approaches for psychotherapy include cognitive-behavioral therapy, interpersonal therapy, and mindfulness interventions [54–60]. Although selective serotonin reuptake inhibitors are considered safest for adults with cardiovascular disease [61, 62], these have not been studied specifically in adults with CHD. It has been suggested that, "many cardiac patients do not want traditional psychiatric treatment but will accept treatment from a clinician who specializes in working with cardiac patients" [63].

26.2.3 Implications for the ICU Setting

Strategies to effectively integrate behavioral health into cardiovascular care have not been established [63], and this holds true in both outpatient and inpatient settings. Within the ACHD field, most psychosocial research has been conducted in the outpatient setting, and we know little about the experiences of hospitalized patients. It is reasonable to hypothesize, however, that psychosocial challenges are amplified when admitted to critical care units. For example, it is difficult to attend to and retain information when distressed. Further, patients are often restricted from usual coping strategies, such as distraction (e.g., with hobbies and interests), physical activity, spending time with pets, and social support. Given that specialized ACHD care is not available in all institutions, many patients are hospitalized far from home [64], which impacts their ability to have face-to-face contact with supportive family and friends. Differences in the provision of mental health care in outpatient vs. inpatient environments should also be noted. Within the inpatient setting, traditional psychotherapy practices (an initial longer assessment followed by regular 45–60-min sessions) might be less realistic given challenges with patient alertness, fatigue, and pain. ACHD programs are thus encouraged to identify mental health providers (such as psychologists, psychiatrists, counselors, and clinical social workers), palliative care professionals, spiritual care providers, and peer support volunteers who can provide emotional support to patients.

When discussing psychosocial challenges, regarding of the setting, it is advised to normalize experiences in order to reduce the stigma often associated with mental health concerns. For example, a provider can explain that "It's very common and understandable that someone would experience emotional distress in this situation." However, it's also important to avoid assumptions and generalizations. For example, although one-third of North American patients might have clinically significant depression and/or anxiety, the corollary is that two-thirds do not [25, 43, 44]. Thus, resilience factors should be explored and emphasized.

In the inpatient setting, the impact of cognitive deficits on patient adherence and decision-making warrants attention [6]. A lot of information can be gleaned from careful questioning of a patient's academic and employment history (e.g., participation in special education, diagnosis of a learning disability or attention deficit hyperactivity disorder, employment limitations) [2]. It is preferable to know about neurocognitive deficits *prior* to hospitalization (e.g., in the case of elective admissions) so that patient education and support can be modified as appropriate.

26.3 Trauma and Adult Congenital Heart Disease

26.3.1 Posttraumatic Stress Disorder and Cardiovascular Disease

In the fourth edition of the *Diagnostic and Statistical Manual of Mental Disorders* (DSM-IV), PTSD was categorized as an anxiety disorder [65]. In the fifth edition, however, it was reclassified into a new category named trauma- and stressor-related disorders [66]. Current diagnostic criteria include the following: (1) exposure to a traumatic event, (2) intrusion symptoms (e.g., flashbacks), (3) avoidance of stimuli associated with the event, (4) negative cognitions and mood, and (5) increased arousal/reactivity. The symptoms must last longer than 1 month, not be due to the physiological effects of a substance or another medical condition, and cause clinically significant distress and/or functional impairment. The same criteria apply to anyone over the age of 6 years, and there are separate criteria for children 6 years and younger. Shalev et al. explained that "PTSD is characterized by hypervigilance that is inappropriate to the situation and the misreading of cues as threatening despite a safe context" [67]. In the United States, the 12-month prevalence of PTSD is 3.5% [68], and the lifetime prevalence is estimated to be between 7 and 8% [69, 70]. However, published studies that relied on clinical interview methodology most often used older DSM-IV criteria, and the impact of the updated diagnostic criteria on prevalence remains unknown [67, 71].

The inclusion of life-threatening illness, such as cardiovascular disease, as a potentially traumatic event is not without controversy [71]. According to the DSM-V, "A life-threatening illness or debilitating medical condition is not necessarily considered a traumatic event" and "Medical incidents that qualify as traumatic events involve sudden, catastrophic events." However, the sheer number of published studies of PTSD associated with cardiovascular disease warrants consideration of cardiac disease as a qualifying traumatic event. In a 2017 systematic review of 150 studies, the prevalence of cardiac-disease-induced PTSD (CDI-PTSD) ranged from 0 to 38% [71]. The authors found that there were few reliable demographic risk factors, that patient-perceived severity of the illness was more relevant than objective disease severity, and that the most consistent risk factor was psychological functioning (e.g., distress before or during the event or personality difficulties). The authors concluded that CDI-PTSD shares many characteristics of PTSD unrelated to life-threatening illnesses, although there are unique features of CDI-PTSD.

Among adults with acquired heart disease, PTSD is known to have negative implications for health outcomes (e.g., mortality or recurrent cardiac events) [72–74]. The recommended treatment for PTSD is trauma-focused cognitive-behavioral therapy, of which exposure therapy is typically an important component [67]. However, few interventions have been developed for CDI-PTSD [71].

26.3.2 Posttraumatic Stress Disorder and Adult Congenital Heart Disease

In the 2017 systematic review of CDI-PTSD, most studies included patients following acute coronary syndrome/myocardial infarction and none included adults with CHD [71]. Further, in most studies, PTSD was assessed within 18 months of the traumatic event. Although it is natural to extrapolate from what is known about PTSD in acquired heart disease, there are certainly unique circumstances for adults with CHD. For example, traumas such as cardiac surgery might have occurred years or even decades before.

Two studies have investigated PTSD in adults with CHD. In the first, Deng and colleagues investigated the prevalence of self-reported symptoms of PTSD in 134 adults with CHD [75]. They found that over half of patients reported at least one traumatic medical event including cardiac surgery, arrhythmia, heart failure, stroke, cardiac arrest, or non-cardiac events (e.g., motor vehicle accident, cancer). Of patients who had previously had cardiac surgery, approximately one in three identified this as a traumatic event. A likely diagnosis of PTSD was observed in 21% of patients using a measure of global PTSD symptoms and in 11% of patients when using a measure in which patients were asked to focus on CHD as the stressor. Using both measures, elevated PTSD symptoms were associated with lower quality of life.

In a second study of 347 adults with CHD from Iran, Eslami observed that 52% of patients met criteria for a likely diagnosis of PTSD [76]. Although this prevalence appears noticeably higher than that observed in the US study, it should be noted that 48% of adults without CHD also met diagnostic criteria. Eslami thus emphasized the importance of considering contextual factors (e.g., cultural, social, and political variables) in which patients live as they often face additional stressors unrelated to health.

In the Iranian study, PTSD was associated with a history of cardiac surgery, whereas in the US study, an earlier year of most recent surgery was an associated factor [75, 76]. Although these two studies included three different measures of PTSD, a consistent finding was that symptoms of depression were positively associated with PTSD [75, 76]. Thus, we should consider the entire context of psychological well-being without limiting our focus to any one specific diagnosis.

26.3.3 Implications for the ICU Setting

The two studies that investigated PTSD in adults with CHD were conducted in the outpatient clinic or home environment rather than the inpatient setting. Thus, the prevalence of PTSD in adults with CHD in the inpatient setting remains unknown. However, all providers managing patients in the inpatient setting are encouraged to be mindful of two factors. First, most adults with CHD admitted to critical care units will have a history of cardiac interventions which might be perceived as traumatic events by patients. The best way to know this is by asking patients and families. Second, critical care admissions may themselves be perceived as traumatic events. Although we do not know the best strategies to ameliorate the effects of negative inpatient experiences, opportunities to empower and support patients in the ICU are clearly encouraged.

In addition, according to DSM diagnostic criteria, a traumatic event need not be directly experienced by an individual and may also entail learning that a traumatic event occurred to a close family member or friend [66]. Thus, although beyond the focus of this paper, the potential for PTSD among patients' parents and partners should also be recognized [77].

Conclusion

Compared to healthy peers, adults with CHD are at elevated risk of neurocognitive deficits, mood and anxiety disorders, and PTSD. These psychosocial concerns have historically been under recognized and undertreated in the outpatient setting, and we know very little about patient and family experiences in the ICU setting. Table 26.1 provides recommendations to enhance psychosocial care in the inpatient setting, divided into suggestions for (1) outpatient consultations prior to admission (i.e., for patients with planned hospitalizations), (2) during the hospital admission, and (3) in the follow-up period. Comprehensive care for hospitalized patients entails interdisciplinary collaboration to attend to the complex interplay that often exists between physical and psychosocial needs.

Table 26.1 Recommendations to enhance psychosocial care in the inpatient setting

Prior to hospital admission (when possible with planned admissions)	Explain to patients that understanding their cognitive/learning abilities and psychosocial concerns will help the team provide optimal care
	Inquire about education and employment history
	If a patient is receiving disability, ask for the reason(s) they qualify
	Inquire about the degree to which a patient assumes responsibility for health-care oversight
	Inquire whether the patient has been diagnosed with a psychiatric problem and/or has had mental health treatment
	Inquire about the patient's coping with previous hospitalizations and surgeries
	Inquire about planned social support during hospitalization

Table 26.1 (continued)

During hospital admission	Be aware that adults with CHD are at elevated risk of neurocognitive deficits, including difficulties with attention, memory, and executive functions and that these might impact understanding treatment recommendations, adherence, and medical decision-making
	Normalize psychosocial difficulties while also avoid making assumptions or generalizations about patient neurocognitive and psychosocial functioning
	When providing patient education or discussing complex treatments and decision-making, provide information in both verbal and written formats, ideally over multiple occasions, and include family and/or friend supports whenever possible
	Given that many adults with CHD admitted to the ICU will live a significant distance from the hospital, encourage virtual contact with loves ones through telephone and the Internet
	Recognize that inpatient admissions can be extremely difficult for loved ones and explore ways to support family members as much as possible
	Establish resources to identify patients with clinically significant neurocognitive deficits and/or psychosocial distress to whom services should be targeted
	Identify health professionals (e.g., psychiatrists, psychologists, counselors, clinical social workers, palliative care professionals, spiritual care providers, peer support volunteers) who can provide support to patients and families
Following hospital admission	Inquire about adherence and barriers to adherence
	Inquire about post-hospitalization mood, anxiety, and trauma-related distress, with a focus on intensity, duration, and impact of symptoms
	Develop clinical algorithms for major health-related events that would benefit from interdisciplinary assessment and care (e.g., complex cardiac surgery, extended ICU stay, sudden cardiac arrest, implantable cardioverter defibrillator shock)

References

1. Marino BS, Lipkin PH, Newburger JW, Peacock G, Gerdes M, Gaynor JW, et al. Neurodevelopmental outcomes in children with congenital heart disease: evaluation and management: a scientific statement from the American Heart Association. Circulation. 2012;126(9):1143–72.
2. Wilson WM, Smith-Parrish M, Marino BS, Kovacs AH. Neurodevelopmental and psychosocial outcomes across the congenital heart disease lifespan. Prog Pediatr Cardiol. 2015;39:113–8.
3. Utens EM, Verhulst FC, Erdman RA, Meijboom FJ, Duivenvoorden HJ, Bos E, et al. Psychosocial functioning of young adults after surgical correction for congenital heart disease in childhood: a follow-up study. J Psychosom Res. 1994;38(7):745–58.
4. Wernovsky G, Stiles KM, Gauvreau K, Gentles TL, du Plessis AJ, Bellinger DC, et al. Cognitive development after the Fontan operation. Circulation. 2000;102(8):883–9.
5. Daliento L, Mapelli D, Russo G, Scarso P, Limongi F, Iannizzi P, et al. Health related quality of life in adults with repaired tetralogy of Fallot: psychosocial and cognitive outcomes. Heart. 2005;91(2):213–8.
6. Ilardi D, Ono KE, McCartney R, Book W, Stringer AY. Neurocognitive functioning in adults with congenital heart disease. Congenit Heart Dis. 2016;12(2):166–73.

7. Tyagi M, Fteropoulli T, Hurt CS, Hirani SP, Rixon L, Davies A, et al. Cognitive dysfunction in adult CHD with different structural complexity. Cardiol Young. 2017;27(5):851–9.
8. Klouda L, Franklin WJ, Saraf A, Parekh DR, Schwartz DD. Neurocognitive and executive functioning in adult survivors of congenital heart disease. Congenit Heart Dis. 2017;12(1):91–8.
9. Murphy LK, Compas BE, Reeslund KL, Gindville MC, Mah ML, Markham LW, et al. Cognitive and attentional functioning in adolescents and young adults with Tetralogy of Fallot and d-transposition of the great arteries. Child Neuropsychol. 2017;23(1):99–110.
10. Diamond A. Executive functions. Annu Rev Psychol. 2013;64:135–68.
11. Calderon J, Bellinger DC. Executive function deficits in congenital heart disease: why is intervention important? Cardiol Young. 2015;25(7):1238–46.
12. Marino BS, Beebe D, Cassedy A, Riedel M, Burger M, Medek S, et al. Executive functioning, gross motor ability and mood are key drivers of poorer quality of life in child and adolescent survivors with complex congenital heart disease. J Am Coll Cardiol. 2011;57:E421.
13. Cassidy AR, White MT, DeMaso DR, Newburger JW, Bellinger DC. Executive function in children and adolescents with critical cyanotic congenital heart disease. J Int Neuropsychol Soc. 2015;21(1):34–49.
14. Sable C, Foster E, Uzark K, Bjornsen K, Canobbio MM, Connolly HM, et al. Best practices in managing transition to adulthood for adolescents with congenital heart disease: the transition process and medical and psychosocial issues: a scientific statement from the American Heart Association. Circulation. 2011;123(13):1454–85.
15. Kovacs AH, McCrindle BW. So hard to say goodbye: transition from paediatric to adult cardiology care. Nat Rev Cardiol. 2014;11(1):51–62.
16. Kovacs AH, Webb GD. Preparing pediatric patients for adult care: are we ready? J Pediatr. 2015;167(6):1194–5.
17. Duke DC, Harris MA. Executive function, adherence, and glycemic control in adolescents with type 1 diabetes: a literature review. Curr Diab Rep. 2014;14(10):532.
18. Bellinger DC, Wypij D, Rivkin MJ, DeMaso DR, Robertson RL Jr, Dunbar-Masterson C, et al. Adolescents with d-transposition of the great arteries corrected with the arterial switch procedure: neuropsychological assessment and structural brain imaging. Circulation. 2011;124(12):1361–9.
19. Bellinger DC, Rivkin MJ, DeMaso D, Robertson RL, Stopp C, Dunbar-Masterson C, et al. Adolescents with tetralogy of Fallot: neuropsychological assessment and structural brain imaging. Cardiol Young. 2015;25(2):338–47.
20. Geyer S, Norozi K, Buchhorn R, Wessel A. Chances of employment in women and men after surgery of congenital heart disease: comparisons between patients and the general population. Congenit Heart Dis. 2009;4(1):25–33.
21. Karsenty C, Maury P, Blot-Souletie N, Ladouceur M, Leobon B, Senac V, et al. The medical history of adults with complex congenital heart disease affects their social development and professional activity. Arch Cardiovasc Dis. 2015;108(11):589–97.
22. Sluman MA, Apers S, Bouma BJ, van Melle JP, Peels CH, Post MC, et al. Uncertainties in insurances for adults with congenital heart disease. Int J Cardiol. 2015;186:93–5.
23. Bellinger DC. Are children with congenital cardiac malformations at increased risk of deficits in social cognition? Cardiol Young. 2008;18(1):3–9.
24. Bellinger DC. Theory of mind deficits in children with congenital heart disease. Dev Med Child Neurol. 2010;52(12):1079–80.
25. Kovacs AH, Saidi AS, Kuhl EA, Sears SF, Silversides C, Harrison JL, et al. Depression and anxiety in adult congenital heart disease: predictors and prevalence. Int J Cardiol. 2009;137(2):158–64.
26. Apers S, Kovacs AH, Luyckx K, Thomet C, Budts W, Enomoto J, et al. Quality of life of adults with congenital heart disease in 15 countries: evaluating country-specific characteristics. J Am Coll Cardiol. 2016;67(19):2237–45.
27. Moons P, Van Deyk K, Marquet K, Raes E, De Bleser L, Budts W, et al. Individual quality of life in adults with congenital heart disease: a paradigm shift. Eur Heart J. 2005;26(3):298–307.
28. Marelli A, Miller SP, Marino BS, Jefferson AL, Newburger JW. Brain in congenital heart disease across the lifespan: the cumulative burden of injury. Circulation. 2016;133(20):1951–62.

29. Lanz J, Brophy JM, Therrien J, Kaouache M, Guo L, Marelli AJ. Stroke in adults with congenital heart disease: incidence, cumulative risk, and predictors. Circulation. 2015;132(25):2385–94.
30. Eggermont LH, de Boer K, Muller M, Jaschke AC, Kamp O, Scherder EJ. Cardiac disease and cognitive impairment: a systematic review. Heart. 2012;98(18):1334–40.
31. Vogels RL, Oosterman JM, van Harten B, Scheltens P, van der Flier WM, Schroeder-Tanka JM, et al. Profile of cognitive impairment in chronic heart failure. J Am Geriatr Soc. 2007;55(11):1764–70.
32. Vogels RL, Scheltens P, Schroeder-Tanka JM, Weinstein HC. Cognitive impairment in heart failure: a systematic review of the literature. Eur J Heart Fail. 2007;9(5):440–9.
33. Gyurak A, Goodkind MS, Kramer JH, Miller BL, Levenson RW. Executive functions and the down-regulation and up-regulation of emotion. Cogn Emot. 2012;26(1):103–18.
34. Cacciatore F, Abete P, Ferrara N, Calabrese C, Napoli C, Maggi S, et al. Congestive heart failure and cognitive impairment in an older population. Osservatorio Geriatrico Campano Study Group. J Am Geriatr Soc. 1998;46(11):1343–8.
35. Trojano L, Antonelli Incalzi R, Acanfora D, Picone C, Mecocci P, Rengo F, et al. Cognitive impairment: a key feature of congestive heart failure in the elderly. J Neurol. 2003;250(12):1456–63.
36. Pressler SJ. Cognitive functioning and chronic heart failure: a review of the literature (2002–July 2007). J Cardiovasc Nurs. 2008;23(3):239–49.
37. Zuccala G, Onder G, Pedone C, Carosella L, Pahor M, Bernabei R, et al. Hypotension and cognitive impairment: selective association in patients with heart failure. Neurology. 2001;57(11):1986–92.
38. Kalantarian S, Ruskin JN. Cognitive impairment associated with atrial fibrillation—in response. Ann Intern Med. 2013;158(11):849.
39. Newman MF, Kirchner JL, Phillips-Bute B, Gaver V, Grocott H, Jones RH, et al. Longitudinal assessment of neurocognitive function after coronary-artery bypass surgery. N Engl J Med. 2001;344(6):395–402.
40. Pandharipande PP, Girard TD, Jackson JC, Morandi A, Thompson JL, Pun BT, et al. Long-term cognitive impairment after critical illness. N Engl J Med. 2013;369(14):1306–16.
41. Ammash N, Warnes CA. Cerebrovascular events in adult patients with cyanotic congenital heart disease. J Am Coll Cardiol. 1996;28(3):768–72.
42. Jackson JL, Misiti B, Bridge JA, Daniels CJ, Vannatta K. Emotional functioning of adolescents and adults with congenital heart disease: a meta-analysis. Congenit Heart Dis. 2015;10(1):2–12.
43. Horner T, Liberthson R, Jellinek MS. Psychosocial profile of adults with complex congenital heart disease. Mayo Clin Proc. 2000;75(1):31–6.
44. Bromberg JI, Beasley PJ, D'Angelo EJ, Landzberg M, DeMaso DR. Depression and anxiety in adults with congenital heart disease: a pilot study. Heart Lung. 2003;32(2):105–10.
45. White KS, Pardue C, Ludbrook P, Sodhi S, Esmaeeli A, Cedars A. Cardiac denial and psychological predictors of cardiac care adherence in adults with congenital heart disease. Behav Modif. 2016;40(1–2):29–50.
46. Kourkoveli P, Rammos S, Parissis J, Maillis A, Kremastinos D, Paraskevaidis I. Depressive symptoms in patients with congenital heart disease: incidence and prognostic value of self-rating depression scales. Congenit Heart Dis. 2015;10(3):240–7.
47. Kim YY, Gauvreau K, Bacha EA, Landzberg MJ, Benavidez OJ. Resource use among adult congenital heart surgery admissions in pediatric hospitals: risk factors for high resource utilization and association with inpatient death. Circ Cardiovasc Qual Outcomes. 2011;4(6):634–9.
48. Lichtman JH, Bigger JT Jr, Blumenthal JA, Frasure-Smith N, Kaufmann PG, Lesperance F, et al. Depression and coronary heart disease: recommendations for screening, referral, and treatment: a science advisory from the American Heart Association Prevention Committee of the Council on Cardiovascular Nursing, Council on Clinical Cardiology, Council on Epidemiology and Prevention, and Interdisciplinary Council on Quality of Care and Outcomes Research: endorsed by the American Psychiatric Association. Circulation. 2008;118(17):1768–75.
49. Warnes CA, Williams RG, Bashore TM, Child JS, Connolly HM, Dearani JA, et al. ACC/AHA 2008 guidelines for the management of adults with congenital heart disease: a report of the American College of Cardiology/American Heart Association Task Force on Practice

Guidelines (Writing Committee to Develop Guidelines on the Management of Adults with Congenital Heart Disease). Developed in Collaboration with the American Society of Echocardiography, Heart Rhythm Society, International Society for Adult Congenital Heart Disease, Society for Cardiovascular Angiography and Interventions, and Society of Thoracic Surgeons. J Am Coll Cardiol. 2008;52(23):e1–121.

50. Thombs BD, Roseman M, Coyne JC, de Jonge P, Delisle VC, Arthurs E, et al. Does evidence support the American Heart Association's recommendation to screen patients for depression in cardiovascular care? An updated systematic review. PLoS One. 2013;8(1):e52654.
51. Ferguson M, Kovacs AH. An integrated adult congenital heart disease psychology service. Congenit Heart Dis. 2016;11(5):444–51.
52. Kovacs AH, Bendell KL, Colman J, Harrison JL, Oechslin E, Silversides C. Adults with congenital heart disease: psychological needs and treatment preferences. Congenit Heart Dis. 2009;4(3):139–46.
53. Page MG, Kovacs AH, Irvine J. How do psychosocial challenges associated with living with congenital heart disease translate into treatment interests and preferences? A qualitative approach. Psychol Health. 2012;27(11):1260–70.
54. Butler AC, Chapman JE, Forman EM, Beck AT. The empirical status of cognitive-behavioral therapy: a review of meta-analyses. Clin Psychol Rev. 2006;26(1):17–31.
55. Hofmann SG, Smits JAJ. Cognitive-behavioral therapy for adult anxiety disorders: a meta-analysis of randomized placebo-controlled trials. J Clin Psychiatry. 2008;69(4):621–32.
56. Kovacs AH, Bandyopadhyay M, Grace SL, Kentner AC, Nolan RP, Silversides CK, et al. Adult Congenital Heart Disease-Coping And REsilience (ACHD-CARE): rationale and methodology of a pilot randomized controlled trial. Contemp Clin Trials. 2015;45(Pt B):385–93.
57. Morton L. Can interpersonal psychotherapy (IPT) meet the psychosocial cost of life gifted by medical intervention. Couns Psychol Rev. 2011;26(3):75–86.
58. Abbott RA, Whear R, Rodgers LR, Bethel A, Coon JT, Kuyken W, et al. Effectiveness of mindfulness-based stress reduction and mindfulness based cognitive therapy in vascular disease: a systematic review and meta-analysis of randomised controlled trials. J Psychosom Res. 2014;76(5):341–51.
59. Bohlmeijer E, Prenger R, Taal E, Cuijpers P. The effects of mindfulness-based stress reduction therapy on mental health of adults with a chronic medical disease: a meta-analysis. J Psychosom Res. 2010;68(6):539–44.
60. Kabat-Zinn J. Full catastrophe living: using the wisdom of your body and mind to face stress, pain, and illness (15th anniversary ed.). New York: Delta Trade Paperback/Bantam Dell; 2005. 471-xxxiii p.
61. Hare DL, Toukhsati SR, Johansson P, Jaarsma T. Depression and cardiovascular disease: a clinical review. Eur Heart J. 2014;35(21):1365–72.
62. Nezafati MH, Vojdanparast M, Nezafati P. Antidepressants and cardiovascular adverse events: a narrative review. ARYA Atheroscler. 2015;11(5):295–304.
63. Dornelas EA. Behavioral cardiology: toward the development of integrated treatment models. In: Dornelas EA, editor. Stress proof the heart: behavioral interventions for cardiac patients. New York: Springer; 2012. p. 389–400.
64. Soufi A, Colman JM, Li Q, Oechslin EN, Kovacs AH. Review of non-elective hospitalisations of adults with CHD. Cardiol Young. 2017;27(9):1764–70.
65. American Psychiatric Association. Diagnostic and statistical manual of mental disorders. 4th ed., text rev ed. Washington: Author; 2000.
66. American Psychiatric Association. Diagnostic and statistical manual of mental disorders. 5th ed. Washington, DC: Author; 2013.
67. Shalev A, Liberzon I, Marmar C. Post-traumatic stress disorder. N Engl J Med. 2017;376(25):2459–69.
68. Kessler RC, Chiu WT, Demler O, Merikangas KR, Walters EE. Prevalence, severity, and comorbidity of 12-month DSM-IV disorders in the National Comorbidity Survey Replication. Arch Gen Psychiatry. 2005;62(6):617–27.
69. Keane TM, Marshall AD, Taft CT. Posttraumatic stress disorder: etiology, epidemiology, and treatment outcome. Annu Rev Clin Psychol. 2006;2:161–97.

70. Kessler RC, Berglund P, Demler O, Jin R, Merikangas KR, Walters EE. Lifetime prevalence and age-of-onset distributions of DSM-IV disorders in the National Comorbidity Survey Replication. Arch Gen Psychiatry. 2005;62(6):593–602.
71. Vilchinsky N, Ginzburg K, Fait K, Foa EB. Cardiac-disease-induced PTSD (CDI-PTSD): a systematic review. Clin Psychol Rev. 2017;55:92–106.
72. Ladwig KH, Baumert J, Marten-Mittag B, Kolb C, Zrenner B, Schmitt C. Posttraumatic stress symptoms and predicted mortality in patients with implantable cardioverter-defibrillators: results from the prospective living with an implanted cardioverter-defibrillator study. Arch Gen Psychiatry. 2008;65(11):1324–30.
73. Edmondson D, Richardson S, Falzon L, Davidson KW, Mills MA, Neria Y. Posttraumatic stress disorder prevalence and risk of recurrence in acute coronary syndrome patients: a meta-analytic review. PLoS One. 2012;7(6):e38915.
74. Dao TK, Chu D, Springer J, Gopaldas RR, Menefee DS, Anderson T, et al. Clinical depression, posttraumatic stress disorder, and comorbid depression and posttraumatic stress disorder as risk factors for in-hospital mortality after coronary artery bypass grafting surgery. J Thorac Cardiovasc Surg. 2010;140(3):606–10.
75. Deng LX, Khan AM, Drajpuch D, Fuller S, Ludmir J, Mascio CE, et al. Prevalence and correlates of post-traumatic stress disorder in adults with congenital heart disease. Am J Cardiol. 2016;117(5):853–7.
76. Eslami B. Correlates of posttraumatic stress disorder in adults with congenital heart disease. Congenit Heart Dis. 2017;12(3):357–63.
77. Vilchinsky N. Unrecognized, undiagnosed, and untreated: cardiac-disease-induced PTSD among patients' partners. Front Psychol. 2017;8:1265.

27 Transitioning the Adult Congenital Heart Disease Patient from the Cardiovascular Intensive Care Unit to the Ward

Christina Sillman, Anitra Romfh, Rose Tompkins, and Susan M. Fernandes

27.1 Introduction

Health-care transitions are associated with increased risk of morbidity and mortality [1]. Ensuring a smooth transition from the cardiovascular intensive care unit (CVICU) to the ward for the ACHD patient requires a comprehensive approach that involves clinicians with an expertise in congenital heart disease (CHD), postoperative surgical management, and adult comorbidities. There must be formal protocols for provider handoffs, and there must be a clear understanding of the limitations within the postoperative settings. Despite varying opinions, there is no ideal setting for the location of cardiac surgery, CVICU care, and ward management for the ACHD patient. Pediatric institutions have the expertise in CHD yet often lack the expertise and resources to manage adult comorbidities. Adult hospitals often lack the understanding of postoperative CHD physiology but have easier access to obtaining adult subspecialists. In addition, adult hospitals have adult nurses who are trained to manage postoperative pain and pulmonary toilet, skin, hygiene, and ambulation issues in adult cardiac patients. These nurses are also more likely to be tuned in to the emotional issues many adults face following cardiac surgery.

Today there are a wide range of approaches to the location of postoperative care for the adult congenital heart disease (ACHD) patient. Many ACHD patients undergo cardiac surgery in a pediatric hospital by a CHD surgeon given improved outcomes associated with this model [2, 3], while other ACHD patients may undergo cardiac surgery in an adult institution by either a CHD cardiothoracic surgeon or an adult cardiothoracic surgeon. In a few cases, especially when the ACHD patient has both CHD and acquired heart disease issues, finding the CHD surgeon and the adult

C. Sillman (✉) · A. Romfh · R. Tompkins · S. M. Fernandes
Lucille Packard Children's Hospital and Stanford Hospital and Clinics, Palo Alto, CA, USA
e-mail: CSillman@stanfordhealthcare.org

E. da Cruz et al. (eds.), *Intensive Care of the Adult with Congenital Heart Disease*, Congenital Heart Disease in Adolescents and Adults,
https://doi.org/10.1007/978-3-319-94171-4_27

cardiac surgeon working side by side in the operating room (OR) may be beneficial. Where a patient is admitted after leaving the OR is also highly variable. ACHD patients operated in a pediatric hospital may transfer to a pediatric CVICU or an adult CVICU when geographically feasible. The location of care after an ACHD patient leaves the CVICU can also vary similarly. Each of these transitions, from OR to CVICU and from CIVCU to ward, places the ACHD patient at increased risk for a negative outcome.

As we explore how to optimize the transition of the ACHD patient from the CVICU to the ward in this chapter, each reader will need to consider their model of ACHD hospital care. There must be a consideration about how their model of care contributes to the potential risks during care transitions and incorporate changes that will improve patient care within that model. The following chapter will describe ways to optimize the transition of the ACHD patient from the CIVU to the ward and will attempt to consider the more common models of care. In the end, there is one single goal which is to provide high-quality, patient-centered care that results in exceptional outcomes for ACHD patients.

27.2 Readiness for Transfer from Cardiovascular Intensive Care Unit to Ward

Criteria for identifying patients who are ready to transfer from the CVICU to the ward should be developed. Such criteria are important for determining resource utilization and minimizing CVICU length of stay while ensuring patient safety. Patients deemed eligible for the next phase in care benefit from transferring as soon as possible to facilitate a shift in focus from achieving medical stability to promoting wellness, mobility, nutrition, and discharge planning.

Fundamentally, patients need to be stable before discharge from the CVICU can be considered. Given higher patient to nursing ratios on the ward, there is less opportunity to identify and manage acute issues that arise. Thus, the key judgment must be that the patient no longer requires intensive care. This is based as much on the judgment and experience of the team as measurable criteria [4–7]. That said, specific factors to gauge CVICU discharge readiness can be identified for each system.

Cardiovascular: Post-extubation, CVICU patients are weaned off vasoactive medications. Once weaned, the patient needs to be observed for several hours to ensure stability. The CVICU patient will typically have an arterial line for the duration of the vasoactive medication, and this may need to be removed prior to being considered for the ward. From a heart rate and rhythm standpoint, the patient ideally will be observed and monitored via telemetry. If the patient has paroxysms of SVT, for example, it is important to initiate an antiarrhythmic agent while in the CVICU [7]. Along this line, if the patient is at risk for heart block based on the type of surgery performed, he or she will need to be observed prior to removal of the surgically placed temporary wires. It is important also that these wires are removed prior to initiation of anticoagulation, as late removal could result in bleeding and tamponade. The patient should be observed in the CVICU for at least 12 hours after removal to ensure no complications prior to transfer to the ward. Regarding volume management, the surgical patient will likely have expected postoperative heart failure after cardiopulmonary bypass. Thus, diuresis can be managed with loop diuretics with or without sequential blockade. While diuresis to preoperative weight is not a criterion for CVICU discharge, it is a goal prior to going home and this management may continue to require IV diuresis on the ward. Adequate potassium and magnesium supplementation is important, especially since arrhythmias are common in ACHD patients. Central lines may or may not need to be removed prior to ward transfer depending on institutional policy.

Pulmonary: Post-extubation, the patient needs to be encouraged toward improved respiratory function and mobility. Provided the patient does not have escalating oxygen needs, the patient can usually be discharged from the CVICU with oxygen therapy. The presence of effusions by exam or chest x-ray may be identified and can be further medically managed on the ward and does not typically preclude transfer. If the ACHD patient has a prior diagnosis of obstructive sleep apnea and is on a stable support of noninvasive positive pressure ventilation (NIPPV), he or she usually can continue to use this on the ward. However, those patients requiring titration of NIPPV or with increased oxygen requirements are not ideal candidates for transfer. While incentive spirometry is often used in the CVICU and continues on the ward, its efficacy in preventing pulmonary complications is yet unproven [8–10].

Hematology: Some ACHD patients may have platelet [11] or other bleeding abnormalities at baseline, and this should be monitored carefully. Despite these tendencies, all ACHD patients after cardiac surgery at a minimum require DVT prophylaxis from sequential compression devices, which should be continued until the patient is mobile. If patients are higher risk or have a prolonged length of stay, prophylactic fractionated heparin may be used subcutaneously. Anemia is also an important hematologic issue to recognize in the CVICU and may require transfusion or iron therapy for a more gradual remediation of blood loss. Anemia may be under-recognized in cyanotic CHD patients as they may need greater oxygen-carrying capacity commensurate with the degree of cyanosis [12].

For patients requiring anticoagulation (i.e., mechanical valve), clinicians should ideally wait until temporary wires or any intracardiac lines have been removed. This decision should be mutual between the CVICU, ACHD, and surgical teams. There should not be any active bleeding when this is started, and the chest tube output should be observed to be serosanguinous. The patient should be watched carefully on the ward for any bleeding complications. Ideally, antiplatelet medications should wait until further convalescence, due to the risk of bleeding.

Gastroenterology: The patient may have expected postoperative nausea after cardiac surgery. This and other nutritional needs as well as narcotic-induced constipation do not provide a contraindication to discharge from the CVICU and can continue to be managed on the ward. If the patient has had a prolonged OR course, liver enzyme abnormalities may be present and peak later in the hospital course. Ideally there should be a downward trend of this prior to transfer to the ward. Some ACHD patients may have liver abnormalities at baseline, and both CVICU and ward teams should be aware of this [13, 14].

Genitourinary: The Foley catheter, placed at the time of surgery, is usually removed while the patient remains in the CVICU. Urine output should continue to be monitored while the patient is on the ward.

Endocrine: Glucose instability is ideally managed postoperatively with an insulin drip, but serum glucose usually stabilizes unless the patient has underlying glucose intolerance. Awareness of the increased prevalence of glucose intolerance in the ACHD patient population is important [15]. This insulin drip is weaned off while in the CVICU prior to transfer to the ward given the frequent glucose checks required. For those patients who required pharmacological treatment for hyperglycemia prior to admission, they should be restarted on their home regimen once tolerating a regular diet. Adjustments to subcutaneous or pump insulin or oral diabetes medications can be accomplished on the ward, provided the glucose checks do not exceed nursing resources.

Neurological: CVICU delirium is important to identify and the underlying cause should be detected if waxing and waning consciousness is observed in the CVICU. A clear sensorium should be noted prior to transferring the patient to the ward. The same can be said for those patients still under the sedative effects of narcotic or other medications like benzodiazepines. During or after cardiac surgery, ACHD patients are at risk for transient ischemic attacks or cerebral vascular accidents. This is more common during the immediate postoperative periods, while the patient is still in the CVICU. If this occurs, the adult neurologic consult service should help provide guidance as to the needs of the patient prior to transfer to the ward.

Infection: ACHD patients are at risk for postoperative pneumonia and other infections. They may have late readmissions for wound infections or may have had endocarditis as the indication for surgery. Infection may be managed on the ward provided the patient is not trending toward a systemic inflammatory response state. Removal of invasive lines including endotracheal tubes, arterial lines, central venous lines, Foley catheter, nasogastric tubes, pacing wires, and chest tubes in a timely manner helps to decrease the risk of infection. Close monitoring of peripheral intravenous lines to ensure patency and asepsis is another important infection control measure. Daily rounding on sources of infection and an assessment for readiness for line removal is a formalized process essential to infection prevention in the critically ill ACHD patient.

Renal: ACHD patients are at increased risk for renal problems and may have under-recognized renal insufficiency that may impact length of stay. Pharmaceutical analysis of all prescribed medications for renal toxicity can be an important component of daily rounding. ACHD patients requiring robust diuresis for challenging fluid management may need to stay in the CVICU to closely monitor renal function and electrolyte disturbances. Ideally, the kidney function should be stable or trending toward improvement prior to transfer to the ward [16, 17].

27.3 Handoff

The World Health Organization (WHO) and Joint Commission on Accreditation of Healthcare Organizations (JCAHO) have listed the handoffs of patients from one health-care provider to another as a recognized patient safety goal [18, 19].

This patient safety goal requires health-care organizations to implement standardized approaches to handoff communications. In dynamic and variable health-care organizations, handoff, or transfer from one unit to another, is a critical time that has a high potential error rate. Standardized and clear handoff between the CVICU team and the ward team is integral to completing a safe and successful transfer for the ACHD patient.

The handoff should begin with the CVICU team notifying the ward team of potential transfer. Daily updates between CVICU charge nurse, ward charge nurse, and bed control help prepare and plan for timely transfers. Standardized, daily communications between units foster collaboration and care coordination [20].

The CVICU bedside nurse can initiate preparation of transfer to the ward by ensuring all intensive care nursing documentation is complete, clear, and concise. Standard items to update include medication administration records, line/tube documentation, patient events, current vital signs, pain assessment, and a current head-to-toe nursing assessment. An important component of nursing documentation is maintaining legible and clearly written notes or use of electronic charting records. Avoiding excessive use of abbreviations helps to ensure understanding by future readers of documented notes [21].

Documentation method is facility dependent, and in ACHD models of care where an interfacility transfer is occurring it is important to have a clearly established pathway for documentation to flow seamlessly from one institution to another. Bedside nursing staff should be allotted support from the charge nurse or break nurse to allow adequate time to review and amend current documentation in preparation for transfer.

Standardized handoff processes are vital to the successful delivery of information and to prevent omission of essential information. Methods for handoffs include electronic transmission of report, telephone-based report, in-person one-on-one report, and team-based report involving patient and family. Use of two or more methods in combination may provide multiple opportunities to transmit information and improve patient safety. A clear, standardized process for handoff needs to be established for ACHD patients transferring from the CVICU setting to the ward setting and is dependent on the resources available and type of transfer (intrafacility vs. interfacility). Once a ward bed is established by bed control or the patient placement manager, the handoff procedure may start.

Computerized clinical documentation systems used as a handoff method should allow for ease of use, accessibility by both units, and standardization of information documented. Telephonic handoff should be completed at an established time with each clinician having support from their respective team in covering patient care duties to allow complete focus for the handoff process. Telephonic handoff should ideally be performed in a quiet space with minimal background noise or interruptions with a good phone connection. Similarly, in-person one-on-one handoff should be completed in a quiet location free from distraction or interruptions with adequate time to review all documentation.

Perhaps one of the strongest methods of handoff involves the patient as a collaborative member of the process [22]. Patient and family involvement in the handoff process provides opportunity for the patient and family to ask questions, clarify details, and maintain active participation in their care.

The use of an CVICU nurse liaison to oversee the transfer process has been shown to provide a statistically significant effect on continuity of care [20]. The nurse liaison assesses the patient for transfer readiness, coordinates the transfer, fosters communication between the CVICU and ward, and monitors the patient post transfer to provide an additional clinical resource to the ward staff and provide overall continuity of care for the patient. In ACHD patients, the use of an ACHD-dedicated hospital liaison nurse may be especially useful for interfacility transfers.

Various handoff communication tools ranging from written worksheets to electronic medical record flow sheets can play an important part in the delivery of handoff communication [20, 23]. A standardized process for communication ensures that all patients receive high-quality care. For ACHD patients, there are specific aspects that should be included in whichever tool is used as part of the standardized communication process for handoff. Table 27.1 lists the ACHD handoff communication items that are typically utilized by the bedside nurse beyond the standard head-to-toe assessment, medications, lines, patient personal belongings, and critical care history.

Table 27.2 lists the ACHD handoff communication items that are typically utilized by the MD and/or APP. The general core elements [24] of any surgical CVICU to ward handoff should occur in a "send and receive" format. First, the transferring CVICU team "sends" basic information regarding the patient identity, the operation and surgeon, any complications, and the CVICU hospital course. The most recent vitals and physical exam (ideally closest to the time of handoff) as well as any key aberrations from normal are important to relay. An example of this would be baseline cyanosis or a paced rhythm. Next, any relevant past medical history, allergies, and medications should be reviewed. The closing assessment and plan should summarize the status of the patient at that point and the next steps in care. The "receiving" ward team should then verbalize a summary of the information presented, reiterate the plan in the context of ward care, and formally accept the patient.

Table 27.1 Adult congenital heart disease specific handoff communication focuses

Congenital heart defect diagnosis—Diagrams of the heart pre-surgery and with all surgical interventions is especially helpful for health-care staff to conceptualize the cardiac anatomy
Surgical history—Including dates and diagrams of surgical interventions
CHD-specific precautions—Baseline O_2 saturation, home oxygen level, need for IV air filters, limbs to avoid blood pressure or venipuncture on, a physical map of old and new scars, baseline rhythm, and device settings
Psychosocial coping—Anxiety or PTSD triggers, history of mood disorders, pain management approach, patient support/family, neurocognitive delays, and health literacy

Table 27.2 Core elements in team handoff

Patient identification
Operation and surgeon
CVICU hospital course
Most recent exam and vitals
Medications and allergies
Assessment
Plan

These core elements of the handoff may require additional specifics, depending on the locations between which the transfer is occurring. This adds additional complexity to the handoff and presents a risk for medical errors. For example, a patient may have recovered from the CVICU stay but requires intensive rehabilitation at an acute rehabilitation facility, or the patient may require transfer to a different ICU. For example, a situation where a patient suffers a stroke would be better served in a specialized neuro-intensive care unit (ICU) instead of a pediatric or adult postsurgical unit.

Lastly, given the nature of ACHD care, the patient may be operated in the pediatric hospital by the pediatric heart surgeon and be awaiting transfer to the ward from the pediatric CVICU. The patient may transfer to the pediatric ward, depending on the age allowances and neurodevelopmental status. When transferring an ACHD patient to a pediatric ward, it is important to point out any adult comorbid conditions that may not be normally managed in the pediatric ward during the handoff. There should also be a plan in place to address these concerns, ideally an ACHD consult team. In some cases, the patient might transfer from the pediatric CVICU to the adult ward, especially if they need adult subspecialty services. In this case, additional handoff procedures center around providing the background on anatomic and surgical procedures related to ACHD. Anticipatory guidance needs to be provided for the specific types of surgery. In many cases, this type of handoff is to an entirely different hospital. As such, the patient is at risk for errors of omission or loss of information if the receiving team does not have access to the medical record at the transferring hospital [25]. Identifying a point person or mechanism from the transferring team is very important, as the receiving team may not be comfortable reaching out for information. In contrast to the above scenarios, the patient may have the operation done by the pediatric or adult heart surgeon in the adult operating room. In this case, the entirety of care is centered in the adult hospital. While this may appear the most seamless type of handoff, the receiving team may again require additional education around the background on anatomic and surgical procedures related to ACHD. Again, anticipatory guidance surrounding the expected post-recovery course is important. Lastly, the mean age of the ACHD is far younger than that of the typical cardiac patient in an adult hospital so the medical team may feel uncomfortable caring for the younger patient. In addition, the patient may not be equipped to advocate for himself. As is not uncommon in the elderly patient, parents and other family members play an important role. The transferring teams must be sure not to lose the patient autonomy in the process of including parental caregivers. Lastly, ACHD patients may have various syndromes such as Down syndrome that may require special needs that need to be addressed. Decision-making capacity, conservatorship, and advanced directives, ideally established prior to admission, should be reiterated at the time of transfer.

With these core elements and various settings, the ideal handoff format occurs with the physical presence of both "sending" and "receiving" teams in their entirety. While it would be beneficial for any patient, the increased complexity of an ACHD patient demands a more integrated approach across the team [20]. The team approach acknowledges not only RNs, APP, and MDs but also other team members such as respiratory therapists and pharmacists. Arranging the two teams in a huddle-type format can be achieved if the transfer can coincide with morning rounding. Ideally, goal hours of planned transfer facilitate availability and communication. In this way, "one message, one time" can be communicated to all team members.

27.4 Preparing for Hospital Discharge

Discharge planning for ACHD patients begins upon admission as the primary goal destination for admitted patients is a healthy discharge to home. Critically ill patients may have long hospital courses and require complex planning for discharge and services that may not have been needed prior to admission. Starting discharge planning early in the hospital course will help the medical team streamline goals of care, prevent premature discharge, and potentially decrease length of stay and rate of readmission after discharge. Discharge planning for ACHD patients includes a comprehensive medication reconciliation; discussion of wound care, if applicable; review of activity restrictions; evaluation of support systems and home environment; and, most notably, ensuring long-term ACHD cardiology care.

27.4.1 Medication Reconciliation

Discharge preparation for an ACHD patient from the hospital represents a critical time to review that patient's prior medication regimen and presents an opportunity to consider the addition of other medications that may be beneficial for the patient. Discharge planning should consider that some newer medications that are not commonly covered by insurance may require early authorization requests to be started prior to discharge such as PDE5 inhibitors, advanced heart failure medications, and some forms of oral and injectable anticoagulation. Insurance authorization may take several days to be approved; thus, starting this process early during admission may decrease length of hospital stay or prevent readmission. Home medication regimens are frequently discontinued in the acute setting of hospitalization, but it is imperative that these medications also be reviewed and the patients are clearly instructed on whether to resume, discontinue, or adjust their prior medications. With respect to the ACHD patient specifically, it is recommended to review an individual's indications for common cardiac medications, anticoagulation, contraception, and antibiotic prophylaxis prior to discharge to ensure there are no missed opportunities for medication optimization.

27.4.1.1 Cardiac Medications

Typical cardiac medications that are often used among ACHD patients include antihypertensives, neurohormonal blockade, diuretics for heart failure, lipid-lowering agents, and antiarrhythmics. Indication for the use of these medications may involve collaboration with other specialists including advanced heart failure, electrophysiology, and interventional cardiology to determine an optimal cardiac regimen for an ACHD patient being discharged from the hospital.

In general, blood pressure goals are reflected to meet the ACC/AHA and JNC standards [26, 27]. Exception to this would include more stringent blood pressure control for those at risk of aortic dissection or rupture including the aortopathy patients like Marfan syndrome, bicuspid aortic valve, aortic coarctation, or Turner's syndrome. Neurohormonal blockade with beta-blockers and RAAS inhibitors along with diuretics should be considered for patients with a history of congestive heart failure, especially those patients being discharged after an acute heart failure decompensation. Lipid-lowering agents should be prescribed in all patients for secondary prevention if they have already experienced an acquired cardiovascular event like myocardial infarction or stroke with LDL goal adjusted per ACC/AHA guidelines. Lipid-lowering agents for primary prevention, specifically statin therapy, should be considered for any patient with an elevated 10-year risk for an acquired cardiovascular event due to risk factors such as diabetes, advancing age, peripheral vascular disease, hypertension, and tobacco use. This is especially important to consider for the aging ACHD patient who is at risk of acquired heart disease. Lastly, antiarrhythmic therapy should be considered pending the patient's arrhythmia history and may be further guided by recommendations from the electrophysiology team.

27.4.1.2 Anticoagulation

Many ACHD patients are recommended to take antiplatelet therapy with aspirin or systemic anticoagulation with either warfarin or a novel oral anticoagulant for a variety of indications. Common indications for initiating aspirin therapy prior to discharge include a recently placed bioprosthetic valve, annuloplasty ring, extracardiac conduit, intracardiac patch, or septal occluder device. Often the decision to start aspirin therapy will be driven by the surgeon or physician who performed the surgery or procedure. Duration of therapy is also determined by the indication and often by the preference of the surgeon or interventionalist. Systemic anticoagulation is initiated or continued for those congenital patients with a mechanical valve, atrial arrhythmia with high risk of stroke, or known thrombus. Education and establishment of oral anticoagulation management prior to discharge is important to ensure seamless transfer of care and prevent gaps in oral anticoagulation management.

27.4.1.3 Contraception

Women of child-bearing age with CHD carry an increased risk of both maternal and fetal morbidity and mortality. When preparing for discharge from the hospital, especially for an acute clinical decompensation, a woman of child-bearing age should be counseled about contraception.

Detailed counseling regarding a patient's individual pregnancy risk may be deferred to her outpatient ACHD provider; however, at the minimum, the patient should be advised to defer pregnancy until such a discussion has occurred and that under ideal circumstances, pregnancies should be planned and monitored by her ACHD provider in collaboration with an obstetrician.

Table 27.3 Indications for antibiotic prophylaxis prior to dental procedures per the 2008 ACHD guidelines

(a) Prosthetic cardiac valve or prosthetic material used for cardiac valve repair
(b) History of infective endocarditis
(c) Unrepaired and palliated cyanotic congenital heart disease, including surgically constructed palliative shunts and conduits
(d) Completely repaired congenital heart disease with prosthetic material, whether placed surgically or via catheter intervention during the first 6 months following the procedure
(e) Repaired congenital heart disease with residual defects at the site or adjacent to the site of a prosthetic patch or prosthetic device that inhibits endothelialization

27.4.1.4 Antibiotic Prophylaxis

Hospital discharge presents an opportunity to review the indications and appropriateness for infective endocarditis prophylaxis for the ACHD patient, especially those that have been previously lost to medical care and may not be aware whether they do or do not meet indications for prophylaxis or those that recently underwent surgical or catheter-based interventional procedure who may now have an indication.

Antibiotic prophylaxis generally is recommended for prevention of infective endocarditis prior to dental procedures that involve manipulation of the gingival tissue or the periapical region of teeth or perforation of the oral mucosa. Antibiotic prophylaxis is not recommended for other non-dental procedures including esophagogastroduodenoscopy, colonoscopy, or genitourinary procedures without active infection. Exception includes highest-risk patients after membrane rupture during pregnancy, but this is not typically included in general counseling of the patient.

In general, the ACC recommends prescribing amoxicillin unless the patient has a penicillin allergy in which case clindamycin is often recommended (Table 27.3).

27.4.2 Activity Counseling

Early activity is a key component to a post-sternotomy patient's recovery. The ACHD adult patients are often being transitioned from a CVICU setting and ultimately discharged from the ward following a cardiac surgery that often requires a sternotomy. Early activity helps improve recovery time, in addition, minimizes complications associated with surgery and prolonged bed rest including deep venous thrombosis and venous thromboembolic events, pneumonia, and exacerbated deconditioning. Sternal precautions should be maintained for 6–8 weeks postoperatively. Sternal precautions entail no lifting, pushing, or pulling anything weighing greater than 10 pounds. Driving is prohibited, while the patient is taking narcotic medications, and resumption of driving should ideally wait until after sternal precautions are lifted to prevent sternal trauma from the steering wheel or airbag in even a minor collision. Seatbelts are encouraged to maintain proper automobile safety. Resumption of sexual activity is dependent upon patient's overall well-being, activity tolerance, willingness and desire to engage in sexual activity, and diligence in maintaining sternal precautions throughout sexual activity. Inpatient cardiac rehabilitation consultation should be obtained followed by ongoing outpatient rehabilitation if deconditioning is identified. Regular aerobic exercise, advanced based upon the patient's activity tolerance, is encouraged for most ACHD patients and will help with reconditioning and overall well-being post critical care admission.

27.4.3 Pain Management

Successful management of the ACHD patient's pain is an imperative component of the patient care experience and overall patient satisfaction. Uncontrolled pain may prevent the patient from engaging in mobility, pulmonary hygiene, and self-care and can greatly affect the overall coping and emotional well-being. When possible, a preadmission assessment of an ACHD patient's pain management history may be helpful in identifying effective and ineffective approaches to pain management prior to the pain event. An assessment of past or present narcotic or illicit substance abuse helps to identify patients at risk for narcotic abuse. Patients who are experiencing uncontrolled pain or requiring pain management above the standard approach may benefit from consultation with pain management services.

27.4.4 Assessing Patient Support Systems and Home Environment

The ward nurse is key to assessing the patient's support systems prior to discharge. The wide range in age, medical history, neurocognitive functioning, health literacy, and patient autonomy makes the ACHD patient unique and challenging. The personal support systems for ACHD patients are integral in their overall coping, medical compliance, and care autonomy. Martin et al. found that some patients may not be able to maintain a complicated medical regimen without the guidance and prompting of a caretaker or support system [28]. Coaching young adults and adolescents to be autonomous and independent with their medical care remains a challenge with the transition from parental control of medical care to patient control of medical care. Co-dependent dynamics established in childhood may remain well into adulthood and pose a unique challenge with critical care admissions and discharge planning. Evaluation of the patient's personal support team and resources, along with the patient's level of autonomy and health literacy will help determine if intervention and guidance is needed prior to discharge. Patients without a personal support team with anticipated high care needs post critical care admission may require establishment with medical or governmental support services prior to discharge such as outpatient rehabilitation, home health nursing, public health nursing, or in-home support services. Referral to the ACHD social worker or hospital social work services may prove beneficial in evaluating the resources available to the patient and with recruiting new resources for the patient prior to discharge.

Discharge planning for patients who will have physical restrictions, limited mobility, or require assistance with activities of daily living post critical care admission must include an evaluation of the home environment, transportation resources, and mobility assistance needs. Assessment of the home setting for physical barriers such as stairs and heavy gates or for other fall hazards helps anticipate the need for intervention or modification prior to discharge. In-home caretakers and support persons may need to be educated on the physical care needs expected for the patient upon discharge. Verbal instruction, written handouts, and demonstration to patient and caregivers for modifications in physical activity and activities of daily living are important tools that may be delivered by the ACHD nurse liaison, nurse educator, bedside nurse, or nursing discharge planner. Transportation upon discharge for patients with limited resources and driving restrictions may require coordination and advanced planning that is best started early in the hospitalization.

Some patients may already utilize durable medical equipment at home prior to their critical care admission, while others may have new needs identified during admission. Acquiring the necessary durable medical equipment and arranging home delivery prior to discharge requires early coordination within the hospital admission. Common durable medical equipment needs for ACHD patients include oxygen delivery systems and other respiratory care systems, medication infusion pumps and indwelling venous access port care items, mobility assist devices such as walking canes or shower chairs, and pressure garments. Changes in health status may also require updates to the previous orders for durable medical equipment.

27.4.5 End-of-Life Care

Ideally, the ACHD patient would complete an advanced care directive prior to admission, but if one is not on file with admission, an early assessment of patient care wishes before the patient deteriorates to a deleterious neurological status helps to avoid medical-ethical complications and family strain with end-of-life decision-making. Advanced disease process and severity of critical care admission necessitate the consultation of palliative or hospice care early within the admission to ensure patient comfort and to reestablish care goals for palliative and end-of-life care. Multidisciplinary and supportive care conferences involving the patient, when possible, and family help to ensure the patient's wishes regarding code status, escalation of care, and withdrawal of care is clearly communicated. In the event that the critical care admission leads to the patient's demise, the goal of care is focused on patient comfort and family support.

27.4.6 Ensuring Long-Term ACHD Care

Preparing the patient for outpatient care is one of the most important components of discharge planning. If a patient does not already have an outpatient ACHD provider, then the hospital team should help identify such a provider. The critical care hospital admission is an opportunity to reconnect a patient who was lost to follow up with appropriate ACHD care or to increase the surveillance on an established patient who may be overdue for follow-up. Coordination with the outpatient ACHD care team to establish a follow-up appointment prior to discharge helps ensure seamless transfer of care from inpatient setting to the outpatient setting. The utilization of advance practice providers for independent post-discharge outpatient visits can help to provide timely appointments for these vulnerable patients. Care coordination of outpatient appointments can be accomplished by the ACHD nurse liaison, discharge planner, or inpatient ACHD team, and the process should start early in the admission as outpatient needs are identified.

Depending on insurance coverage or where the patient lives, there can exist many barriers that make receiving outpatient ACHD specialty care challenging. ACHD providers can often partner with a local cardiologist to help improve ACHD care. Two resources that may be beneficial in identifying a local or regional ACHD provider is available via the Adult Congenital Heart Association (ACHA) and International Society for Adult Congenital Heart Disease (ISACHD) websites.

Conclusion

The critical care admission for the ACHD patient can be a time of vulnerability. Transition from the CVICU to the ward, although a milestone in the process of recovery, can also be associated with negative outcomes. A team-based approach that includes standardizing assessment of readiness to transfer out of the CVICU, formalizing the handoff process, and comprehensive assessment, planning, and teaching before discharge can ensure a seamless transition that results in high-quality, patient-centered care with exceptional outcomes.

References

1. Rennke S, Shoeb MH, Nguyen OK, Magan Y, Wachter RM, Ranji SR. Interventions to improve care transitions at hospital discharge (NEW) in: making health care safer II: an updated critical analysis of the evidence for patient safety practicesRockville (MD): Agency for Healthcare Research and Quality (US); 2013 (Evidence Reports/Technology Assessments, No. 211.) Chapter 37.
2. Karamlou T, Diggs BS, Person T, Ungerleider RM, Welke KF. National practice patterns for management of adult congenital heart disease: operation by pediatric heart surgeons decreases in-hospital death. Circulation. 2008;118:2345–52.
3. Karamlou T, Diggs BS, Ungerleider RM, Welke KF. Adults or big kids: what is the ideal clinical environment for management of grown-up patients with congenital heart disease? Ann Thorac Surg. 2010;90:573–9.
4. Nates JL, et al. ICU admission, discharge, and triage guidelines. A framework to enhance clinical operations, development of institutional policies, and further research. Crit Care Med. 2016;44(8):1553–602.
5. Baslaim G, Bashore JA. A unique milieu for perioperative care of adult congenital heart disease patients at a single institution. Thorac Cardiovasc Surg. 2009;15(3):150–4.
6. Badawi O, Breslow MJ. Readmissions and death after ICU discharge: development and validation of two predictive models. PLoS One. 2012;7(11):e48758.
7. Kumar S, Tedrow UB, Triedman JK. Arrhythmias in adult congenital heart disease: diagnosis and management. Cardiol Clin. 2015;33(4):571–88, viii. https://doi.org/10.1016/j.ccl.2015.07.007.

8. Krastins I, Corey ML, McLeod A, Edmonds J, Levison H, Moes F. An evaluation of incentive spirometry in the management of pulmonary complications after cardiac surgery in a pediatric population. Crit Care Med. 1982;10(8):525–8.
9. Pasquina P, Tramér MR, Walder B. Prophylactic respiratory physiotherapy after cardiac surgery: systematic review. BMJ. 2003;327(7428):1379.
10. Pasquina P, Tramèr MR, Walder B. Incentive spirometry for preventing pulmonary complications after coronary artery bypass graft. Cochrane Database Syst Rev. 2012;(9):CD004466.
11. Peters AM, Rozkovec A, Bell RN, et al. Platelet kinetics in congenital heart disease. Cardiovasc Res. 1982;16(7):391–7.
12. Broberg CS, Jayaweera AR, Diller GP, Prasad SK, Thein SL, Bax BE, Burman J, Gatzoulis MA. Seeking optimal relation between oxygen saturation and hemoglobin concentration in adults with cyanosis from congenital heart disease. Am J Cardiol. 2011 Feb 15;107(4):595–9.
13. Adachi K, Toyama H, Kaiho Y, Adachi O, Hudeta H, Yamauchi M. The impact of liver disorders on perioperative management of reoperative cardiac surgery: a retrospective study in adult congenital heart disease patients. J Anesth. 2017;31(2):170–7. https://doi.org/10.1007/s00540-017-2308-4.
14. Price S, Jaggar SI, Jordan S, Trenfield S, Khan M, Sethia B, Shore D, Evans TW. Adult congenital heart disease: intensive care management and outcome prediction. Intensive Care Med. 2007;33(4):652–9.
15. Deen JF, Krieger EV, Slee AE, Arslan A, Arterburn D, Stout KK, Portman MA. Metabolic syndrome in adults with congenital heart disease. J Am Heart Assoc. 2016;5(2):e001132.
16. Cedars A, Benjamin L, Burns SV, Novak E, Amin A. Clinical predictors of length of stay in adults with congenital heart disease. Heart. 2017;103(16):1258–63.
17. Kwiatkowski DM, Price E, Axelrod DM, Romfh AW, Han BS, Sutherland SM, Krawczeski CD. Incidence, risk factors, and outcomes of acute kidney injury in adults undergoing surgery for congenital heart disease. Cardiol Young. 2016;21:1–8.
18. Communication during patient hand-overs. In: World Health Organization (WHO) Collaborating Centre for Patient Safety Solutions. 2007. http://www.who.int/patientsafety/solutions/patientsafety/PS-Solution3.pdf. Accessed 4 Apr 2017.
19. Joint Commission 2008. National Patient Goals PowerPoint Presentation. http://www.jointcommission.org/NR/rdonlyres/7079B888-7C6F-4D5B-9AEF-56F5AFB034ED/0/08_NPSG_general_presentation.ppt [Reference list]. Accessed 4 Apr 2017.
20. Sluisveld NV, Hesselink G, Hoeven JG, Westert G, Wollersheim H, Zegers M. Improving clinical handover between intensive care unit and general ward professionals at intensive care unit discharge. Intensive Care Med. 2015;41(4):589–604. https://doi.org/10.1007/s00134-015-3666-8.
21. Friesen MA, White SV, Byers JF. Handoffs: implications for nurses. In: Hughes RG, editor. Patient safety and quality: an evidence-based handbook for nurses. Rockville (MD: Agency for Healthcare Research and Quality (US); 2008.
22. Grewves C. Patients' perceptions of bedside handover. Nurs Stand. 1999;14(12):32–5.
23. Graan SM, et al. Nursing handover from ICU to cardiac ward: standardised tools to reduce safety risks. Aust Crit Care. 2016;29(3):165–71.
24. Wohlauer M. Fragmented care in the era of limited work hours: a plea for an explicit handover curriculum. BMJ Qual Saf. 2012;21(Suppl 1):i16–8.
25. Ong MS, Coiera E. A systematic review of failures in handoff communication during intrahospital transfers. Jt Comm J Qual Patient Saf. 2011;37(6):274–84.
26. James JA, et al. 2014 evidence-based guideline for the management of high blood pressure in adults: report from the panel members appointed to the eighth joint national committee (JNC 8). JAMA. 2014;311(5):507–20.
27. Go AS, et al. An effective approach to high blood pressure control. J Am Coll Cardiol. 2014;63(12):1230–8.
28. Martin LR, Williams SL, Haskard KB, DiMatteo MR. The challenge of patient adherence. Ther Clin Risk Manag. 2005;1(3):189–1.

Thrombosis and Modern Anticoagulation Options for the Adult with Congenital Heart Disease

28

Therese M. Giglia, Char M. Witmer, and Yuli Y. Kim

28.1 Propensity to Thrombosis in Adults with Congenital Heart Disease

It has long been recognized that adults with congenital heart disease (CHD), in particular cyanotic congenital heart disease (CCHD), are prone to thrombosis whether or not they have Eisenmenger physiology [1–3]. Although cerebrovascular events and pulmonary embolism (PE) are the most widely discussed, thrombosis of additional sites in the single-ventricle population, namely, the Fontan pathway [3–19] and deep veins of the lower extremities [20], may be equally devastating.

It is not surprising that adult congenital heart disease (ACHD) patients are prone to thrombosis. Throughout their lifetime, they have been exposed to the triad of risk factors for thrombosis initially described by Virchow in 1856 [21], namely, (a) stasis of blood, (b) hypercoagulability, and (c) endothelial injury. As in pediatric heart disease [14, 22, 23], an expansion of Virchow's triad [24] appears warranted:

1. **Altered blood flow (an expansion of "stasis of blood")**
   In addition to stasis of blood, ACHD patients have the potential to be exposed to "altered blood flow":
   (a) **Stasis of blood** may occur in dilated heart chambers as well as in dilated native or prosthetic outflow tracts. These areas of stasis may serve as a nidus for thrombus formation.
   (b) **Turbulent flow** may occur across stenotic native or prosthetic heart valves, intracardiac devices/leads, stents, and/or obstructed native or prosthetic outflow tracts activating platelets either directly [25, 26] or by increasing sheer

T. M. Giglia (✉) · C. M. Witmer · Y. Y. Kim
Children's Hospital of Philadelphia, Philadelphia, PA, USA
e-mail: gigliat@email.chop.edu

E. da Cruz et al. (eds.), *Intensive Care of the Adult with Congenital Heart Disease*, Congenital Heart Disease in Adolescents and Adults,
https://doi.org/10.1007/978-3-319-94171-4_28

stress that can result in platelet activation independent of endothelial damage [27]. Activated platelets adhere to these "abnormal," artificial vascular surfaces and may result in thrombus formation. The same mechanisms are involved in the turbulent flow of mechanical support (cardiopulmonary bypass (CPB), extracorporeal membrane oxygenation (ECMO), ventricular assist devices (VAD)) where thrombosis can occur despite systemic anticoagulation. Platelets are activated. Thrombin generation is increased via the extrinsic system in response to cytokines, ischemia, sheer stress, and activated platelets and via the contact system in response to contact of blood with the circuit. A profound derangement in the coagulation/fibrinolytic balance occurs with an ineffective counterbalance by anticoagulant factors such as antithrombin III. The procoagulant state may persist well past decannulation [28–31]. Although children, especially infants with their immature coagulation system, may be more prone to such effects, it seems most likely that at least some of these factors are at play in ACDH patients as well.

2. **Blood component abnormalities (expansion of hypercoagulability)**
   Blood component abnormalities have been described in children with acyanotic, acquired, as well as single-ventricle heart disease and include altered anticoagulation protein levels, increased thrombin generation potential, decreased endogenous inhibitors of coagulation, and decreased fibrinolytic proteins, among others. Such coagulopathies were first identified in children and adolescents with a Fontan circulation but more recently have been described through all stages of single-ventricle palliation, i.e., even before the Fontan completion [32–41]. Coagulopathies in Fontan patients are further described in the section on Fontans below.

   As is well known to physicians caring for adults with CHD, erythrocytosis and hyperviscosity associated with chronic cyanosis are risk factors for thrombosis as well. This may be exacerbated by iron deficiency anemia which makes red cells more rigid and less deformable as well as by dehydration [3, 14, 34, 42].
3. **Endothelial injury and dysfunction**
   Turbulent flow along normal vascular endothelial surfaces results in endothelial injury and dysfunction which is a precursor to thrombosis. Endothelial injury exposes tissue factor and subendothelial collagen-stimulating platelet aggregation and coagulation at the site of injury. Altered levels of endothelial markers in plasma have been found to precede intravascular coagulation and thrombosis in one study of patients with functionally univentricular hearts [43]. In addition, adults with CHD most likely have had numerous cardiac catheterizations, exposure to CPB, and central lines throughout their medical history that have the potential of further damaging an already compromised endothelium.
4. **Inflammation and bloodstream infection**
   Adults with CHD are at risk for exposure to inflammation and blood stream infections which pose further risk for thrombosis. In addition to creating turbulent flow and endothelial disruption, mechanical support (CPB, ECMO, VAD) results in an inflammatory state [29–31], activating platelets and exposing tissue factor by cytokine release [26]. Recent pediatric studies have implicated sepsis

with increased thrombus formation especially in the presence of an indwelling central venous line [44–46].

Patients with CHD often have one or more of these thrombosis risk factors at play, while during mechanical circulatory support (CPB, ECMO, VAD), all four of these conditions coexist.

28.1.1 Eisenmenger Physiology

A special note should be made about patients with Eisenmenger physiology who have a well- known risk of bleeding as well as clotting, thereby making anticoagulation controversial and often contradicted [Giannakoulas 2015]. In addition to the four factors described above, pulmonary hypertension in and of itself may result in endothelial dysfunction in the pulmonary arteries increasing the risk of pulmonary emboli. Cell aggregation secondary to decreased pulmonary blood flow may also be a thrombotic risk [10, 47]. On the other side of the spectrum, pulmonary hemorrhage from rupture of one of the pulmonary vessels is often the cause of death in this patient population [48–50].

This chapter will discuss common thrombotic concerns in the adult with CHD, namely, deep venous thrombosis (DVT), pulmonary embolism (PE), arrhythmias as a risk factor for stroke, and special concerns in the Fontan patient. We will conclude with a discussion of both currently available and "under-investigation" antithrombotic therapies.

28.2 Deep Venous Thrombosis and Pulmonary Embolism in Adults with Congenital Heart Disease

A recent editorial by Giannakoulas and Boutsikou [51] reviewed the prevalence of thrombosis in adults with CCHD from ten studies over the past 25 years. The prevalence of arterial cerebral thrombosis ranged from 0 to 47%, whereas the prevalence of pulmonary thrombosis ranged from 13.2 to 35%. Only two studies looked at both cerebral and pulmonary thromboses, and as expected, the studies differed in whether they were prospective/retrospective and most importantly in whether the thrombosis was clinically evident or clinically silent and documented on screening studies only. The most recent of the included studies by Jensen [52] documented cerebral thrombosis at 47% and pulmonary thrombosis at 31% in a prospective study and commented that the large discrepancy between clinical history and imaging findings suggests a high prevalence of silent thrombotic events.

Although single-ventricle anatomy and cyanosis are significant risk factors for early postoperative thrombosis in infants and children (especially DVT associated with central venous lines) [53, 54], there is limited data on the significance of these risk factors in the adult with CHD.

It is estimated that just over half of all medical patients in US acute care hospitals are at risk for venous thromboembolism (VTE) including DVT and PE [55] with those in the critical care setting at particularly increased risk [56]. Pulmonary embolism is considered the most common preventable cause of hospital death [57], and the Institute of Medicine defines the failure to provide adequate thromboprophylaxis to hospitalized, at-risk patients a medical error [58]. Although the prevalence of VTE in critically ill adults with CHD in the ICU is not known, based on the propensity for thrombosis in adults with CHD and the increased risk of VTE with age, it can be inferred that adults with CHD incur as much or more risk for VTE than those without CHD.

28.2.1 Risk Assessment and VTE Prophylaxis in Hospitalized Patients

Hospitalized patient characteristics considered high risk for VTE are malignancy, stroke, major general surgery and orthopedic surgery, trauma and fractures, spinal cord injury, obesity, pregnancy, heart failure, myocardial infarction, sepsis, respiratory failure, renal disease, older age, prolonged immobility >3 days, hypercoagulable states, and history of previous VTE [59, 60]. Although there are a number of schemes devised to assess thrombosis risk in the non-congenital heart disease population [61–63], they are not validated in those with CHD, and in general, we recommend that all adults with CHD in the ICU receive prophylactic anticoagulation unless they are at increased risk for bleeding (i.e., acute gastrointestinal or intracerebral bleed, profound thrombocytopenia).

Pharmacologic VTE prophylaxis is recommended over mechanical means (i.e., sequential compression devices) with the agent of choice being low molecular weight heparin (LMWH), though unfractionated heparin (UFH) can be used for those with renal failure. If the patient is at high risk for bleeding, sequential compression devices and elastic graduated compression stockings are recommended over no prophylaxis. Thromboprophylaxis should continue until the patient is ambulatory or discharged.

In the general population, prophylaxis has been found to decrease the risk of VTE in acutely ill medical patients, but there is no proven mortality benefit in medical patients [64]. In contrast, mortality benefit has been seen in surgical patients [65], although the reasons for this difference are not known. Outcomes for VTE prophylaxis in the adult with CHD are yet to be defined.

28.2.2 Management of Deep Venous Thrombosis and Pulmonary Embolism in ACHD

The mainstay of deep vein thrombosis treatment is anticoagulation in the absence of contraindications (i.e., active hemorrhage, recent intracerebral bleed, trauma, thrombocytopenia). The purpose of anticoagulation is to prevent complications such as clot extension, acute pulmonary embolism, and recurrent DVT. Anticoagulation is specifically indicated for proximal DVT which has a higher risk of embolization and death compared to distal (e.g., below the knee) DVT [66] as well as for symptomatic distal DVTs. Other factors should be considered when deciding between surveillance and anticoagulation of asymptomatic distal DVTs such as high D-dimer levels, clot burden and extent, prior DVT, prolonged immobility, as well as bleeding risk. Inferior vena cava filter can be considered for those with a lower extremity proximal DVT and an absolute contraindication to anticoagulation [67]. Thrombolytic therapy or catheter-based extraction is reserved for rare cases such as those with massive ilio-femoral DVT (phlegmasia cerulea dolens).

The diagnosis of PE in the single-ventricle patient by conventional means such as computed tomography with contrast or ventilation-perfusion scans is limited by the alteration in pulmonary arterial blood flow (lack of a systemic venous mixing chamber), and thus the diagnosis may rely on pulmonary angiography. The treatment of acute PE is guided by severity, hemodynamic stability, and bleeding risk. Therapeutic anticoagulation is indicated for patients with confirmed PE and no contraindications to anticoagulation. In general, those with hemodynamic instability with concern for massive PE should be considered for more aggressive therapies such as thrombolysis and/or mechanical embolectomy [68, 69].

The choice of anticoagulation for the treatment of VTE must take into account a number of factors including liver disease, renal disease, route of administration and dosing, compliance, and reversibility, keeping in mind that the critically ill patient in the ICU may have a predisposition toward hemorrhage. Direct oral anticoagulants (DOACs) are safe and effective alternatives to standard anticoagulation (heparin and warfarin). Table 28.1 summarizes factors to consider in selecting anticoagulation for patients with acute VTE [68]. Extensive discussion regarding diagnosis and treatment of VTE is beyond the scope of this chapter, and management should follow recommendations from clinical guidelines [68, 69].

28.3 Arrhythmia and Thromboembolic Stroke in Adults with Congenital Heart Disease

Atrial arrhythmias such as intra-atrial reentry tachycardia, typical atrial flutter, and atrial fibrillation occur in 15% of adult patients with congenital heart disease [70]. The incidence of atrial arrhythmias increases with age and underlying disease complexity, representing a major source of morbidity for adults with CHD including thromboembolic stroke [70, 71]. In the critical care setting, there is an increased risk of atrial tachyarrhythmias due to inflammation, surges in catecholamines, ischemia, volume shifts, and atrial stretch [72]. Additional superimposed risk factors include immobility, presence of prosthetic material, indwelling leads, intracardiac shunts or septal patch margin defects, sluggish flow and venous stasis, cyanosis, and hypercoagulability [3, 12], making the risk of stroke considerable.

The presence of atrial fibrillation increases the risk of thromboembolic stroke by fivefold, but stroke risk also depends on the presence of other risk factors [73]. The anticoagulation management of atrial fibrillation or atrial flutter in the critically ill adult with CHD must balance the risk of bleeding against the risk of stroke. The

Table 28.1 Factors affecting choice of treatment for acute VTE [68]

Factor	Preferred anticoagulant	Qualifying remarks
Cancer	LMWH	More so if: just diagnosed, extensive VTE, metastatic cancer, very symptomatic; vomiting; on cancer chemotherapy
Parenteral therapy to be avoided	Rivaroxaban; apixaban	VKA, dabigatran, and edoxaban require initial parenteral therapy
Once daily oral therapy preferred	Rivaroxaban; edoxaban; VKA	
Liver disease and coagulopathy	LMWH	NOACs contraindicated if INR raised because of liver disease; VKA difficult to control, and INR may not reflect antithrombotic effect
Renal disease and creatinine clearance <30 mL/min	VKA	NOACs and LMWH contraindicated with severe renal impairment. Dosing of NOACs with levels of renal impairment differs with the NOAC and among jurisdictions
Coronary artery disease	VKA, rivaroxaban, apixaban, edoxaban	Coronary artery events appear to occur more often with dabigatran than with VKA. This has not been seen with the other NOACs, and they have demonstrated efficacy for coronary artery disease. Antiplatelet therapy should be avoided if possible in patients on anticoagulants because of increased bleeding
Dyspepsia or history of GI bleeding	VKA, apixaban	Dabigatran increased dyspepsia. Dabigatran, rivaroxaban, and edoxaban may be associated with more GI bleeding than VKA
Poor compliance	VKA	INR monitoring can help to detect problems. However, some patients may be more compliant with a NOAC because it is less complex
Thrombolytic therapy use	UFH infusion	Greater experience with its use in patients treated with thrombolytic therapy
Reversal agent needed	VKA, UFH	
Pregnancy or pregnancy risk	LMWH	Potential for other agents to cross the placenta
Cost, coverage, licensing	Varies among regions and with individual circumstances	

CHA2DS2-VASc score and the HAS-BLED score are means of assessing stroke and bleeding risk, respectively. The CHA2DS2-VASc score is a risk stratification scheme for adults with non-valvular atrial fibrillation to assess stroke risk which considers the following: age, gender, heart failure, hypertension, history of stroke or transient ischemic attack, vascular disease, and diabetes [74] (Table 28.2). Those with CHA2DS2-VASc score ≥ 2 are considered at high risk for stroke and in whom benefit from anticoagulation exceeds bleeding risk. Though not necessarily meant to be used in the ICU setting, it can potentially help determine overall stroke risk. HAS-BLED is a risk score intended to assess bleeding risk which must always be considered when placing a patient on anticoagulation therapy [74]. The HAS-BLED

Table 28.2 CHA_2DS_2-VASc score and stroke risk [145]

	Risk factor	Points
C	Congestive heart failure (or left ventricular dysfunction)	1
H	Hypertension	1
A_2	Age ≥ 75 years	2
D	Diabetes	1
S_2	Stroke or transient ischemic attack history	2
V	Vascular disease (e.g., peripheral arterial disease, myocardial infarction)	1
A	Age 65–74 years	1
Sc	Sex category (i.e., female gender)	1

CHA_2DS_2-VASc score	Unadjusted ischemic stroke rate (% per year)
0	0.2%
1	0.6%
2	2.2%
3	3.2%
4	4.8%
5	7.2%
6	9.7%
7	11.2%
8	10.8%
9	12.2%

score assigns 1 point for the presence of each of the following bleeding risk factors: **h**ypertension, **a**bnormal renal and/or liver function, previous **s**troke, **b**leeding history, **l**abile INR, **e**lderly and concomitant **d**rugs, and/or alcohol abuse with a score of ≥3 indicating a high risk of bleeding (Table 28.3).

The applicability of both schemes in ACHD has been examined [75–77]. The Anticoagulation Therapy in Congenital Heart Disease (TACTIC) study was a retrospective multicenter trial examining the incidence of thromboembolic events in adults with CHD and atrial arrhythmias and the predictive capacity of the CHA2DS2-VASc and HAS-BLED scores [75]. There were 482 patients managed on a variety of antiplatelet/anticoagulation schemes, including no therapy. The thromboembolic event rate was 8.7% over an average follow-up time of 11.3 ± 9.4 years after the qualifying arrhythmia. The CHA2DS2-VASc score was not predictive of thromboembolism, but higher congenital heart lesion complexity correlated with higher thromboembolic risk. Bleeding events occurred in 8.3% of patients, and HAS-BLED was an independent predictor of major bleed on multivariable analysis.

That the CHA2DS2-VASc score did not adequately predict thromboembolic risk in adults with CHD may be a reflection of a distinct, heterogeneous patient population with wide variation of underlying lesions and younger age. The average age of ACHD patients who experience atrial arrhythmias and the age at which they present with stroke are significantly younger than that of the general population [70, 78, 79]. The authors suggest the CHA2DS2-VASc score could be modified to include disease complexity as defined by the Bethesda criteria [80] which is consistent with recent guidelines on arrhythmia management in ACHD that recommend disease complexity be considered in guiding anticoagulation strategy. In this document, long-term

Table 28.3 HAS-BLED score and risk of bleeding [146]

	Risk factor	Points
H	Hypertension	1
A	Abnormal renal and/or liver function	1 or 2
S	Stroke	2
B	Bleeding predisposition or diathesis	1
L	Labile INR	2
E	Elderly age > 65 years	1
D	Drugs (aspirin or NSAIDs) and/or excessive alcohol	1 or 2

HAS-BLED score	Bleeds per 100 patient-years
0	1.13
1	1.02
2	1.88
3	3.74
4	8.70
5–9	Insufficient data

INR international normalized ratio, *NSAIDs* nonsteroidal anti-inflammatory drugs
Hypertension is defined as systolic blood pressure >160 mmHg. Abnormal renal function is defined as the presence of chronic dialysis, renal transplantation, or serum creatinine ≥200 micromol/L. Abnormal liver function is defined as chronic hepatic disease (e.g., cirrhosis) or biochemical evidence of significant hepatic derangement (e.g., bilirubin more than two times the upper limit of normal, plus one or more of aspartate transaminase, alanine transaminase, and/or alkaline phosphatase more than three times the upper limit normal). Bleeding predisposition includes chronic bleeding disorder or previous bleeding requiring hospitalization or transfusion. Labile INRs for a patient on warfarin include unstable INRs, excessively high INRs, or <60% time in therapeutic range

anticoagulation is a Class I recommendation for intra-atrial reentry tachycardia or atrial fibrillation in patients with highly complex CHD and Class IIA recommendation for those with moderate forms of CHD. For patients with simple non-valvular forms of CHD with intra-atrial reentry tachycardia or atrial fibrillation, anticoagulation, aspirin, or no thromboprophylaxis is a Class IIB recommendation [81].

In practice, there is no risk stratification scheme that completely captures stroke risk for adults with CHD and atrial arrhythmias, especially in the ICU setting, but underlying disease complexity and risk factors as described by the CHA2DS2-VASc score as well as HAS-BLED score can be used in guiding therapy especially as the patient transitions out of the ICU setting and into ambulatory care. In general, if a new-onset atrial fibrillation or flutter continues for more than 48 h in the ICU, anticoagulation is recommended, and any attempt at rhythm control should be preceded by transesophageal echocardiography to rule out intracardiac thrombosis. Anticoagulation should be instituted and continued for at least 4–6 weeks afterward. However, bleeding risk in the ICU patient may be prohibitive due to platelet dysfunction from renal failure, thrombocytopenia, liver disease/cirrhosis, coagulopathy, etc., and benefit must be balanced against risk.

Patients who are admitted to the ICU on anticoagulation for stroke prophylaxis in the setting of atrial arrhythmias should have anticoagulation continued. Consideration should be made to switching to a reversible short-acting agent such as intravenous heparin if invasive procedures are anticipated. Gaps in anticoagulation can be managed for short periods of time as day-to-day stroke risk is relatively low.

28.4 Prosthetic Valves in Adults with Congenital Heart Disease

Valve replacement surgery is one of the most common types of cardiac surgery in ACHD [82]. Thromboembolic complications and anticoagulation-related bleeding are major contributors to morbidity and mortality after valve replacement surgery [83].

Management of patients with prosthetic valves in the ICU may involve the postoperative management of those who undergo valve replacement or long-term complications such as valve thrombosis, embolic phenomenon, or infective endocarditis. Furthermore, the anticoagulation management of patients with mechanical valve prostheses can post special challenges for patients in the ICU who are admitted for noncardiac reasons, and interruption of anticoagulation may be necessary.

28.4.1 Thromboembolism Prophylaxis

The highest risk of thromboembolic complications occurs within the first 3 months of surgery for both bioprosthetic and mechanical valve prostheses [84]. Atrial arrhythmias, a common comorbidity found in conjunction with valvular heart disease, can further increase the risk of thromboembolic stroke. After implantation of a mechanical prosthetic valve, anticoagulation with warfarin, a vitamin K antagonist, is recommended which has been proven to decrease risk of thrombosis and thromboembolism [85]. The addition of antiplatelet therapy can decrease the risk of systemic embolism or death in patients with mechanical heart valves [86]. The American College of Cardiology (ACC)/American Heart Association (AHA) recommends anticoagulation in patients with mechanical valve prostheses with warfarin at a target INR of 2.5 in the aortic and 3.0 in the mitral positions in the absence of other risk factors (Class I Ib) as well as a low-dose antiplatelet agent (Class IA) [87]. The On-X mechanical prosthesis (On-X Life Technologies Inc., Austin, Texas) in the aortic position can be maintained at a lower target INR 1.5–2.0 (Class IIb) after 3 months of standard therapy [88]. Direct oral anticoagulants (DOACs) should not be used in patients with mechanical valves. A recent trial investigating dabigatran vs. warfarin after aortic or mitral mechanical valve replacement was terminated early after demonstrating excess thromboembolic events and bleeding in the dabigatran arm [89].

The risk of thromboembolism after bioprosthetic valve surgery is not as high as mechanical valve replacement surgery, but there is an increased risk of events in the first 3–6 months after surgery [84, 90]. Early thrombogenicity of bioprosthetic valves can be attributed to incomplete endothelialization [91], so therefore some form of antiplatelet and/or antithrombotic therapy is recommended after bioprosthetic valve surgery. Anticoagulation with a warfarin for 3 months after bioprosthetic mitral or aortic valve replacement surgery with a target INR 2.5 is considered a reasonable strategy (IIa recommendation) to address risk of early postoperative thrombotic risk [88]. The role of DOACs in the anticoagulation management of patients with bioprosthetic valves is not yet defined.

28.4.2 Bridging Anticoagulation Therapy

Anticoagulation management including cessation and bridging therapy when there is interruption should take into account the type of procedure for which interruption is being considered, bleeding risk, as well as type, location, and number of prosthetic heart valves [88]. Minor procedures such as cataract removal, cutaneous biopsy, or dental procedures generally do not require cessation of anticoagulation. Critically ill patients in the ICU may have predisposition toward hemorrhage as discussed above including sepsis, thrombocytopenia, and renal and/or liver failure. The ACC/AHA guidelines do not recommend bridging when anticoagulation is interrupted in patients with mechanical aortic valves and no other risk factors for thrombosis [87].

When oral anticoagulation with warfarin is temporarily interrupted, bridging therapy with intravenous UFH or subcutaneous LMWH can be considered for higher-risk patients including those with mechanical mitral valve prostheses or patients with aortic mechanical valve prosthesis and an additional risk factor (e.g., atrial fibrillation, previous thromboembolism, hypercoagulable state, older-generation mechanical valve, left ventricular systolic dysfunction, or >1 mechanical valve) [92], but decisions should be made on an individual basis. Data supports the use of LMWH for bridging as safe and effective in mechanical heart valves [93, 94] although intravenous unfractionated heparin UFH may be preferable in the ICU setting given its short half-life. Figure 28.1 summarizes the ACC/AHA recommendations for antithrombotic therapy in prosthetic valves [87].

28.4.3 Prosthetic Valve Thrombosis and Stenosis

Mechanical prosthetic valve obstruction can be caused by thrombosis, pannus, or a combination thereof and can present as progressive dyspnea or in extremis with severe pulmonary edema [95]. Transthoracic echocardiogram is the first-line imaging modality (including Doppler gradient across the valve), but transesophageal echocardiography is often necessary to assess leaflet motion. Computed tomography and fluoroscopy are useful to evaluate for thrombosis, but differentiation between thrombosis and pannus is challenging and can be difficult to distinguish [96]. Clinical history is important in the evaluation including time from surgery, history of inadequate anticoagulation, and acuity of symptoms as thrombosis more often presents acutely compared to pannus. Infective endocarditis must be excluded. Once thrombosis is diagnosed, anticoagulation should be instituted. Mechanical

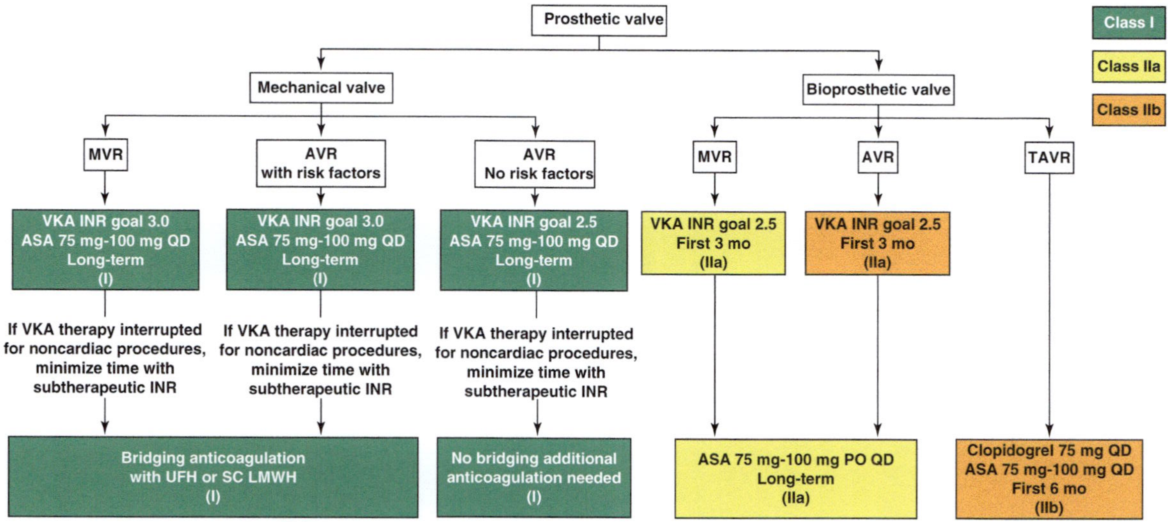

Risk factors include AF, previous thromboembolism, LV dysfunction, hypercoagulable condition, and older-generation mechanical AVR. For the strength of recommendations: Class I means the procedure/treament should be performed/administered. Class IIa means it is reasonable to perform the procedure/administer treatment. Class IIb means the procedure/treatment may be considered. Class III means that the procedure ro treatment is not useful/effective and may be harmful.
For the level of evidence: Level A means multiple populations evaluated; data derived from multiple randomized clinical trails or meta-analyses. Level B means limited populations evaluated; data derived from a single randomized trial or nonrandomized studies. Level C means very limited populations evaluated; only consensus opinion of experts, case studies, or standard of care.

AF: atrial fibrillation; ASA: aspirin; AVR: aortic valve replacement; INR: international normalized ratio; LMWH: low-molecular-weight heparin; MVR: mitral valve replacement; PO: by mouth; QD: every day; SC: subcutaneous; TAVR: transcatheter aortic valve replacement; UFH: unfractionated heparin; VKA: vitamin K antagonist.

Fig. 28.1 ACC/AHA recommendations for anticoagulation of prosthetic heart valves [87, 88]. *Note*: Updates in 2017 include [88]: • IIa recommendation from IIb for VKA after bioprosthetic AVR, • On-X AVR without risk factors target INR 1.5–2.0 (IIb, LOE B-R), and • IIb recommendation for VKA INR target 2.5 for 3 months after TAVR

left-sided prosthetic valve obstruction has a high mortality rate and requires urgent therapy including fibrinolysis or surgery (Class Ib) [88].

Bioprosthetic valve thrombosis usually presents in a more subacute manner with progressive stenosis and can occur years after surgery [97]. Evaluation is similar as above with the use of transesophageal echocardiography to better evaluate for thrombosis. Again, infective endocarditis must be ruled out. Bioprosthetic valve thrombosis has been shown to respond to warfarin [98] which can be considered as an initial treatment in patients who are hemodynamically stable (Class IIa) [88].

Patients with a prosthetic valve and stroke should undergo work-up for cardio-embolic stroke including evaluation of the prosthetic valve by echocardiogram. Specifically, transesophageal echocardiography is recommended to better evaluate valve function, evidence of thrombosis or vegetation, or any other source of embolism including a careful interrogation of the left atrium, left atrial appendage, and aorta for atherosclerotic plaque. If thromboembolism occurred in the setting of inadequate antithrombotic therapy, institution of adequate therapy is the first step [87]. If thromboembolism occurred despite adequate antithrombotic therapy, consideration should be given to augmenting therapy which includes the addition of low-dose aspirin if maintained only on therapeutic warfarin, increasing the goal INR, or adding warfarin for those who were maintained on aspirin alone (i.e., bioprosthetic valves) [87].

28.5 Special Consideration of Thrombosis in Adult Patients with Fontan Circulation

It has long been recognized that thrombosis in the patient with Fontan circulation is associated with significant mortality and morbidity. A recent systemic review by Alsaied in 2017 of 28 studies, 6707 patients, and a mean follow-up time from Fontan of 8.23 ± 5.42 years found thrombosis and bleeding to be the fifth most common cause of death accounting for 10% of the 1000 deaths reported [19].

The overall incidence of thrombosis in the patient with Fontan circulation is about 12% in recent reports [15, 18] and 5.2% in a meta-analysis looking at extracardiac Fontans only [13]. Earlier reports describe a 3–33% incidence with stroke in 1.4–3.6% [14]. The discrepancy in reported incidence is secondary to the variability in the population studied, the time from the Fontan procedure, the method of thrombosis detection, the location of the thrombosis investigated (i.e., all thrombosis vs. pulmonary emboli vs. cerebral vascular event), and whether the study investigated clinically evident or silent thrombosis. Although these reviews are an important source of observational data, their heterogeneous designs limit the ability to draw conclusions from which clinical practice guidelines can be generated. They have, however, generated the following important observations:

- There appears to be two peaks in the incidence of thrombosis post Fontan: early (0–6 months) [99] and late (5–15 years post Fontan) [4–6, 9, 11, 16].
- Thrombosis post Fontan is most commonly found in the Fontan itself, intracardiac (systemic venous atrium, pulmonary venous atrium, hypoplastic ventricle)

and pulmonary arteries, although it has been reported as well in the ligated pulmonary artery stump, hypoplastic aortic root, and coronary arteries and associated with heparin-induced thrombocytopenia (HIT) [7, 15, 17]. Silent pulmonary emboli have also been described [8].

- Risk factors supported by focused retrospective observational studies include atriopulmonary type of Fontan connection, bilateral bidirectional cavopulmonary anastomoses, hypoplastic cardiac chambers with flow stasis, presence of a blind-ended pulmonary artery stump, and a history of previous thrombosis. Additional potential factors supported by general retrospective observational studies or expert opinion include protein-losing enteropathy, prolonged pleural effusions, prolonged immobilization, ventricular dysfunction, arrhythmia, presence of thrombogenic foreign material, atrial-level fenestration, Kawashima connection, and an abnormal thrombophilia profile [14]. Additional risk factors for stroke identified in adults with CHD that include the Fontan include systemic arterial hypertension, atrial fibrillation, iron deficiency anemia, microcytosis, and prior phlebotomy [3]. Additional risk factors for pulmonary embolus include age, female gender, low oxygen saturation, ventricular dysfunction, and low systolic flow velocities in the pulmonary arteries [10, 47].

It is not surprising that the adult with Fontan circulation has a propensity to thrombosis, especially in the ICU setting. The factors described above of altered blood flow, blood component abnormalities, and endothelial dysfunction are intrinsic to the Fontan. Several studies have evaluated coagulation proteins in single-ventricle patients and have shown an infantile pattern, namely, lower levels of both pro- and anticoagulant proteins, namely, low protein C and suppression of the thrombomodulin-protein C-protein S pathway [32, 35, 36, 40]. In addition several studies have documented elevated factor VIII after the Fontan [34, 37, 41]. Odegard in 2009 showed lower than control levels of both pro- and anticoagulation proteins from Norwood stage I up to Fontan [39]. After the Fontan protein C stayed low, and factor VIII was found to be significantly higher than controls; 42% of Fontan patients had F VIII >160%. There was no correlation with hemodynamics, hepatic synthetic function, or hepatocellular dysfunction. The speculation is that high factor VIII, low protein C plus Fontan physiology puts patients at risk of thrombosis over a lifetime.

Knowing that the Fontan patient is prone to thrombosis, what data is available regarding thromboprophylaxis? Two recent meta-analyses warrant mention. In 2011 Marrone reviewed 20 studies, 1075 patients who had extracardiac Fontans [13]. The average time from Fontan in the studies was 2 months to 12 years. The overall thrombotic rate was 5.2%, 4.5% in those who received aspirin alone and 5% in those receiving warfarin with or without aspirin. Alsaied in 2015 reviewed 10 studies, 1200 patients with all types of Fontans [15]. The average time from Fontan in the combined studies was 7.1 years. The overall thrombotic rate was 11.3%: 18.6% in those receiving no thromboprophylaxis, 8.6% in those receiving aspirin only, and 9% in those receiving warfarin. From these meta-analyses, it appears that some form of thromboprophylaxis is protective but that warfarin is not superior to aspirin. Whether or not thrombosis is less frequent in the extracardiac Fontan warrants further investigation.

When considering the adult Fontan patient, several limitations in these meta-analyses must be acknowledged. The average follow-up from the Fontan in the two meta-analyses was less than 15 years, giving little information about the risk of thrombosis and effect of thromboprophylaxis in the third and fourth decade of life. Second, the studies address neither time in therapeutic range for warfarin patients nor aspirin resistance in the patients receiving aspirin. Third, additional risk factors for thrombosis were not address in either meta-analysis.

Carefully considering the currently available, albeit limited, data, the American Heart Association's 2013 Scientific Statement on Prevention and Treatment of Thrombosis in Pediatric and Congenital Heart Disease makes the following recommendations regarding prevention and treatment of thrombosis in the patient with a palliated single ventricle at all stages [14]:

1. Patients with a palliated single ventricle should undergo clinical assessment for the anatomic and hemodynamic risk factors for thrombus. Risk factors for thrombus (as listed earlier in this chapter) should be ameliorated (i.e., arrhythmias, ventricular dysfunction, prolonged immobilization) and minimized (blind-ended pulmonary artery stump, prolonged immobilization) when possible (Class I; Level of Evidence B).
2. For patients with a palliated single ventricle, serial clinical assessment and monitoring for changes in anatomic and hemodynamic thrombotic risk factor are indicated because risk factors may change over time (Class I; Level of Evidence C). New risk factor for thrombus should be ameliorated (i.e., arrhythmias, ventricular dysfunction, prolonged immobilization) and minimized (prolonged immobilization) when possible (Class I; Level of Evidence C).
3. Patients with a palliated single ventricle should be monitored for thrombosis with periodic transthoracic echocardiography (with focused attention to the identification of thrombi) as part of routine follow-up assessments (Class I; Level of Evidence C).
4. For patients with a palliated single ventricle, if thrombosis is suspected on clinical grounds or from transthoracic echocardiography, diagnostic confirmation with transesophageal echocardiography, MRI, computed tomography, computed tomographic angiography, nuclear medicine lung perfusion scan, or venography/angiography can be useful (Class IIa; Level of Evidence C).
5. For patients with a palliated single ventricle, other imaging modalities (in addition to echocardiography) used to detect thrombosis such as transesophageal echocardiography or MRI may be considered for surveillance for patients with anatomic or hemodynamic risk factors (Class IIb; Level of Evidence C).
6. Initiation of antithrombotic therapy or an increase in the magnitude of antithrombotic therapy for prophylaxis (change in agent, i.e., from antiplatelet to anticoagulant or higher target levels) is probably reasonable if anatomic or hemodynamic risk factors become present at any stage in the single-ventricle pathway (Class IIa; Level of Evidence C).

   And in addition specifically for Fontan patients:
7. Long-term antiplatelet therapy for prevention of thrombosis is reasonable after the Fontan procedure (Class IIa; Level of Evidence C).

8. Prophylaxis with warfarin or LMWH may be reasonable in infants and children for 3–12 months after the Fontan procedure (Class IIb; Level of Evidence C).
9. Long-term therapy with warfarin may be reasonable after the Fontan procedure for patients with anatomic or hemodynamic risk factors (Class IIb; Level of Evidence C).

Several additional comments are warranted regarding thromboprophylaxis in the Fontan patient. No method of thromboprophylaxis is 100% effective with a thrombosis rate of currently about 12% [15, 18]. Thrombosis prevention in the Fontan patient is more than pharmacotherapy. Understanding and mitigating risk factors as well as diagnosing and treating thrombosis as early as possible are essential. Thrombosis risk in the Fontan patient is not constant over time. As risk factors increase, antithrombotic therapy should be reassessed and readjusted. Continued assessment of risk over time [9] with adjustment of antithrombotic therapy based on current risk assessment is essential. Finally, as is well known to ACHD physicians, warfarin is a medication with a narrow therapeutic window and many drug-drug interactions. The DOACs are discussed below. They may have promise in the adult with Fontan circulation [100], but safety and efficacy have not yet been established especially in the Fontan with liver disease, thrombocytopenia, and/or protein-losing enteropathy where concerns of bleeding are real.

28.6 Anticoagulant Therapy

The following section will provide specific information regarding mechanism of action, pharmacokinetics, dosing, monitoring, and associated harms for commonly used anticoagulants. It is important to note that the predominant risk associated with anticoagulation therapy is hemorrhage. To minimize this bleeding risk, concurrent antiplatelet therapy should be avoided, if possible.

28.6.1 Unfractionated Heparin

Unfractionated heparin (UFH) is extracted from bovine lung or porcine intestine and is composed of a heterogeneous mixture of highly sulfated glycosaminoglycans [101]. UFH itself has no intrinsic anticoagulant effect but instead acts through the binding of antithrombin (AT) potentiating the AT anticoagulant activity over 1000-fold inactivating coagulant factors IIa (thrombin), Xa, XIa, and XIIa [102–105]. UFH is parentally available as either a continuous intravenous infusion or a subcutaneous injection. The half-life is short and estimated at 1.5 ± 0.5 h [106]. Unfortunately, UFH interacts with other plasma proteins, endothelial cells, and macrophages which can alter the pharmacokinetics with a resultant high inter- and intra-patient dose response.

Intravenous UFH therapy is typically started as a bolus (80 units/kg, maximum bolus 4000–5000 units) followed by the initiation of a continuous infusion (18 units/

kg/h, maximum initial infusion 1000–2000 U/h). If a patient has a low AT level (i.e., congenital deficiency, acquired deficiency secondary to losses from nephrotic syndrome, draining chylous effusion, consumption, or asparaginase therapy), higher UFH doses may be required. The two most common assays used to monitor UFH include the aPTT and the UFH anti-Xa level. Both tests have pitfalls when used to monitor UFH as well as poor correlation. The therapeutic goal for the aPTT is 1.5–2.5 times control (60–85 seconds), and the UFH anti-Xa goal is 0.3–0.7 units/mL. See Table 28.4 for the dose titration of UFH using these laboratory markers.

The aPTT is not a direct measure of the UFH effect and can be impacted by many other parameters that could result in either an over or underestimation of the true UFH effect. For example, an elevated factor VIII or fibrinogen (acute phase reactants) will shorten the aPTT making it appear that the patient is heparin resistant. Alternatively a deficiency in a coagulation factor (i.e., from liver failure or consumption) or the presence of an antiphospholipid antibody will prolong the aPTT making it appear that the patient is therapeutic on UFH. The UFH anti-Xa level provides a more direct measure that is not impacted by the above factors, although the UFH anti-Xa level does not reflect additional anticoagulant targets of UFH. The activated clotting time (ACT) is used to monitor higher heparin doses given to patients undergoing cardiopulmonary bypass or cardiac catheterization. The ACT is a whole-blood clotting time that is simple to perform with a rapid turnaround time. It is more sensitive to a wider range of heparin doses than the PTT and is impacted by the same factors as the PTT, and additionally thrombocytopenia prolongs the ACT.

Table 28.4 The 4T's clinical probability score for heparin-induced thrombocytopenia [120]

	Score = 2	Score = 1	Score = 0
Thrombocytopenia	Platelet count fall >50% and platelet nadir ≥20 × 10^9/L	Platelet count fall 30–50% or nadir 10–19 × 10^9/L	Platelet count fall <30% or a platelet nadir <10 × 10^9/L
Timing of platelet count fall	Clear onset 5–10 days post-heparin or within 1 day with a prior heparin exposure within 30 days	Consistent with days 5–10 fall but not clear (missing data), onset post day 10; or fall within 1 day with a prior heparin exposure 30–100 days	Platelet count fall <4 days without recent heparin exposure
Thrombosis	New confirmed thrombosis can be venous or arterial, skin necrosis at heparin injection site, anaphylactic reaction to IV heparin bolus	Progressive or recurrent thrombosis, suspected thrombosis, erythematous skin lesions at heparin injection sites	None
Other causes for thrombocytopenia	None apparent	Possible	Definite

HIT probability score: low, ≤3 points; intermediate, 4–5 points; high, 6–8 points
Adapted from Lo GK et al. [120]

Full reversal of heparin can be obtained with the use of protamine sulfate, a basic protein that binds heparin and forms a salt [105]. Approximately 1 mg of protamine will neutralize 100 units of UFH [105]. Calculations should be made based on the total amount of heparin received in the prior 2–2.5 h [105]. Adverse events such as hypotension and bradycardia can be minimized with slow administration of protamine.

The benefits of UFH include the short half-life and the ability to completely reverse the anticoagulation effect. Additionally UFH can be used in the setting of renal failure where LMWHs cannot. In clinically unstable patients at risk for hemorrhage who require anticoagulation, UFH should be strongly considered. Transition to an alternative anticoagulant should occur once the patient is clinically stable. Nonhemorrhagic complications associated with UFH include HIT/HITT (see separate section) and osteopenia with long-term use [107, 108].

28.6.2 Low Molecular Weight Heparin

Low molecular weight heparins (LMWH) are derived from UFH by chemical or enzymatic depolymerization and contain shorter-length polysaccharide chains. Similar to UFH, LMWH exert an anticoagulant effect through binding AT and potentiating the AT anticoagulant activity, but as compared to UFH, there is a reduced inhibitory activity against factor IIa (thrombin) relative to factor Xa. LMWH are administered as a subcutaneous injection. The PK properties are more stable as compared to UFH. The half-life is 3–6 h and the LMWH anti-Xa levels peak 3–5 h after dosing. LMWH is predominantly cleared by the kidneys.

Dosing will vary based on the exact LMWH that is used. Common preparations include enoxaparin, 1 mg/kg/dose every 12 h, or 1.5 mg/kg once daily; in obesity, use ideal body weight to calculate the dose and tinzaparin 175 anti-Xa IU/kg daily . Additionally, similar to UFH if a patient has a low AT level, higher doses of the LMWH may be required.

Routine monitoring is not recommended except for extreme obesity or in the setting of renal insufficiency. When monitoring the LMWH, anti-Xa peak level is used with a goal of 0.5–1 units/mL (drawn 4–6 h postinjection). LMWH can be partially reversed (approximately 70%) with protamine. LMWH should not be used in the setting of renal failure. Nonhemorrhagic complications associated with LMWH are similar to UFH. HIT has been reported with the use of LMWH, but it is thought to be less frequent than UFH [109]. Long-term LMWH use is associated with less bone loss than UFH [105].

28.6.3 Heparin-Induced Thrombocytopenia

Heparin-induced thrombocytopenia (HIT) is an immunologic complication of heparin therapy. Antibodies are formed against complexes of heparin and an endogenous platelet protein, platelet factor 4 (PF4) [110]. It is postulated that the binding of antibodies to the heparin-PF4 complex results in increased platelet reactivity with a resultant prothrombotic state [110]. This disorder is characterized by thrombocytopenia (HIT) and sometimes thrombosis (HITT) that can occur in any vascular bed and can be catastrophic. Interestingly, while the immune reaction is relatively common post-heparin exposure (8–50%), with the highest in those undergoing cardiac surgery (25–50%), only a small portion of patients will actually develop the clinical consequences of thrombocytopenia and thrombosis [111, 112]. Overall the incidence of HIT is estimated to be approximately 0.02–3% of patients [111–114]. The incidence is influenced by the clinical setting, type of heparin used, and dose [115]. Prophylactic dose UFH has a higher risk of HIT versus prophylactic LMWH [114]. Untreated HIT has a mortality of 20–30% [116, 117].

The diagnosis of HIT is based on clinical criteria. Multiple scoring systems have been developed [118–120]. The most commonly used is the 4T's clinical probability score (Table 28.5) [120]. Classically, HIT is characterized by symptoms appearing 5–10 days post-heparin exposure with a 50% fall in the platelet count (rarely is the platelet count <50,000/μL), and there can be venous or arterial thrombosis. Laboratory testing can be supportive in making the diagnosis and includes ELISA for the heparin-P4 antibodies and the serotonin-releasing assay. The ELISA is readily available with a fast turnaround time. This test is highly sensitive but has a significant false-positive rate. The ELISA is most helpful in ruling out the diagnosis with a negative assay. The serotonin-releasing assay is highly specific and sensitive; it measures platelet reactivity in the presence of the patient's plasma. Unfortunately, it is only performed in a few highly specialized laboratories so is not readily available for most clinicians.

The treatment of HIT includes the removal of all heparin from the patient including from central lines and avoidance of LMWH. Anticoagulation should be initiated (even without thrombosis) with a non-heparin anticoagulant such as a direct thrombin inhibitor (i.e., bivalirudin or argatroban) [121]. In this setting, warfarin should never be initiated by itself due to an increased risk of skin necrosis and further thrombotic events. Warfarin can be initiated once the platelet count has normalized and overlapped with the non-heparin anticoagulant until the INR is therapeutic. The median time for platelet recovery is approximately 4 days. Fondaparinux, a synthetic pentasaccharide LMWH, is also commonly used off-label for the treatment of

Table 28.5 Unfractionated heparin dose titration [147]

aPTT (s)	UFH Anti-Xa (units/mL)	Dose adjustment	Lab monitoring
<50	<0.1	Bolus: 50 IU/kg Increase infusion rate by 10%	4 h post rate change
50–59	0.1–0.29	Increase infusion rate by 10%	4 h post rate change
60–85	0.3–0.7	No change	4 h then q24 hours
86–95	0.71–0.9	Decrease infusion rate by 10%	4 h post rate change
96–120	0.91–1	Hold infusion for 30 min Decrease infusion rate by 10%	4 h post rate change
>120	>1	Hold infusion for 60 min Decrease infusion rate by 15%	4 h post rate change

Adapted from Monagle P et al. [147]

HIT. Although rarely HIT has been reported with the use of fondaparinux [122]. The direct oral anticoagulants (DOACs) have not been studied in HIT, so their use in this clinical setting would be considered off-label and without sufficient clinical supporting data.

The duration of anticoagulation in HIT is determined by the presence of thrombosis. For those patients with only thrombocytopenia, there remains a high risk of thrombosis for 2–4 weeks after developing HIT. Anticoagulation should be continued during this high-risk time [121]. For patients with a thrombosis, anticoagulation should be continued for 3 months [121]. In general, HIT antibodies are transient with a median time of disappearance of 50–85 days without clear evidence of an amnestic immune response with reexposure [123]. In general, patients with a history of HIT should not be reexposed to UFH or LMWH. The one exception is for procedures where the use of UFH is favored over other anticoagulants like CPB if repeat HIT antibody testing is negative. In those patients with a history of HIT who have demonstrated resolution of the HIT antibodies, a short exposure to UFH during CPB is considered acceptable [121]. This strategy does not apply to those patients with persistent antibodies, however.

28.6.4 Direct Thrombin Inhibitors: Argatroban or Bivalirudin

Argatroban and bivalirudin are parenteral direct thrombin inhibitors and are typically used in the setting of HIT/HITT when heparin needs to be avoided. Bivalirudin reversibly binds the active catalytic and substrate binding site of thrombin. It has a half-life of 25 min and has approximately 20% renal clearance. The initial dose is 0.15–0.2 mg/kg/h. It is typically monitored by the aPTT titrated to 1.5–3 times control, but the ACT has also been used. A limited number of laboratories are running direct thrombin inhibitor assays, although this has not yet become standard of care.

Argatroban reversibly binds the active catalytic site of thrombin. It also has a very short half-life of 45 min. It is predominantly metabolized in the liver so should not be used in the setting of hepatic failure. The initial dose is 2 mcg/kg/min. It is titrated via the aPTT to 1.5–3 times control; the ACT has also been used. No antidote exists for the reversal of bivalirudin or argatroban, but both have very short half-lives, so discontinuation of the infusion should be sufficient for most forms of bleeding.

28.6.5 Fondaparinux

Fondaparinux is a synthetic analog of the AT-binding pentasaccharide found in heparin and LMWH. The structure was modified to enhance its affinity for AT increasing the specific activity and half-life. Unlike UFH or LMWH, fondaparinux has no inhibitory activity against factor IIa (thrombin) and only inactivates factor Xa.

Fondaparinux is administered via a subcutaneous injection. The half-life is longer than LMWH at 17 h. There is minimal binding to other proteins. The clearance is exclusively renal. A steady state is reached after the third or fourth daily dose. Dosing is guided by weight: <50 kg 5 mg daily, 50–100 kg 7.5 mg daily, and >100 kg 10 mg daily. Routine coagulation monitoring is not recommended. If a level is needed, specific assays calibrated for fondaparinux should be used [124]. Similar to LMWH, monitoring is achieved by measuring fondaparinux anti-Xa peak level with a goal of 0.5–1 mg/L (drawn 4 h post).

There are no reversal agents available for fondaparinux. Unlike other forms of heparin, protamine does not bind fondaparinux. There are reports of using various hemostatic therapies (prothrombin complex concentrates, activated prothrombin complex concentrates, or recombinant factor VIIa) to treat life-threatening bleeding secondary to fondaparinux [125]. Due to the long half-life and lack of a reversal agent, this medication should only be utilized in patients who are clinically stable with a low risk of hemorrhage. It should not be used in patients with renal insufficiency.

28.6.6 Warfarin

Warfarin is a vitamin K antagonist and interferes with the cyclic conversion of vitamin K through the inhibition of vitamin K epoxide reductase. This results in a decrease in the posttranslational γ-carboxylation of vitamin K-dependent clotting factors which is imperative for biologic function. This impacts coagulation factors II, VII, IX, and X and anticoagulant proteins C and S [126]. Warfarin absorption is primarily gastric and is complete within 4 h of administration. It has a very long half-life of 36–42 h. In general, warfarin is initiated with an anticoagulation "bridge" because patients are initially prothrombotic due to the variable half-lives of anti- and procoagulant proteins lowered by warfarin.

Initial dosing is individualized considering the patient's cardiac function, nutritional status, prior warfarin dosing, current medications, and hepatic function. Typical maintenance dosing is 2–5 mg/day. Patients with Fontan circulation may require less warfarin. Patients >60 years of age may require less warfarin due to changes in warfarin metabolism. The warfarin dose is titrated via the international normalized ratio (INR). The INR goal is dictated by the clinical indication for warfarin but is commonly 2–3.

There are multiple choices available for warfarin reversal including vitamin K (oral, intravenous, or subcutaneous), non-activated prothrombin complex concentrate (PCC, Kcentra), or fresh frozen plasma. How warfarin reversal is completed is determined by the severity of bleeding and the patient's thrombotic risk associated with reversal [127]. In the setting of severe, life-threatening bleeding, vitamin K replacement should be augmented with the use of either Kcentra or fresh frozen plasma. Kcentra contains concentrated non-activated coagulation factors II, VII, IX, and X and anticoagulant proteins C and S and is FDA approved for the urgent reversal of warfarin. Kcentra dosing is determined by the INR and the patient's body weight: INR 2–<4, 25 units FIX/kg (maximum 2500 units); INR 4–6, 35 units FIX/kg (maximum 3500 units); and INR 6, 50 units FIX/kg (maximum 5000 units). The benefit to using a Kcentra as opposed to fresh frozen plasma is that a much smaller volume is given to the patient and replaces only those coagulation and anticoagulation proteins impacted by warfarin.

28.6.7 Direct Oral Anticoagulants

The first direct oral anticoagulant (DOAC) received FDA approval in 2010. All of the DOACs bind directly to a key coagulant protein to inhibit fibrin formation. There are two broad categories for mechanism of action including direct anti-Xa inhibitors (rivaroxaban, apixaban, and edoxaban) and direct thrombin (IIa) inhibitors (dabigatran). The advantage to all of the DOACs is more predictable pharmacokinetics with a wide therapeutic window and limited drug-drug interactions as compared to warfarin. They also have a relative rapid onset of action and shorter half-lives as compared to warfarin. Dosing of DOACs varies by the specific drug.

Table 28.6 provides general dosing schema for each DOAC. For all of the DOACs, dosing needs to be adjusted in the setting of impaired renal clearance, and in significant renal impairment, DOAC use is not recommended.

The key advantage to predictable pharmacokinetics and a wide therapeutic window for DOACs is that routine therapeutic monitoring is not needed [128]. The disadvantage is that methods to monitor these medications are not readily available [128]. There are times when drug monitoring might be needed including in the setting of emergency surgery, breakthrough thrombosis, renal insufficiency, or bleeding [129]. Specialized laboratory assays for DOACs have been developed including a dilute thrombin time for dabigatran and anti-Xa assays that are drug calibrated for the anti-Xa inhibitors. The PT or PTT cannot reliably be used to monitor these medications.

In the setting of bleeding, all of the DOACs have relatively short half-lives of 10–12 h, so supportive care can be given, while the medication is wearing off in most cases. In the setting of life-threatening hemorrhage, reversal for dabigatran or consideration for other hemostatic therapies for oral Xa inhibitors needs to be considered. Currently, idarucizumab is the only FDA-approved DOAC reversal agent, and it is specific for dabigatran. Idarucizumab is a monoclonal antibody fragment

Table 28.6 Direct oral anticoagulant dosing

	Acute VTE	Atrial fibrillation	VTE prophylaxis
Rivaroxaban	15 mg twice daily for 21 days, followed by 20 mg daily	20 mg once daily	10 mg once daily
Apixaban	10 mg twice daily for 7 days, followed by 5 mg twice daily	5 mg twice daily	2.5 mg twice daily
Edoxaban	60 mg once daily after 5–10 days of initial therapy with a parenteral anticoagulant	60 mg once daily	
Dabigatran	150 mg twice daily, after 5–10 days of initial therapy with a parenteral anticoagulant	150 mg twice daily	220 mg once daily

All of the direct oral anticoagulants require dose adjustment for renal insufficiency

that binds dabigatran with an affinity that is 350 times greater than thrombin [130]. It can bind both free and thrombin-bound dabigatran and neutralizes its activity [130]. Clinically it is given as a one-time intravenous infusion with a complete reversal of the anticoagulant effect in minutes [131]. A rebound anticoagulant effect after the initial idarucizumab transfusion has been reported and needs to be considered in the setting of renal failure [132, 133]. Dabigatran can also be partially removed with hemodialysis [134]. For the Xa inhibitors, there is a reversal agent in development, andexanet alfa. It is a human factor Xa decoy protein but is not currently FDA approved [135]. There are reports of using various hemostatic therapies (prothrombin complex concentrates, activated prothrombin complex concentrates, or recombinant factor VIIa) to treat life-threatening bleeding secondary to DOACs [136, 137].

DOACs have been demonstrated to be efficacious and in the USA are approved for the use in stroke prevention from non-valvular atrial fibrillation, the treatment of DVT and PE, secondary prevention of DVT, and DVT prevention post-elective knee and hip surgery [138]. As mentioned above, at this time DOACs should not be used in the setting of mechanical heart valves. A clinical trial comparing dabigatran to warfarin in patients with either an aortic or mitral mechanical heart valve was halted early secondary to increased thrombotic and bleeding events in those patients receiving dabigatran as compared to warfarin [89]. A phase 2 clinical trial is currently underway using rivaroxaban in the setting of mechanical aortic valve replacement (ClincalTrials.gov Identifier: NCT02128841). There is no data to support the routine use of DOACs for thrombosis prevention in Fontan patients though case reports have been published and a multicenter trial is underway.

28.7 Thrombolytic Therapy

The strongest indication for thrombolytic therapy includes either a life- or limb-threatening thrombotic event including stroke, prosthetic valve thrombosis, or a massive pulmonary embolism [139–144]. Significant bleeding (including intracranial hemorrhage) and thromboembolism are known complications of thrombolysis. Thrombolysis can be performed locally or systemically. Contraindications to thrombolytic therapy generally include active bleeding, an inability to maintain the platelet count >75,000/μL or fibrinogen >100 mg/dL, a major operation or site of hemorrhage within 7–10 days, seizures within 48 h, central nervous system surgery/ischemia/trauma/hemorrhage within 30 days, or uncontrolled hypertension. These contraindications are not absolute, and the relative risks of thrombolytic therapy should be weighed against the potential benefits in each clinical situation.

When instituting thrombolytic therapy, baseline laboratory values should be obtained (CBC, PT, PTT, fibrinogen, and D-dimer) to assess for additional bleeding risks. For systemic sustained thrombolysis, these labs should be obtained prior to therapy and followed every 4–6 h during therapy. An increase in the D-dimer and a drop in the fibrinogen level are indicative of a "lytic" state. To minimize the risk of bleeding, if the fibrinogen level drops below 100 mg/dL, consider either holding thrombolytic therapy or infusing cryoprecipitate as an external source of fibrinogen. The platelet count should be kept >75,000/μL. Tissue plasminogen activator (tPA) is currently the only thrombolytic agent available in the USA. Concomitant use of heparin has been used at either low or therapeutic dosing with therapeutic heparin usually continued after the thrombolytic is stopped. Due to the very high risk of hemorrhage during and immediately after thrombolysis, invasive procedures should be minimized.

References

1. Ihenacho HN, Fletcher DJ, Breeze GR, Stuart J. Consumption coagulopathy in congenital heart-disease. Lancet. 1973;1:231–4.
2. Perloff JK, Marelli AJ, Miner PD. Risk of stroke in adults with cyanotic congenital heart disease. Circulation. 1993;87:1954–9.
3. Ammash N, Warnes CA. Cerebrovascular events in adult patients with cyanotic congenital heart disease. J Am Coll Cardiol. 1996;28:768–72.
4. Rosenthal DN, Friedman AH, Kleinman CS, Kopf GS, Rosenfeld LE, Hellenbrand WE. Thromboembolic complications after Fontan operations. Circulation. 1995;92:II287–93.
5. Coon PD, Rychik J, Novello RT, Ro PS, Gaynor JW, Spray TL. Thrombus formation after the Fontan operation. Ann Thorac Surg. 2001;71:1990–4.
6. Seipelt RG, Franke A, Vazquez-Jimenez JF, et al. Thromboembolic complications after Fontan procedures: comparison of different therapeutic approaches. Ann Thorac Surg. 2002;74:556–62.
7. Porcelli R, Moskowitz BC, Cetta F, et al. Heparin-induced thrombocytopenia with associated thrombosis in children after the Fontan operation: report of two cases. Tex Heart Inst J. 2003;30:58–61.
8. Varma C, Warr MR, Hendler AL, Paul NS, Webb GD, Therrien J. Prevalence of "silent" pulmonary emboli in adults after the Fontan operation. J Am Coll Cardiol. 2003;41:2252–8.
9. Kaulitz R, Ziemer G, Rauch R, et al. Prophylaxis of thromboembolic complications after the Fontan operation (total cavopulmonary anastomosis). J Thorac Cardiovasc Surg. 2005;129:569–75.
10. Broberg CS, Ujita M, Prasad S, et al. Pulmonary arterial thrombosis in eisenmenger syndrome is associated with biventricular dysfunction and decreased pulmonary flow velocity. J Am Coll Cardiol. 2007;50:634–42.
11. Khairy P, Fernandes SM, Mayer JE Jr, et al. Long-term survival, modes of death, and predictors of mortality in patients with Fontan surgery. Circulation. 2008;117:85–92.
12. Khairy P. Thrombosis in congenital heart disease. Expert Rev Cardiovasc Ther. 2013;11:1579–82.
13. Marrone C, Galasso G, Piccolo R, et al. Antiplatelet versus anticoagulation therapy after extracardiac conduit Fontan: a systematic review and meta-analysis. Pediatr Cardiol. 2011;32:32–9.
14. Giglia TM, Massicotte MP, Tweddell JS, et al. Prevention and treatment of thrombosis in pediatric and congenital heart disease: a scientific statement from the American Heart Association. Circulation. 2013;128:2622–703.
15. Alsaied T, Alsidawi S, Allen CC, Faircloth J, Palumbo JS, Veldtman GR. Strategies for thromboprophylaxis in Fontan circulation: a meta-analysis. Heart. 2015;101:1731–7.
16. Ohuchi H, Yasuda K, Miyazaki A, et al. Prevalence and predictors of haemostatic complications in 412 Fontan patients: their relation to anticoagulation and haemodynamics. Eur J Cardiothorac Surg. 2015;47:511–9.
17. Keraliya AR, Murphy DJ, Steigner ML, Blankstein R. Thrombus in hypoplastic aorta: an uncommon cause of acute myocardial infarction. J Cardiovasc Comput Tomogr. 2016;10:263–4.

18. Atz AM, Zak V, Mahony L, et al. Longitudinal outcomes of patients with single ventricle after the Fontan procedure. J Am Coll Cardiol. 2017;69:2735–44.
19. Alsaied T, Bokma JP, Engel ME, et al. Factors associated with long-term mortality after Fontan procedures: a systematic review. Heart. 2017;103:104–10.
20. Valente AM, Bhatt AB, Cook S, et al. The CALF (congenital heart disease in adults lower extremity systemic venous health in Fontan patients) study. J Am Coll Cardiol. 2010;56:144–50.
21. Virchow R. Thrombose und Embolie. Gefässentzündung und septische Infektion. Gesammelte Abhandlungen zur wissenschaftlichen Medicin. 1856. pp. 219–752.
22. Giglia TM, Witmer C. Bleeding and thrombosis in pediatric cardiac intensive care. Pediatr Crit Care Med. 2016;17:S287–95.
23. Giglia TM, Witmer C. Hematologic aspects of pediatric and adolescent heart disease: bleeding, clotting and blood component abnormalities in Moss & Adams Heart Disease in Infants, Children, and Adolescents: Including the Fetus and Young Adult, 9th ed. In: Allen HDS, Robert E, Penny DJ, Feltes TF, Cetta F, editors. Moss & Adams' heart disease in infants, children, and adolescents, including the fetus and young adult. Philadelphia: Lippincott Williams & Wilkins; 2016. p. 1900.
24. Wolberg AS, Aleman MM, Leiderman K, Machlus KR. Procoagulant activity in hemostasis and thrombosis: Virchow's triad revisited. Anesth Analg. 2012;114:275–85.
25. Waniewski J, Kurowska W, Mizerski JK, et al. The effects of graft geometry on the patency of a systemic-to-pulmonary shunt: a computational fluid dynamics study. Artif Organs. 2005;29:642–50.
26. Ravn HB, Hjortdal VE, Stenbog EV, et al. Increased platelet reactivity and significant changes in coagulation markers after cavopulmonary connection. Heart. 2001;85:61–5.
27. Savage B, Saldivar E, Ruggeri ZM. Initiation of platelet adhesion by arrest onto fibrinogen or translocation on von Willebrand factor. Cell. 1996;84:289–97.
28. Jaggers JJ, Neal MC, Smith PK, Ungerleider RM, Lawson JH. Infant cardiopulmonary bypass: a procoagulant state. Ann Thorac Surg. 1999;68:513–20.
29. Guay J, Ruest P, Lortie L. Cardiopulmonary bypass induces significant platelet activation in children undergoing open-heart surgery. Eur J Anaesthesiol. 2004;21:953–6.
30. Heying R, van Oeveren W, Wilhelm S, et al. Children undergoing cardiac surgery for complex cardiac defects show imbalance between pro- and anti-thrombotic activity. Crit Care (London England). 2006;10:R165.
31. Jaggers J, Lawson JH. Coagulopathy and inflammation in neonatal heart surgery: mechanisms and strategies. Ann Thorac Surg. 2006;81(6):S2360.
32. Tomita H, Yamada O, Ohuchi H, et al. Coagulation profile, hepatic function, and hemodynamics following Fontan-type operations. Cardiol Young. 2001;11:62–6.
33. Jahangiri M, Shore D, Kakkar V, Lincoln C, Shinebourne E. Coagulation factor abnormalities after the Fontan procedure and its modifications. J Thorac Cardiovasc Surg. 1997;113:989–92; discussion 92–3
34. Jahangiri M, Kreutzer J, Zurakowski D, Bacha E, Jonas RA. Evaluation of hemostatic and coagulation factor abnormalities in patients undergoing the Fontan operation. J Thorac Cardiovasc Surg. 2000;120:778–82.
35. Odegard KC, McGowan FX Jr, DiNardo JA, et al. Coagulation abnormalities in patients with single-ventricle physiology precede the Fontan procedure. J Thorac Cardiovasc Surg. 2002;123:459–65.
36. Odegard KC, McGowan FX Jr, Zurakowski D, et al. Coagulation factor abnormalities in patients with single-ventricle physiology immediately prior to the Fontan procedure. Ann Thorac Surg. 2002;73:1770–7.
37. Odegard KC, McGowan FX Jr, Zurakowski D, et al. Procoagulant and anticoagulant factor abnormalities following the Fontan procedure: increased factor VIII may predispose to thrombosis. J Thorac Cardiovasc Surg. 2003;125:1260–7.
38. Odegard KC, Zurakowski D, Hornykewycz S, et al. Evaluation of the coagulation system in children with two-ventricle congenital heart disease. Ann Thorac Surg. 2007;83:1797–803.

39. Odegard KC, Zurakowski D, DiNardo JA, et al. Prospective longitudinal study of coagulation profiles in children with hypoplastic left heart syndrome from stage I through Fontan completion. J Thorac Cardiovasc Surg. 2009;137:934–41.
40. Horigome H, Murakami T, Isobe T, Nagasawa T, Matsui A. Soluble P-selectin and thrombomodulin-protein C-Protein S pathway in cyanotic congenital heart disease with secondary erythrocytosis. Thromb Res. 2003;112:223–7.
41. Rask O, Hanseus K, Ljung R, Strandberg K, Berntorp E. Lower incidence of procoagulant abnormalities during follow-up after creation of the Fontan circulation in children. Cardiol Young. 2009;19:152–8.
42. Levin E, Wu J, Devine DV, et al. Hemostatic parameters and platelet activation marker expression in cyanotic and acyanotic pediatric patients undergoing cardiac surgery in the presence of tranexamic acid. Thromb Haemost. 2000;83:54–9.
43. Binotto MA, Maeda NY, Lopes AA. Evidence of endothelial dysfunction in patients with functionally univentricular physiology before completion of the Fontan operation. Cardiol Young. 2005;15:26–30.
44. Thornburg CD, Smith PB, Smithwick ML, Cotten CM, Benjamin DK Jr. Association between thrombosis and bloodstream infection in neonates with peripherally inserted catheters. Thromb Res. 2008;122:782–5.
45. Randolph AG, Cook DJ, Gonzales CA, Andrew M. Benefit of heparin in peripheral venous and arterial catheters: systematic review and meta-analysis of randomised controlled trials. BMJ. 1998;316:969–75.
46. O'Connor MJ, Ravishankar C, Ballweg JA, et al. Early systemic-to-pulmonary artery shunt intervention in neonates with congenital heart disease. J Thorac Cardiovasc Surg. 2011;142:106–12.
47. Silversides CK, Granton JT, Konen E, Hart MA, Webb GD, Therrien J. Pulmonary thrombosis in adults with Eisenmenger syndrome. J Am Coll Cardiol. 2003;42:1982–7.
48. Saha A, Balakrishnan KG, Jaiswal PK, et al. Prognosis for patients with Eisenmenger syndrome of various aetiology. Int J Cardiol. 1994;45:199–207.
49. Daliento L, Somerville J, Presbitero P, et al. Eisenmenger syndrome. Factors relating to deterioration and death. Eur Heart J. 1998;19:1845–55.
50. Niwa K, Perloff JK, Kaplan S, Child JS, Miner PD. Eisenmenger syndrome in adults: ventricular septal defect, truncus arteriosus, univentricular heart. J Am Coll Cardiol. 1999;34:223–32.
51. Giannakoulas G, Boutsikou M. The Gordian knot of thromboembolism in congenital heart disease. Heart. 2015;101:1523–4.
52. Jensen AS, Idorn L, Thomsen C, et al. Prevalence of cerebral and pulmonary thrombosis in patients with cyanotic congenital heart disease. Heart. 2015;101:1540–6.
53. Manlhiot C, Menjak IB, Brandao LR, et al. Risk, clinical features, and outcomes of thrombosis associated with pediatric cardiac surgery. Circulation. 2011;124:1511–9.
54. Giglia TM, Petrosa WL, Veneziale K, et al. Use of PC4 database in a prospective cohort study of hospital-acquired thrombosis in pediatric cardiac in-patients. J Am Coll Cardiol. 2016;67:976.
55. Anderson FA Jr, Zayaruzny M, Heit JA, Fidan D, Cohen AT. Estimated annual numbers of US acute-care hospital patients at risk for venous thromboembolism. Am J Hematol. 2007;82:777–82.
56. Lim W, Meade M, Lauzier F, et al. Failure of anticoagulant thromboprophylaxis: risk factors in medical-surgical critically ill patients*. Crit Care Med. 2015;43:401–10.
57. Horlander KT, Mannino DM, Leeper KV. Pulmonary embolism mortality in the United States, 1979–1998: an analysis using multiple-cause mortality data. Arch Intern Med. 2003;163:1711–7.
58. The Surgeon General's Call to Action to Prevention Deep Vein Thrombosis and Pulmonary Embolism. In: Services UDoHaH, editor. http://www.surgeongeneral.gov/topics/deepvein/calltoaction/call-to-action-ondvt-2008.pdf.2008.
59. Anderson FA Jr, Spencer FA. Risk factors for venous thromboembolism. Circulation. 2003;107:I9–16.

60. Di Nisio M, van Es N, Buller HR. Deep vein thrombosis and pulmonary embolism. Lancet. 2016;388:3060–73.
61. Barbar S, Noventa F, Rossetto V, et al. A risk assessment model for the identification of hospitalized medical patients at risk for venous thromboembolism: the Padua Prediction Score. J Thromb Haemost. 2010;8:2450–7.
62. Spyropoulos AC, Anderson FA Jr, FitzGerald G, et al. Predictive and associative models to identify hospitalized medical patients at risk for VTE. Chest. 2011;140:706–14.
63. Nendaz M, Spirk D, Kucher N, et al. Multicentre validation of the Geneva Risk Score for hospitalised medical patients at risk of venous thromboembolism. Explicit ASsessment of Thromboembolic RIsk and Prophylaxis for Medical PATients in SwitzErland (ESTIMATE). Thromb Haemost. 2014;111:531–8.
64. Kakkar AK, Cimminiello C, Goldhaber SZ, Parakh R, Wang C, Bergmann JF. Low-molecular-weight heparin and mortality in acutely ill medical patients. N Engl J Med. 2011;365:2463–72.
65. Collins R, Scrimgeour A, Yusuf S, Peto R. Reduction in fatal pulmonary embolism and venous thrombosis by perioperative administration of subcutaneous heparin. Overview of results of randomized trials in general, orthopedic, and urologic surgery. N Engl J Med. 1988;318:1162–73.
66. Galanaud JP, Sevestre-Pietri MA, Bosson JL, et al. Comparative study on risk factors and early outcome of symptomatic distal versus proximal deep vein thrombosis: results from the OPTIMEV study. Thromb Haemost. 2009;102:493–500.
67. White RH, Brunson A, Romano PS, Li Z, Wun T. Outcomes after vena cava filter use in non-cancer patients with acute venous thromboembolism: a population-based study. Circulation. 2016;133:2018–29.
68. Kearon C, Akl EA, Ornelas J, et al. Antithrombotic therapy for VTE disease: CHEST guideline and expert panel report. Chest. 2016;149:315–52.
69. Jaff MR, McMurtry MS, Archer SL, et al. Management of massive and submassive pulmonary embolism, iliofemoral deep vein thrombosis, and chronic thromboembolic pulmonary hypertension: a scientific statement from the American Heart Association. Circulation. 2011;123:1788–830.
70. Bouchardy J, Therrien J, Pilote L, et al. Atrial arrhythmias in adults with congenital heart disease. Circulation. 2009;120:1679–86.
71. Engelfriet P, Boersma E, Oechslin E, et al. The spectrum of adult congenital heart disease in Europe: morbidity and mortality in a 5 year follow-up period. The Euro Heart Survey on adult congenital heart disease. Eur Heart J. 2005;26:2325–33.
72. Walkey AJ, Hogarth DK, Lip GYH. Optimizing atrial fibrillation management: from ICU and beyond. Chest. 2015;148:859–64.
73. Pisters R, Lane DA, Marin F, Camm AJ, Lip GY. Stroke and thromboembolism in atrial fibrillation. Circulation. 2012;76:2289–304.
74. Lip GY, Nieuwlaat R, Pisters R, Lane DA, Crijns HJ. Refining clinical risk stratification for predicting stroke and thromboembolism in atrial fibrillation using a novel risk factor-based approach: the euro heart survey on atrial fibrillation. Chest. 2010;137:263–72.
75. Khairy P, Aboulhosn J, Broberg CS, et al. Thromboprophylaxis for atrial arrhythmias in congenital heart disease: a multicenter study. Int J Cardiol. 2016;223:729–35.
76. Masuda K, Ishizu T, Niwa K, et al. Increased risk of thromboembolic events in adult congenital heart disease patients with atrial tachyarrhythmias. Int J Cardiol. 2017;234:69–75.
77. Heidendael JF, Bokma JP, de Groot JR, Koolbergen DR, Mulder BJ, Bouma BJ. Weighing the risks: thrombotic and bleeding events in adults with atrial arrhythmias and congenital heart disease. Int J Cardiol. 2015;186:315–20.
78. Lanz J, Brophy JM, Therrien J, Kaouache M, Guo L, Marelli AJ. Stroke in adults with congenital heart disease: incidence, cumulative risk, and predictors. Circulation. 2015;132:2385–94.
79. Mandalenakis Z, Rosengren A, Lappas G, Eriksson P, Hansson PO, Dellborg M. Ischemic stroke in children and young adults with congenital heart disease. J Am Heart Assoc. 2016;5:e003071.

80. Warnes CA, Williams RG, Bashore TM, et al. ACC/AHA 2008 guidelines for the management of adults with congenital heart disease: a report of the American College of Cardiology/American Heart Association Task Force on Practice Guidelines (Writing Committee to Develop Guidelines on the Management of Adults With Congenital Heart Disease). Developed in Collaboration With the American Society of Echocardiography, Heart Rhythm Society, International Society for Adult Congenital Heart Disease, Society for Cardiovascular Angiography and Interventions, and Society of Thoracic Surgeons. J Am Coll Cardiol. 2008;52:e143–263.
81. Khairy P, Van Hare GF, Balaji S, et al. PACES/HRS Expert Consensus Statement on the Recognition and Management of Arrhythmias in Adult Congenital Heart Disease: developed in partnership between the Pediatric and Congenital Electrophysiology Society (PACES) and the Heart Rhythm Society (HRS). Endorsed by the governing bodies of PACES, HRS, the American College of Cardiology (ACC), the American Heart Association (AHA), the European Heart Rhythm Association (EHRA), the Canadian Heart Rhythm Society (CHRS), and the International Society for Adult Congenital Heart Disease (ISACHD). Heart Rhythm. 2014;11:e102–65.
82. Holst KA, Dearani JA, Burkhart HM, et al. Reoperative multivalve surgery in adult congenital heart disease. Ann Thorac Surg. 2013;95:1383–9.
83. Brennan JM, Edwards FH, Zhao Y, et al. Long-term safety and effectiveness of mechanical versus biologic aortic valve prostheses in older patients: results from the Society of Thoracic Surgeons Adult Cardiac Surgery National Database. Circulation. 2013;127:1647–55.
84. Heras M, Chesebro JH, Fuster V, et al. High risk of thromboemboli early after bioprosthetic cardiac valve replacement. J Am Coll Cardiol. 1995;25:1111–9.
85. Cannegieter SC, Rosendaal FR, Briet E. Thromboembolic and bleeding complications in patients with mechanical heart valve prostheses. Circulation. 1994;89:635–41.
86. Massel DR, Little SH. Antiplatelet and anticoagulation for patients with prosthetic heart valves. Cochrane Database Syst Rev. 2013;(7):CD003464.
87. Nishimura RA, Otto CM, Bonow RO, et al. 2014 AHA/ACC guideline for the management of patients with valvular heart disease: a report of the American College of Cardiology/American Heart Association Task Force on Practice Guidelines. Circulation. 2014;129:e521–643.
88. Nishimura RA, Otto CM, Bonow RO, et al. AHA/ACC focused update of the 2014 AHA/ACC guideline for the management of patients with valvular heart disease: a report of the American College of Cardiology/American Heart Association Task Force on clinical practice guidelines. Circulation. 2017;135:e1159–e95.
89. Eikelboom JW, Connolly SJ, Brueckmann M, et al. Dabigatran versus warfarin in patients with mechanical heart valves. N Engl J Med. 2013;369:1206–14.
90. Russo A, Grigioni F, Avierinos JF, et al. Thromboembolic complications after surgical correction of mitral regurgitation incidence, predictors, and clinical implications. J Am Coll Cardiol. 2008;51:1203–11.
91. Roudaut R, Serri K, Lafitte S. Thrombosis of prosthetic heart valves: diagnosis and therapeutic considerations. Heart. 2007;93:137–42.
92. Douketis JD, Spyropoulos AC, Spencer FA, et al. Perioperative management of antithrombotic therapy: antithrombotic therapy and prevention of thrombosis, 9th ed: American College of Chest Physicians Evidence-Based Clinical Practice Guidelines. Chest. 2012;141:e326S–50S.
93. Seshadri N, Goldhaber SZ, Elkayam U, et al. The clinical challenge of bridging anticoagulation with low-molecular-weight heparin in patients with mechanical prosthetic heart valves: an evidence-based comparative review focusing on anticoagulation options in pregnant and nonpregnant patients. Am Heart J. 2005;150:27–34.
94. Spyropoulos AC, Turpie AG, Dunn AS, et al. Perioperative bridging therapy with unfractionated heparin or low-molecular-weight heparin in patients with mechanical prosthetic heart valves on long-term oral anticoagulants (from the REGIMEN registry). Am J Cardiol. 2008;102:883–9.
95. Barbetseas J, Nagueh SF, Pitsavos C, Toutouzas PK, Quinones MA, Zoghbi WA. Differentiating thrombus from pannus formation in obstructed mechanical prosthetic valves: an evaluation of

clinical, transthoracic and transesophageal echocardiographic parameters. J Am Coll Cardiol. 1998;32:1410–7.
96. Tanis W, Habets J, van den Brink RB, Symersky P, Budde RP, Chamuleau SA. Differentiation of thrombus from pannus as the cause of acquired mechanical prosthetic heart valve obstruction by non-invasive imaging: a review of the literature. Eur Heart J Cardiovasc Imaging. 2014;15:119–29.
97. Egbe AC, Pislaru SV, Pellikka PA, et al. Bioprosthetic valve thrombosis versus structural failure: clinical and echocardiographic predictors. J Am Coll Cardiol. 2015;66:2285–94.
98. Pislaru SV, Hussain I, Pellikka PA, et al. Misconceptions, diagnostic challenges and treatment opportunities in bioprosthetic valve thrombosis: lessons from a case series. Eur J Cardiothorac Surg. 2015;47:725–32.
99. Manlhiot C, Brandao LR, Kwok J, et al. Thrombotic complications and thromboprophylaxis across all three stages of single ventricle heart palliation. J Pediatr. 2012;161:513–9.e3.
100. Pujol C, Niesert AC, Engelhardt A, et al. Usefulness of direct oral anticoagulants in adult congenital heart disease. Am J Cardiol. 2016;117:450–5.
101. Linhardt RJ, Gunay NS. Production and chemical processing of low molecular weight heparins. Semin Thromb Hemost. 1999;25(Suppl 3):5–16.
102. Damus PS, Hicks M, Rosenberg RD. Anticoagulant action of heparin. Nature. 1973;246:355–7.
103. Rosenberg RD, Lam L. Correlation between structure and function of heparin. Proc Natl Acad Sci U S A. 1979;76:1218–22.
104. Lindahl U, Backstrom G, Hook M, Thunberg L, Fransson LA, Linker A. Structure of the antithrombin-binding site in heparin. Proc Natl Acad Sci U S A. 1979;76:3198–202.
105. Garcia DA, Baglin TP, Weitz JI, Samama MM. Parenteral anticoagulants: antithrombotic therapy and prevention of thrombosis, 9th ed: American College of Chest Physicians Evidence-Based Clinical Practice Guidelines. Chest. 2012;141:e24S–43S.
106. Estes JW. The kinetics of heparin. Ann N Y Acad Sci. 1971;179:187–204.
107. Murphy MS, John PR, Mayer AD, Buckels JA, Kelly DA. Heparin therapy and bone fractures. Lancet. 1992;340:1098.
108. Sackler JP, Liu L. Heparin-induced osteoporosis. Br J Radiol. 1973;46:548–50.
109. Warkentin TE, Levine MN, Hirsh J, et al. Heparin-induced thrombocytopenia in patients treated with low-molecular-weight heparin or unfractionated heparin. N Engl J Med. 1995;332:1330–5.
110. Warkentin TE, Hayward CP, Boshkov LK, et al. Sera from patients with heparin-induced thrombocytopenia generate platelet-derived microparticles with procoagulant activity: an explanation for the thrombotic complications of heparin-induced thrombocytopenia. Blood. 1994;84:3691–9.
111. Warkentin TE, Sheppard JA, Horsewood P, Simpson PJ, Moore JC, Kelton JG. Impact of the patient population on the risk for heparin-induced thrombocytopenia. Blood. 2000;96:1703–8.
112. Pouplard C, May MA, Iochmann S, et al. Antibodies to platelet factor 4-heparin after cardiopulmonary bypass in patients anticoagulated with unfractionated heparin or a low-molecular-weight heparin : clinical implications for heparin-induced thrombocytopenia. Circulation. 1999;99:2530–6.
113. Smythe MA, Koerber JM, Mattson JC. The incidence of recognized heparin-induced thrombocytopenia in a large, tertiary care teaching hospital. Chest. 2007;131:1644–9.
114. Martel N, Lee J, Wells PS. Risk for heparin-induced thrombocytopenia with unfractionated and low-molecular-weight heparin thromboprophylaxis: a meta-analysis. Blood. 2005;106:2710–5.
115. Arepally GM. Heparin-induced thrombocytopenia. Blood. 2017;129:2864–72.
116. Ahmed I, Majeed A, Powell R. Heparin induced thrombocytopenia: diagnosis and management update. Postgrad Med J. 2007;83:575–82.
117. Warkentin TE, Greinacher A. Heparin-induced thrombocytopenia and cardiac surgery. Ann Thorac Surg. 2003;76:2121–31.
118. Cuker A, Arepally G, Crowther MA, et al. The HIT Expert Probability (HEP) Score: a novel pre-test probability model for heparin-induced thrombocytopenia based on broad expert opinion. J Thromb Haemost. 2010;8:2642–50.

119. Lillo-Le Louet A, Boutouyrie P, Alhenc-Gelas M, et al. Diagnostic score for heparin-induced thrombocytopenia after cardiopulmonary bypass. J Thromb Haemost. 2004;2:1882–8.
120. Lo GK, Juhl D, Warkentin TE, Sigouin CS, Eichler P, Greinacher A. Evaluation of pretest clinical score (4 T's) for the diagnosis of heparin-induced thrombocytopenia in two clinical settings. J Thromb Haemost. 2006;4:759–65.
121. Linkins LA, Dans AL, Moores LK, et al. Treatment and prevention of heparin-induced thrombocytopenia: antithrombotic therapy and prevention of thrombosis, 9th ed: American College of Chest Physicians Evidence-Based Clinical Practice Guidelines. Chest. 2012;141:e495S–530S.
122. Bhatt VR, Aryal MR, Shrestha R, Armitage JO. Fondaparinux-associated heparin-induced thrombocytopenia. Eur J Haematol. 2013;91:437–41.
123. Warkentin TE, Kelton JG. Temporal aspects of heparin-induced thrombocytopenia. N Engl J Med. 2001;344:1286–92.
124. Paolucci F, Frasa H, Van Aarle F, et al. Two sensitive and rapid chromogenic assays of fondaparinux sodium (Arixtra) in human plasma and other biological matrices. Clin Lab. 2003;49:451–60.
125. Elmer J, Wittels KA. Emergency reversal of pentasaccharide anticoagulants: a systematic review of the literature. Transfus Med (Oxford, England). 2012;22:108–15.
126. Furie B, Bouchard BA, Furie BC. Vitamin K-dependent biosynthesis of gamma-carboxyglutamic acid. Blood. 1999;93:1798–808.
127. Ansell J, Hirsh J, Hylek E, Jacobson A, Crowther M, Palareti G. Pharmacology and management of the vitamin K antagonists: American College of Chest Physicians Evidence-Based Clinical Practice Guidelines (8th). Chest. 2008;133:160S–98S.
128. Baruch L. Laboratory monitoring of anticoagulant medications: focus on novel oral anticoagulants. Postgrad Med. 2013;125:135–45.
129. Wright C, Brown R, Cuker A. Laboratory measurement of the direct oral anticoagulants: indications and impact on management in clinical practice. Int J Lab Hematol. 2017;39 Suppl 1:31–6.
130. Schiele F, van Ryn J, Litzenburger T, Ritter M, Seeliger D, Nar H. Structure-guided residence time optimization of a dabigatran reversal agent. MAbs. 2015;7:871–80.
131. Pollack CV Jr, Reilly PA, Eikelboom J, et al. Idarucizumab for dabigatran reversal. New Engl J Med. 2015;373:511–20.
132. Stecher A, Vene N, Mavri A, Mijovski MB, Krevel B, Gradisek P. Late rebound of dabigatran levels after idarucizumab reversal in two patients with severe renal failure. Eur J Anaesthesiol. 2017;34:400–2.
133. Simon A, Domanovits H, Ay C, Sengoelge G, Levy JH, Spiel AO. The recommended dose of idarucizumab may not always be sufficient for sustained reversal of dabigatran. J Thromb Haemost. 2017;15:1317–21.
134. Khadzhynov D, Wagner F, Formella S, et al. Effective elimination of dabigatran by haemodialysis. A phase I single-centre study in patients with end-stage renal disease. Thromb Haemost. 2013;109:596–605.
135. Connolly SJ, Milling TJ Jr, Eikelboom JW, et al. Andexanet alfa for acute major bleeding associated with factor Xa inhibitors. N Engl J Med. 2016;375:1131–41.
136. Yates S, Sarode R. Novel thrombin and factor Xa inhibitors: challenges to reversal of their anticoagulation effects. Curr Opin Hematol. 2013;20:552–7.
137. Siegal DM, Garcia DA, Crowther MA. How I treat target-specific oral anticoagulant-associated bleeding. Blood. 2014;123:1152–8.
138. Cowell RP. Direct oral anticoagulants: integration into clinical practice. Postgrad Med J. 2014;90:529–39.
139. Sun JC, Davidson MJ, Lamy A, Eikelboom JW. Antithrombotic management of patients with prosthetic heart valves: current evidence and future trends. Lancet. 2009;374:565–76.
140. Whitlock RP, Sun JC, Fremes SE, Rubens FD, Teoh KH. Antithrombotic and thrombolytic therapy for valvular disease: Antithrombotic Therapy and Prevention of Thrombosis, 9th ed: American College of Chest Physicians Evidence-Based Clinical Practice Guidelines. Chest. 2012;141:e576S–600S.

141. Desai S, Kavinsky C. Localized left atrial administration of tPA for the treatment of mechanical mitral valve thrombosis. Catheter Cardiovasc Interv. 2008;72:151–5.
142. Johnson JA, Rauh RA, Phillips SD, Cetta F. Thrombolytic therapy in the treatment of right-sided prosthetic valve thrombosis in adults with congenital heart disease. Congenit Heart Dis. 2011;6:266–8.
143. Taherkhani M, Hashemi SR, Hekmat M, Safi M, Taherkhani A, Movahed MR. Thrombolytic therapy for right-sided mechanical pulmonic and tricuspid valves: the largest survival analysis to date. Tex Heart Inst J. 2015;42:543–7.
144. Ozturk S, Erdem F, Ozturk S, Ayhan S. Successful thrombolytic therapy in a patient with congenital corrected transposition of the great arteries. Acta Med Acad. 2016;45:158–62.
145. Friberg L, Rosenqvist M, Lip GY. Evaluation of risk stratification schemes for ischaemic stroke and bleeding in 182 678 patients with atrial fibrillation: the Swedish Atrial Fibrillation cohort study. Eur Heart J. 2012;33:1500–10.
146. Pisters R, Lane DA, Nieuwlaat R, de Vos CB, Crijns HJ, Lip GY. A novel user-friendly score (HAS-BLED) to assess 1-year risk of major bleeding in patients with atrial fibrillation: the Euro Heart Survey. Chest. 2010;138:1093–100.
147. Monagle P, AKC C, Goldenberg NA, et al. Antithrombotic therapy in neonates and children: Antithrombotic Therapy and Prevention of Thrombosis, 9th ed: American College of Chest Physicians Evidence-Based Clinical Practice Guidelines. Chest. 2012;141:e737S–801S.

ACHD Advanced Directives and Discontinuation of Life in the Critical Care Environment

29

Matthias Greutmann and Daniel Tobler

29.1 Introduction and Scope of the Problem

With the introduction of open heart surgery and improved cardiology care, most complex congenital heart defects have transformed from deadly diseases into well-treatable conditions with survival to adulthood being the rule for the majority of affected patients [1]. This leads to rapidly growing novel cohorts of adults with congenital heart disease, most of them requiring lifelong specialist care [2, 3]. These adults are not cured, and many remain at high risk of cardiovascular complications and premature death as young adults [4]. The majority of patients die from their cardiac disease with perioperative death, sudden cardiac death, and death from heart failure being the most common causes [5, 6]. Care for survivors of childhood congenital heart disease in end-stage heart failure has become everyday reality in specialist centers for adult congenital heart disease. Many of these patients are dying from their disease as young and middle-aged adults. As these patient cohorts are still rapidly growing and as for many patients, the risk for complications will substantially increase within their third, fourth, and fifth decade of life, the burden of care for adult congenital heart disease patients with end-stage disease is expected to markedly increase over the next few decades with growing and aging of contemporary cohorts [3, 4].

M. Greutmann (✉)
University Heart Center, Cardiology, University Hospital Zurich, Zurich, Switzerland
e-mail: matthias.greutmann@usz.ch

D. Tobler
Department of Cardiology, University Hospital Basel, Basel, Switzerland
e-mail: daniel.tobler@usb.ch

E. da Cruz et al. (eds.), *Intensive Care of the Adult with Congenital Heart Disease*, Congenital Heart Disease in Adolescents and Adults,
https://doi.org/10.1007/978-3-319-94171-4_29

29.2 Current Practice of End-of-Life Care in Adults with Congenital Heart Disease

Although the need for comprehensive care, including multidisciplinary end-of-life care is well recognized, little is known about current practice in centers for adults with congenital heart disease [7]. One study explored the provision of end-of-life care in a cohort of adults with congenital heart disease dying from their disease between 2000 and 2009 at a large tertiary care center in Canada. A total of 48 patients were identified that died from their cardiac disease during the study period [8]. Patients dying in the perioperative period or dying from non-cardiac disease were excluded.

Table 29.1 illustrates the disease characteristics of these, mainly young adults.

Despite clear evidence of advanced/end-stage disease in a large number of these patients, only five patients (10%) had documented discussions about end-of-life care prior to their death, only three of them as outpatients during a cardiology visit. The majority of patients had aggressive medical treatment up to their demise with two thirds dying on the intensive care unit and more than half under attempted resuscitation [8]. Although this study is not designed to elucidate the appropriateness of medical treatment in individual patients, given the clear evidence of end-stage disease in many of these patients, there is a high suspicion that at least in some individuals, care may have been overly aggressive or even futile. Palliative care teams were involved in a minority of patients only (19%) [8]. None of these patients died under attempted resuscitation.

Better exploration of patients' wishes regarding end-of-life care and promotion of structured advance care planning may prevent overaggressive treatment at the end of life and may enhance patient autonomy and self-determination at their end of life.

Table 29.1 Sociodemographic and medical characteristics of 48 patients who died from their congenital heart disease between 2000 and 2009 at a single tertiary center

Male, *n* (%)	28 (58)
Age at death, years ± SD (range)	37 ± 14 (18–68)
Sociodemographic characteristics, n (%)	
Married/living with partner	20 (42)
Had at least one child	11 (23)
Medical background, n (%)	
Moderate or great disease complexity	45 (94)
Previous cardiac surgery	38 (79)
Implanted cardiac defibrillator	5 (10)
NYHA class III or IV at last clinic visit	29 (60)
Previous major adverse cardiac events[a]	43 (90)
Prior admission due to heart failure[b]	27 (56)
Prior heart transplant assessment	20 (42)
On active heart transplant waiting list	4 (8)

Modified Tobler et al. with permission [8]

NYHA New York Heart Association

[a]Defined as heart failure, arrhythmias, myocardial infarction, endocarditis, pulmonary emboli, or severe hemoptysis

[b]Defined as pulmonary edema or decompensation of chronic heart failure

29.3 Patient Perspective and Barriers to End-of-Life Discussions

In contrast to the lack of end-of-life discussions in clinical practice, a substantial number of patients seem to wish such discussions becoming part of routine clinical care. In a survey of 200 adult congenital heart disease outpatients and 48 health-care providers, three quarters of patients stated that end-of-life discussions should be part of routine clinic visits [9]. This was independent of the underlying disease severity and socioeconomic characteristics of the patients (Fig. 29.1). In contrast to the patients' expectations, health-care providers stated they would tailor such discussions in respect to the complexity of their patients underlying heart defect and the presence or absence of major cardiovascular complications. Furthermore, most patients preferred to have such discussions starting early in the disease course, before life-threatening complications occur, while most health-care providers would reserve such discussions toward the later stages of the disease, when life-threatening complications are imminent or when patients have to be admitted to hospital for such complications. Interestingly, when asked who should initiate end-of-life discussions during outpatient visits, patients reported that they expected the medical team to raise these discussions, while physicians would reserve such discussions rather for patients who brought them up by themselves. Health-care providers reported uncertainty about patients' wishes and readiness for end-of-life discussions and major uncertainties about the individual patient's prognosis as major obstacles to start such discussions [9].

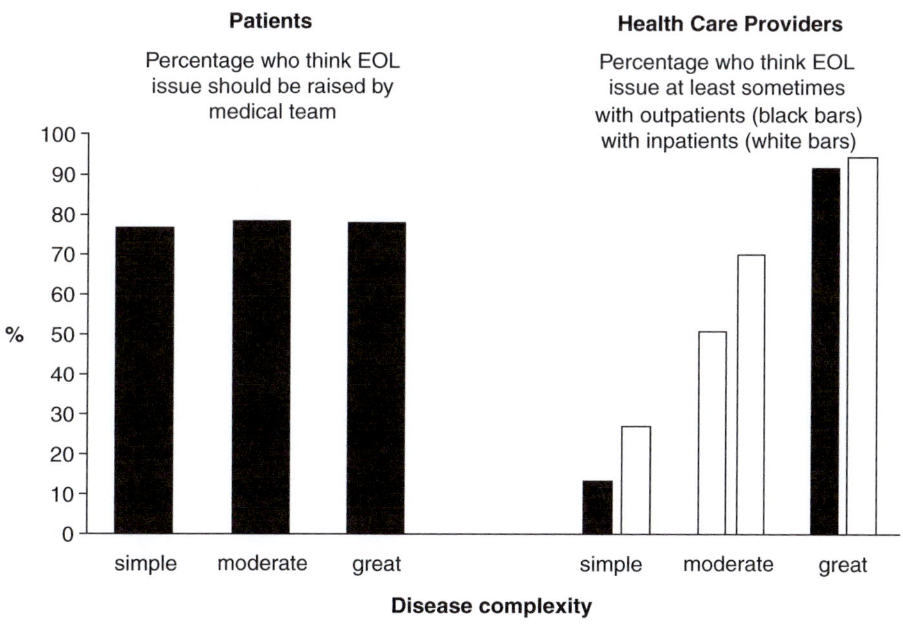

Fig. 29.1 Preferences of patients and health-care providers for end-of-life discussions stratified by disease complexity (from Tobler et al. with permission) [9]

29.4 Advance Care Planning in Adult Congenital Heart Disease

Although guidelines for the care of adults with congenital heart disease encourage promoting early advance care planning, surveys suggest that only a small minority of adult congenital heart disease patients had completed advance directives or formally identified a substitute decision-maker [10, 11].

Advance care planning in a broader sense is part of the routine clinical work we provide to all our patients. This includes, for example, counseling about recreational sports, appropriate career decisions (choice of profession), or counseling about pregnancy risks. These aspects of counseling have been adopted in a widely accepted model of comprehensive care in patients with congenital heart disease. This comprehensive care model integrates the provision of cardiac care and includes supportive as well as palliative care, adapted to the lifetime disease stages of the individual patient (Fig. 29.2, adapted from Sarah Goodlin, a pioneer in palliative care for patients with heart failure [12, 13]). Unfortunately, important aspects of such a comprehensive care model are still regarded as taboos in our day-to-day clinical routine practice.

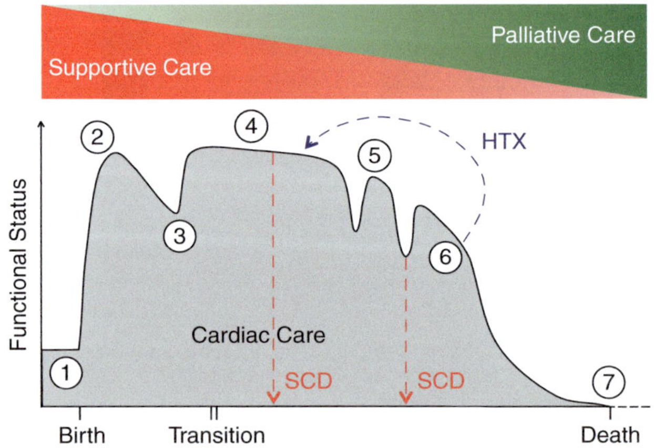

Fig. 29.2 Illustration of the comprehensive care model with stages of disease in patients with congenital heart disease (Modified from Greutmann et al. with permission) [13]. Disease stages in congenital heart disease covering the entire life span (*x*-axis). The *y*-axis depicts the functional status along the different disease stages. Numbers *1–7* represent the several stages of comprehensive care in patients with congenital heart disease: (*1*) Parental prenatal support. (*2*) Initial surgical repair/palliation. (*3*) Re-interventions during childhood or adolescence. (*4*) Plateau of variable lengths in adulthood. (*5*) Variable adverse cardiac events and functional decline with variable slope, intermittent exacerbations that respond to rescue efforts, and/or adult re-interventions or procedures. (*6*) Refractory symptoms and limited function. (*7*) End-of-life care including bereavement care. Dotted line with arrowhead represents possible occurrence of sudden cardiac death events. *SCD* sudden cardiac death, *CHD* congenital heart disease, *HTX* heart transplantation. These taboos include discussions about end-of-life issues and advance care planning, i.e., planning of care for end-of-life situations. In a survey of 200 adult outpatients with congenital heart disease, more than half had never heard about the principles of advance care planning

As physicians caring for adults with congenital heart disease, we follow our patients often for years or even decades. Given that for many patients with complex defects, medical care is centered around their heart defect, their cardiologist is their main caregiver knowing not only the medical situation but also their social situation very well. It is thus no surprise that most patients prefer to discuss sensitive issues about end-of-life care or advance care planning with their cardiologists, with whom they often have a long-standing and trusting relationships. On the physicians' side, one of the main barriers for discussions about end-of-life care or advance care planning relates to uncertainties about prognostication in individual patients [13].

We should remind ourselves, however, that open discussions about patient preferences for end-of-life care, identification of a substitute decision-maker, and completion of advance directives will greatly enhance patient autonomy. Advance care planning is a formalized process. Many resources are available to support the creation of advance directives (e.g., https://agingwithdignity.org and http://adcanceca-replanning.ca). Such a document enables the patient to express his or her personal wishes, views, and values about life and death that will help to guide care if the patient becomes unconscious and is no longer able to speak for himself or herself. As adult congenital heart disease cardiologists, we may offer to assist our patients regarding questions around specific medical aspects of advance directives. In the authors' own experience, it is important to emphasize to our patients that the goal of the advance directive must not be to define management directives for all potential medical situation, but rather to give the medical team and the patient's relatives a framework of values and views toward life that allows to estimate the patient's presumed wishes, should she or he not be able to speak for himself or herself.

Importantly, wishes and views may change over time, and thus, discussions about end-of-life care and advance care planning are not a single-step procedure but rather a continuous endeavor in our patient care. To "normalize" these discussions as part of routine clinical care—in analogy to other preventive measures such as prevention of infective endocarditis—may greatly facilitate these discussions. How best to implement such "normalization" of these discussions needs to be further explored (e.g., by physicians, specialist nurses, or other members of the medical team) and is certainly dependent on local resources and organization of care at individual centers. To delegate general information about advance care planning and documents for advance directives to specialist nurses may, however, facilitate "normalization" of these discussions in day-to-day practice.

29.5 Providing End-of-Life Care on the ICU

Most in-hospital deaths in congenital heart disease occur in the ICU [14]. In-hospital deaths frequently come along with technical support and aggressive therapy such as extracorporeal membrane oxygenation (ECMO), mechanical ventilation, and cardiopulmonary resuscitation [8]. According to the guidelines for palliative care in pediatric oncology, curative treatment should be avoided when cure is no longer possible [15]. A similar concept seems meaningful in congenital heart disease. The Academy of Pediatrics emphasizes that technology should only be used when the benefits outweigh the harms and this principle certainly should be adopted to adults [16].

Comprehensive end-of-life care toward the end stage of congenital heart disease is a multidisciplinary endeavor. It often requires involvement of multiple subspecialties, including not only cardiologists and intensivists but many other subspecialties such as palliative care specialists, spiritual care, or social workers to support relatives and families. A particular emphasis must be made on the support of caring families and friends of our patients. After a patient's death, follow-up debriefing with the family in person or by phone call or a condolence card is important. In our experience it is often very helpful for families to schedule an appointment a few weeks after the patient's death to offer the opportunity to discuss unresolved issues and remaining questions.

References

1. Moons P, Bovijn L, Budts W, Belmans A, Gewillig M. Temporal trends in survival to adulthood among patients born with congenital heart disease from 1970 to 1992 in Belgium. Circulation. 2010;122(22):2264–72.
2. Marelli AJ, Ionescu-Ittu R, Mackie AS, Guo L, Dendukuri N, Kaouache M. Lifetime prevalence of congenital heart disease in the general population from 2000 to 2010. Circulation. 2014;130(9):749–56.
3. Padrutt M, Bracher I, Bonassin F, Santoslopes B, Gruner C, Stampfli SF, et al. Impact of growing cohorts of adults with con-genital heart disease on clinical workload: a 20-year experience at a tertiary care Centre. Swiss Med Wkly. 2017;147:w14443.
4. Greutmann M, Tobler D, Kovacs AH, Greutmann-Yantiri M, Haile SR, Held L, et al. Increasing mortality burden among adults with complex congenital heart disease. Congenit Heart Dis. 2015;10(2):117–27.
5. Oechslin EN, Harrison DA, Connelly MS, Webb GD, Siu SC. Mode of death in adults with congenital heart disease. Am J Cardiol. 2000;86(10):1111–6.
6. Nieminen HP, Jokinen EV, Sairanen HI. Causes of late deaths after pediatric cardiac surgery: a population-based study. J Am Coll Cardiol. 2007;50(13):1263–71.
7. Bowater SE, Speakman JK, Thorne SA. End-of-life care in adults with congenital heart disease: now is the time to act. Curr Opin Support Palliat Care. 2013;7(1):8–13.
8. Tobler D, Greutmann M, Colman JM, Greutmann-Yantiri M, Librach LS, Kovacs AH. End-of-life care in hospitalized adults with complex congenital heart disease: care delayed, care denied. Palliat Med. 2012;26(1):72–9.
9. Tobler D, Greutmann M, Colman JM, Greutmann-Yantiri M, Librach LS, Kovacs AH. End-of-life in adults with congenital heart disease: a call for early communication. Int J Cardiol. 2012;155(3):383–7.
10. Warnes CA, Williams RG, Bashore TM, Child JS, Connolly HM, Dearani JA, et al. ACC/AHA 2008 guidelines for the management of adults with congenital heart disease: a report of the American College of Cardiology/American Heart Association Task Force on Practice Guidelines (Writing Committee to Develop Guidelines on the Management of Adults With Congenital Heart Disease). Developed in Collaboration With the American Society of Echocardiography, Heart Rhythm Society, International Society for Adult Congenital Heart Disease, Society for Cardiovascular Angiography and Interventions, and Society of Thoracic Surgeons. J Am Coll Cardiol. 2008;52(23):e143–263.
11. Tobler D, Greutmann M, Colman JM, Greutmann-Yantiri M, Librach SL, Kovacs AH. Knowledge of and preference for advance care planning by adults with congenital heart disease. Am J Cardiol. 2012;109(12):1797–800.

12. Goodlin SJ. Palliative care in congestive heart failure. J Am Coll Cardiol. 2009;54(5):386–96.
13. Greutmann M, Tobler D, Colman JM, Greutmann-Yantiri M, Librach SL, Kovacs AH. Facilitators of and barriers to advance care planning in adult congenital heart disease. Congenit Heart Dis. 2013;8(4):281–8.
14. Morell E, Wolfe J, Scheurer M, Thiagarajan R, Morin C, Beke DM, et al. Patterns of care at end of life in children with advanced heart disease. Arch Pediatr Adolesc Med. 2012;166(8):745–8.
15. Masera G, Spinetta JJ, Jankovic M, Ablin AR, D'Angio GJ, Van Dongen-Melman J, et al. Guidelines for assistance to terminally ill children with cancer: a report of the SIOP Working Committee on psychosocial issues in pediatric oncology. Med Pediatr Oncol. 1999;32(1):44–8.
16. American Academy of Pediatrics. Committee on Bioethics and Committee on Hospital Care. Palliative care for children. Pediatrics. 2000;106(2 Pt 1):351–7.

MIX
Papier aus verantwortungsvollen Quellen
Paper from responsible sources
FSC® C105338

If you have any concerns about our products,
you can contact us on
ProductSafety@springernature.com

In case Publisher is established outside the EU,
the EU authorized representative is:
Springer Nature Customer Service Center GmbH
Europaplatz 3, 69115 Heidelberg, Germany

Printed by Libri Plureos GmbH
in Hamburg, Germany